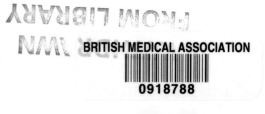

Neonatal Cerebral Investigation

SECOND EDITION

Edited by

JANET M. RENNIE

CORNELIA F. HAGMANN

NICOLA J. ROBERTSON

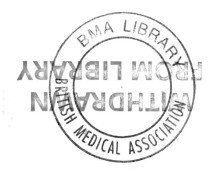

Neonatal
Cerebral
Investigation

SECOND EDITION

Edited by

JANET M. RENNIE
Consultant and Senior Lecturer in Neonatal Medicine

CORNELIA F. HAGMANN
Clinical Lecturer and Honorary Consultant Neonatologist

NICOLA J. ROBERTSON
Senior Lecturer in Neonatology and Honorary Consultant Neonatologist

UCL Elizabeth Garrett Anderson Institute for Women's Health
University College London Hospitals
London UK

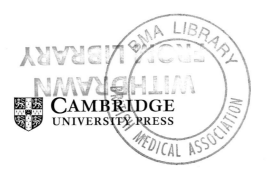

CAMBRIDGE
UNIVERSITY PRESS

CAMBRIDGE UNIVERSITY PRESS
Cambridge, New York, Melbourne, Madrid, Cape Town, Singapore, São Paulo, Delhi

Cambridge University Press
The Edinburgh Building, Cambridge CB2 8RU, UK

Published in the United States of America by Cambridge University Press, New York

www.cambridge.org
Information on this title: www.cambridge.org/9780521838481

First published 2008

Printed in the United Kingdom at the University Press, Cambridge

A catalog record for this publication is available from the British Library

Library of Congress Cataloging in Publication data
Neonatal cerebral investigation / editors, Janet M. Rennie, Cornelia F. Hagmann, Nicola J. Robertson.
p. ; cm.
Rev. ed. of: Neonatal cerebral ultrasound / Janet M. Rennie. 1997.
Includes bibliographical references.
ISBN-13: 978-0-521-83848-1
1. Pediatric neurology – Diagnosis. 2. Newborn infants – Diseases – Diagnosis. 3. Brain – Imaging.
[DNLM: 1. Cerebrovascular Disorders – diagnosis. 2. Electroencephalography. 3. Infant, Newborn. 4. Magnetic Resonance
Imaging. 5. Ultrasonography. WL 355 N438 2008] I. Rennie, Janet M. II. Hagmann, Cornelia F. III. Robertson, Nicola J.
IV. Rennie, Janet M. Neonatal crebral ultrasound.
RJ488.N46 2008
618.92′8047543–dc22

                                                                                                        2007051667

ISBN 978-0-521-83848-1 hardback

Contents

Contributors

JANET M. RENNIE MA MD FRCP FRCPCH DCH
Consultant and Senior Lecturer in Neonatal Medicine
UCL Elizabeth Garrett Anderson Institute for Women's Health
University College London Hospitals
London UK

CORNELIA F. HAGMANN MD FMH PAEDIATRICS AND
NEONATOLOGY
Clinical Lecturer and Honorary Consultant Neonatologist
UCL Elizabeth Garrett Anderson Institute for Women's Health
University College London Hospitals
London UK

NICOLA J. ROBERTSON PHD FRCPCH
Senior Lecturer in Neonatology and Honorary Consultant Neonatologist
UCL Elizabeth Garrett Anderson Institute for Women's Health
University College London Hospitals
London UK

GERALDINE B. BOYLAN PHD
Senior Lecturer in Medical Education and Paediatrics
School of Medicine
University College Cork
Ireland

ERNEST B. CADY FINSTP
Clinical Scientist and Section Head MR Physics UCLH NHS Trust
Director Bloomsbury Centre for Magnetic Resonance Spectroscopy
Honorary Lecturer UCL
Department of Medical Physics and Bioengineering
UCLH NHS Foundation Trust
London UK

ENRICO DE VITA PHD
Magnetic Resonance Physicist
Department of Medical Physics and Bio-Engineering
University College London Hospitals NHS Foundation Trust
London UK

JEREMY C. HEBDEN PHD
Professor of Medical Physics and Bioengineering
University College London
London UK

ANDREW B. KAPETANAKIS MBBS MRCP MRCPCH
Imaging Fellow and Neonatologist
UCLH NHS Foundation Trust
London UK

DEIRDRE M. MURRAY MBBS MRCPI
Research Fellow
Department of Paediatrics and Child Health
University College Cork
Ireland

Preface

The natural anxiety experienced by all new parents about the well-being and future of their child is increased when the baby is born small or ill, and is further heightened if there is any concern about the function of the brain. As clinicians involved in the care of newborns with neurological problems, and who are often asked to advise parents whose fetus is thought to have a neurological abnormality, we have considerable experience with the situations we describe in this book. Over the years we have sought advice from others, searched the literature, and consulted and read widely in order to solve clinical problems on a daily basis. This book represents a summary of the results of our knowledge and experience, and we have started with the clinical presentation of neonatal neurological disease rather than using a pathological or end-stage neuroimaging classification. We describe our approach to the problem and the way we interpret the results of the investigations we request, and hope others will find this approach useful as they strive to provide the best possible care to their vulnerable patients.

By the time this book is published it will be almost 30 years since the first ultrasound images of the neonatal brain were made at University College London Hospital and published in the *Lancet*. There have been huge advances since then, and the field has moved on considerably in the decade since the first edition of this book was published, as *Neonatal Cerebral Ultrasound* written by Janet M. Rennie. The wealth of detailed information that modern imaging produces has far exceeded the expectations which were envisaged in the early days of ultrasound imaging in the 1980s. Magnetic resonance imaging (MRI) is much more readily obtainable, and digital technology allows prolonged electroencephalogram (EEG) recordings to be made at the cotside. Ultrasound is still an important tool, but we have expanded the scope and the material to include the full range of investigations now available, and we have indicated when MRI and EEG are particularly helpful.

For convenience, we have adopted masculine pronouns when referring to babies, and feminine when referring to neonatologists. We hope that this will not offend anyone who reads the book.

JANET RENNIE, CORNELIA HAGMANN, NICOLA ROBERTSON

Acknowledgements

Peter Silver never gave up hoping and believing that a second edition of *Neonatal Cerebral Ultrasound* would eventually appear, and since his departure from Cambridge University Press Deborah Russell and her team have been unfailingly enthusiastic and supportive. We thank Deborah for her patience and for remaining cheerful as each new deadline came and went without sight of any material, and for her tolerance as the count of words and figures steadily rose. Doreen Robertson has redrawn many of the figures, and we are very grateful to her for giving so freely of her time and skill.

The literature and knowledge base have exploded in the last 10 years, and we are eternally grateful to our contributors. Their expertise on specific topics is greater than our own, and we very much appreciate the time they gave up to help us in this enterprise. We have received much help and advice from Rox Gunny, our neuroradiologist, and her colleagues at Great Ormond Street Children's Hospital and the National Hospital for Neurology and Neurosurgery Queen Square; also Ronit Pressler, pediatric neurophysiologist at Great Ormond Street Children's Hospital. Dr Lyn Chitty, in fetal medicine, made very helpful comments on the appropriate parts of the text and lent us several images, for which we are grateful. Many of the images could not have been obtained without the help of our nursing staff, whose dedicated care ensures that we can perform MRI on even the sickest baby safely. We could not have made such rapid progress in imaging quality without the help of a superb NHS medical physics department, and we would like to thank all those involved.

This work was undertaken at University College London Hospital (UCLH)/University College London (UCL) who received a proportion of funding from the Department of Health's National Institute for Health Research (NIHR) Biomedical Research Centres funding scheme. The views expressed in this publication are those of the authors and not necessarily those of the Department of Health.

The cover photograph of Elliot Bowden, a very special baby to us all, is reproduced with grateful thanks to his parents. He represents many others, and we take this opportunity to extend our thanks to the parents of all our patients, who have allowed us to share their hopes and fears, to advise and inform them, and to walk with them on what is so often a difficult and stressful journey. In particular, we would like to acknowledge all those parents who have allowed us to enrol their babies into research studies over the years; without them, the advances which we report in this book would not have been possible.

We cannot finish the acknowledgements without thanking our partners: Ian Watts, Jürg Schlumpf, and Dominique Acolet. They have patiently endured many broken social engagements and evenings alone, and shouldered more than their share of household chores during the hours we have spent with our computers. We dedicate this book to them, with gratitude and much love.

Glossary and abbreviations

Acoustic impedance A fundamental property of tissue. Ultrasound is reflected at boundaries between tissues of different impedance

Acoustic shadow An area that is poorly visualized with ultrasound due to the fact that most of the beam energy has been reflected by a boundary above it

Adenosine diphosphate (ADP) Produced in energy reactions when ATP monodephosphorylates

Adenosine triphosphate (ATP) The key metabolite in biological energy reactions

Advanced method for accurate, robust, and efficient spectral fitting (AMARES) A magnetic resonance spectroscopy analysis technique based on time-domain data fitting

Aliasing Ambiguity resulting in an erroneous representation of the signal. Results from inadequate sampling, e.g., the fastest velocities appear in the reverse channel when all the flow is forward. In MRI, due to tissue outside the field of view

Anisotropy Anisotropy is the property of being directionally dependent, as opposed to *isotropy*, which means homogeneity in all directions

Apparent diffusion coefficient (ADC) An MRI parameter related to water diffusion properties. To obtain pure diffusion information a diffusion map can be calculated by combining at least two diffusion-weighted images that are differently sensitized to diffusion but remain identical with respect to the other parameters, spin density, T1, T2, TR, and TE. A parametric image containing these data is called an apparent diffusion coefficient (ADC) map

Attenuation Loss of energy from the ultrasound beam (leading to heating of tissue) during its passage

Axial resolution The ability to separate two targets at different depths along the axis of the beam

Bilirubin-induced neuronal dysfunction (BIND)

Blood oxygen level dependent (BOLD) Contrast mechanism based on blood oxygenation level frequently employed in functional MRI experiments

Cavitation The production and subsequent oscillation and collapse of bubbles in tissues subjected to high-intensity ultrasound

Cerebral metabolic rate (CMR)

Chemical shift imaging (CSI) In MRI a method for separately imaging water or fat: in MRS a multi-voxel localization technique

Chemical shift selective (CHESS) An MRS RF pulse sequence often used for water suppression

Choline (Cho) Commonly observed by MRS: includes membrane-related metabolites

Congenital heart disease (CHD)

Continuous wave (CW) Type of Doppler study in which ultrasound is transmitted and received continuously (in contrast to pulsed wave)

Creatine (Cr) Commonly observed by MRS: often co-existing with phosphocreatine in living tissue.

Demodulation Computerized process whereby frequency information is extracted from complex multifrequency signals – used in Doppler

Diffuse excessive high signal intensity (DEHSI) Qualitative MRI finding on T_2-weighted images: abnormally high signal intensity in white matter seen frequently in ex preterm infants at term-equivalent age

Diffusion-weighted imaging (DWI) MRI method demonstrating changes in tissue water transport; useful for demonstrating cerebral damage very early after an injury

Doppler effect A change in frequency of an ultrasound pulse reflected from moving tissue (e.g., fast flowing blood)

Duplex system The combination of range-gated Doppler velocity measurement with real-time imaging

Echo The portion of an ultrasound pulse that is reflected at a boundary and subsequently detected by the transducer

Echo time (TE) In an MRI or MRS spin-echo study the total time from excitation pulse to the echo

Exponential decay time constant of the observed FID (T_2^*) Effective time constant for MRI magnetization decay in the plane orthogonal to B_0 including local magnetic-field inhomogeneity effects: always $\leq T_2$

Extracorporeal membrane oxygenation (ECMO) An advanced intensive care technique available in very few centers, which involves oxygenation of the baby's blood outside the body

Fourier transform A mathematical technique which analyzes the different frequencies present in a signal

Fractional anisotropy (FA) Fractional anisotropy is calculated from the eigenvalues λ_1, λ_2, λ_3 of the diffusion tensor:

$$FA = \frac{\sqrt{3}}{\sqrt{2}} \frac{\sqrt{(\lambda_1 - \lambda)^2 + (\lambda_2 - \lambda)^2 + (\lambda_3 - \lambda)^2}}{\sqrt{\lambda_1^2 + \lambda_2^2 + \lambda_3^2}}$$

λ is the mean diffusivity (trace/3); and λ_1, λ_2, λ_3 diffusion tensor eigenvalues. FA is between 0 (perfect isotropic diffusion) and 1 (the hypothetical infinite cylinder – unidirectional) and subject intercomparable

Fraunhofer zone A region of an ultrasound beam furthest from a transducer where the beam becomes too broad to be useful for imaging

Free induction decay (FID) The exponentially decaying MRI RF signal from the flipped nuclear magnetization

Frequency Number of times per second that a change occurs; refers to the transducer vibration in ultrasound and precession rate of nuclear magnetization in MRI

Fresnel zone A region of an ultrasound beam nearest a transducer where the beam is narrowest and most useful for imaging

Germinal matrix–intraventricular hemorrhage (GMH-IVH) Bleeding that is isolated to the germinal matrix or associated with uncomplicated intraventricular hemorrhage – where there is blood in the ventricular cavity but no ventriculomegaly. This terminology clearly separates GMH-IVH from parenchymal lesions

Half-Fourier acquisition single shot turbo spin echo (HASTE) Very fast MRI technique based on the acquisition of a whole image following a single excitation. Often used when the organ of interest is subject to motion

Hypoplastic left heart syndrome (HLHS)

International Commission on Non-ionizing Radiation Protection (ICNIRP) International organization assessing risks and producing safety guidelines relevant to MRI

International Electrotechnical Commission (IEC) International body assessing risks and producing safety guidelines relevant to MRI

Inorganic phosphate (P$_i$) The orthophosphate in biological tissues: exists as the rapidly exchanging species HPO_4^{2-} and $H_2PO_4^{-}$

Intensity A measure of the strength of an ultrasound beam, equal to the energy (joules) traveling through the tissue per second per square meter of area (or watts per square meter)

Intracellular pH (pH$_i$) Estimable via MRS using many metabolite resonances (P$_i$ often used)

Inversion recovery (IR) MRI technique providing T_1 contrast

Larmor frequency The frequency of precession of the nuclear magnetic vector about the static magnetic field; in other words the resonance frequency (in Hz) of a peak

Lateral resolution The ability to distinguish between two closely spaced objects located at the same depth

Lenticulostriate vasculopathy (LSV)

Linear array An ultrasound probe consisting of a large number (up to 300) of small transducers arranged in a row

Line density Number of scan lines per unit distance or degree of arc

Longitudinal or spin-lattice relaxation time constant (T$_1$) Time constant for MRI magnetization recovery parallel to B_0

Magnetic resonance angiography (MRA) MRI technique imaging the vascular system

Magnetic resonance imaging (MRI) Imaging modality using magnetic and RF fields and obtaining contrast via tissue-water characteristics

Magnetic resonance spectroscopy (MRS) Informs about tissue metabolite composition and other biophysical attributes including pH

Magnetic resonance spectroscopy imaging (MRSi) Multi-voxel MRS localization method

Magnetization transfer (MT) MRI method relying on transfer of nuclear magnetization to adjacent, otherwise unimaged, molecules

Medicines and Healthcare Products Regulatory Agency (MHRA) United Kingdom government-sponsored body providing MRI safety guidance

N-Acetyl aspartate (Naa) A predominantly neuronal metabolite

National Radiological Protection Board (NRPB) United Kingdom government-sponsored body providing MRI safety guidance

Net sample magnetization (M_0) The magnetization induced in a tissue sample by B_0 and utilized by MRI and MRS

Nuclear magnetic resonance (NMR) The phenomenon of a resonance signal detectable from certain isotopes when in a strong magnetic field

Number of phase encoding steps (N$_{pe}$) An MRI and MRSi parameter that is linked to spatial resolution in one of the dimensions

Noise An unwanted signal contaminating the signal of interest, which is usually random and will have a variety of causes

N-Methyl-D-aspartate (NMDA) An *amino acid* derivative that mimics the action of the *neurotransmitter glutamate* on NMDA receptors

Nucleotide triphosphate (NTP) Gives three prominent signals in phosphorus brain MRS: mainly attributable to ATP

Nyquist limit The maximum measurable Doppler shift frequency, equal to half the pulse repetition frequency

Outer volume suppressed image related in vivo spectroscopy (OSIRIS) MRS localization method: often used for phosphorus MRS

Phased array A compact linear array that produces a beam which is steered electronically, forming a sector scan image

Phosphocholine (PCho) Membrane-related metabolite

Phosphoethanolamine (PEt) Membrane-related metabolite: prominent in neonatal brain phosphorus MRS

Phosphocreatine (PCr) Detectable by phosphorus brain MRS: contributes to creatine signal in proton MRS

Phosphorus MRS (^{31}P MRS) MRS detecting metabolites containing phosphorus atoms

Piezoelectric A physical property of certain crystals which can generate sound waves when an electrical current is applied, and can generate a current when vibrated by a sound wave

Pixel A "picture element". Every electronic image is made up of a large array of (usually square) pixels

Point resolved spectroscopy (PRESS) MRS single-voxel localization method: often used for proton MRS

Polymerase chain reaction (PCR) Method of "amplifying" small amounts of cellular components in order to establish their identity. Used in the diagnosis of viral infection, for example

Pourcelot Index (PI) Doppler-derived measure calculated from flow velocity trace

Proton MRS (^{1}H MRS) MRS detecting metabolites containing hydrogen atoms

Pulsatility index (Pul or PI) Doppler-derived measure calculated from flow velocity trace

Pulse-echo principle The measurement of the time taken for pulses to arrive back from reflecting boundaries as a means of determining their distance

Pulse repetition frequency (PRF) The number of ultrasound pulses generated each second

Pulsed wave (PW) Used to refer to Doppler studies where the velocity information is obtained by analyzing data from "packets" or "pulses" of sound waves sent intermittently from the transducer, in contrast to continuous wave studies

Radiofrequency (RF) The oscillation frequency of the electromagnetic waves used by MRI

Real-time imaging The display of continuously updated images during a scan which will reveal any changes in the tissues immediately as they occur

Refraction A phenomenon that can cause an ultrasound pulse to change direction when it passes across a boundary between tissues with a different velocity of sound, resulting in a distorted ultrasound image

Repetition time (TR) In MRI or MRS the delay between consecutive RF pulse sequences

RF pulse magnetic field (B$_1$) The magnetic component of the RF pulses used in MRI

Scattering Random and/or variable reflection of ultrasound by smaller tissue structures which can contribute background noise to an image

Single ventricle (SV)

Spin echo (SE) The MRI signal obtained by refocussing the FID generated by an excitation RF pulse

Signal-to-noise ratio (SNR) Information quality improves as this increases

Spatial resolution A measure of the ability of a system to distinguish between two closely spaced objects

Speckle A random pattern of bright and dark spots which occur when echoes from small scattering structures interfere with each other when they arrive at the transducer at the same time

Spectral analysis The display of the frequencies contained within Doppler ultrasound signals

Static magnetic field (B$_o$) The main, homogeneous magnetic field of an MRI scanner

Stimulated echo acquisition mode (STEAM) MRS single-voxel localization method: often used for proton MRS

Sturge Weber Syndrome (SWS)

Subependymal pseudocyst (SEPC)

T$_2$ relaxometry MRI and MRS methods to measure tissue-water and metabolite T$_2$ values

T$_1$-weighted MRI contrast weighted according to longitudinal or spin-lattice relaxation

T$_2$-weighted MRI contrast weighted according to transverse or spin-spin relaxation

Tesla (T) Unit of magnetic field strength (1 T = 10 000 Gauss). For comparison, the Earth's magnetic field at its surface is between 20 and 70 μT.

Time-gain compensation (TGC) The electronic enhancement of signals obtained from deeper regions to compensate for loss of signal by attenuation

Transducer A (normally piezoelectric) device which converts electrical signals to sound energy, and vice versa

Transposition of the great arteries (TGA)

Transverse or spin-spin relaxation time constant (T$_2$) Time constant for MRI magnetization decay in the plane orthogonal to B_o

Twin-to-twin transfusion syndrome (TTTS) Syndrome that occurs in 15% of monochorionic twin pregnancies and results from the shunting of blood from one twin (the donor) to the other twin (the recipient). The donor becomes hypovolemic and oliguric whereas the recipient becomes hypervolemic and polyuric

Unconjugated bilirubin (UCB)

Uridine diphosphoglucuronyl transferase (UDPGT)

Volume of interest (VOI) The volume of tissue for analysis as represented on an image

Voxel Volume element, used in MRI and MRS to indicate the tissue contributing to an image pixel or an MR spectrum

Wall-thump filter Circuitry which eliminates low (<100 Hz) frequencies from Doppler signals produced by pulses reflected off the walls of blood vessels

Wavelength Distance between two consecutive peaks in an ultrasound or electromagnetic wave (abbreviated λ)

JEREMY C. HEBDEN *and*
JANET M. RENNIE

Discovery of ultrasound

The term ultrasound refers to sound with a frequency above that which can be detected by the human ear. The audible frequency range lies between 20 Hz and 20 kHz (one hertz equals one cycle per second, one kilohertz equals one thousand cycles per second), whereas the frequencies of sound waves used for diagnostic applications in medicine are of the order of one thousand times higher than this, with a range between 1 and 10 MHz (megahertz = one million hertz). Ultrasound imaging relies on the so-called pulse echo principle, which involves emitting a short burst of ultrasound and then listening for the returning "echo" after the sound has been reflected off appropriate surfaces. This is exactly the mechanism which has been employed by bats for millions of years to navigate their way around dark caves and to catch flying insects. Human interest in navigation using sound waves was significantly enhanced (if not initially inspired) by the sinking of the Titanic, which occurred when the ship collided with an iceberg in April 1912. Within a few years, ships were widely equipped with SONAR (Sound Navigation And Ranging) devices, which emit sound waves beneath the surface of the sea, and detect echoes from large objects within a radius of several miles. The technology advanced considerably during both world wars as it was utilized to detect submarines and mines. Ultrasound imaging of patients began to evolve in the late 1940s, and over the following decade simple (A-mode) systems were developed that could detect midline shift in head injury and the presence of foreign bodies in the orbit. These devices emitted ultrasound pulses and detected echoes along a single line through the tissue. To generate two-dimensional images, however, echoes must be acquired over multiple lines. Various methods of scanning the beam were explored, and Holmes [1] describes how some early imaging systems required subjects to be immersed in a water bath for the duration of the scan.

Reflection of sound from a moving object gives rise to a change in the observed frequency. This phenomenon, known as the Doppler effect, was first described by Austrian physicist Christian Doppler in 1842. By measuring the change in frequency one can estimate the velocity of the moving object. That this is possible with some accuracy is well known to those who have been caught driving above the legal speed limit by police officers armed with a speed gun. Doppler measurement of blood flow has now become a standard feature of ultrasound systems, which commonly use color to display the velocity and direction of blood superimposed on conventional anatomical ultrasound images.

Ultrasound waves: basic principles

Diagnostic ultrasound uses a device known as a transducer, which can both emit and detect ultrasound waves. Transducers are made from a material known as a piezoelectric crystal, which vibrates millions of times per second when a short burst of electric current is applied to it. These crystals also have the property of detecting ultrasound by converting vibrations back into electrical energy. Piezoelectric properties occur in some naturally occurring crystals such as quartz, although most clinical transducers are based on a synthetic piezoelectric substance known as lead zirconate titanate (PZT). For imaging applications, the same crystal is used to transmit and receive, sending small bursts (pulses) of sound energy into the tissue and then "listening" for the returning echoes.

Ultrasound energy spreads by means of rapid alternate compression and expansion of the matter through which it travels, and therefore it cannot pass through a vacuum. Ultrasound passes through most biological tissues with a roughly constant speed (c) of 1540 metres per second. As shown in Fig. 1.1a, the distance between two consecutive peaks in an ultrasound wave is known as the wavelength (λ), and each pulse typically consists of a few wavelengths. The wavelength depends on the frequency (f) and speed of sound (c) according to the following equation:

$$c = \lambda f. \tag{1.1}$$

The *intensity* of ultrasound is equal to the energy (in joules, J) transmitted each second per unit area, and is expressed in

Neonatal Cerebral Investigation, eds. Janet M. Rennie, Cornelia F. Hagmann and Nicola J. Robertson. Published by Cambridge University Press. © Cambridge University Press 2008.

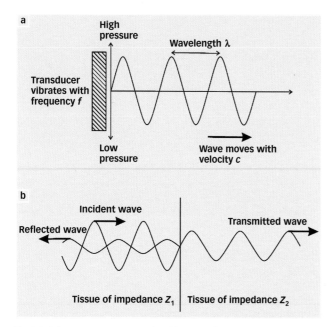

Fig. 1.1. **(a) A pressure wave emitted by a continuously vibrating ultrasound transducer; (b) the partition of an incident wave into transmitted and reflected waves at a boundary between tissues of different acoustic impedance.**

units of watts (W) per square metre (1 W = 1 J per second). However, as ultrasound travels through tissue its intensity is steadily decreased as the sound energy is converted into heat. The attenuation causes the intensity I to decrease according to a so-called exponential function:

$$I = I_0 \exp(-\alpha x),\qquad\text{1.2}$$

where I_0 is the initial intensity, x is the distance traveled by the beam, and α is the *attenuation coefficient* of the tissue. The attenuation coefficient is strongly dependent on frequency, and rises roughly linearly between 1 MHz and 10 MHz.

When ultrasound passes through tissue, the most important interaction is reflection, which occurs when the beam encounters a boundary between two tissues having a different *acoustic impedance* (Z). This is illustrated in Fig. 1.1b. The greater the difference, the more the beam is reflected back towards the transducer. When a beam encounters bone, which has a much higher impedance than any soft tissue, almost all the ultrasound energy is reflected. Thus it is very difficult to view tissues directly beneath bones, and images display an artifact known as an acoustic shadow (see Fig. 4.23). Likewise, air has a much lower impedance than biological tissues, and virtually all ultrasound energy is reflected at an air/tissue boundary. Consequently it is necessary to use coupling gel to eliminate air between the transducer and the patient's skin during an ultrasound examination.

Other interactions between ultrasound and tissue include *refraction*, which occurs when the beam encounters a boundary between two tissues having a different speed of sound and *scatter*, which occurs when the beam encounters features with a size much smaller than the ultrasound wavelength.

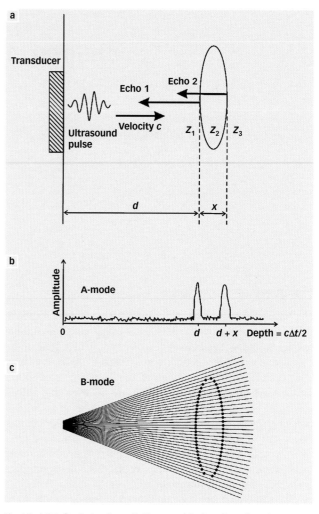

Fig. 1.2. **(a) Reflected pulses of ultrasound (echoes) produced at boundaries between tissues of different acoustic impedance; (b) A-mode display of echo amplitudes as a function of depth below the surface; (c) B-mode display of echo amplitudes obtained from multiples lines through the tissue.**

Further reading on the fundamental physics of ultrasound can be found in Hedrick, Hykes, and Starchman [2].

Echo location

The diagnostic use of ultrasound involves measuring and displaying the depths of boundaries between tissues of different acoustic impedance. This is achieved by determining the time taken (Δt) for the pulse to travel down to the boundary and for the echo to travel back up to the transducer (Fig. 1.2a). Since the velocity of sound (c) is fairly constant, the depth of the reflecting boundary (d) can be obtained from the following equation:

$$d = c\,\Delta t\,/2.\qquad\text{1.3}$$

When a pulse of ultrasound energy is transmitted into tissue it is likely that several echoes will be detected at different times, due to reflections occurring at different depths within the beam. The maximum depth that can be interrogated will depend on the time available before the next pulse is emitted.

Methods of displaying located echo information

A-mode

The earliest form of diagnostic ultrasound involved displaying echo strength as a function of depth along a single "line of sight" through the tissue. A single fixed transducer was employed, and the echo amplitudes were displayed on the screen of a cathode ray oscilloscope. This was known as "amplitude mode" or "A-mode," and is illustrated in Fig 1.2b. Among its first uses was the detection of midline shift. Although A-mode is rarely used now, many modern commercial systems include an option to display the signal strength along a selected line of sight as a function of time (known as "M-mode").

B-mode

To produce a two-dimensional (2D) ultrasound image it is necessary to acquire signals along multiple lines of sight through the tissue. For each line, the detected echoes are converted into bright spots on a screen, whose brightness depends on the echo amplitude and whose position depends on the echo arrival time and the direction of the beam (Fig 1.2c). This is consequently known as "brightness mode" or "B-mode." A full 2D gray scale picture is formed by displaying the spots acquired from a series of successive lines of sight simultaneously. B-mode imaging therefore involves sweeping the beam across a plane through the tissue. The earliest imaging systems required the beam to be swept manually, with the transducer mounted on a device which continuously recorded its position and orientation as it was moved back and forth by the operator. Thus the picture was built up gradually. Thereafter, mechanical scanning systems were developed which used electric motors to translate or rotate one or more transducers across the tissue surface. By displaying many images (or frames) per second, diagnostic ultrasound became a *real-time* imaging technique. Modern ultrasound systems scan the beam without moving parts by employing an array of small transducers. *Linear arrays* use a row of up to 300 transducers, which are pulsed in small groups to emit a beam that travels perpendicular to the array. By selecting different groups, the beam is translated back and forth, sampling a rectangular slice across the tissue. *Phased arrays* consist of a much smaller row of transducers that are pulsed (almost) together. By introducing slight delays between the pulsing of neighboring transducers within the array, the beam can be steered, covering a sector of a circle. The angle of the sector depends on the scan depth and the number of distinct lines sampled by the scanner. The number of pulses generated per second (equal to the number of lines of sight sampled per second) is known as the pulse repetition frequency (PRF). Because of the finite speed of sound (*c*), the PRF limits the maximum depth from which echoes can be detected (d_{max}):

$$PRF = c/2d_{max}. \qquad 1.4$$

The depth d_{max} is therefore the depth of the displayed image. The maximum number of frames displayed per second (*F*) is given by the following equation:

$$F = PRF/N, \qquad 1.5$$

where *N* is the number of sampled lines per frame. To avoid the perception of flicker, *F* is always more than about 20 frames per second. Higher values of *F* provide better images of rapidly moving objects such as heart valves. However, increasing *F* means increasing PRF or decreasing *N*, both of which mean reducing the size of the scanned area.

The small size (or "footprint") of phased arrays makes them particularly suitable for neonatal examinations, where the curvature of the head makes it difficult to keep a larger array in contact.

3D imaging

Some commercial ultrasound imaging systems offer the facility to construct and display three-dimensional (3D) images. In principle, these enable the operator to determine spatial relationships in all three dimensions more accurately and more efficiently. There are two basic 3D scanning mechanisms. One involves mechanical scanning of a linear or phased array to acquire consecutive 2D slice images (which are then combined into a 3D image), while the other utilizes a static 2D transducer array that produces a beam which is steered electronically in three dimensions. Because of the significantly larger volume of tissue being scanned, 3D ultrasound imaging is inevitably slower than conventional 2D imaging. The principles and technology involved in 3D ultrasound imaging are described in detail by Fenster *et al.* [3].

Time-gain compensation

The attenuation of ultrasound as it passes through tissues means that echoes obtained from deep structures are much weaker than those obtained from more superficial tissues. Ultrasound intensity decreases exponentially with depth as described above. To compensate for this effect, the amplitudes of returning echoes are therefore multiplied by a number that *increases* exponentially with time. This has the effect of amplifying the echoes that originate at increasing depth. This is known as "time-gain compensation" (TGC), and allows similar features at different depths to give a similar appearance in the ultrasound image. The degree of compensation required (known as the "gain") depends on the attenuation coefficient (α) of the tissue. Since α can vary depending on the tissue type, most ultrasound systems allow the operator to adjust the gain at different depths to give the best possible image. Some systems allow TGC to be estimated automatically according to the strength of the returning echoes.

Very weak echoes can be rejected entirely by setting an appropriate intensity threshold (before or after TGC is applied). This helps to suppress noise in the image. When setting up the sensitivity controls at the start of imaging, the

TGC and rejection threshold are best set to low levels. They can then be adjusted to give a suitable contrast for the main object of interest, and then refined to suppress unwanted small echoes. Many systems offer the ability to store the combinations of settings in the computer's memory which produce the best result for a given examination.

Resolution

The quality of an ultrasound image is determined by a broad variety of operational and systematic factors. The operator plays a vital role in choosing the best transducer for the job, in setting appropriate sensitivity and gain controls, and using coupling gel correctly. The image sector angle can be made narrower to increase the line density and/or the image depth. Overall performance can be checked with various commercially produced phantoms and test objects.

Spatial resolution is defined as the ability of an imaging system to distinguish between two closely spaced objects. For ultrasound imaging, this is characterized in terms of two independent measures: the axial resolution and the lateral resolution.

Axial resolution

Axial resolution refers to the ability of a system to distinguish between two objects that are separated by a small distance along the axis of the beam. In an ideal system the minimum resolving distance is equal to half the pulse length. Therefore, to achieve better axial resolution requires shorter pulses, which in turn requires smaller ultrasound wavelengths. The velocity of ultrasound in biological tissue is approximately constant, therefore to obtain a smaller wavelength requires higher frequency transducers. The wavelength of ultrasound transmitted through the body from a 1-MHz transducer is 1.5 mm, and from a 10-MHz transducer is 0.15 mm. However, in biological soft tissue the attenuation coefficient α is roughly proportional to the frequency, and thus higher frequency ultrasound is not able to penetrate as deeply as lower frequency ultrasound. In practice, therefore, the choice of probe is a compromise between the required depth of the image and the need for good spatial resolution. For imaging the neonatal brain a 7.5-MHz transducer is now usually chosen, and most of the pictures in this book were taken using a probe of this frequency. There are occasions in neonatal cranial ultrasound imaging when a 5- or 10-MHz transducer is required and most machines do offer a choice.

Lateral resolution

Lateral resolution is a measure of the ability to distinguish between two objects at the same depth. This is dependent on the width of the beam as it is scanned across the image plane. To distinguish between two objects they must not lie within the beam at the same time, and therefore their minimum separation is equal to the beam width. The narrowest region of the beam nearest the transducer where lateral resolution is good is termed the Fresnel zone, while the region further from the transducer where the beam broadens significantly is known as the Fraunhofer zone. Lateral resolution within the Fresnel zone can be enhanced by focussing the beam, either by using an acoustic lens or by giving the transducer a concave surface. Lateral resolution is always worse than axial resolution. To achieve good lateral resolution it is essential to have a long Fresnel zone, which in turn needs higher frequencies. Again a compromise exists between requirements for high resolution and good penetration.

Contrast resolution

Contrast resolution is the ability of an ultrasound system to display different shades of gray corresponding to subtle changes in tissue reflectivity. This is largely determined by the energy of each pulse emitted into the tissue and by the amount of electronic noise contaminating the signals, although contrast resolution can be improved by averaging over signals from successive pulses emitted along the same line of sight. Contrast is also degraded by "speckle," which is a random pattern of bright and dark spots that occur when echoes from small scattering structures interfere with each other when they arrive at the transducer at the same time. Again, the effects of speckle can be significantly reduced by averaging successive images, although at a cost of reduced temporal resolution (see below).

The capability of the equipment as a whole must be considered; the measured signals undergo much processing before the image is presented on a video monitor. At this point the number of pixels, or dots, which make up the screen is also factor in the ability of a system to display small objects and distinguish them from each other. The quality of signal processing affects speckle reduction and interference from noise. In practice a good-quality 7.5-MHz imaging transducer operating on the infant head is capable of achieving a lateral resolution of about 1 or 2 mm, a performance a good deal worse than the limit imposed by the ultrasound wavelength alone. For comparison, magnetic resonance imaging or a good quality computerized tomography (CT) image with 512 pixels would achieve a resolution of about 0.5 mm.

Temporal resolution

Temporal resolution is defined as the ability of a system to distinguish between the times of occurrence of two separate events. Any tissue movement that occurs during the acquisition of a single ultrasound frame will appear blurred, and therefore to improve temporal resolution, the frame rate F must be increased. As described above, this requires the depth of the image and/or the number of lines in each frame to be reduced.

Doppler ultrasound

So far we have considered the behavior of ultrasound waves with regard to static boundaries within tissues. However, living tissues are not static, and some tissues, such as flowing blood, can move quite rapidly. In 1842 Christian Doppler first reported his observation that sound waves emitted by a source moving towards an observer have their wavelengths compressed, which raises the pitch (frequency). Meanwhile, for a source moving away from the observer the wavelengths are stretched, which reduces the pitch. This "Doppler effect" is the cause of the familiar change in pitch of a train speeding through a station or of an ambulance siren as it passes by. The same phenomenon occurs with light waves, and is exploited by astronomers to determine the velocity of stars and galaxies relative to the Earth.

When ultrasound is reflected by moving tissues, a change occurs in the frequency of the reflected wave. A measurement of this change enables the velocity of moving tissues (and of flowing blood in particular) to be measured. In so-called color-flow Doppler imaging, blood flow information is superimposed in color onto the real-time gray-scale image.

The Doppler equation

When an ultrasound beam of transmitted frequency f encounters a target (such as a region of flowing blood) moving with a velocity v, the frequency of the reflected wave f_r is different by an amount f_d, given by the following equation:

$$f_d = (f - f_r) = f \frac{2v \cos \theta}{c}, \qquad 1.6$$

where θ is the angle between the ultrasound beam and the direction of motion of the target and c is the velocity of sound in the tissue. Assuming both f and c are known and θ can be estimated, the velocity v can be obtained from a measurement of f_r. Estimating θ can be difficult, although when Doppler measurements of flow are combined with imaging, the orientation of the vessel of interest can be determined reasonably accurately, enabling good estimates of velocity to be obtained.

Continuous wave Doppler probes

A *continuous wave* (CW) Doppler probe consists of two transducer crystals: one to emit a continuous beam of ultrasound and one to detect the waves reflected back to the probe. The detected signals are amplified and filtered to reduce the effects of noise, and the shifts in the frequency are extracted by a process known as *demodulation*. For typical blood flow velocities and probe frequencies the Doppler shifts (f_d) happen to occur within the audible range of frequencies (i.e., a few kilohertz). Consequently they are commonly presented as an audio signal. The human ear is a sensitive instrument and the fact that Doppler signals can be heard in this way has undoubtedly helped the success of the method, as a trained operator can gain a great deal of information just by listening. Blood flowing in a vessel does not all flow at the same velocity and the changes induced by diseased or stenosed segments often produce a characteristic signal that can be detected by ear. However, a more objective analysis and the conversion of the information into a form that can be represented pictorially requires *spectral analysis*.

Pulsed Doppler instruments

A continuous beam of ultrasound does not allow the locations of reflecting structures to be determined, and therefore CW Doppler probes cannot identify the depths of blood vessels or even establish if the acquired signal originates from more than one vessel within the beam. However, these limitations are overcome by pulsed Doppler instruments, which use a single transducer crystal to both transmit and detect. The Doppler shift frequency is determined by monitoring successive echoes obtained from reflecting structures at a given depth. If those structures move, those echoes will exhibit a small shift in their short waveform profile, from which the Doppler shift frequency can be derived. By selecting echoes arriving at a specific time following the emitted pulse, the instrument can extract the flow velocity information at a specific depth. Scanning the beam then allows a 2D map of flow information to be displayed. This Doppler map is normally combined with real-time B-mode imaging in a device sometimes known as a *duplex system*. This is a powerful investigative tool, as velocities can be sampled from known anatomical locations (see Fig. 1.3). The ability to view the orientation of blood vessels allows the velocities to be determined quite accurately.

Aliasing

Pulsed Doppler systems are only able to detect velocities unambiguously up to a finite maximum. The so-called sampling theorem [4] states that a continuous signal must be sampled at least twice at the highest frequency present in order to accurately recover the signal. This implies that to determine a Doppler shift frequency from a series of discrete measurements (i.e., from successive pulses) without ambiguity it is necessary that the PRF is at least twice that frequency. The maximum measurable frequency (= PRF/2) is known as the Nyquist frequency. If the Doppler shift frequency exceeds the Nyquist, then a phenomenon known as aliasing will occur, and the frequency is falsely recognized as being a lower frequency. The corresponding flow velocity, obtained by inserting the frequency into the Doppler equation, will be lower than its true value, and the flow direction can appear reversed (Fig. 1.4). Obviously if estimates of flow velocity are incorrect this can have negative clinical consequences.

A familiar example of aliasing is the curious apparent rotation of cartwheels recorded on film, which can often appear to be rotating much more slowly than they really are, or even in the reverse direction. This occurs when the film frame rate (the sampling rate) is insufficient to represent the true rotation rate of the wheel.

The example represented in Fig. 1.4 would be fairly easy to spot, but if the aliasing is very marked the Doppler signal can "wrap around" the forward and reverse channels making the resulting display appear like that of turbulent flow. If there is a possibility that aliasing is occurring, then this should be checked, either by using a CW Doppler probe (for which aliasing cannot occur), or by increasing the PRF. However, increasing the PRF decreases the maximum depth at which echoes can originate. As the maximum depth is reduced, it becomes increasingly feasible that late arriving echoes (from deeper structures) due to an emitted pulse can arrive during the measurement cycle for echoes produced by the following pulse (i.e., echoes are obtained simultaneously from two sampling volumes). The resulting ambiguity in sampling location can be

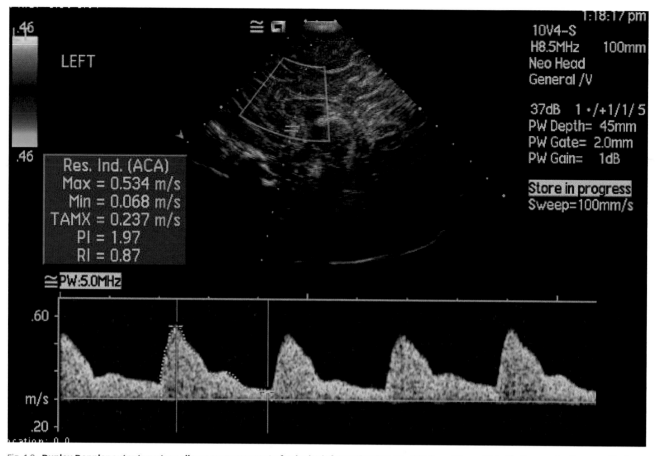

Fig. 1.3. **Duplex Doppler output; system allows measurement of velocity information in a specified position within the image depth. Note display of the information as a sonogram after signal processing.**

avoided if one of the potential sampling volumes is strategically placed within a region of no flow.

Doppler signal processing

The origin of the echoes used to determine blood flow is the back-scatter of the ultrasound by red blood cells. Since blood cells within a typical vessel are traveling with a broad range of velocities, echoes return with a range of Doppler-shifted frequencies. The complexity of the returned signal requires signal processing, both for audio interpretation and for visual presentation. Demodulation circuitry extracts the Doppler frequency signal, and amplifies it to an appropriate level. It is customary to subject the signal to a filter (known as a *wall-thump filter*) to remove a high-amplitude, low-frequency component due to reflection off the blood vessel walls. Wall thump filters are usually set for frequencies below 200 Hz, and therefore produce a gap in the velocity spectrum around zero. This can give rise to inaccuracies when distinguishing between minor degrees of reversed diastolic flow, and for neonatal cerebral work it is important to set the filter as low as possible. Further electronic circuitry is involved in distinguishing between forward and reverse flow, and in generating a sonogram.

A circuit known as a zero-crossing detector is sometimes used to quantify the principal Doppler frequency (and therefore the

dominant flow velocity), although its performance is unreliable when a large range of frequencies are involved or when the signal is particularly noisy. The best method of displaying and quantifying flow characteristics is spectral analysis. This involves performing a *Fourier transform* of the Doppler signals acquired over successive short windows of time (typically a few milliseconds). Although various display modes are used, the frequency content (i.e., the velocity content) is commonly exhibited as a function of time, with time updated continuously along the horizontal axis.

Color flow Doppler

The combination of pulsed Doppler and real-time imaging enables velocity information to be superimposed on the anatomical representation, and the concept of color coding the velocity information was first proposed in 1981 [5]. Real-time color flow mapping (CFM) systems are now commonplace. The usual pulse-echo B scan is used to provide a gray-scale image and multiple Doppler interrogations are performed in order to add information about the direction and velocity of blood flow within a selected region of the B scan.

Color flow mapping is perhaps of most use in cardiology, although the combination of Doppler and real-time imaging allows the location of vessels to be identified easily and significantly reduces the time required to examine flow in

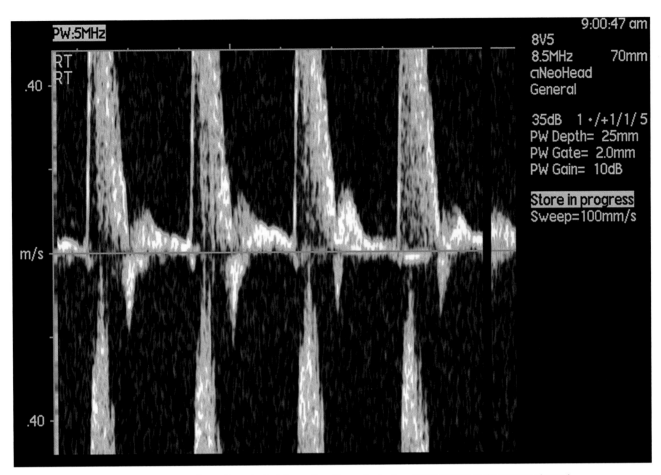

Fig. 1.4. **Example of aliasing of range-gated Doppler velocity information. Tops of velocity profiles appear in the reverse channel.**

neonatal cranial arteries (Fig. 1.5). Abnormal vascular leashes can be seen, allowing the diagnosis of arterio-venous malformations. Typically the velocities are displayed in shades of red through yellow for flow toward the transducer, and shades of blue through purple for flow away from the transducer. However, the scale is only approximately quantitative, mostly because of the averaging performed over a finite volume and period of time. Turbulent flow is typically represented as green, although color aliasing can occur with very high velocities in the same way as described for pulsed Doppler earlier. Aliasing can result in fast flow being coded as green (turbulent) when in fact the Doppler frequency has exceeded the Nyquist limit. Turbulent jets should therefore be checked, as advised for possible aliasing, with CW Doppler ultrasound.

Safety of ultrasound

Sound waves are a form of energy, and the amount of energy emitted by a typical ultrasound system is similar to that generated by the human voice during normal conversation. Nevertheless, exposure of tissue to very high levels of ultrasound is known to cause harmful biological effects. Given the possibility that diagnostic ultrasound may not be completely safe, regulatory authorities frequently examine the potential risks, and have occasionally issued guidelines for the prudent use of ultrasound imaging. There is a general consensus that the potential for risk continues to grow as a result of the tendency for commercial scanners to provide an increasing level of exposure. This is a consequence of the manufacturers' quest to develop systems that deliver further improvements in diagnostic information and image quality. For example, achieving a higher spatial resolution requires higher frequencies, and therefore higher intensities to overcome the greater attenuation. Although a variety of potential harmful effects of diagnostic levels of ultrasound have been postulated, only two are generally considered to be of significant concern: thermal damage due to heating of tissue, and mechanical damage due to a phenomenon known as cavitation.

During a clinical ultrasound examination, almost all the energy in the ultrasound beam ends up being absorbed and therefore heats the tissue. The ability of the tissue to dissipate the heat depends on a variety of factors such as thermal conductivity and blood flow, but at typical diagnostic exposure levels the likely maximum rise in tissue temperature is generally considered too low to be a significant hazard.

Cavitation is the name given to the phenomenon that can cause sound waves to produce bubbles of gas in tissue. Tissues, like most liquids at normal pressures and temperatures, contain dissolved gas. During the negative pressure phase of an ultrasound wave, the dissolved gas can spontaneously come

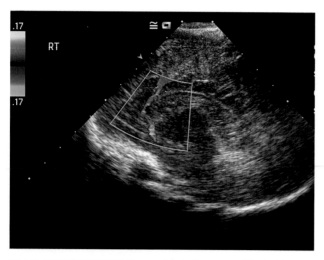

Fig. 1.5. **Example of color flow mapping in the neonatal brain. The anterior cerebral artery appears red; flow towards the transducer.**

out of solution producing microscopic bubbles. Once formed, these bubbles have a tendency to grow. If they reach a certain size they can vibrate in resonance with the ultrasound, producing violent forces within the immediate vicinity of the bubbles. This can lead to a phenomenon known as *microstreaming*, where high-velocity currents are established that are potentially damaging to biological molecules and structures. If the ultrasound intensity were to become sufficiently high (well above diagnostic levels) the bubbles can collapse destructively, producing exceedingly high local temperatures and pressures, leading to a variety of highly destructive effects.

As described by Wells [6], the authorities that regulate use of diagnostic ultrasound in some countries now require system manufacturers to provide an on-screen indication of the relative risk in terms of a "thermal index" (related to likelihood of thermal damage) and a "mechanical index" (related to risk of damage due to cavitation).

The overwhelming conclusion of the leading professional clinical and scientific organizations concerned with the use of the modality is that there are no confirmed harmful effects of diagnostic ultrasound. Nevertheless, it is recommended that the prudent operator will attempt to limit the exposure of his or her patient to a minimum, and a significant reduction can be achieved by following these simple suggestions (modified from Evans *et al.* [7], with permission):

1. Use the lowest transmitted power that will give a result.
2. Keep the duration of the examination to a minimum.
3. Use CW Doppler rather than pulsed wave if it will give a result.
4. Use the lowest PRF of pulsed Doppler that will allow the highest velocity to be measured.
5. Do not leave the Doppler beam irradiating a particular region for longer than is necessary. Switch back to imaging mode as soon as the Doppler examination is complete.
6. Use color Doppler only when necessary to make the diagnosis.

Note that the Royal College of Radiologists [8] has produced specific guidelines on cranial ultrasound in infants that are available on their website: www.rcr.ac.uk/docs/radiology/pdf/ultrasound.pdf.

References

1. Holmes JH. Ultrasound during the early years of AIUM. *J Clin Ultrasound* 1980; **8**: 299–308.
2. Hedrick WR, Hykes DL, Starchman DE. *Ultrasound Physics and Instrumentation*, 4th edn. St. Louis, MO: Mosby-Year Book, 2005.
3. Fenster A, Downey DB, Cardinal H N. Three-dimensional ultrasound imaging. *Phys Med Biol* 2001; **46**: R67–R99.
4. Shannon CE. Communications in the presence of noise. *Proc IRE* 1949; **37**: 10–21.
5. Eyer MK, Brandestini MA, Phillips DJ, Baker DW. Colour digital echo/Doppler image presentation. *Ultrasound Med Biol* 1981; **7**: 21–31.
6. Wells PNT. Ultrasound imaging. *Phys Med Biol* 2006; **51**: R83–R98.
7. Evans DH, McDicken WN, Skidmore R, Woodcock JP. *Doppler Ultrasound: Physics, Instrumentation and Clinical Applications.* Chichester: John Wiley, 1989.
8. Royal College of Radiologists. Appendix 8: Cranial ultrasound in infants. In: *Ultrasound Training Recommendations for Medical and Surgical Specialities.* London: Royal College of Radiologists, 2004.

Chapter 2 | Principles of EEG

GERALDINE B. BOYLAN

Introduction

Electroencephalography (EEG) monitors the function of the neonatal brain and provides a sensitive real-time measure of cerebral activity. The neonatal brain is particularly vulnerable to changes in oxygenation and blood pressure and the effects of these physiological changes can often be detected by the EEG. In addition, it is now clear that clinical seizure expression in neonates is ambiguous and most seizures can only be detected by the EEG, which can also provide helpful information regarding the differential diagnosis (Chapter 7). Electroencephalography is also the most sensitive tool available for predicting neurodevelopmental outcome in neonates with early neonatal encephalopathy, particularly that due to hypoxic ischemia, and can provide this information much earlier than any other method. Many units use continuous amplitude integrated EEG (aEEG) to monitor cerebral activity. This provides a more limited measure of cerebral activity but nonetheless can be very useful, particularly if no other monitoring is available. Continuous monitoring with EEG is becoming a standard of care in many neonatal intensive care units (NICUs) around the world.

The aim of this chapter is to describe principles of EEG and aEEG recording. At the end of this chapter the reader should feel confident enough to record either the EEG or an aEEG from a newborn baby in the NICU. They will appreciate the characteristics of different recording devices, recognize the difficulties that are particular to the NICU environment which can impede recordings, recognize common sources of artifact that often mimic events such as seizures, and appreciate the difference between EEG and aEEG. Information on the appearances of the normal neonatal EEG and aEEG can be found in Chapter 6.

The electroencephalogram

The EEG is a measure of the electrical activity of the brain. Hans Berger first recorded this electrical activity from the scalp in humans in 1929. It is now known that EEG activity recorded from the scalp arises from ionic currents generated by postsynaptic potentials caused by changes in the membrane permeability of dendrites and neuronal bodies. The electrical activity recorded from the scalp has a frequency range from 0.1 Hz to approximately 100 Hz and the amplitude is typically less than 200 μV. Electrodes are used to make connections between the biological tissue (scalp generally in neonates) and a recording device (EEG machine). Unfortunately one electrode is not enough to measure the EEG; it has to be measured between two points on the scalp.

Technology of EEG recording

The EEG voltage recorded at the scalp is of low amplitude, being attenuated by the meninges, skull and scalp, and is of the order of microvolts (μV; one millionth of a volt). The EEG activity is measured from metal electrodes that are fixed to the scalp using adhesive conductive paste and connected to a recording device that amplifies the tiny signals. Different regions of the brain generate different types of activity; therefore, electrodes have to be applied in a systematic fashion so that each area of the brain is studied.

The need for a general electrode placement format led the International Federation of Societies for Electroencephalography and Clinical Neurophysiology (IFSECN) to recommend a specific system of electrode placement for use in all laboratories under standard conditions. This is referred to as the 10–20 system of electrode placement. Specific measurements from bony landmarks (nasion, inion and left and right preauricular points) are used to determine the placement of electrodes. The term 10–20 is used because electrodes are placed at points 10% and 20% along lines between these bony landmarks (Fig. 2.1). The standard numbering system places even-numbered electrodes on the right side of the head and odd-numbered electrodes on the left with a letter designating the anatomical area. Midline electrodes are designated with the letter "z." Therefore, an electrode on the left central region would be designated C_3; an electrode on the right parietal region, P_4; and an electrode on the mid frontal region, F_z (Fig. 2.1).

The way in which the EEG activity is displayed on the screen is dependent on a "montage." A montage is a pattern of

Neonatal Cerebral Investigation, eds. Janet M. Rennie, Cornelia F. Hagmann and Nicola J. Robertson. Published by Cambridge University Press. © Cambridge University Press 2008.

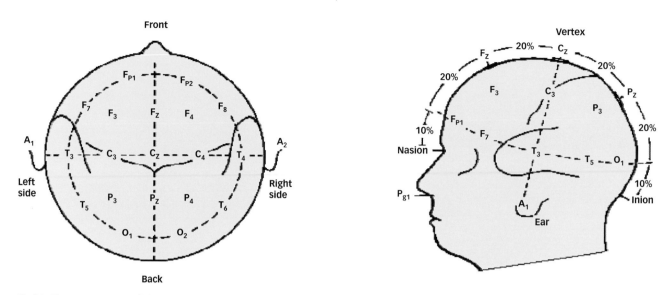

Fig. 2.1. **The 10–20 system of electrode placement showing right and left designation and measurement landmarks. Fp, prefrontal; F, frontal; C, central; T, temporal; A, auricular; P, parietal; O, occipital.**

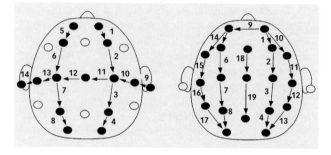

Fig. 2.2. **Examples of EEG montages. This is the arrangement in which electrodes are linked for display. It makes EEG interpretation simpler.**

electrode arrangement used for EEG display. Montages are generally selected so that recordings are made from rows of equidistant electrodes running from the front to the back of the head or transversely across it. Examples of montages are illustrated in Fig. 2.2.

Recording arrangements can be varied so that the potential difference is measured between pairs of scalp electrodes (bipolar) or between individual electrodes and a common reference point. In the latter arrangement the reference site can be either a relatively inactive site (such as linked ears) or a point connected to all the electrodes in use so that it reflects the average of the potentials at these electrodes. Most modern digital EEG machines use the common reference method for EEG signal acquisition, but have the ability to redisplay the EEG in any montage required termed "re-montaging."

Recording the neonatal EEG

Recording the neonatal EEG requires certain modifications to allow for the fact that babies on the NICU are often very sick and incredibly small. The NICU environment is electrically very noisy and it can be difficult to extract small-amplitude EEG signals from a tiny baby who is often attached to lots of other monitoring equipment.

Full-term babies should ideally have a full set of electrodes applied to the scalp using the 10–20 system of electrode placement. However, it may not always be possible to apply a complete set of EEG electrodes to a premature or very sick unstable baby. The extra time involved in trying to achieve this is likely to worsen the baby's condition. It is far more important to apply a fixed minimum number of electrodes as carefully and as efficiently as possible, ensuring that there is good contact and symmetry. Once a good recording has been obtained using these, it may be possible to apply more electrodes if required. Once electrode application has started there may be frequent interruptions for nursing/medical procedures such as suctioning and blood gas measurement. It can take over an hour to apply a complete set of electrodes carefully, particularly if the baby is ventilated. Quite often, electrodes become dislodged during the procedure and require re-application.

It is important to record from other non-cerebral channels during EEG monitoring. Electrocardiography or ECG is mandatory for neonatal EEG due to the frequent presence of ECG artifact, which may mimic stereotyped neonatal seizure patterns. There is also an increased risk of picking up pulse artifact through the fontanelles, which have not closed. Premature babies often have bradycardias and it is important to note this for optimum EEG interpretation. Any baby can have a bradycardia associated with a seizure. It is also important to record a respiration trace in the neonate because of the frequency of apneas during seizures, particularly in full-term babies. Rhythmic delta activity (slow wave activity) recorded in the neonatal EEG can often simply be respiration artifact since babies have high respiration rates of up to 100 breaths per min. Eye movement or electrooculogram (EOG) and muscle tone (EMG) channels are extremely useful to help determine sleep state in the baby.

Stockard-Pope et al. [1] in their excellent atlas of neonatal EEG recommend that at least eight scalp and two ear mastoid electrodes, covering all major areas of the brain, are used in

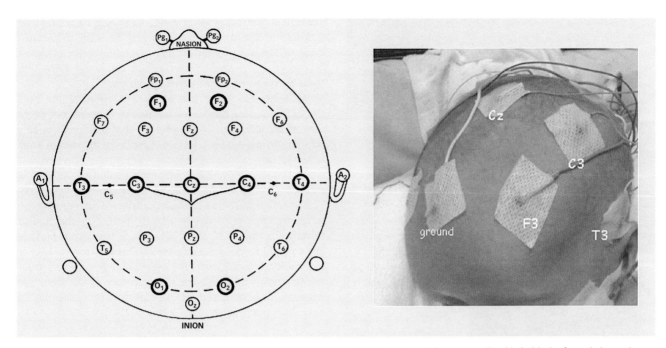

Fig. 2.3. **Recommended neonatal EEG recording positions [3]. The recommended electrode positions are outlined in bold. The frontal electrodes F4 and F3 can be used, or they can be positioned midway between the usual prefrontal and frontal electrode positions (F1 and F2).**

preterm and low-birth-weight babies. There are no UK guidelines on neonatal EEG recording. American guidelines suggest that 16 channel instruments should be used to record at least 8 channels of EEG and other non-cerebral signals, e.g., ECG, EMG, etc. [2]. The minimum array acceptable according to these guidelines is Fp_1, Fp_2, C_3, C_z, C_4, T_3, T_4, O_1, O_2, A_1, A_2. Mizrahi and Kellaway [3] recommend the use of nine EEG positions and these are illustrated in Fig. 2.3.

Whatever montage is adopted, the following areas require monitoring in preterm and full-term babies so that all the specific waveforms that occur at different conceptional ages are recorded: right and left frontal, temporal, occipital, central (or parietal), and the mid central region. Midline electrodes are useful for the recognition of developmental patterns, neonatal seizures (may only be in the midline), interictal patterns in encephalopathy, neonatal myoclonus, cerebrovascular accidents, and congenital anomalies [4].

Electrode application

The most important factor to consider when applying neonatal EEG electrodes is undoubtedly preparation of the electrode sites. Babies are usually admitted to the NICU before they have been washed and with blood and vernix adhering to the scalp. This is particularly the case when the baby has required resuscitation after birth. The scalp should be cleaned with an alcohol wipe if possible to remove all traces of blood and birth residues. Each site should then be rubbed gently (cotton buds are ideal) with a slightly abrasive conducting gel (such as NuPrep®) and the electrode then applied using a fixative paste (Table 2.1). It is important to rub the electrode site until the impedance (resistance to current flow) of the skin has been

reduced to below $5\,k\Omega$ (displayed as an output on most EEG machines). For optimum EEG recording electrode impedances should be low, equal, and stable. Equal impedances ensure rejection of common-mode signals such as 50-Hz mains interference, a problem generally encountered in the NICU. Once electrode application has started there may be frequent interruptions for nursing/medical procedures such as suctioning and blood gas measurement. It is often useful to secure all the electrodes on the scalp using a soft net, similar to those used to keep dressings in place after surgery (Table 2.1). If a baby is in an incubator, the electrode leads can be fed through the incubator access ports and then to the amplifier headbox of the EEG system. Electrode leads should be bunched together and secured so that they do not hinder any other tubes or lines. Securing the electrode leads together also reduces lead movement artifact on the EEG and also mains interference pick-up.

Measurement of the electrocardiogram

Lead 1 ECG should be recorded simultaneously with the EEG in all neonatal recordings. It is best to record this from the shoulders or forearms as the lower arms frequently have drips sited. The recording parameters of the EEG machine should be adjusted to capture this signal, which is of the order of millivolts and therefore much larger than the EEG signals. A sensitivity of 1 mV is generally recommended. The right arm and left leg can also be used but this is susceptible to movement artifact.

Measurement of respiration

Respiration can be measured using nasal or oral airflow but this method is not possible in ventilated babies. Commercially

Table 2.1. EEG electrode application. Before EEG electrodes are attached to the scalp, the head should be cleaned thoroughly with an alcohol wipe. The head should then be measured and the electrode positions marked on the scalp using a suitable skin pencil.

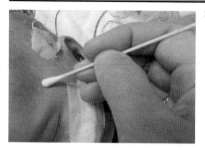

Step 1: Prepare the electrode site by rubbing the skin gently but firmly with a cotton bud and electrode prepping gel such as NuPrep®. If the baby has hair it should be separated out to expose the scalp.

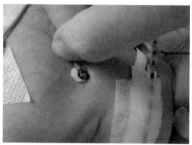

Step 2: Scoop some sticky conductive electrode paste into the cup of the electrode and stick on to the prepared site. Conductive paste is available from most EEG system distributors. If the baby has hair, it can be smoothed over the electrode to help it stay in place.

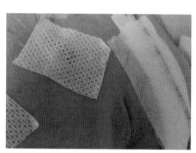

Step 3: Cover the electrode with sticky tape such as Mefix®. It can be difficult to get tape to stay on over hair and in some cases a little more conductive paste on top of the electrode helps.

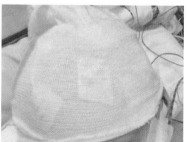

Step 4: When all electrodes have been applied to the scalp a soft net hat can be used to keep the electrodes in place if long-term recording is anticipated.

available chest wall movement detectors can be used but the band should be placed at the level of the end of the sternum in order to pick up respiration movement in premature babies, who are generally abdominal breathers. An effective method is to use impedance measurement of respiration. This method measures the impedance changes caused by thoraco-

abdominal ventilatory movements of the baby. In babies with a history of apnea, an attempt should be made to measure nasal airflow using a thermistor.

Measurement of the electrooculogram

Ag/AgCl disc electrodes can be used to measure the EOG. Disposable surface electrodes are not recommended or necessary as considerable skin abrasion is often required to reduce impedance, and Ag/AgCl electrodes applied with paste or a *little* adhesive tape such as Micropore® are just as effective (and much less expensive). Two channels should be devoted to recording the EOG if available. An electrode should be placed 1 cm lateral to and below the outer canthus of each eye and this is referred to an electrode slightly lateral to the nasion. However, if time or number of channels is a constraint then one channel works quite effectively. One electrode is applied to the left upper canthus of the left eye and the other electrode to the cheek just below the lateral corner of the right eye. Adequate documentation of eye movements is essential for sleep state recognition.

Measurement of the electromyogram

The EMG (surface EMG) is a measure of the electrical activity of muscle and in neonates is often recorded from the submental region (i.e., over the right and left sides of the inferior edge of the mandible). As the EMG is a high-frequency signal it is best to set the high-frequency filter as high as possible, or, better still, off. The EEG electrodes are perfectly acceptable for recording the EMG. The submental EMG is useful for sleep state documentation in term babies, as a high level of tonic activity is present during quiet sleep. Quite often, in neonates with abnormal movements, it is useful to record EMG activity from a limb in order to determine the relationship between EEG and EMG activity.

Neonatal EEG acquisition

Modern EEG machines convert the EEG signal into digital form and display it on a standard computer screen. The EEG signals recorded at the surface of the scalp by the electrodes are then fed to a headbox device. The headbox is the patient interface and the EEG electrodes are plugged into predetermined input terminals on this headbox and then referred to a reference, which is usually an additional scalp EEG electrode (Fig. 2.4). These input terminals are often displayed on a head diagram on the headbox. The signals from each headbox socket are amplified, filtered, digitized and then transmitted through a cable to an interface card in the computer. Synchronized digital video recording is very useful for neonates, particularly for long-term monitoring as frequent interruptions occur during the course of a baby's care and it is useful to correlate these interruptions with the EEG. In addition, video is invaluable for accurate seizure identification (Chapter 7).

When the electrodes have been attached to the scalp and plugged into the EEG headbox the next step involves an impedance check to ensure integrity of all the electrodes and connections. The user then needs to select how the EEG is going to be displayed. In most modern EEG systems, a set of protocols can be set up soon after the machine is purchased and these rarely need to be changed thereafter. In the protocol for neonatal EEG monitoring the display amplitude, filter settings, display speed, and display montage can be selected so that the system defaults to this when a new recording begins. However, when a recording commences this can be altered usually from a panel on the screen (Fig. 2.5). The recommended settings for neonatal EEG are displayed in Table 2.2. Most digital EEG machines have a notch or 50-Hz filter. This is a sharply tuned bandstop filter that is centered at the frequency of mains interference (50 or 60 Hz depending on location). This filter should always be considered a last resort filter and should only be used after all other methods have been utilized to eliminate mains interference. This includes procedures such as reduction of electrode impedances, bunching electrodes together, and repositioning of other mains power equipment. Given the technologically intensive environment of the NICU it is often very difficult to eliminate all mains interference and the notch filter is essential (Fig. 2.6).

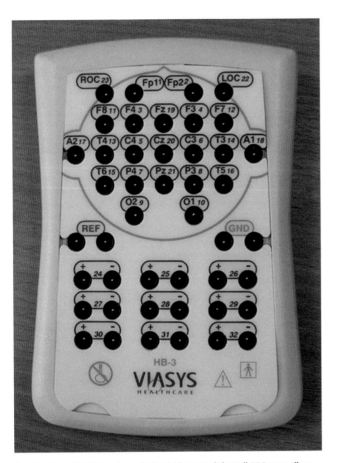

Fig. 2.4. **Typical EEG headbox. It should be noted that all EEG recordings require a reference (REF – in red) and ground or earth (GND – in green) input.**

Table 2.2. Recommended neonatal EEG recording parameters.

Display sensitivity (amplification)	50–100 µV/cm
High-frequency filter	70 Hz
Time constant (low-frequency filter)	0.3 s (0.5 Hz)
Display speed	30 mm or 15 mm/s

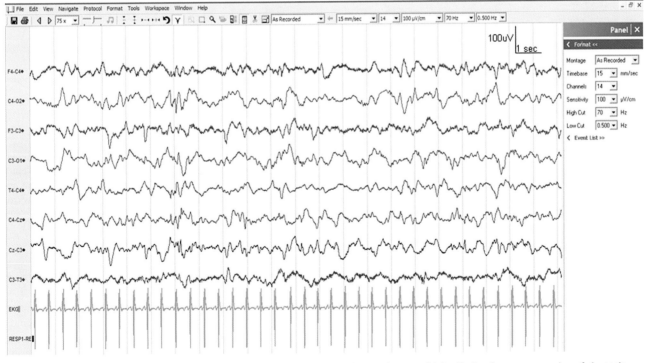

Fig. 2.5. **Typical EEG display screen showing panel that allows alteration of settings such as sensitivity display, frequency, number of channels, and montage.**

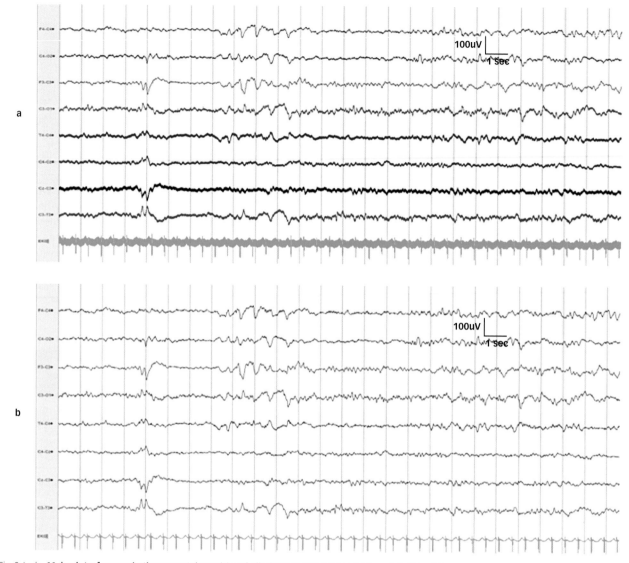

Fig. 2.6.a,b. **Mains interference in the neonatal EEG (a) and elimination after the use of a notch filter (b).**

Artifacts

Artifacts on the neonatal EEG are signals that contaminate the EEG and make it difficult to interpret. They can arise from biological and non-biological sources. The NICU environment itself can make it technically demanding to record the tiny amplitude signals of the neonatal EEG. The amplifiers in modern digital EEG machines are improving all the time and the susceptibility to electrically noisy environments is becoming less of a problem. A more detailed review of artifacts in the neonatal EEG is available in the excellent *Atlas of Neonatal Electroencephalography* by Mizrahi *et al.* [5].

Biological artifacts

Biological artifacts in the neonatal EEG are artifacts that arise from the baby and are most commonly due to ECG, respiration, and movement. It is often very difficult to distinguish respiration artifact from a stereotyped seizure discharge; hence, the need for respiration monitoring in any EEG recording. Table 2.3 shows a list of the most common biological artifacts encountered in neonatal EEG recording.

Non-biological artifacts

The most common non-biological artifact encountered in neonatal EEG recordings is mains interference. As already discussed, all EEG machines have a specific filter available to eliminate this type of interference if it is excessive and cannot be removed by bunching electrodes together and switching off any unnecessary mains-powered equipment. Infusion pumps can cause a repetitive artifact on the neonatal EEG and it is always worth switching these to battery power if possible

Table 2.3. Common biological artifacts in the neonatal EEG.

Source	Type	
Cardiac	ECG artifact is the most common but pulse (fontanelle-related pulsations) and ballistocardiographic (movement of head with heartbeat) can also be seen	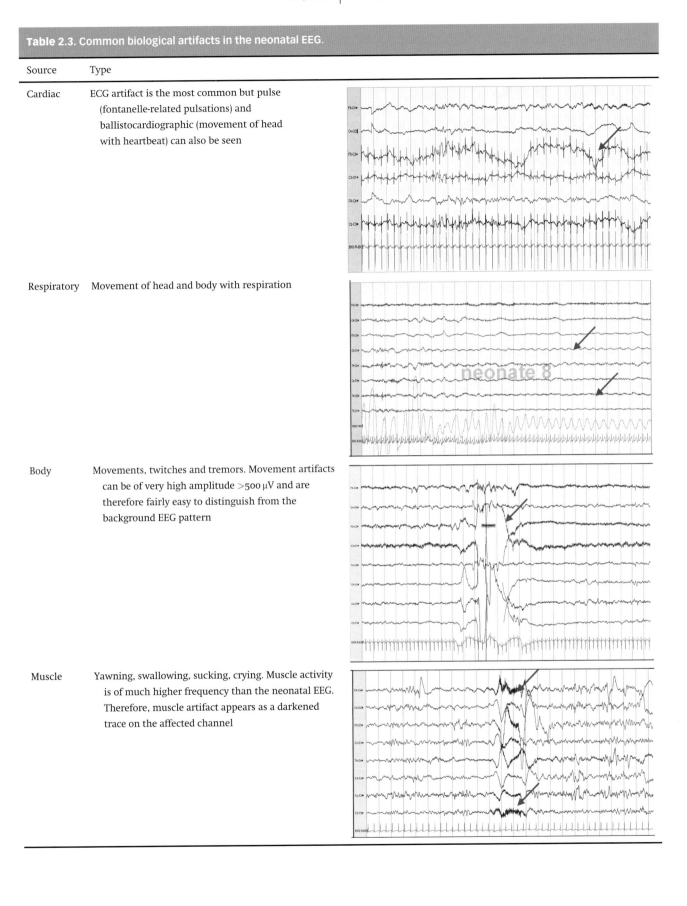
Respiratory	Movement of head and body with respiration	
Body	Movements, twitches and tremors. Movement artifacts can be of very high amplitude >500 μV and are therefore fairly easy to distinguish from the background EEG pattern	
Muscle	Yawning, swallowing, sucking, crying. Muscle activity is of much higher frequency than the neonatal EEG. Therefore, muscle artifact appears as a darkened trace on the affected channel	

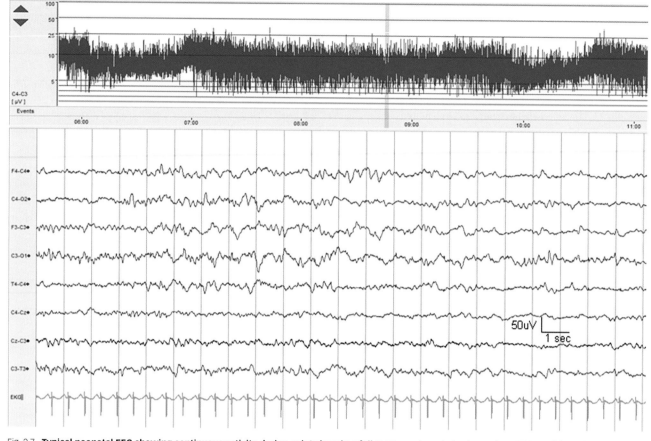

Fig. 2.7. **Typical neonatal EEG showing continuous activity during quiet sleep in a full-term newborn baby. In modern EEG machines the aEEG (top trace) can also be displayed with the multi channel EEG.**

during the EEG recording session to see if it improves the recording. Ventilators often produce an artifact on the EEG but in most cases this is due to head movement at the ventilator rate frequency. High frequency oscillation ventilation is particularly problematic.

EEG phenomenology

Figure 2.7 shows a typical neonatal EEG from a full-term baby during sleep. The full-term neonatal EEG generally contains mixed-frequency continuous activity that is symmetric and synchronous between the right and left hemispheres.

EEG frequencies

The frequency of the EEG is described in hertz (Hz) or the number of times a wave repeats itself within a second. Therefore, to calculate the frequency of the activity in the EEG it is necessary to examine how many repetitions of a wave are seen in a 1-s period. On most EEG systems, a 1-s marker is visible (generally a vertical line). There are four main types of EEG frequencies:

Activity	Frequency (Hz)
Beta	>13
Alpha	8–13
Theta	5–7
Delta	0–4

The commonest types of activity seen in the neonatal EEG are theta and delta activity; beta activity may be seen more infrequently (Fig. 2.8). Alpha frequency components are also seen and seizures on the neonatal EEG can have alpha frequency. The EEG is also described in terms of amplitude or power. The EEG signal is in the order of microvolts and is generally measured from the peak of the top of the waveform to its trough (Fig. 2.8).

In limited channel aEEG systems (see "The CFM and amplitude integrated EEG (aEEG)"), information on frequency is not available, and the original analog cerebral function monitor (CFM), designed for use in adults, was limited to a single channel. In preterm neonates, asymmetry and asynchrony are seen at various stages of development. Most of the background or "ongoing" activity of the neonatal EEG lies in the frequency range of 0.5–12 Hz. Most EEG systems display 1-s markers on the screen, making frequency easy to estimate by eye. Alternatively the amplitude and frequency of the EEG can usually be measured on screen using a waveform measurement tool (Fig. 2.9).

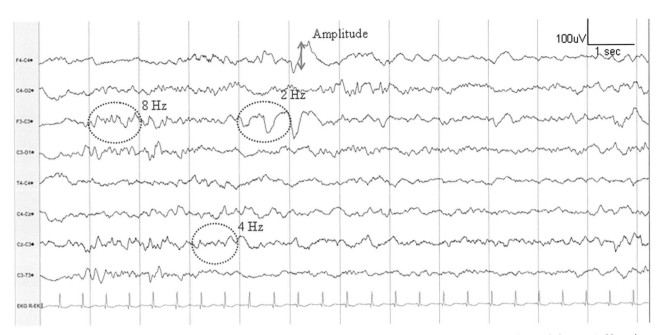

Fig. 2.8. Illustrating two of the more common EEG interpretation criteria: frequency and amplitude measurement. The EEG is interpreted based on frequency, amplitude, waveform morphology, state differentiation, and reactivity. The display montage used is featured on the gray bar to the left of the waveform. Each vertical line represents 1 s.

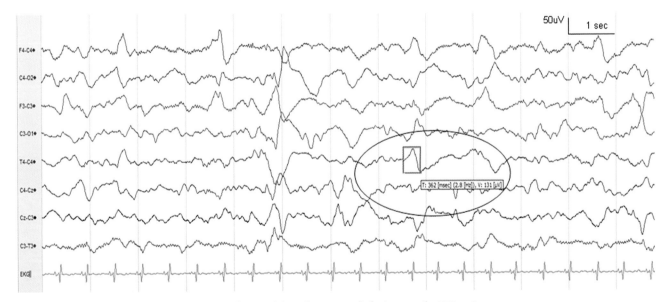

Fig. 2.9. **Amplitude and frequency measurement of EEG activity using automatic features on the EEG system.**

Abnormal waveforms

To the novice, a 30-s window of EEG in a full-term baby looks like a series of random varying lines without any obvious pattern. This is probably one of the most important features of the EEG; the absence of obvious patterns when the EEG is normal. The EEG becomes abnormal when specific wave patterns become repetitive, when the amplitude is low and lacks variability, or when other patterns emerge such as burst suppression (Fig. 2.10).

The CFM and amplitude integrated EEG (aEEG)

The cerebral function monitor (CFM), which displays a single channel of aEEG, is still quite widely used in the NICU despite the fact that it was originally designed for use in adults. It is used for the assessment of brain activity in both term and preterm neonates, for seizure detection, prognosis, and to assess the severity of encephalopathy in trials of therapeutic hypothermia [6,7,8]. The single channel CFM recording is generally based on one channel from the

Generalized Suppression

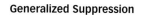

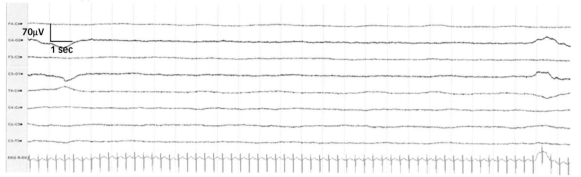

Seizures

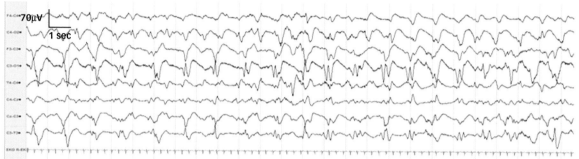

Burst Suppression

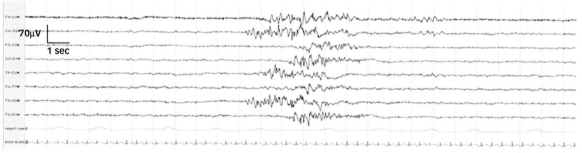

Fig. 2.10. **Abnormal patterns in the neonatal EEG.**

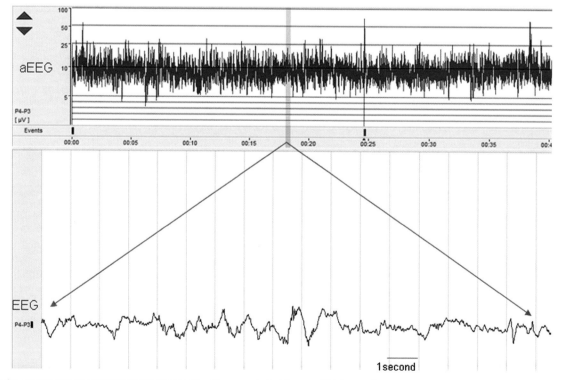

Fig. 2.11. **The aEEG over a 40-min period (top trace) and a 17-s snapshot of the raw EEG (arrows).**

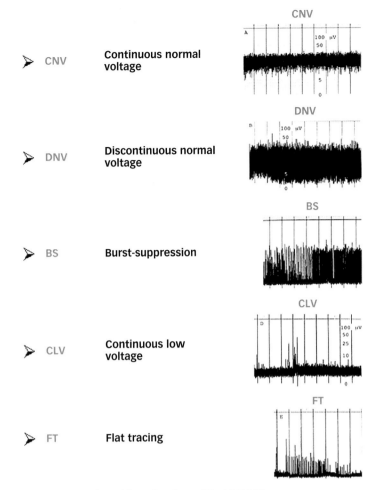

➤	CNV	Continuous normal voltage
➤	DNV	Discontinuous normal voltage
➤	BS	Burst-suppression
➤	CLV	Continuous low voltage
➤	FT	Flat tracing

Fig. 2.12. **The normal background aEEG patterns. Adapted from de Vries and Toet 2006 [6].**

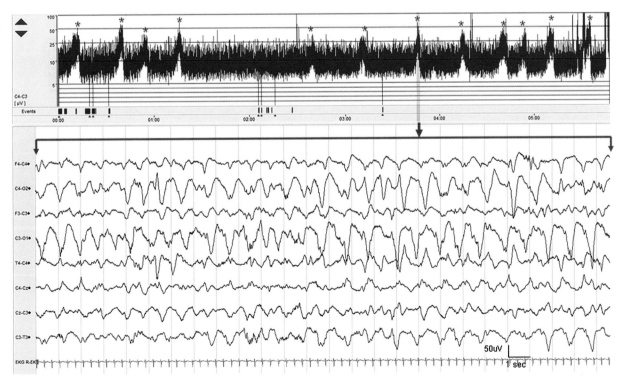

Fig. 2.13. **Seizure on the aEEG (*) and the corresponding EEG segment on a multichannel EEG recording. These seizures were of high amplitude and obvious on the aEEG recording.**

19

parietal region (P4 and P3). The aEEG is recorded using EEG electrodes applied to the scalp in the same way as for routine EEG recording. However, the process is then different as it is not the raw EEG signal that is displayed. The aEEG is calculated by band-pass filtering the signal between 2 and 15 Hz, amplifying the higher frequency components, rectifying the signal and then submitting it to a part-linear, part-logarithmic amplitude compression, "peak-smoothing" and time-compression. The resultant trace is very different to a "raw" EEG signal (Fig. 2.11). The overall amplitude of the EEG is assessed by the aEEG pattern and a number of normal background aEEG patterns have been described (Fig. 2.12). Interpretation of the aEEG is based on pattern recognition and, like EEG, requires considerable experience before it can be used competently.

The original CFM system has been criticized because of its limitation to a single EEG channel (plus a simultaneous "artifact detection" channel) and the lack of detailed information compared with the conventional multichannel EEG, especially when used for the detection of neonatal seizures [9,10,11,12]. However, newer aEEG systems are now available, which offer more than a single channel and also allow interrogation of the simultaneous "raw" EEG. These systems do offer more information than previous versions but again are limited in comparison to EEG and suffer from a lack of spatial information. Seizures can be detected if they are of high amplitude, generalized and of more than 1 min in duration (Fig. 2.13). Spatial information is often lost and it is impossible to assess background EEG synchrony and symmetry (Fig. 2.14). Information such as the interburst interval, which is important in prognosis, cannot be obtained from the aEEG due to compression of the EEG signal, but may be available on some of the newer monitors when using a simultaneous EEG display. Table 2.4 compares the type of information that can be obtained from both multichannel EEG recording and aEEG.

Technology is developing rapidly in the field of EEG and modern systems are now capable of displaying both the multichannel EEG and a number of other quantitative features

Table 2.4. Showing the type of information available from multichannel EEG compared to CFM/aEEG.

Cerebral activity	EEG	aEEG
Amplitude measurement	Yes	Yes
Frequency measurement	Yes	No
Synchrony assessment	Yes	No
Symmetry assessment	Yes	No
Interburst interval measurement	Yes	No
Sleep wake cycling	Yes	Yes
Specific maturational features	Yes	No
Spatial information	Yes	No
Generalized seizures	Yes	Yes[a]
Focal seizures	Yes	No
Artifact identification	Yes	No

[a] Only if high amplitude, see Rennie et al. [12]

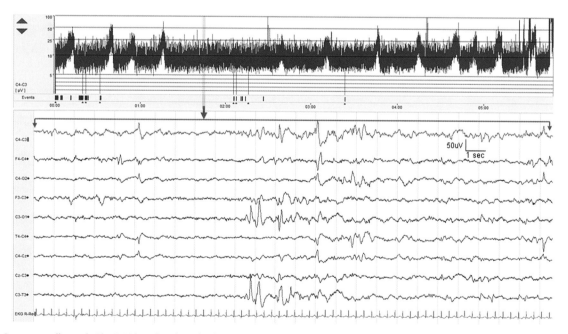

Fig. 2.14. **Same recording as in Fig. 2.13 but showing a background EEG segment (non-seizure). The single channel EEG from the same electrodes as the aEEG recording is displayed on top (red channel). At the same time the multichannel EEG is displayed, which clearly shows an asynchronous background EEG pattern. This information is lost in the single channel recording.**

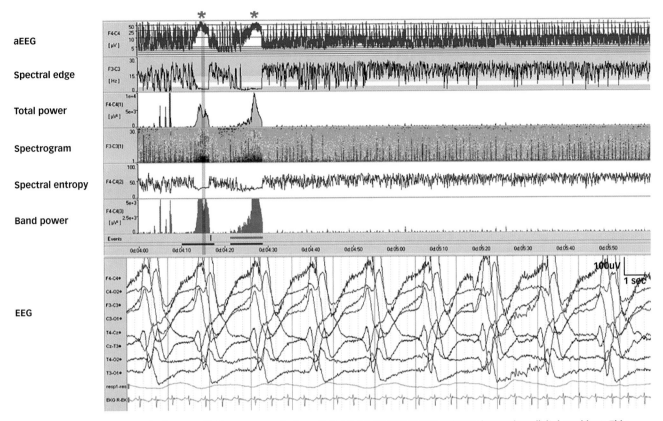

Fig. 2.15. **Simultaneous EEG and other quantitative summary features that can be calculated in real time using modern digital machines. This example shows two clear seizures (*) during a 6-h recording.**

(Fig. 2.15). Automated EEG interpretation remains elusive but must surely be on the horizon in the near future.

References

1. Stockard-Pope J, Werner S, Bickford G. *Atlas of Neonatal Electroencephalography*, 2nd edn. New York: Raven Press, 1992.
2. American EEG Society. Guidelines in EEG 1–7. *American EEG Society Ad Hoc Committee on Techniques*. 1985.
3. Mizrahi EM, Kellaway P. Neonatal electroencephalography. In: Mizrahi EM, Kellaway P, eds. *Diagnosis and Management of Neonatal Seizures*. Philadelphia: Lipincott-Raven, 1998; 99–144.
4. Scher MS. Midline electrographic abnormalities and cerebral lesions in the newborn brain [published erratum appears in *J Child Neurol* 1988 Jul; 3(3): 229]. *J Child Neurol* 1988; **3(2)**: 135–146.
5. Mizrahi EM, Hrachovy RA, Kellaway P. *Atlas of Neonatal Electroencephalography*. Philadelphia: Lippincott Williams & Wilkins, 2003.
6. de Vries LS, Toet MC. Amplitude integrated electroencephalography in the full-term newborn. *Clin Perinatol* 2006; **33(3)**: 619–32, vi.
7. Hellstrom-Westas L, Rosen I. Electroencephalography and brain damage in preterm infants. *Early Hum Dev* 2005; **81(3)**: 255–61.
8. Gluckman PD, Wyatt JS, Azzopardi D, *et al.* Selective head cooling with mild systemic hypothermia after neonatal encephalopathy: multicentre randomised trial. *Lancet* 2005; **365(9460)**: 663–70.
9. Eaton DM, Toet M, Livingston J, Smith I, Levene M. Evaluation of the Cerebro Trac 2500 for monitoring of cerebral function in the neonatal intensive care. *Neuropediatrics* 1994; **25(3)**: 122–8.
10. Klebermass K, Kuhle S, Kohlhauser-Vollmuth C, Pollak A, Weninger M. Evaluation of the cerebral function monitor as a tool for neurophysiological surveillance in neonatal intensive care patients. *Childs Nerv Syst* 2001; **17(9)**: 544–50.
11. Toet MC, van der MW, de Vries LS, Uiterwaal CS, van Huffelen KC. Comparison between simultaneously recorded amplitude integrated electroencephalogram (cerebral function monitor) and standard electroencephalogram in neonates. *Pediatrics* 2002; **109(5)**: 772–9.
12. Rennie JM, Chorley G, Boylan GB, Pressler R, Nguyen Y, Hooper R. Non-expert use of the cerebral function monitor for neonatal seizure detection. *Arch Dis Child Fetal Neonatal Ed* 2004; **89(1)**: F37–F40.

Chapter 3 | Principles of magnetic resonance imaging and spectroscopy

NICOLA J. ROBERTSON, ENRICO
DE VITA, *and* ERNEST B. CADY

Nuclear magnetic resonance – a historical perspective

Magnetic resonance imaging (MRI) is the most important medical diagnostic development since the discovery of X-rays by Roentgen in 1895. Professor Paul Lauterbur obtained the world's first MRI scan in the USA in 1973, but many techniques empowering the modality were invented in the UK at Aberdeen, Nottingham, and Oxford Universities. The main historical highlights are summarized in Fig. 3.1 and Table 3.1.

In 1952 Felix Bloch of Stanford and Edward Purcell of Harvard Universities shared the Nobel Prize for observing nuclear magnetic resonance (NMR) [1, 2] (see below). Following this, the imaging applications of NMR evolved independently of metabolic uses and the terms MRI and magnetic resonance spectroscopy (MRS) came into use (clinical MRI primarily detects hydrogen (^{1}H) nuclei (protons) in water and MRS detects protons and other nuclei in more complicated metabolites).

Magnetic resonance imaging

In 1971 Raymond Damadian showed differences in NMR water characteristics between normal and abnormal tissues as well as between different types of normal tissue [3]. Contemporaneously, Paul Lauterbur superimposed small magnetic field gradients on the highly uniform magnetic field required for NMR spectroscopy: the NMR resonant frequency, of water for example, is directly proportional to the local magnetic field strength and thus location can be encoded. Signal intensity at a particular radio frequency (RF) was then proportional to the water concentration at the corresponding location. Lauterbur's technique ("Back Projection") produced a two-dimensional image and its publication in *Nature* [4] included the first ever images (of two tiny, water-filled tubes). This was innovational as many scientists then thought NMR diagnostic imaging unlikely because existing instruments were mainly chemist's tools with magnets that could contain a sample only the size of a pen. Peter Mansfield further developed the utilization of magnetic-field gradients and mathematical processing of MRI signals culminating in 1977 with the development of echo-planar imaging (EPI), which reduced acquisition and processing time from almost an hour to a fraction of a second [5]. Some 10 years later EPI enabled real-time "movie" imaging of a single cardiac cycle and is now also used in functional brain MRI [6]. Paul Lauterbur and Peter Mansfield shared the 2003 Nobel Prize in Medicine.

The first MRI scanner for human application completed construction in 1977 and others were soon developed commercially (Fig. 3.2). Other researchers soon made their mark on the field. Lauterbur's original method encoded spatial information by rotating a magnetic-field gradient around the sample. Richard Ernst simplified the process by using orthogonal gradients and fast Fourier transform (FFT) reconstruction to form an image on a rectangular grid [7]: this method is still the basis of MRI today. Ernst was awarded the Nobel Prize for Chemistry in 1991. The Aberdeen research group described the "spin warp" technique, which is a practical implementation of Ernst's FFT method [8].

The first transverse human head image was obtained in 1978 [9]. In 1980, the Aberdeen group and a collaboration between Electromusical Industries Ltd and Hammersmith Hospital separately optimized image contrast using water-relaxation differences. Important developments have been superconductors, which enable generation of very strong magnetic fields uniform over a volume encompassing the whole body, and faster computing resulting in almost instantaneous image visualization. In 1987 Charles Dumoulin developed magnetic resonance angiography (MRA), which imaged flowing blood without contrast agents [10]. In 1990, it was shown that MRI of water diffusion depicted ischemic cat-brain regions before any changes could be visualized on conventional MRI [11]; studies have suggested that a reduced apparent diffusion coefficient (ADC) during ischemia is associated with disrupted ion homeostasis and cell swelling [12]. Diffusion-weighted imaging (DWI) has significantly increased MRI's utility in non-invasive pathophysiology studies particularly in stroke. In 1992, functional MRI was developed utilizing EPI to image small regional brain blood-oxygen-level-dependent (BOLD) changes in response to photic stimulation [13].

Neonatal Cerebral Investigation, eds. Janet M. Rennie, Cornelia F. Hagmann and Nicola J. Robertson. Published by Cambridge University Press. © Cambridge University Press 2008.

Table 3.1. Main historical landmarks in the history of nuclear magnetic resonance (NMR), magnetic resonance imaging (MRI) and in vivo magnetic resonance spectroscopy (MRS). The discoveries of computerized tomography (CT) and ultrasound examination of the newborn brain are included in the context of developments in the field of brain imaging in the 1970s and 1980s.

	Date	Event	People involved	Where
Nuclear magnetic resonance	1882	Rotating magnetic field work: magnetic-field strength unit (Tesla; T) named after him ($\sim$20 000 × Earth's field)	Nikola Tesla	Budapest, Paris, and (mainly) Strasbourg Railway Station
	1937	Radiowave absorption and emission by atomic nuclei in a magnetic field	Isidor Rabi Nobel Prize 1944	Columbia University, New York City
	1946	Discovery of nuclear magnetic resonance (NMR), birth of NMR spectroscopy	Felix Bloch and Edward Purcell Nobel Prizes 1952	Stanford and Harvard Universities
MRI	Early 1970s	Demonstration that T_1 relaxation can identify tissue abnormality and differentiate tissues	Raymond Damadian [3]	State University of New York
	1973	Back-projection MRI	Paul Lauterbur [4] Nobel Prize 2003	State University of New York
	1975	Phase and frequency encoding, Fourier transform use	Richard Ernst Nobel Prize (Chemistry) 1991	Swiss Federal Institute of Technology, Zurich
	1977	Echo-planar imaging described	Peter Mansfield Nobel Prize 2003	Nottingham University
		First in vivo human MRI (finger cross-section)	Mansfield and Maudsley	Nottingham University
		First MRI system (Fig. 3.2)	Damadian	State University of New York
	1978	First transverse human head image	Clow and Young [9]	ElectroMusical Industries Ltd., UK
	1980	2-min whole-body imaging (Ernst's technique)	Edelstein et al. [8]	University of Aberdeen, Scotland
	1987	MRI angiography	Dumoulin et al. [10]	New York
	1990	Diffusion-weighted imaging detects feline brain ischemic regions before conventional MRI	Moseley et al. [11]	University of California
	1992	Functional MRI – imaging local brain changes coincident with and caused by activation, e.g., visual or motor	Belliveau et al. [88]	Massachusetts General Hospital, USA
Ultrasound	1979	First ultrasound detection of brain damage in preterm infants	Pape et al. [16]	University College London
		Linear-array real-time scanner (5 MHz) was used (Fig. 3.3)		
		Lesion type and extent confirmed by CT and post-mortem		
		Before 1979, preterm brain hemorrhage was diagnosed by CT		
In vivo MRS		MRS mainly in vitro to study soluble proteins, metabolites		
		In vivo MRS concept developed more slowly		
	1973	Adenosine triphosphate, inorganic phosphate, intracellular pH measurement in red blood cells	Moon and Richards [19]	California Institute of Technology, Pasadena
	1974	Phosphorus MRS detects metabolites in fresh excised muscle – scene set for MRS as non-invasive energy-metabolism probe (Fig. 3.4)	Hoult et al. [20]	Oxford University
	1977	Proton MRS of red blood cells (glucose, lactate, alanine, creatine detected)	Brown et al. [26]	Oxford University
	1980	In vivo phosphorus MRS (surface coil) of rat brain	Ackerman et al. [22]	Oxford University
	1982	In vivo phosphorus MRS of gerbil-brain ischemia	Thulborn et al. [23]	Oxford University
	1982	First in vivo MRS (phosphorus) of human brain (preterm birth asphyxia)	Cady et al. [24]	University College london
	1984	MRS shows biphasic energy failure during and after brain hypoxia-ischemia – concept of "therapeutic window"		University College London
	1989	Phosphorus MRS prognostic in neonatal encephalopathy	Azzopardi et al. [89]	
Computed X-ray tomography (CT)	1972	The discovery of CT has been described as the greatest legacy of the Beatles pop group – profits from record sales funded the research	Godfrey Hounsfield Hounsfield shared the 1979 Nobel Prize for Medicine	Thorn Research Laboratories, Hayes, UK

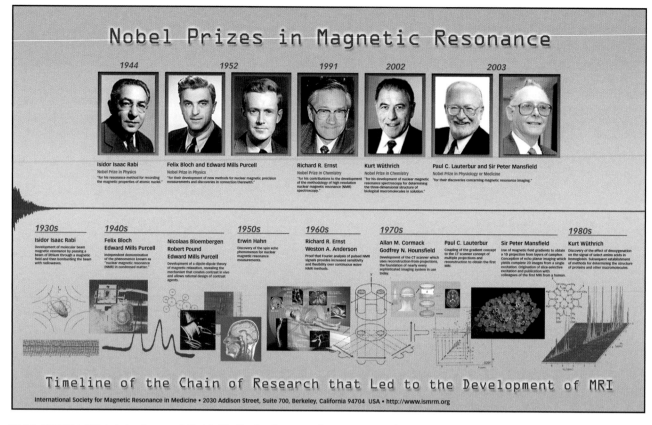

Fig. 3.1. **Timeline of the chain of research that led to the development of MRI. Courtesy of International Society for Magnetic Resonance in Medicine (http://www.ismrm.org).**

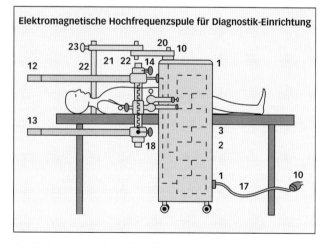

Fig. 3.2. **An example of one of the first NMR whole-body machines. This machine was designed to measure the NMR signal of flowing blood at different vessel locations using a series of small coils. A patent for a whole-body NMR machine to measure blood flow in the human body was filed by Alexander Ganssen in early 1967. Such measurements were not introduced into common medical practice until the mid 1980s. This NMR system could be described as the first scanner, however it is not an imager.**

Clinical MRI is based on many faculties including medicine, chemistry, physics, and computer science, therefore groups with multidisciplinary input have been most successful. Magnetic resonance imaging has become the main routine clinical diagnostic tool in many diseases: it is particularly useful for imaging brain and spine, soft tissues of joints, bone internal structure, and liver. Particular advantages are that MRI is non-invasive (non-ionizing radiation), provides good contrast between various soft tissues, and images can have any orientation. Magnetic resonance imaging has revolutionized knowledge about the developing brain and perinatal brain injury, has unprecedented sensitivity to gray and white matter abnormalities, and can differentiate myelinated from unmyelinated white matter.

During the 1970s and 1980s other brain imaging modalities were being developed. X-ray computerized tomography (CT) became available in 1972 [14] and was later used to diagnose preterm brain hemorrhage [15]. In 1979, the first ultrasound detection of brain hemorrhage was reported at University College Hospital (Fig. 3.3) [16]; in the 1980s cranial ultrasound imaging became a useful, safe cotside tool for the diagnosis of hemorrhage and cystic white matter injury, allowing serial scanning of brain injury evolution. There has been recent awareness of unnecessary CT X-ray dose and specific cancer risks in the pediatric population [17]. In children the lifetime risk of cancer mortality attributed to CT is 10 times higher than in adults [18]: neonatal sensitization factors include: (1) increased radio-sensitivity of certain tissues (thyroid, breast, gonads), (2) longer lifetime for radiation-related cancer development, and (3) lack of body-size-based technique adjustments. It was realized that neonatal MRI access should be improved to avoid routine CT use, but if CT is specifically required, the radiation dose must be reduced according to patient size. This is termed the ALARA concept – to reduce the CT dose "as low as reasonably achievable."

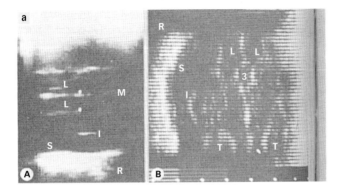

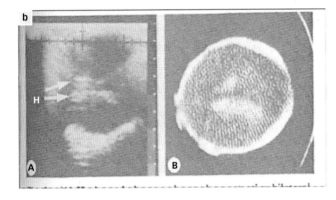

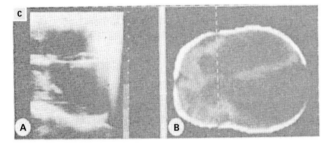

Fig. 3.3. **The first ultrasound brain image was acquired in 1979 at University College London using a linear-array real-time scanner with a 5-MHz probe [16]. The type and extent of lesions were confirmed by CT and at necropsy. (a) Normal scans. A: Horizontal view through the lateral ventricles (anterior to the left). The probe was placed against the right side of the head (top of figure). Reverberant echoes are seen adjacent to the probe and also on the opposite side of the head (R). S, inner skull table; I, sulcus of insula; M, midline; L, lateral ventricles. The two dots are the electronic measuring calipers: the upper one is just to the right of the midline and the lower one is at the lateral wall of the left lateral ventricle. B: Coronal view at right angles to the mid-point of the canthomeatal line. 3, 3rd ventricle; L, bodies of lateral ventricles; T, temporal horns of ventricles. (b) A: Horizontal scan demonstrating bilateral intraventricular hemorrhages (H). B: CT scan of the same infant. (c) A: Horizontal scan showing enlarged posterior poles of the lateral ventricles. B: CT scan of the same infant.**

Magnetic resonance spectroscopy

Magnetic resonance spectroscopy (MRS) combines the spatial properties of MRI with metabolite specificity. A pioneering event in 1973 was Moon and Richard's use of high-resolution phosphorus (^{31}P) MRS to study intact red blood cells [19]. In addition to observing signals from 2,3-diphosphoglycerate, inorganic phosphate (P_i) and adenosine triphosphate (ATP), Moon and Richards demonstrated that several metabolite signals could be used to determine intracellular pH (pH_i). In 1974, ^{31}P MRS was used to detect phosphocreatine (PCr), ATP and P_i in intact, freshly excised rat skeletal muscle: pH_i was estimated from the P_i signal [20] (Fig. 3.4). Over 2 h there was gradual PCr loss followed by ATP reduction. This and another study [21] demonstrated the value of ^{31}P MRS for investigation of tissue energy metabolism. In 1980 ^{31}P spectra were obtained from living rat brain using a surface coil [22]. Studies on experimental brain pathophysiology followed rapidly as the potential importance of ^{31}P MRS had become obvious; the first such study was of ischemia in gerbils [23]. The first in vivo MRS studies of human brain were performed in term and preterm infants with a history of perinatal hypoxia-ischemia [24]. The development of 1.5-tesla (T) whole-body scanners enabled the first MRS observations of adult human stroke [25].

Although ^{1}H is the commonest biological nucleus and provides the highest sensitivity, in vivo application of ^{1}H MRS was delayed compared to ^{31}P MRS. In vivo ^{1}H MRS is a technical challenge for several reasons:
1. The water signal is 10 000 times larger than metabolite signals
2. Metabolites resonate within a narrow frequency range causing peak overlap
3. Magnetic field homogeneity must be extremely good

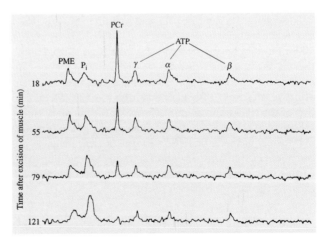

Fig. 3.4. [^{31}P] spectra of intact, excised, rat hind-leg muscle. The signals are assigned to the α-, β-, and γ-phosphates of nucleotide triphosphate (NTP) (predominantly ATP), phosphocreatine (PCr), inorganic phosphate (P_i) and the phosphomonoesters (PME). [^{31}P] MRS is a non-invasive probe of tissue energy metabolism: a gradual breakdown of high-energy phosphates and a fall in intracellular pH resulting from the accumulation of lactic acid is shown in this series of spectra. From Hoult *et al.*, 1974, *Nature*, 252: 285–7 [20]; reproduced with permission.

4. Interaction between adjacent molecular protons (spin-spin coupling) can engender doublet, triplet, and more complicated spectrum peaks
5. The lipid signal is often ~100 times larger than metabolite signals and overlaps and obscures the latter.

However, in 1977 proton signals were observed from, for example, glucose, lactate (Lac), pyruvate, alanine and total creatine (i.e., creatine plus PCr; Cr) in a suspension of red blood cells [26]. The first studies demonstrating the feasibility of ^{1}H MRS for study of living brain used water suppression techniques and documented reversible Lac elevation caused by transient hypoxia and ischemia in rats and rabbits [27]. The demonstration that fundamental biochemical processes could be monitored non-invasively was of major importance. Once the feasibility of water-suppressed cerebral ^{1}H MRS was established in animals, implementation on whole-body MRI scanners followed rapidly [28].

Today ^{1}H MRS has important clinical uses; for example, providing information on tumor biochemistry and classification [29], early diagnosis of Alzheimer's disease [30], as a cognitive research tool [31], and in the diagnosis and monitoring of hepatic encephalopathy [32]. In neonatology, ^{1}H MRS has a particularly important prognostic role during the first and second weeks after birth asphyxia [33] and also can diagnose specific metabolic diseases, such as non-ketotic hyperglycinemia. More recent applications include non-invasive regional-brain temperature measurement [34], imaging brain metabolite (instead of water) distributions [35], and postmortem examinations [36].

The fundamentals of magnetic resonance

Nuclear magnetic resonance (NMR) depends on certain isotopic nuclei possessing "spin" of which ^{1}H, carbon (^{13}C), and ^{31}P have greatest biomedical importance. (Nitrogen (^{14}N and ^{15}N), oxygen (^{17}O), fluorine (^{19}F), and sodium (^{23}Na) are also of interest but will not be dealt with here.) ^{1}H is obviously of great MRI interest because tissue water is visualized. The combination of the nucleus's positive charge with spin turns the nucleus into a small magnet. For conceptual clarity we will utilize a "classical," instead of quantum mechanical, description of the NMR phenomenon. Normally the magnetic nuclei are oriented randomly. However, if for example a ^{1}H sample is in a strong magnetic field (B_0) then the nuclear magnets precess about B_0 similarly to a child's spinning top gyrating in the Earth's gravitational field (Fig. 3.5 a). The precession rate is given by the Larmor equation [37, 38]:

$$\nu = \gamma B_0/2\pi, \qquad (3.1),$$

where ν is the precession frequency (Hz), γ is an isotope-specific constant called the gyromagnetic ratio, and B_0 has units of T. Table 3.2 gives the Larmor frequencies at the common clinical field strength of 1.5 T for various biomedically interesting isotopes: they are in the radio range.

In a sample there are many nuclear magnets precessing about B_0 at the Larmor frequency (Fig. 3.5a): their precession

axis can be parallel or anti-parallel to B_0 ("spin up" and "spin down"). There is a small difference in the numbers of spin-up and spin-down nuclei (N_2 and N_1 respectively) given by the Boltzmann equation:

$$N_2/N_1 = \exp(\gamma\hbar B_0/k_B T_S), \qquad (3.2)$$

where $\hbar$ is Planck's constant/2π, k_B is Boltzmann's constant, and T_S is sample temperature. Because $N_2 - N_1$ is small the net sample magnetization (M_0) is also small: for this reason NMR is intrinsically "insensitive."

Signal generation and detection

Magnetic resonance imaging scanners include a strong magnet (often superconducting, but resistive and permanent are also used) producing a uniform constant B_0 and a radio transmitter

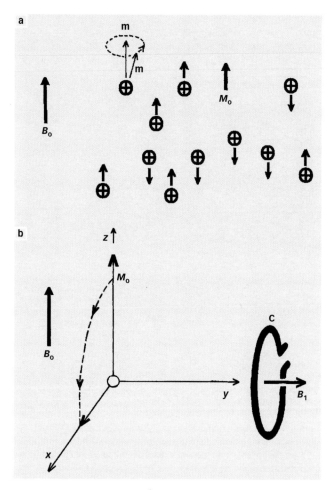

Fig. 3.5. **(a)** A representation of ^{1}H nuclei (+) in a static magnetic field (B_0). Individual nuclei precess about B_0 at the Larmor frequency (top left): some parallel to B_0, the rest anti-parallel. The difference between the numbers of parallel and anti-parallel nuclei gives the net detectable magnetization (M_0). **(b)** The effect of a radiofrequency (RF) pulse. For simplicity the MRI probe (a tuned surface coil C) transmits an RF pulse at the Larmor frequency during which M_0 precesses through angle θ about the RF pulse's magnetic component (B_1). It is often arranged that at the pulse end $\theta = 90°$ M_0 will then be in the xy plane, which is perpendicular to B_0. M_0 now precesses again about B_0 (i.e., about the z axis) inducing a sinusoidal RF signal in the coil.

and receiver. In order to gain useful information M_0 is first perturbed by applying a brief radiofrequency (RF) pulse at the Larmor frequency of the isotope concerned. Radio waves are electromagnetic: M_0 begins precessing around the RF pulse's magnetic component (B_1) similar to the previous precession around B_0 (Fig. 3.5b). However, because the RF pulse is brief, this precession soon terminates. The angle through which M_0 "flips" is effectively proportional to the RF pulse's duration and strength. If the flip angle θ is 90°, M_0 ends up in the "xy" plane (perpendicular to B_0; Fig. 3.5b) and now precesses only around B_0 again effectively creating a magnetic field varying sinusoidally at the Larmor frequency. If the sample is in an MRI probe tuned to the Larmor frequency, this varying magnetic field induces an RF signal in the probe (the free induction decay or FID), which is then detected by the radio receiver and digitized for further computer processing.

Relaxation

At the end of the RF pulse relaxation processes eventually return M_0 to the "equilibrium" situation existing beforehand. "Longitudinal" (or "spin-lattice") relaxation results in energy loss and consequent regeneration of M_0 parallel to B_0 with exponential time constant T_1. After $\sim 5T_1$, sample magnetization has essentially recovered its equilibrium state (Fig. 3.6a–d). "Transverse" (or "spin-spin") relaxation occurs simultaneously:

Table 3.2. Characteristics of some isotopes of biomedical interest.

Isotope	Relative sensitivity[a]	Natural abundance(%)[b]	Absolute sensitivity[c](%)	1.5-T Larmor frequency (MHz)
^{1}H	1.00	99.98	1.00	63.9
^{13}C	0.016	1.11	1.76×10^{-4}	16.1
^{19}F	0.83	100	0.83	60.1
^{23}Na	0.093	100	0.093	16.9
^{31}P	0.066	100	0.066	25.9

[a] The signal obtainable per nucleus relative to ^{1}H.

[b] The natural isotope percentage of all nuclei.

[c] Relative sensitivity × natural abundance (i.e., sensitivity obtained in practice without isotopic enhancement normalized; to ^{1}H).

perturbations from neighboring nuclei randomly accelerate or retard precession and M_0 "dephases" in the xy plane resulting in signal decaying exponentially with time constant T_2 (Fig. 3.6a–d). (If B_0 varies spatially in the sample, some nuclei precess faster and others slower, increasing the observed rate of signal decay.) T_2 is always shorter than T_1: for mobile molecules in tissue T_1 may be $\sim$1–2 s whereas T_2 may be $\sim$100–200 ms. Biophysical factors can influence relaxation; for example, T_2 shortens as viscosity increases. A major consequence of longitudinal relaxation is that without allowing $\sim 5T_1$ delay after an RF pulse, M_0 will not have recovered its unperturbed status and the next RF pulse will flip magnetization less than M_0 giving a smaller signal. However, this situation is partially offset by rapid pulsing enabling more summed acquisitions per unit time. The delay between consecutive RF pulses (or pulse sequences) is the repetition time (TR).

The spin echo

To obtain images or localize spectra to a particular tissue region it is often necessary to generate a spin echo (see, e.g., [39]). This requires an initial excitation pulse (often giving 90° flip) followed after delay τ by a refocussing pulse (180° flip): after a further delay τ a spin echo is detected. After the excitation pulse, transverse relaxation during τ fans out M_0 in the xy plane (Fig. 3.7). The 180° pulse then flips this magnetization fan into the xy plane on the opposite side of the z axis. The magnetization fan is now a mirror image of that before the 180° pulse: magnetization previously precessing faster still does and magnetization formerly precessing slower maintains this. However, instead of fanning out, faster and slower precessing magnetizations now do the opposite and after a further delay, τ, the magnetization "refocusses," generating a spin echo. The total time from excitation pulse to echo (2τ) is the echo time (TE). Spin-echo generation is analogous to a race in which after the start (90° pulse) the runners, each having a different constant speed, spread out around the circuit. After τ the runners are signalled (180° pulse) to return to the start: if the runners maintain their individual speeds they all arrive back at the start simultaneously (echo) 2τ after the race began. One spin-echo application is to provide image contrast; for example, the echo from water with $T_2 <$ TE will have decayed more than that of water with $T_2 >$ TE.

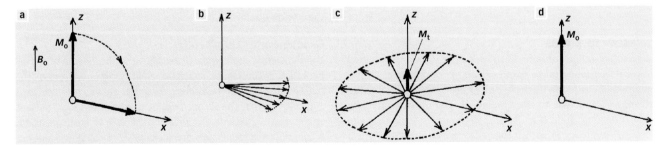

Fig. 3.6. **Transverse ("spin-spin") and longitudinal ("spin-lattice") relaxation. (a)** M_0 is flipped 90° into the xy plane (for simplicity only the x axis shown). **(b)** Transverse relaxation fans out ("dephases") the magnetization in the xy plane. **(c)** After time t the xy-plane magnetization has now completely dephased (no net xy-plane magnetization and, hence, no signal) and by longitudinal relaxation M_0 has partly recovered its equilibrium state along the z axis (M_t, parallel to B_0). **(d)** More than $5T_1$ after (a) M_0 has essentially recovered its equilibrium (pre RF pulse) state.

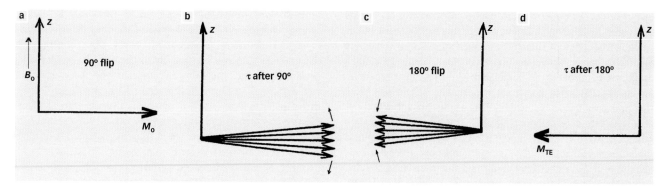

Fig. 3.7. Spin echo generation. (a) The sample magnetization (M_0) is firstly flipped from its original orientation along the z axis (parallel to B_0) through 90° into the xy plane (for clarity x and y axes not shown). (b) Random perturbations by neighboring nuclei and B_0 inhomogeneity modulate the Larmor frequencies of individual nuclei during delay τ and the flipped sample magnetization fans out in the xy plane. (c) At the end of delay τ a 180° pulse flips the sample magnetization fan again into the xy plane but on the opposite side of the z axis. (d) Components of the sample magnetization fan that precessed faster or slower in (b) now continue to do so with preserved precession directions so that after a further delay τ magnetization fanned out due to constant effects (e.g., B_0 inhomogeneity) "refocuses" and a "spin echo" is detected centered at 2τ (the echo time; TE) after the 90° pulse. However, random effects are irreversible; hence, echo magnetization (M_{TE}) is $< M_0$.

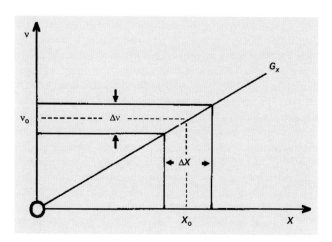

Fig. 3.8. Slice selection using a "selective" RF pulse and a magnetic field gradient. The magnetic gradient (G_x) increases the Larmor frequency linearly across the sample. A selective RF pulse is effective over only a narrow frequency bandwidth (Δv) centered on frequency v_0. A selective pulse only flips sample magnetization in a slice centered on the spatial location (x_0) at which the gradient value plus static magnetic field gives Larmor frequency v_0 and between slice edges at $x_0 - \Delta x/2$ and $x_0 + \Delta x/2$ corresponding respectively to Larmor frequencies $v_0 - \Delta v/2$ and $v_0 + \Delta v/2$. Outside the slice the selective pulse ideally has no effect.

Selective RF pulses

A selective pulse contains RF power only within a specified narrow frequency range (bandwidth). In combination with a magnetic-field gradient these pulses only flip M_0 in a tissue slice (perpendicular to the gradient direction) in which the local magnetic field (i.e., B_0 plus gradient) is such that the Larmor frequency is within the pulse bandwidth (Fig. 3.8). If the RF pulse is designed well, no signal originates outside the slice. Slice position depends on the pulse center frequency and slice thickness depends on bandwidth. Selective pulses are important for both MRI and localized MRS.

Instrumentation

Clinical MRI scanners are mostly "whole-body" (any adult body part can be imaged); however, other types exist (e.g., head only). A scanner has several components (see, e.g., [38]).

Magnets

Since images improve with stronger B_0 many clinical scanners use superconducting magnets (Fig. 3.9a): these contain a superconducting wire coil in liquid helium ($\sim -269°C$); once energized no further power is required (caution: the magnet is always on). A further advantage of superconducting magnets is B_0 has good homogeneity over a large volume. Helium evaporation is reduced by thermal shielding and high-vacuum containment. Occasionally, the magnet may cease superconductance and contained energy is released as heat (a "quench") with copious expulsion of helium gas, which should be conveyed safely outside the building by a quench pipe. Permanent and resistive magnets are sometimes used in lower field strength imagers: the former is always on; the latter can be switched off.

Many clinical MRI scanners now operate at 1.5 T but 3-T systems are becoming affordable. Currently the highest field whole-body scanner is the 9.4-T research system at the University of Illinois; however, an 11.4-T imager is planned for Orsay, France. Some small-bore scanners for in vivo experimentation operate at 14 T.

Gradient and "shim" coils

Gradient coils are required for MRI and localized MRS: they generate orthogonal magnetic field gradients across the patient. In a superconducting magnet, these coils are in a cylinder inside the bore, which slightly reduces patient space: the z gradient is along the bore, y is vertical, and x horizontal. Gradient coils are often water cooled. By generating additional weak magnetic fields, "shim" coils optimize B_0 uniformity thereby reducing image distortions and, in MRS, nuclei resonate at more similar Larmor frequencies giving narrower peaks (better spectral resolution). In superconducting

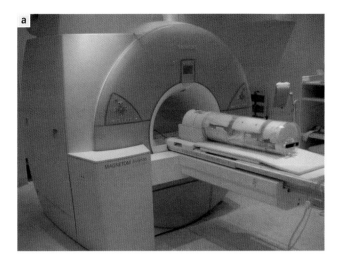

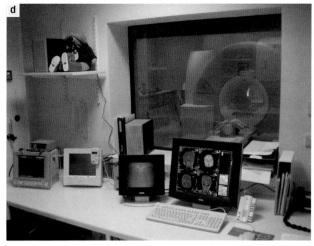

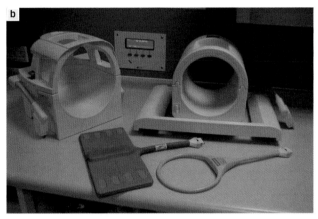

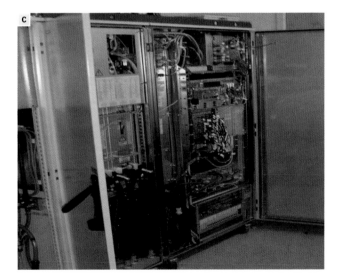

Fig. 3.9. **(a) A 1.5-T whole-body superconducting magnet. The patient couch is to the right. The patient is positioned using laser reference markers: the couch and patient then move automatically into the magnet until the patient is located correctly for imaging. In this picture a protective plastic pod designed to contain a newborn infant is on the couch: at the left of the pod is an "extremity" coil (in this instance used for neonatal brain MRI and MRS). (b) MRI probeheads and coils. At the back left and right are respectively adult head and extremity probeheads: the top halves are removable to facilitate patient positioning. At the front left and right are respectively an "array" coil and a standard surface coil for imaging organs close to the body surface (e.g., heart). (c) The racks of electronic hardware located in an air-conditioned room adjacent to the scanner room: these contain the RF transmitter and receiver, gradient power amplifiers, data acquisition computer, and other essential items. (d) The radiographer's console. Behind the MRI monitor is an RF-screened window which enables visualization of the scanner room without introduction of RF interference: the couch is set up for a "phantom" study. To the immediate left of the MRI monitor is a screen visualizing the patient. Further to the left are physiological-monitoring screens.**

involves maximizing the water FID duration (equivalent to minimizing water-peak width).

MRI probeheads (coils)

The probehead has to be designed and "tuned" to the resonant frequency given by the Larmor equation for the magnetic field strength and the isotope of interest (e.g., 64.5 MHz for ^{1}H at 1.5 T). There are various types (see Fig. 3.9b and, e.g., [40]). Some surround the body part (e.g., head): these are "volume" coils and often quasi-cylindrical (e.g., birdcage design). Some are placed against the skin near the target tissue (e.g., a surface coil; in simplest form an insulated wire loop tuned to the Larmor frequency; sometimes surface-coil arrays are used). Coil combinations can be employed depending on the type of investigation; for example, for brain a single volume coil could transmit and receive whereas for joint imaging a volume coil could transmit and a smaller surface coil receive (the volume coil gives a very uniform flip angle with good depth penetration, whereas a surface coil has poor depth penetration but gives stronger signals from adjacent tissue). In order to optimize image intensity and

magnets some shim coils are superconductive and used to coarsely adjust B_0 uniformity at scanner installation: others are resistive and can be adjusted automatically or manually to further optimize B_0 homogeneity for each study. "Shimming"

spatial resolution MRI of newborn brain should use the smallest volume coil that can encompass the head (often an "extremity" coil). Recently, dedicated coils for newborn infants have become commercially available and satisfy the needs for head access, physiological monitoring, and artificial ventilation (e.g., see Lammers Medical Technology http://www.lammersmedical.com).

If an RF pulse flips M_0 towards the xy plane through angle θ, M_0 can be resolved into two components: $M_0\cos\theta$ parallel to B_0 and $M_0\sin\theta$ in the xy plane (perpendicular to B_0). Because it is only $M_0\sin\theta$ that induces probe signal, to maximize signal it is essential that B_1 is perpendicular to B_0 (e.g., surface-coil loops must be parallel to B_0 if they are perpendicular to B_0 no signal will be detected!

Preamplifiers

To minimize signal contamination by RF noise the MRI probe is connected to an adjacent preamplifier at the magnet. This provides initial signal amplification before long cables convey the signal to the RF receiver outside the scanner room. Many scanners will only have ^{1}H preamplification; however, if the scanner is multinuclear, at least one additional preamplifier (e.g., ^{31}P) will be necessary.

Scanner room

Potential hazards mean that the scanner room must be a controlled area which only authorized staff may enter. To eliminate RF interference the room is lined with earthed conducting sheet (usually copper) creating a Faraday cage: all cabling through the cage must pass through RF filters. A few special tubes (waveguides) passing through the Faraday cage are provided for optical fibers and non-conductive clinical tubing (electrical wiring through a waveguide introduces interference). The cage should include an RF window that allows visual access. It is desirable that the 0.5-mT "fringe" field is contained in the room: external areas at ≥ 0.5 mT must be controlled (no public access). It is often necessary to restrict the 0.5-mT fringe field by steel sheeting in the walls, floor, and ceiling.

Radiofrequency power amplifier and gradient amplifier and RF receiver

These items are normally racked in an air-conditioned room next to the scanner room (Fig. 3.9c). Low-voltage RF pulses are input to the RF amplifier which generates several kilowatts of power. The high-voltage RF output is fed to the MRI probehead: between pulses a blanking signal nulls the output, which might otherwise generate interference. The gradient amplifiers supply high current pulses to the gradient coils to generate magnetic field gradients. In older scanners the RF signal from the preamplifier is input to the RF receiver and converted to audio frequency followed by digitization; however, in many modern scanners audio-frequency conversion is unnecessary because of advanced digital technology.

Operator console

Many older systems had dedicated, manufacturer-designed consoles. Modern scanners are often based on personal computers or workstations with dedicated software running on commercially available operating systems (Fig. 3.9d).

Magnetic resonance imaging

The term "imaging" in MRI results from its ability to discriminate between signals arising from nuclei (generally ^{1}H) at different positions. The next sections describe how this is achieved and how MRI can be tailored for different applications by modifying parameters determining spatial resolution and image contrast.

Spatial discrimination

As Larmor frequency increases linearly with B_0 spatial discrimination can be obtained by superimposing a small magnetic field increasing linearly in a particular direction during signal acquisition. The higher the total magnetic field the higher the Larmor frequency; hence, nucleus positions will be linearly related to their Larmor frequencies. After an excitation RF pulse the scanner receiver will detect a combination of signals each with amplitude proportional to the number of nuclei at each location along the magnetic field gradient and Larmor frequency proportional to their position along the gradient. These frequencies and amplitudes can be extracted by FFT. This mechanism for spatial discrimination is termed "frequency encoding."

MRI pulse sequences and spatial encoding

Since thousands of different types of MRI studies are possible, they are referred to by specifying the associated "pulse sequence," which is a sequential cycle of signal excitation, manipulation, and acquisition repeated a number of times followed by image reconstruction.

Magnetic field gradient pulses can be applied throughout a sequence along three mutually orthogonal axes termed "read," "phase," and "slice"; signal manipulation can consist of additional excitation and/or magnetic field gradient pulses. Image reconstruction is achieved by appropriately amplifying, processing, and recombining the coil signal(s) from each pulse-sequence cycle according to the spatial-encoding protocol employed.

Many MRI sequences give two-dimensional (2D) spatial discrimination and provide images of thin tissue "slices." The simplest way to achieve this is:

1. To use frequency-selective RF pulses to excite the signal within a single slice (see "Selective RF pulses" section above and Fig. 3.8).
2. To use "frequency-encoding" gradients before and during signal acquisition to provide spatial discrimination in the "read" direction within the selected slice.
3. To use "phase encoding" in the "phase" direction: this is basically a frequency encoding prior to signal acquisition and is achieved with short gradient pulses applied between signal excitation and detection and incremented in strength at each of N_{pe} successive pulse-sequence cycles.

To image a whole organ (instead of a single slice) further pulse-sequence cycles can be applied during TR with each selective pulse designed for a separate parallel slice (multi-slice imaging): this obtains many parallel images separated by a specified interslice gap. Typical clinical 2D sequences have in-plane spatial resolution ~0.5–1.5 mm and slice thickness ~2–6 mm.

Some MRI sequences are three-dimensional (3D): the whole volume of interest is excited by each RF pulse ("non-selective") and phase encoding is applied sequentially in two directions orthogonal to the read (frequency encoding) direction. The pulse sequence is repeated $N_{pe1} \times N_{pe2}$ times (covering all possible combinations of phase-encoding gradient amplitudes) with N_{pe1} and N_{pe2} dependent on the desired spatial resolution. In 3D sequences spatial resolution is often isotropic with ~1 mm now common for the brain. The choice of imaging sequence and parameters determines the resulting tissue contrast and spatial resolution.

The basic 2D MR sequences are:

1. Spin echo (SE): the basic SE sequence is described earlier (see "The spin echo" section and Fig. 3.7). A slice-selective 90° pulse is followed after TE/2 by a 180° pulse (also slice selective) and a spin echo is acquired TE/2 later. The SE sequence has N_{pe} phase-encoding steps at intervals TR (total acquisition time (AT) = TR $\times N_{pe}$). If TE is short, TR can be adjusted to give T_1-weighted tissue contrast; if TR is long compared to T_1, then TE can be adjusted to provide T_2-weighted contrast.

2. Gradient echo (GE): following a single slice-selective RF pulse (flip angle generally <90°) gradients both dephase and subsequently refocus the sample magnetization to give a "gradient echo" TE after the initial pulse. Again AT = TR $\times N_{pe}$ though TR is generally much shorter.

3. Multi-echo sequences: two or more echoes can often be acquired during each pulse-sequence cycle, thus reducing patient study time. Echoes can be generated as either gradient echoes (as in EPI) or spin echoes, using more refocussing RF pulses (as in "fast spin echo" or "HASTE" methods), or by combining the gradient and spin-echo methods (as in "GRASE").

4. Inversion recovery (IR): this consists of an "inversion pulse" (180°) followed by a delay (the "inversion time", TI) after which the preferred single or multi-echo sequence is applied. TI can be varied to modulate T_1-weighted tissue contrast; indeed, TI can be adjusted such that tissues with a certain T_1 give little if any signal (as in fluid attenuated inversion recovery methods).

Spatial resolution and sensitivity

One of MRI's beautiful aspects is its provision of spatial information unrelated to the RF wavelength. The spatial detail of MRI is only limited by the available study time; theoretically, the longer the total AT the better are the images. However, in real life there are economic and patient-endurance considerations that limit scan sessions to ~30 min to 2 h at the most. Furthermore, a single scan taking >10–15 min is unlikely to succeed without subject immobilization. It is important to note that image signal-to-noise ratio (SNR; mean signal intensity/local variability (background noise); an image "graininess" measure) is proportional to $\sqrt{AT}$; hence, AT must quadruple to double SNR.

Digital images are displayed as a rectangular "pixel" (picture cell) lattice with each pixel assigned an intensity related to the signal from the corresponding small volume of sample (voxel). Hence, SNR is also proportional to pixel volume (in-slice read-direction × phase-direction pixel dimensions × slice thickness). For example, compared to a 2-mm cubic voxel (volume 8 mm³) a 1-mm cubic voxel (volume 1 mm³) will give 1/8th the signal: to regain the 8-mm³ voxel SNR, AT must be 64 times longer! The SNR also depends on the isotope imaged (normally ¹H; see Table 3.2), B_0, receive-coil efficiency ("sensitivity"), the pulse sequence and its parameters, the tissue studied (see following section "Image contrast"), and temperature (lower tissue and RF-receiver temperatures give a higher signal).

Image contrast

Contrast is fundamentally important for diagnosis and is simply the difference in signal strength observed from different tissues or pathological conditions. In X-ray and CT images contrast relates to tissue density and characteristic attenuation: the operator has little control. However, MRI contrast can be manipulated over a wide range: images can be sensitized to a multitude of bio-characteristics, e.g., blood oxygenation, water relaxation, diffusion, and perfusion. By selecting appropriate pulse sequences and acquisition parameters (e.g., TE or TR) contrast can be optimized for each particular application, e.g., by acquiring T_2- or T_1-weighted images; "weighting" alters signal intensity according to the chosen MRI characteristic and can provide tissue and pathology contrast. To optimize visual distinction between tissues a and b, it is important to maximize the contrast-to-noise ratio; $(S_a - S_b)/N = SNR_a - SNR_b$, where S is signal intensity. Some common contrast parameters are now discussed.

Proton density (PD)

Simply the number density of the imaged isotope's nuclei in the tissue (e.g., ¹H). Purely PD-weighted images must have TR $\approx 5T_1$ and TE $\ll T_2$; ¹H PD-weighted images ideally directly reflect free water content since strongly bound protons (e.g., in cell membranes and macromolecules) are not visualized easily with conventional sequences due to their extremely short T_2.

T_1

In SE/GE sequences T_1-weighted images are obtained by adjusting the RF-pulse flip angle and TR relative to T_1: pulse-sequence cycles are repeated without M_0 regaining equilibrium. For "pure" T_1-weighted images TE $\ll T_2$. In IR sequences, T_1-weighted contrast is also modulated by TI. The more the weighting the brighter the appearance of short-T_1 tissues. T_1-weighted sequences are often used to study vascular and tissue permeability to specific substances.

T_2

In SE sequences T_2-weighting is modulated by adjusting TE relative to T_2. For pure T_2-weighted images TR $\approx 5T_1$. The more the weighting the darker the appearance of short-T_2 tissues.

T_2^*

T_2^* is the time constant of the observed exponential FID decay and is always $< T_2$: $T_2 - T_2^*$ depends on the refocussable dephased component of the sample magnetization. Intrinsic B_0 inhomogeneity, iron, deoxyhemoglobin, or contrast agents (e.g., containing gadolinium) decrease T_2^*. In GE images T_2^*-weighting is modulated by adjusting TE relative to T_2^*. Functional MRI exploiting BOLD (visualizing brain activation) and blood-perfusion measurements after contrast-agent administration are T_2^*-weighted.

Magnetization transfer (MT)

The coupling and exchange between free-water protons and those motion-restricted or in macromolecules and membranes can also provide contrast. If selective RF pulses with a frequency offset relative to water are applied before an imaging sequence, it is possible to saturate less mobile protons. This saturation transfers (preferentially by chemical exchange) to the more mobile protons: consequentially signal from the latter is decreased. The reduction depends, for example, on relaxation times and the bound and free proton fractions. Magnetization transfer contrast could be used to study myelination.

Flow

In conventional MRI flow (e.g., of blood) can cause undesirable artifacts. However, MRI's inherent motion sensitivity can be exploited to visualize vessel blood flow. When employed with 3D-GE sequences, contrast agents can reduce T_1 and produce angiograms. Alternatively there are non-invasive, angiogram methods, e.g., time-of-flight and phase contrast. Neonatal applications remain rare [41].

Diffusion

The term diffusion refers to thermal Brownian molecular motion. In biological systems water diffusion occurs within and around cells and can also involve exchange between intra- and extracellular compartments. Tissue-water diffusion is restricted by intracellular structures and cell membranes (Fig. 3.10a). The easiest way to diffusion weight images is by pairs of gradient pulses. The first gradient pulse gives the water magnetization a location-dependent phase: after a "diffusion time" a further equivalent gradient pulse refocuses the magnetization of all static molecules. However, diffused molecules experience the second gradient pulse at a new location (with a different local magnetic field strength) and their refocussing is incomplete, resulting in signal reduction. Diffusion weighting increases with stronger gradient pulses and longer diffusion times and is characterized by the "b" factor, which depends on the diffusion-sensitizing gradients' amplitude, duration, and relative position in the sequence. MRI diffusion is quantified by the ADC (as opposed to a "pure" diffusion coefficient, which is also sometimes termed mean or average "diffusivity"). A lower ADC gives a higher DWI signal.

Quantitative MRI

Technology improvements continuously enhance MRI's spatial resolution and contrast. MRI has now become a standard

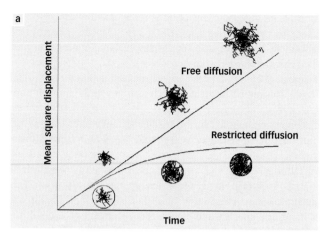

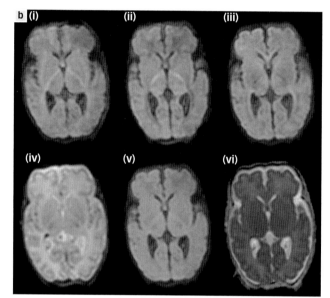

Fig. 3.10. **(a) Free and restricted diffusion. With free diffusion (e.g., as in a pure water sample) the mean square displacement increases linearly with time. If diffusion is restricted (e.g., the water is contained in an impermeable cell membrane), the measured diffusion coefficient depends on the length of time for which the molecules can diffuse before encountering a barrier (image courtesy of Dr D. Tournier). (b) Diffusion-weighted images and ADC map. Shown are: axial neonatal brain images diffusion sensitized in the (i) left–right, (ii) anterior–posterior, and (iii) cephalo–plantar directions; (iv) a corresponding diffusion-weighted image ($b = 0 \, \text{s/mm}^2$); (v) a direction-averaged diffusion-weighted image; and (vi) an ADC map (vi). Note the reversed contrast between (v) and (vi).**

imaging modality for premature babies as well as term infants with neonatal encephalopathy [42]. Clinical MRI reporting remains mostly qualitative (subjective and observer dependent) by visual assessment of images acquired with various contrast weightings. However, MRI techniques can now provide many objective, quantitative, scanner- and sequence-independent measures associated with brain maturation and pathology. Such quantitative MRI (qMRI) [43] may prove more sensitive than visual assessments to subtle tissue changes. It is thus possible to develop a large database containing quantitative, normative developmental cerebral MRI information (the National Institutes of Health MRI study of normal brain development represents an effort in this direction [44]). In future it may be possible to compare a pediatric qMRI measurement to age-equivalent normative ranges similarly to the current use of height or head circumference.

DWI and diffusion tensor imaging

The simplest pulse sequence sensitizing MRI to one-dimensional (1D) water diffusion has been outlined above. By applying only 1D diffusion-weighting gradients and collecting at least two images (one having $b = 0$, i.e., no diffusion-weighting gradient), a 1D ADC estimate can be obtained for each pixel: $ADC = -\ln[S(b)/S(0)]/b$. However, this ADC would depend on the chosen sensitizing-gradient direction within the subject. To obtain an ADC independent of patient and scanner orientation, DWI must use at least three orthogonal directions (e.g., x, y, z) to give the directionless mean $= (ADC_x + ADC_y + ADC_z)/3$ (only correct if negligible diffusion weighting is incurred by the other "imaging" gradient pulses in the sequence). If a single b is used, the greatest SNR is for $b \times ADC \sim 1.1$ [45]; for neonatal brain typical optimum $b = 600–800$ s/mm² (1000 s/mm² for adult brain). Typical diffusion-weighted images are shown in Fig. 3.10b with the corresponding ADC map.

Theoretically ADC gives direct insight into brain microstructure; however, ADC can depend on measurement method (pulse sequence, and diffusion time in particular, see Fig. 3.10a): multicenter intercomparisons require particular care. Another noteworthy aspect is that the relation between DWI signal intensity and b is not mono-exponential in many tissues (e.g., cerebral white matter or prostate). Bi-exponential fits are sometimes more appropriate: slow- and fast-diffusion components can be discerned and, although historically identified with intra- and extracellular compartments, recent evidence suggests that the slow component may pertain to motionally restrained water irrespective of location [46].

The diffusion tensor

Diffusion anisotropy was first observed in cerebral white matter: diffusion was faster parallel to axons [11]. The scalar ADC is inadequate for characterization of 3D water diffusion that is hindered by, for example, axonal membranes, myelin, and neurofilaments: molecular motion is biased towards particular directions. The diffusion-tensor (DT) model uses a 3×3 symmetric "tensor" to characterize the diffusion properties of a medium. A minimum of six independent measurements are needed for its complete definition: DWI must use at least six different gradient directions (DT imaging – DTI). The "diffusion ellipsoid" helps DT visualization, showing the isoprobability surface of the mean water-molecule displacement (Fig. 3.11a) [47].

For isotropic diffusion the ellipsoid is spherical with radius proportional to the average diffusivity, and reducing with increasing motion-hindering structure density. For cerebral white matter, which contains directionally ordered axonal tracts, the ellipsoid is prolate with its major axis parallel to the tracts: membrane permeability and tract disposition determine DT magnitude and anisotropy. The DT is fully described

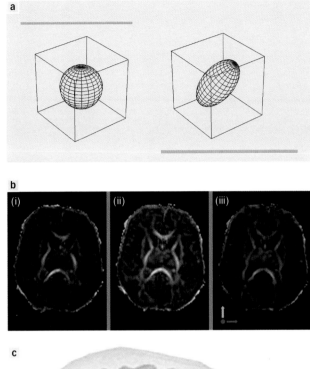

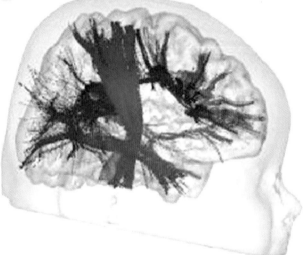

Fig. 3.11. **(a) The diffusion ellipsoid. Diffusion characteristics can be described by a diffusion ellipsoid: if spherical, diffusion is isotropic; if there is a preferred diffusion direction (e.g., as in white matter) the ellipsoid will appear prolate (image courtesy of Dr D. Tournier). (b) Visualizing diffusion anisotropy. Maps of (i) relative anisotropy and (ii) fractional anisotropy from the brain of a newborn infant. The color-coded fractional-anisotropy image (iii) shows the direction of the main eigenvector (direction of highest diffusivity). (c) Major white matter fiber tracts in a 3-month-old infant. The corpus callosum (red), the corticospinal (blue) and spinothalamic (light green) tracts, the inferior longitudinal (deep green) and uncinate (pink) fascicles are highlighted. From: Huppi P. S. and Dubois J.,** *Semin Fetal Neonatal Med.* **2006; 11(6): 489–497.**

by its "eigenvectors" (the orientation of the diffusion ellipsoid axes for which water displacements are uncorrelated) and "eigenvalues" (squared length of each ellipsoid axis) and directly relates to tissue microstructure.

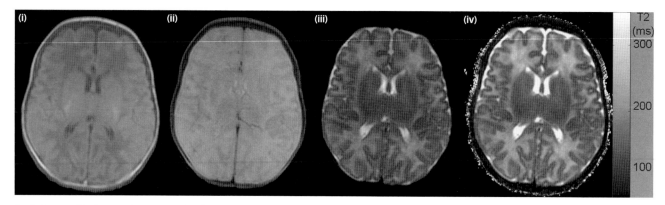

Fig. 3.12. Quantitative T$_2$ relaxometry. The displayed spin-echo images of neonatal brain were acquired with TE 11 ms (i), 100 ms (ii), and 300 ms (iii). A quantitative T$_2$ image generated from images (i), (ii), and (iii) is also shown (iv). Note the relatively low white- to grey-matter contrast with TE 100 ms and the contrast reversal between TE 11 ms and 300 ms.

Diffusion tensor measures independent of patient and scanner orientation are [48]: mean diffusivity (average of the three eigenvalues, equivalent to ADC), relative anisotropy (RA), and fractional anisotropy (FA). The terms FA and RA describe the deviation of the diffusion process from an isotropic diffusion case. Other anisotropy indices have been suggested that explicitly include eigenvector orientation, or depend on the DT in neighboring pixels (e.g., lattice anisotropy). Colors are often superimposed on anisotropy images which encode the main diffusion direction and visualize diffusion directionality (Fig. 3.11b). Anisotropy measures can help identify subtle brain pathologies that are subjectively assessed with only moderate success by conventional MRI (e.g., [49]). A shortcoming of the DT model is its inability to assess correctly pixels containing several differently oriented axonal tracts: when this occurs, the diffusion ellipsoid has little relation to microstructure. Diffusion-weighted imaging problems have been reviewed and models that overcome single DT limitations have been recently summarized [50].

Fiber tracking
Diffusion-tensor imaging also enables 3D delineation of specific neural pathways [51,52,53]. One approach uses the direction of greatest diffusion for each pixel, or the whole DT, to follow white-matter axonal tracts through the brain: "fiber assignment by continuous tracking" (FACT) is one of the simplest methods. Starting pixels are chosen and tract trajectories are defined to match the direction of greatest diffusion at that position; on entering a neighboring pixel the trajectory direction is altered to that of the new pixel's direction of greatest diffusion. Termination criteria are defined which end the tract if: the pixel-to-pixel direction deviation is excessive (e.g., >50°–60°); the tract enters a very low anisotropy region (e.g., FA < 0.1–0.2); or the tract leaves the brain. Alternative "probabilistic" tracking methods are becoming popular [54]. For each starting pixel, many trajectories are launched: the directions for each pixel are determined by its main diffusion axis and degree of anisotropy. As the trajectories fan out, the fraction passing through each pixel defines a probabilistic connectivity index and gives a

confidence figure for including that pixel in the trajectory. These methods have enabled quantification of neonatal white-matter tract maturation [55,56] (Fig. 3.11c).

T$_2$ relaxometry
In 1971 excised normal and cancerous tissue were distinguished by T$_1$ and T$_2$ [3]: NMR systems then did not include imaging capability. Today, quantitative relaxation-time imaging is relatively easy and T$_2$ measurement (relaxometry) in particular has identified subtle abnormalities not obvious on conventional MRI [57, 58].

T$_2$ relaxometry only requires two or more SE images with differing TE: using $S_{TE} = S_o \exp(-TE/T_2)$ gives S_o (the signal intensity extrapolated to TE = 0 ms) and T$_2$. T$_2$-weighted images and the corresponding T$_2$ image are shown in Fig. 3.12. The problem with T$_2$ relaxometry is obtaining scanner- and imaging-sequence-independent measurements in an acceptable time. The above approach may take too long if many slices are imaged with many TEs. A multi-echo, spin-echo sequence is often used. However, B_1 non-uniformity is a problem: slight deviation of the multiple refocussing-pulse flip angles from the ideal 180° will induce more signal decay between successive echoes making the apparent T$_2$ smaller than the true value. This effect is always present in the "through slice" direction due to the fact that the slice excitation profile is never ideal; variations across the slice can also occur (especially at high fields) due to B_1 non-uniformity.

The wider availability of fast imaging sequences such as SE EPI enables T$_2$ relaxometry to be acquired in a reasonable time with full brain coverage: a disadvantage is the lower spatial resolution and larger geometric distortions. Similarly to diffusion, transverse relaxation is not always mono-exponential and more TEs and higher SNR are necessary to distinguish compartments with discrete T$_2$ values or characterize a continuous T$_2$ distribution [59]. T$_2$ generally decreases with neonatal brain maturation [60, 61]. There is also evidence that early T$_2$ relaxometry is prognostic in neonatal encephalopathy [62] and may detect diffuse white matter damage at term-corrected age in infants born prematurely. Knowledge of the expected regional relaxation times at the B_0 used is also necessary for optimizing conventional MRI [63].

Magnetic resonance spectroscopy

Whereas MRI provides information about anatomical structure and also about the biophysical state of tissue water, MRS obtains mainly chemical and biophysical information and can be used in vitro or in vivo [38]. In vitro studies utilize very high B_0 (e.g., 14.1 T) to obtain exquisite spectroscopic resolution and probe body fluids, cellular extracts, and even cell cultures. In vivo MRS utilizes lower B_0 (e.g., 1.5 T is often used clinically), but is uniform over a much larger volume in order to encompass the head, for example, and probes intracellular metabolites with tissue concentrations $\sim$10 mM (much less than that of tissue water, e.g., $\sim$50 M in neonatal brain). Hence, metabolite signals are much weaker than that of water, and for certain isotopes (e.g., ^{31}P), signal weakness is further reduced by low absolute sensitivity (Table 3.2). As a result MRS is often time consuming to allow for build up of signal.

Chemical shift

Nuclei of a particular isotope in different molecular species, and also in different locations in the same molecule, experience a perturbed local magnetic field due to the molecular electron cloud screening B_0: the screening is metabolite specific. The Larmor equation now becomes:

$$\nu = \gamma B_0 (1 - \sigma)/2\pi, \qquad (3.3)$$

where σ is the screening factor. Because σ is very small, metabolite resonant frequencies cluster closely; e.g., for ^{1}H $\sigma < 10^{-5}$ and for ^{31}P and ^{13}C $\sigma < 5 \times 10^{-3}$.

In order to compare directly spectra acquired in differing B_0, resonant frequency is quoted as "chemical shift" (δ) measured in parts per million (ppm) of B_0. Thus:

$$\delta = 10^6 (\nu - \nu_S)/\nu_S \, ppm, \qquad (3.4)$$

where ν_S is the resonant frequency (Hz) of a reference peak (in ^{31}P MRS the singlet PCr resonance at 0 ppm is often used; see Fig. 3.13).

Free induction decay and spectrum

The raw RF signal detected by the receiver is the FID: this includes an exponentially decaying sinusoidal signal for each resonance from the sample. One method for extracting metabolic information from the FID is the FFT which converts the original time-dependent FID into a frequency-dependent spectrum (Fig. 3.13). (Analogous to the way the brain interprets a musical chord by analyzing for the notes present.)

Cerebral metabolites detectable by ^{1}H MRS

The major peaks in a human-brain ^{1}H spectrum (Fig. 3.14) are singlets originating from choline-containing compounds (Cho; at $\sim$3.2 ppm), Cr ($\sim$3.0 ppm; containing unresolved resonances from creatine and PCr), and N-acetylaspartate (Naa; $\sim$2.0 ppm). Lactate (Lac) is sometimes detected in normal neonatal brain

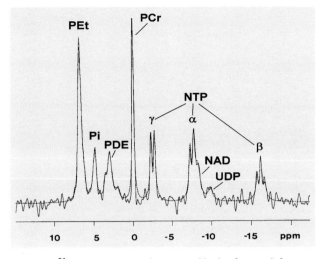

Fig. 3.13. A ^{31}P PRESS spectrum from central brain of a term infant studied because of perinatal hypoxia-ischemia, who survived with minor neurodevelopmental impairment. Resonance identifications: PEt, phosphoethanolamine; Pi, inorganic phosphate; PDE, phosphodiesters; PCr, phosphocreatine; NTP, nucleotide triphosphates (mainly adenosine triphosphate); NAD, nicotinamide dinucleotide; UDP, uridine diphosphosugars. NTP multiplet structure can be clearly seen (γ and α doublets, β a triplet). Acquisition conditions: 2.4 T, TE 10 ms, TR 12 s, 160 summed echoes, 5 cm cubic voxel. The dashed line is the result of analysis using statistical fitting of Lorentzian peaks to the spectrum.

but at a low level; however, following severe hypoxia-ischemia the Lac methyl doublet ($\sim$1.3 ppm) can become very prominent. Numerous other less prominent resonances are often present including glutamate, glutamine, *myo*-inositol, and γ-aminobutyrate. (For a list of ^{1}H-MRS neonatal brain metabolites see [64]; [65] also contains useful information including exemplary metabolite spectra.) Of the major ^{1}H resonances Naa and Lac are particularly important in hypoxic-ischemic injury. N-Acetylaspartate (Naa) is predominantly neuronal [66] and decreased Naa can represent neuronal loss; furthermore, the Naa signal increases with neuronal development. Lactate (Lac) is produced by anaerobic glycolysis: increased Lac may represent impaired cerebral energy production by oxidative phosphorylation. Because of high absolute sensitivity and resonances often originating from several equivalent nuclei (e.g., 3 for Cr, Naa, and Lac, and 9 for Cho), ^{1}H spectra can be acquired more rapidly and from smaller tissue volumes than ^{31}P spectra.

Cerebral metabolites detectable by ^{31}P MRS

Most peaks in a brain ^{31}P spectrum (Fig. 3.13) are singlets: the γ-, α-, and β-nucleotide triphosphate (NTP) resonances are an exception being two doublets and a triplet respectively. The NTP resonances originate predominantly from ATP but include minor guanosine-, uridine-, and cytidine-triphosphate contributions [67]. After NTP, phosphoethanolamine (PEt) is the most prominent neonatal-brain peak: PEt declines with development and is thought to be involved in membrane (e.g., axonal) development. Adjacent to PEt is a smaller peak from phosphocholine (PCh; also thought to be associated with

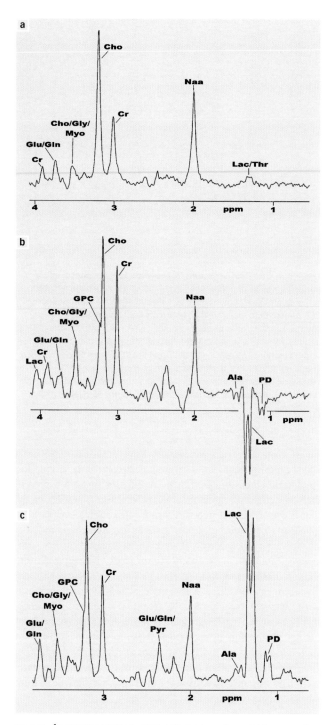

Fig. 3.14. **¹H PRESS spectra from the thalamic regions of (a) a normal term infant (TE 270 ms); and (b) and (c) a term infant who died as a result of neonatal encephalopathy consequential to perinatal hypoxia-ischemia (TE 135 ms and TE 270 ms respectively). Resonance identifications: Ala, alanine; Cho, choline; Cr, creatine (including PCr); Gln, glutamine; Glu, glutamate; Gly, glycine; GPC, glycerophosphocholine; Lac, lactate; Myo, *myo*-inositol; Naa, *N*-acetylaspartate; PD, propan-1,2-diol (an anticonvulsant injection medium); Pyr, pyruvate; Thr, threonine. In (b) phase modulation at TE 135 ms inverts the Ala, Lac, and PD doublets (between 1.5 and 1.0 ppm). Acquisition conditions: 2.4 T, TR 2 s, 128 summed echoes, 2 cm cubic voxel.**

membrane development). Pi is also near PEt. PCr resonates adjacent to γ-NTP: PCr rephosphorylates adenosine diphosphate (ADP) via the creatine-kinase reaction in order to maintain ATP. In hypoxic-ischemic neonatal encephalopathy, increased Pi and reduced PCr, and in severe cases reduced NTP, convey unfavorable outcome [68]. Other resonances include phosphodiesters, nicotinamide adenine diphosphate, and uridine diphosphosugars. (For ³¹P brain-metabolite chemical shifts see references [69, 70]; the latter includes ¹H and ¹³C.) Because ³¹P peaks originate from single molecular nuclei (unlike ¹H) and ³¹P has intrinsically poor sensitivity, acquisition times and localized volumes have to be larger in order to obtain signal comparable to ¹H.

Homonuclear and heteronuclear coupling

If a molecule contains only a single nucleus of the isotope of interest, MRS detects one singlet peak from the metabolite concerned; however, if more than one such nucleus is present, "homonuclear coupling" can occur between the nuclear magnets. For example, a ³¹P brain spectrum (e.g., Fig. 3.13) has three prominent resonances originating predominantly from ATP denoted as γ, α, and β: γ and α are doublet peaks; β is a triplet. These originate from three chained phosphate groups as shown:

$$\text{Adenosine - O -} \underset{\underset{O}{\|}}{\overset{\overset{OH}{|}}{P_\alpha}} \text{- O} \sim \underset{\underset{O}{\|}}{\overset{\overset{OH}{|}}{P_\beta}} \text{- O} \sim \underset{\underset{O}{\|}}{\overset{\overset{OH}{|}}{P_\gamma}} \text{- OH}$$

The α and γ ³¹P nuclei "sense" the possible spin orientations of the interstitial β nucleus (up or down) with almost equal probability; hence, α and γ can each experience two possible slightly different local magnetic field strengths: consequently α and γ each have two possible slightly different Larmor frequencies making them doublet resonances. The β ³¹P nucleus "senses" α and γ, both of which can be spin up or down; hence, the four possible α and γ spin combinations (again with approximately equal probabilities) are α and γ up, α and γ down, α up and γ down, and α down and γ up (the latter two are magnetically equivalent). Hence, the β peak is a triplet with outer components of approximately equal amplitude and the central component (originating from the last two combinations) is approximately twice the outer component amplitude. Multiplet component separation is B_0 independent and called "J" (~16 Hz for ATP in vivo). Many ¹H MRS peaks exhibit splitting due to homonuclear coupling, of which that of Lac is probably the most important in neonatal brain studies. Lactate has the following molecular structure:

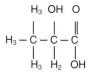

The three methyl protons (H₃) are magnetically equivalent (identical spatial probability distributions). The adjacent solitary methene proton (H_2) experiences eight possible H_3 spin combinations: all up, all down, three equivalent two up and one down combinations, and three equivalent one up and two down combinations. Hence, the Lac methene resonance (at ~4.1 ppm [65]) is a quartet with the two inner-component amplitudes equal and ~3 times those of the outer components. The H_3 protons only significantly "sense" the H_2 spin, which can be up or down with approximately equal probabilities; hence, the methyl resonance (~1.3 ppm) is a doublet with $J \sim 7$ Hz.

In addition to coupling to nuclei of the same isotope it is possible to couple to nuclei of different isotopes (heteronuclear coupling) of which adjacent hydrogen nuclei are the most important biomedically. In ^{13}C MRS such coupling causes peak splitting resulting in multiplet overlap and difficult spectrum analysis and interpretation. It is possible to negate heteronuclear coupling by irradiating the sample at the ^{1}H frequency (decoupling) but great care is necessary to avoid overheating. ^{31}P resonances also couple to ^{1}H, however, this peak splitting is unresolvable in vivo. In addition to simplifying, for example ^{13}C, spectra (the multiplets coalesce to form singlets), decoupling can also induce the nuclear Overhauser effect (NOE) further increasing peak amplitudes [38].

Spectrum acquisition and localization

There are many spectrum acquisition methods. The current localization techniques of choice combine "selective" RF pulses and pulsed magnetic-field gradients. There are two approaches: single voxel, which acquires a spectrum only from one tissue region; and MRS imaging (MRSi), which collects information from the whole field of view (FOV) and then determines a spectrum for each square on a "checker-board" grid thereby giving a metabolite image albeit with much worse spatial resolution than MRI.

Pulse acquire

This is the simplest acquisition method: a single RF pulse is applied n times at intervals TR and successive FIDs are added in computer memory. Because of low metabolite concentrations, and other reasons, e.g., for ^{31}P also because of factors including low absolute sensitivity, many FIDs must be added to get an acceptable spectrum. Signal builds up proportional to n and the noise as $\sqrt{n}$; hence, SNR increases as $\sqrt{n}$. Pulse acquire has most often been used with a surface coil [38] on the skin adjacent to the target organ (e.g., skeletal muscle) and with the coil designed to exclude unwanted signal from other tissues. Surface-coil signal is acquired from an approximately hemispheric sensitive volume centered on the coil and of similar radius. This approach obviously has limited application: ideally one wants to localize signal to a specific region inside the body.

Single-voxel localization

^{1}H single-voxel methods now almost universally use PRESS or STEAM, which are spin- and stimulated-echo methods respectively [38, 71]. Theoretically PRESS provides twice the STEAM signal. PRESS is a double spin-echo technique: M_0 is firstly

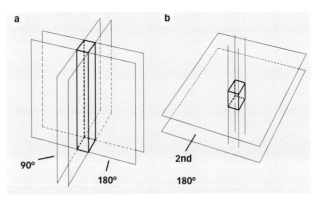

Fig. 3.15. **PRESS localization. (a) Firstly, combined with a magnetic field gradient, a 90° selective RF pulse flips M_0 only within a tissue slice containing the volume of interest (VOI). A 180° selective pulse with a gradient parallel to the 90° slice is then applied after delay τ_1: again this flips sample magnetization only within an orthogonal slice containing the VOI and which defines a column at the intersection of the 90° and 180° slices; τ_1 later, a normal spin echo (not acquired) refocusses originating only from the column. (b). After a further delay τ_2, during which columnar magnetization fans out again, a final 180° pulse flips sample magnetization only within a slice orthogonal to the column and containing the VOI: this produces a final refocussing and an echo τ_2 later originating exclusively from the cuboidal VOI defined by the intersection of all three slices. Because PRESS is a spin-echo method, only VOI signal refocusses: external signal decays by transverse relaxation before echo acquisition at TE = $2\tau_1 + 2\tau_2$ after the 90° pulse.**

flipped into the xy plane by a 90° selective RF pulse (this defines a slab of tissue passing through the region of interest) (Fig. 3.15a). After a short delay τ_1 a 180° selective pulse is applied with a gradient perpendicular to that of the 90° pulse: this defines a column of tissue at the intersection of the 90° and 180° slabs (Fig. 3.15a); τ_1 after this 180° pulse a spin echo would refocus. However, in PRESS after a further delay τ_2 a final 180° pulse with gradient orthogonal to both the previous gradients is applied: the intersection of the final slab with the tissue column defines a cuboidal region of interest (voxel) (Fig. 3.15b). During τ_2 the spin-echo magnetization fans out again and the last 180° pulse flips this enabling a second refocussing to give a final echo τ_2 later. Because PRESS is a spin-echo method magnetization is only refocussed in the voxel: external magnetization decays before acquiring the echo TE = $2(\tau_1 + \tau_2)$ after the 90° pulse.

OSIRIS [72] has found some use for ^{31}P: this combines suppression of external signal with voxel localization from a combination of selective inversion (180°) pulses. ^{31}P has only ~6% of ^{1}H absolute sensitivity and ^{1}H resonances often originate from three or more equivalent nuclei; therefore, to attain comparable SNR ^{31}P voxels must be much larger than for ^{1}H. For example, whereas ^{1}H MRI can provide pixel resolution <1 mm, ^{1}H MRS voxel dimensions need to be ~1.5 cm, and ^{31}P ~5 cm.

Water suppression

In ^{1}H MRS tissue water creates a problem. Metabolites of interest have concentrations ~10 mM, whereas there is a water concentration of ~50 M in the neonatal brain, giving a concentration ratio of ~5000. The water signal thus dwarfs those of the metabolites rendering digitization of the latter difficult. One common solution is saturating the water signal by several selective RF pulses (chemical shift selective or "CHESS" pulses; centered on the water peak with bandwidth narrow enough to only affect water) accompanied by "spoiler" magnetic gradients: water magnetization becomes mostly randomly orientated with greatly reduced signal.

MRS imaging (MRSi)

This localization modality, also known as chemical-shift imaging (CSI), can be applied with pulse-acquire, spin- and stimulated-echo sequences [38]. For 2D MRSi a tissue slice is defined by a selective RF pulse and a magnetic gradient: for spin-echo MRSi phase-encoding gradient pulses are applied between the 90° and 180° pulses; starting as a negative gradient these are incremented at each sequence application until an equal positive gradient is reached. Phase-encoding gradients in orthogonal directions and all incremental combinations are applied. Whilst the phase-encoding gradient is on, nuclei at each location have a unique Larmor frequency perturbation and, similar to MRI, the echo acquired from each sequence application has a unique "phase." Unlike MRI, gradients are off during data acquisition thus preserving chemical-shift information: Fourier transformation gives a spectrum located appropriately at each of the "squares" in the "checkerboard" which typically may be 16×16 1-cm squares (Fig. 3.16). 3D MRSi uses three orthogonal phase-encoding gradients (without slice selection) and can cover the whole brain, for example. However, many more phase-encoding steps are needed (e.g., $16 \times 16 \times 16$), which takes a lot longer to acquire.

Phase modulation

If a multiplet resonance is studied using a spin-echo sequence, "phase modulation" occurs [73]. This is of particular importance for ^{1}H MRS because of the numerous multiplets; however, ^{31}P ATP resonances also modulate. The Lac methyl doublet (~1.3 ppm) is of prognostic importance in brain MRS. When using PRESS or STEAM Lac appearance depends on TE: with PRESS the Lac doublet is normal at TE 288 ms (Fig. 3.14) but inverted (often with reduced amplitude) at 144 ms [71]; with STEAM a normal Lac signal is seen with TE 288 ms whereas at 144 ms the signal is small and appearance depends on the precise "mixing time."

Phase modulation is caused by the multiplet components precessing separately in the xy plane during TE. For example, the Lac doublet has J ~7 Hz and during TE the two components separate at $7 \times 360°$/s. In PRESS with TE 144 ms during TE each component precesses by 180° (but in opposite directions) so Lac magnetization is now in the opposite direction to that of a singlet peak (which does not phase modulate) and, hence, Lac appears inverted; with TE 288 ms each component precesses through 360°, which brings the Lac magnetization back to its original orientation and the doublet now appears normal. The TE dependences of many multiplets are complex: Ernst and Hennig [71] describe PRESS and STEAM phase modulation in many cerebral metabolites.

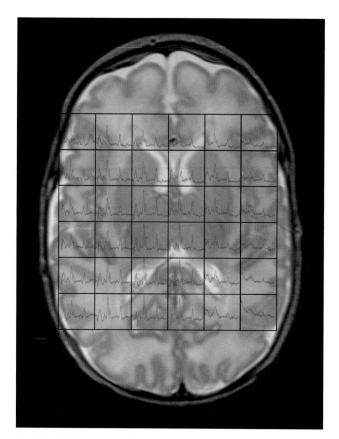

Fig. 3.16. **MRS imaging of the brain of a term infant. This method can display spatial metabolite distributions; however, SNR and spectral resolution may be less satisfactory than provided by single-voxel MRS. PRESS was used to reduce fat contamination by exciting only a selected region within brain followed by 2D MRS imaging. Acquisition conditions were: TE 144 ms, TR 2.14 s, seven summations, in-plane resolution 8.75 mm × 8.75 mm, slice thickness 15 mm.**

Spectrum analysis

The aim of spectrum analysis is mainly to obtain peak areas (proportional to metabolite concentration) and chemical shifts. The method must be resilient to peak overlap and poor SNR. There are two main approaches: computerized fitting of simulated peaks to the actual spectrum (frequency domain) and fitting of exponentially decaying sinusoids to the FID or echo (time domain). The latter approach is becoming more common since, in addition to determining chemical shifts, decay time constants, and resonance amplitudes (in time-domain analysis amplitude is proportional to concentration), this method also finds resonance phase (in the frequency domain this is determined by other means – often manually). Furthermore, broad underlying signals can be removed simply by omitting the first few data points. AMARES is such a time-domain method [74] and has been implemented in the magnetic resonance user interface (MRUI; [75]).

The information obtainable

A prime aim is to obtain measures proportional to metabolite concentration such as peak areas (frequency-domain analysis) and signal amplitudes (time-domain analysis): if $TR < 5T_1$ these are reduced by $\sin(\theta)[1 - \exp(-TR/T_1)]/[1 - \cos(\theta)\exp(-TR/T_1)]$; if using a spin-echo method these additionally decrease as TE increases according to $\exp(-TE/T_2)$. Hence, unless TR (if $<5T_1$) and TE corrections are applied, metabolite ratios will depend on T_1 and T_2: the latter are peak specific and may be altered by pathology. Metabolite ratios, e.g., Lac/Naa and PCr/Pi, have demonstrated significant prognostic benefit. However, pathology could be concealed if, for example, both metabolite concentrations changed similarly. Hence, a further goal has been to estimate "absolute" metabolite concentrations, i.e. mmol/kg wet weight tissue. To achieve this, in addition to correcting for T_1, T_2, and numbers of equivalent nuclei, metabolite signals must be compared with that of an external or internal standard [38]. If an external vial of standard solution is used at the time of study, then a correction may be necessary for B_1 inhomogeneity; if at a different time, then it is also necessary to correct for coil-efficiency differences between reference and in vivo studies. Neonatal brain water has a fairly uniform concentration in both white and gray matter and in ^1H studies has been used as an internal reference. (It is often necessary to determine metabolite T_1 and T_2 for absolute quantitation: these may themselves be of interest [33].)

Resonance chemical shifts are also of interest. PEt [76], P_i [77], and ATP [78] ^{31}P chemical shifts can be used to estimate internal pH or pH_i. There are subtle differences in the information obtained: pH_{PEt} is exclusively intracellular whereas P_i includes an extracellular component which may bias pH_{P_i} slightly alkaline; pH_{ATP} exclusively probes intracellularly and only in "viable" cells (i.e., those retaining ATP). ATP chemical shifts can also be used to estimate Mg_{free} concentration [78]: only $ATPMg^{2-}$ participates in transport and other important cellular processes; increased Mg_{free} may suggest reduced ATP. The ^1H-MRS water chemical shift is temperature dependent and, with suitable calibration, can be used to estimate local brain temperature non-invasively and even to generate maps of cerebral temperature.

Advantages and disadvantages of increasing magnetic field strength

The main benefits of stronger B_0 are: higher SNR, greater susceptibility-related contrast, and increased MRS peak resolution. These advantages drive the commercial race to develop and optimize scanners with ever increasing B_0. The increased SNR (approximately proportional to B_0) can be utilized to reduce examination time but more often is devoted to improve data quality. In MRI better quality means increased spatial resolution and tissue contrast. In MRS higher SNR means: reduced chemical-shift and peak-area random errors; detection of metabolites with little signal due to low concentration or phase modulation (e.g., γ-aminobutyrate, glutamate, and glutamine); and the possibility of smaller voxels (to acquire spectra exclusively from smaller anatomical structures). Increased susceptibility contrast also benefits BOLD functional MRI and venography.

However, the following effects occur at higher B_0: B_1 non-uniformity is worse, resulting in reduced image-intensity uniformity; susceptibility artifacts (geometric distortions or signal loss) increase; and T_1 lengthens, while T_2 and T_2^* shorten, giving altered tissue contrast. Some of these issues can be addressed by modifying the transmit and receive RF coils, or by employing special RF pulses and sequences. The theoretical potential of higher B_0 is limited by safety aspects: higher B_0 incurs increased RF power deposition and more acoustic noise, (the latter from pulsed magnetic-field gradients). Realizing the advantages of higher B_0 safely is thus costly and technically challenging, requiring substantial pulse-sequence modification and reassessment of normal tissue contrast and normative quantitative values. For example, T_2-weighted images with submillimeter spatial resolution have revealed substantial signal heterogeneity in adult white matter at 4.7 T and above: with lower spatial resolution and B_0 this was only apparent with mild to severe atrophy [79]. Benefits and limitations of high B_0 and acquisition conditions have thus to be carefully reassessed for each specific clinical application.

Research scanners operating at 7 T and 8 T have been used to study adult brain for several years and approximately a dozen such systems are now operational. The recent optimization of whole-body applications is currently making 3-T scanners more attractive than the 1.5-T systems, which were the clinical state-of-the-art over the last decade. The use of $B_0 \geq 3$ T for neonatal brain is relatively recent [41, 63] and the highest used so far is 4.7 T [80]. The high-B_0 study of neonatal brain has been delayed by the necessary submission to more conservative safety limits. However, results of initial studies are extremely encouraging.

Common artifacts on magnetic resonance imaging

In order to interpret an image appropriately it is important to be aware of the possibility of unwanted image features (artifacts) unrelated to the target anatomy. The most common are due to: loss of the spatial conformity of target anatomy and imaged position (signal mispositioning); signal-intensity and contrast variations across an image; body-fluid flow and tissue motion; inappropriate pulse sequence; or hardware failure (Fig. 3.17).

Signal mispositioning

Geometric distortions
Correct spatial encoding, e.g., good correspondence between anatomical locations and their image positions, can only be assured if B_0 is acceptably uniform before applying imaging gradients. However, magnetic susceptibility differences create local B_0 inhomogeneities giving geometric distortions at interfaces between, for example, tissue and air or bone. Failure of a "shim" coil or ferromagnetic material within tissue can produce gross distortion. Through-slice local magnetic-field gradients affect all imaging sequences, in-slice (in-plane) gradients only affect GE sequences.

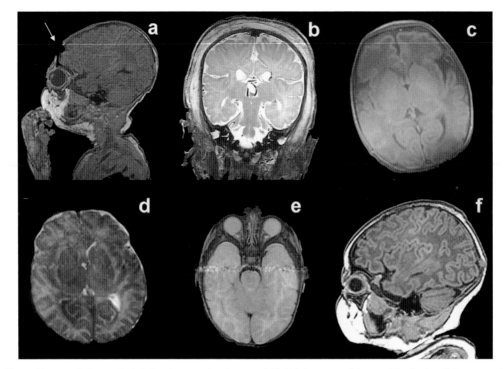

Fig. 3.17. **MRI artifacts. (a)** A metal clip on a baby's head creates local magnetic field inhomogeneities resulting in signal drop-out, which appears as a dent in the skull (arrow) on a 1.5-T 3D-FLASH image. **(b)** B_1 inhomogeneity causes contrast variation across this coronal 4.7-T fast SE image. **(c)** Coil malfunctioning causes smooth image brightness variations across this T_2-weighted SE image acquired with an extremity coil at 1.5 T. **(d)** Motion-corrupted infant brain image: 1.5-T T_2-weighted SE. **(e)** A horizontal band of increased signal is a flow artifact arising from a blood vessel anterior to the brain stem (T_2-weighted SE, 1.5 T). **(f)** Gibbs ringing conformal with the skull curvature and arising from the high scalp signal intensity can be seen near the top of the brain in this 1.5-T 3D-FLASH image.

Chemical-shift artifact

Unless more sophisticated methods are used conventional MRI actually visualizes a combined fat and water image. The predominant fat-proton resonance has a different chemical shift to water; consequentially, the fat image will be shifted spatially in the imaging plane relative to the water image. Furthermore, the phase of fat relative to that of water will be TE dependent: for certain TEs the shifted fat image will cancel the water signal in the same pixels producing a "black-line" artifact.

Gradient non-linearity

If the MRI system has been installed properly and the gradient coils designed appropriately, substantial distortions should only occur if target anatomy is a large distance from the magnet center where the gradients are not within the manufacturer's linearity specification.

Aliasing

Incorrect FOV setting can result in some imaged anatomy appearing on the opposite side of the image (in the phase-encode direction) compared to its physical location and thus overlapping the main image.

Solutions

Geometric shift due to chemical shift differences or distortion due to local magnetic-field inhomogeneities can be minimized by increasing signal acquisition speed (readout bandwidth); however, SNR reduces as $1/\sqrt{}$(bandwidth). In vivo B_0 maps can be obtained and used to partially correct in-plane image distortion. Special acquisition protocols that segment image collection can also minimize geometric distortions. Aliasing can be avoided by appropriate choice of phase and read direction and/or by application of signal saturation bands.

Signal-intensity and contrast variations

Signal drop out

Total signal loss can occur when local intrapixel signals are dephased by local B_0 inhomogeneities and cancel each other at the time of echo formation (Fig. 3.17a).

Partial volume effects

The final signal intensity in each pixel is determined by the averaged signals from all anatomical structures in the corresponding volume. If a pixel contains half gray and half white matter, the corresponding pixel intensity will be the average for these tissues (partial volume effect). Image spatial resolution (typically defined as in-plane resolution and slice thickness for a 2D protocol) determines the significance of the partial volume effect: the worse the spatial resolution the larger the effect, which impairs visualization of well-defined anatomical boundaries.

Coil inhomogeneity

Excitation and receive coils typically have non-uniform spatial sensitivities: if the flip angle is non-uniform over the image, both contrast and SNR will vary. Moreover, non-uniform, receive-coil spatial sensitivity will by itself also incur inhomogeneous image signal intensity (typically brighter closer to the coil). Non-uniform flip angle can be addressed by special sequences (e.g., with adiabatic pulses) or coils providing uniform excitation over the target anatomy. Non-uniform, receive sensitivity can be partially addressed by measuring it spatially and correcting image signal intensity; however, this does not correct for SNR variation across the image (Fig. 3.17b). Coil malfunctioning may also cause severe signal intensity variations across the image (Fig. 3.17c).

Motion and flow artifacts

Motion artifacts are very common and can be a particular problem in pediatric, neonatal, and fetal MRI. Tissue movement during acquisition results in image blurring (appearance similar to long-exposure photographs) or "ghosting." The latter refers to signals from the same anatomical source appearing at different image locations, typically shifted in the phase-encoding direction (Fig. 3.17d). These artifacts are due to tissue motion between different phase-encoding steps or between excitation and echo acquisition. If stationary tissue is unattainable (e.g., the awake fetus), one option is to employ very rapid MRI sequences (AT 50–200 ms) to collect a few slices and subsequently realign them. Respiratory and cardiac motion are cyclical and artifacts can often be mimimized by triggering ("gating") the pulse sequence by a physiological signal (e.g., electrocardiogram). Optimal conditions for studying newborn infants are during natural sleep or slightly sedated with gentle but efficient head restraint.

Flow

The pulsatile nature of blood and cerebrospinal fluid flow is another artifact cause (Fig. 3.17e). In GE images blood vessels usually appear bright because new blood is excited by each pulse. In SE images vessels appear dark because blood flows through the slice too fast to experience both the excitation and refocussing pulses. Furthermore, the range of flow velocities encountered during the cardiac cycle will result in phase shifts differing between phase-encoding steps and will produce ghosting artifacts. Electrocardiogram gating significantly obviates this problem. An alternative approach is to use special "flow-compensating" gradient schemes that null the phase shifts.

Other artifacts

Gibbs ringing

This looks like pond ripples and appears near anatomical boundaries where there are large signal intensity changes: it is caused by insufficient data sampling and can be reduced by applying a smoothing filter to the acquired signal although this also blurs the final image (Fig. 3.17f).

RF interference

The scanner is surrounded by a Faraday cage which should stop external RF interference from entering the scan room. All electrical cables entering the scan room must pass through appropriate filters. Bright bands in the phase-encoding direction are characteristic of "spot-frequency" interference.

RF spikes

Occasionally, bands of rapidly alternating signal intensity at a particular inclination appear across the whole image; this is typically caused by RF spikes (e.g., a sudden signal increase detected by the receiver coil). The scanner manufacturer should be contacted if this occurs.

Safety of patients and staff

There are several potential MRI-associated risks including those pertaining to B_0, pulsed magnetic gradients, RF power, and acoustic noise. There are also additional risks specific to neonatal studies. In the United Kingdom (UK) the Medicines and Healthcare Products Regulatory Agency (MHRA) publishes clinical MRI safety guidelines [81] based on guidelines set by the UK National Radiological Protection Board (NRPB) [82], the International Commission on Non-Ionising Radiation Protection [83], and the International Electrotechnical Commission [84].

Static magnetic field

There are several potential B_0 risks including biological effects: above 4 T there may be vertigo, nausea, reduced aortal flow, and increased blood pressure. For brain the NRPB guideline is $B_0 < 2.5$ T for "uncontrolled" studies (IEC < 2 T): between 2.5 T and 4 T (upper level) subjects must have appropriate physiological monitoring (IEC level 1 "controlled" mode: $2 T < B_0 < 4$ T); above 4 T ethics committee approval is essential (research/experimental mode; IEC level 2 "controlled" mode).

Ferromagnetic items will be attracted to the magnet causing injury ("projectile effect"; the force is about inversely proportional to distance cubed, increasing ~8 times at half the distance; a single step and an item may be wrenched from the hand). This risk must be reduced by rigorous patient screening, thorough staff training, and removal of ferromagnetic scan-room equipment. Newborn infants can be further protected by an enveloping pod. Implanted medical devices (e.g., cardiac pacemakers, arterial clips) could be compromised functionally or moved on entering the magnet: metal fragments in situ after prior injury may also move. Thorough clinical-history inspection is essential before entering the magnet. Furthermore, essential medical equipment may malfunction, e.g., MRI-compatible mechanical ventilators may need adjustment near the magnet. In addition to screening patients, staff such as neonatologists, nurses, and MRI physicists who enter the "controlled" area (where $B_0 > 0.5$ mT) must be similarly screened (even footwear should be closely inspected, e.g., for loose nails).

Table 3.3. National Radiological Protection Board (NRPB) gradient slew-rate exposure limits.

Duration of field change (t)	Uncontrolled level (T/s)	Upper level (T/s)
<2.5 μs	950	1300
2.5–45 μs	$2.4 \times 10^{-3}/t$	1300
45–120 μs	$2.4 \times 10^{-3}/t$	$60 \times 10^{-3}/t$
120 μs to 3 ms	20	$60 \times 10^{-3}/t$
>3 ms	20	20

Table 3.4. NRPB RF power limits (W/kg) assuming relative humidity <60% and ambient temperature <24 °C.

Exposure dura-tion (t; min)	Whole-body uncontrolled[a]	Whole-body controlled[a]	Head/ fetus[b]
<15 min	2	4	4
15–30 min	30/t	60/t	60/t
>30 min	1	2	2

[a] Averaged over any 15-min period.

[b] Averaged over any 6-min period.

Pulsed magnetic gradients

Magnetic-field gradient pulses have short rise and fall times: as a consequence the rate of change of magnetic field ("slew" rate) can be large. Possible risks are peripheral nerve and muscle stimulation (particularly cardiac), and acoustic noise (gradient pulses effectively make the magnet a loudspeaker driven by the gradient amplifiers). Table 3.3 gives guidelines.

RF power

Although brief, the RF pulses are generated by powerful amplifiers. The potential hazards are tissue heating (the RF heats tissue water like a microwave oven), burns from current induced in conductive loops formed by body parts, and burns at points of contact with metal items (e.g., monitoring probes, clothing fasteners, etc.).

Tissue heating

The RF power deposited in tissue is expressed as the specific absorption rate (SAR; W/kg tissue). For neonatal studies different exposure limits will apply depending on whether effectively the whole body is exposed (e.g., if using an adult head coil or a body coil for transmission) or just the head (e.g., using a smaller dedicated probehead). Table 3.4 gives NRPB limits. Particular care must be taken for tissues with poor blood flow (e.g., the eye lens) and in pathologies with compromised thermoregulation or blood flow.

Burns

It is safer to study newborn infants with a dedicated small head coil which minimizes RF exposure of torso and limbs and monitoring cabling. To minimize risk it is necessary to avoid limb loops around which induced RF current can flow; thus, legs (including thighs) should be isolated from each other by foam pads; the infant should also be isolated from monitoring cabling, which should run centrally parallel to the magnet bore. MHRA (2002) gives comprehensive precautions [81].

Acoustic noise

For neonatal studies the American Academy of Pediatrics [85] recommends <90 dB peak sound level in the ear (quieter than the IEC adult limit). Before neonatal investigations noise must be measured in the magnet for every pulse sequence to be used: if >90 dB, reduction methods must be employed such as trimmed adult ear plugs, small ear muffs, and even the study pod can incorporate a sound-absorbent lining.

Emergency evacuation

Emergency evacuation may be essential in certain situations including cardiac arrest, fire, or magnet quench (superconductors may suddenly de-energize leading to copious expulsion of helium gas, which should be conveyed safely out of the building by a quench pipe). Procedures for rapid infant evacuation to a safe place must be developed with training of staff concerned and practiced regularly. Appropriate facilities should be available at the "safe place" for clinical emergency.

Physiological monitoring and fluids

Newborn infants should be physiologically monitored during study including electrocardiogram (ECG), skin (and maybe rectal) temperature, pulse oximetry, and possibly apnea sensing. Unless they are MRI-compatible, ECG, temperature, and pulse oximetry monitors must be outside the Faraday cage with electrical cabling entering only via RF filters. Pulse oximetry has optical transmission and optical fibers can pass through a "waveguide" (a special tube through the Faraday cage). Similarly syringe drivers, unless MRI-compatible, must be outside the Faraday cage with fluid tubing entering through a waveguide.

Oxygen

There is significant risk associated with excess oxygen combined with flammable material (e.g., fabric) and an ignition mode: with precautions this risk is negligible. During mechanical ventilation expelled oxygen vents via the ventilator and conveys no increased risk. However, some non-ventilated infants may need enhanced respiratory oxygen levels. Clothing, etc. should be kept clear of the oxygen source and the study pod should be continuously flushed with ambient air (positive pressure). MRI probes should be external to the pod thereby excluding an ignition candidate (RF "arcing"). Monitoring cabling should be well insulated and regularly checked.

Contrast agents

Contrast agent should only be administered at the request of, and under the supervision of, a registered medical practitioner. Care must be taken to ensure no contraindications such as impaired kidney function. MRI centers should have local neonatal contrast-agent policies and on-site facilities to deal with adverse reactions including anaphylactic shock.

Staff exposure

For neonatal studies staff exposure can be important, e.g., if a neonatologist remains in the scanner room during study or significant patient preparation is close to the magnet. The hazards are similar to those for the patient but guidelines differ because of increased exposure frequency. Staff exposure can be minimized by performing all patient preparation outside the scanner room. If staff remain in the scanner room during study, acoustic noise reducers (e.g., ear plugs) should be used. The reader is directed to publications by NRPB [86] and ICNIRP [87] for guidance on staff exposure to, e.g., B_0 and RF power.

References

1. Purcell EM, Torrey HC, Pound RV. Resonance absorption by nuclear magnetic resonance moments in a solid. *Phys Rev* 1946; **69**: 37–8.
2. Bloch F, Hansen WW, Packard M. The nuclear induction experiment. *Physics Rev* 1946; **70**: 474–85.
3. Damadian RV. Tumour detection by nuclear magnetic resonance. *Science* 1971; **171**: 1151–53.
4. Lauterbur PC. Image formation by induced local interactions: examples of employing nuclear magnetic resonance. *Nature* 1973; **242**: 190–1.
5. Mansfield P. Multi-planar image formation using NMR spin echoes. *J Phys C: Solid State Phys* 1977; **10**: L55–L58.
6. Bandettini PA, Wong EC, Hinks RS, Tikofsky RS, Hyde JS. Time course EPI of human brain function during task activation. *Magn Reson Med* 1992; **25**(5): 390–7.
7. Kumar A, Welti D, Ernst RR. NMR Fourier Zeumatography. *J Magn Reson* 1975; **18**: 69–83.
8. Edelstein WA, Hutchison JM, Johnson G, Redpath T. Spin warp NMR imaging and applications to human whole-body imaging. *Phys Med Biol* 1980; **25**(4): 751–6.
9. Clow H, Young IR. Britain's brains produce first NMR scans. *New Sci* 1978; **80**: 588.
10. Dumoulin CL, Souza SP, Hart HR. Rapid scan magnetic resonance angiography. *Magn Reson Med* 1987; **5**(3): 238–45.
11. Moseley ME, Cohen Y, Kucharczyk J, *et al.* Diffusion-weighted MR imaging of anisotropic water diffusion in cat central nervous system. *Radiology* 1990; **176**(2): 439–45.
12. Benveniste H, Hedlund LW, Johnson GA. Mechanism of detection of acute cerebral ischemia in rats by diffusion-weighted magnetic resonance microscopy. *Stroke* 1992; **23**(5): 746–54.
13. Kwong KK, Belliveau JW, Chesler DA, *et al.* Dynamic magnetic resonance imaging of human brain activity during primary sensory stimulation. *Proc Natl Acad Sci USA* 1992; **89**(12): 5675–79.
14. Ambrose J, Hounsfield G. Computerized transverse axial tomography. *Br J Radiol* 1973; **46**(542): 148–9.
15. Krishnamoorthy KS, Fernandez RA, Momose KJ, *et al.* Evaluation of neonatal intracranial hemorrhage by computerized tomography. *Pediatrics* 1977; **59**(2): 165–72.
16. Pape KE, Blackwell R, Cusick G, *et al.* Ultrasound detection of brain damage in preterm infants. *Lancet* 1979; **1**(8129): 1261–64.
17. Brenner DJ, Elliston CD, Hall EJ, Berdon WE. Estimates of the cancer risks from pediatric CT radiation are not merely theoretical: comment on "point/counterpoint": in x-ray computed tomography, technique factors should be selected appropriate to patient size. *Med Phys* 2001; **28**(11): 2387–88.
18. Slovis TL. The ALARA concept in pediatric CT: myth or reality? *Radiology* 2002; **223**(1): 5–6.
19. Moon RB, Richards JH. Determination of intracellular pH BY 31P magnetic resonance. *J Biol Chem* 1973; **248**: 7276–8.
20. Hoult DI, Busby SJ, Gadian DG, Radda GK, Richards RE, Seeley PJ. Observation of tissue metabolites using ^{31}P nuclear magnetic resonance. *Nature* 1974; **252**: 285–7.
21. Burt CT, Glonek T, Barany M. Analysis of phosphate metabolites, the intracellular pH, and the state of adenosine triphosphate in intact muscle by phosphorus nuclear magnetic resonance. *J Biol Chem* 1976; **251**: 2584–91.
22. Ackerman J, Grove T, Wong G, Gadian D, Radda G. Mapping of metabolites in whole animals by ^{31}P NMR using surface coils. *Nature* 1980; **283**: 167–170.
23. Thulborn K, du Boulay G, Duchen L, Radda G. A ^{31}P nuclear magnetic resonance in vivo study of cerebral ischaemia in the gerbil. *Cereb Blood Flow Metab* 1982; **2**(3): 299–306.
24. Cady E, Costello A, Dawson M, *et al.* Non-invasive investigation of cerebral metabolism in newborn infants by phosphorus nuclear magnetic resonance spectroscopy. *Lancet* 1983; **1**(8333): 1059–62.
25. Bottomley P, Drayer B, Smith L. Chronic adult cerebral infarction studied by phosphorus NMR spectroscopy. *Radiology* 1986; **160**(3): 763–6.
26. Brown F, Campbell I, Kuchel P, Rabenstein D. Human erythrocyte metabolism studies by ^{1}H spin echo NMR. *FEBS Lett* 1977; **82**: 12–16.
27. Behar K, den Hollander J, Stromski M, *et al.* High-resolution ^{1}H nuclear magnetic resonance study of cerebral hypoxia in vivo. *Proc Natl Acad Sci USA* 1983; **80**(16): 4945–48.
28. Bottomley P, Edelstein W, Foster T, Adams W. In vivo solvent-suppressed localized hydrogen nuclear magnetic resonance spectroscopy: a window to metabolism? *Proc Natl Acad Sci USA* 1985; **82**(7): 2148–52.
29. Howe F, Opstad K. ^{1}H MR spectroscopy of brain tumours and masses. *NMR Biomed* 2003; **16**(3): 123–31.
30. Soher B, Doraiswamy P, Charles H. A review of ^{1}H MR spectroscopy findings in Alzheimer's disease. *Neuroimaging Clin N Am* 2005; **15**(4): 847–52.
31. Ross A, Sachdev P. Magnetic resonance spectroscopy in cognitive research. *Brain Res Brain Res Rev* 2004; **44**(2–3): 83–102.
32. Grover V, Dresner M, Forton D, *et al.* Current and future applications of magnetic resonance imaging and spectroscopy of the brain in hepatic encephalopathy. *World J Gastroenterol* 2006; **12**(19): 2969–78.
33. Cheong J, Cady E, Penrice J, Wyatt J, Cox I, Robertson N. Proton MR spectroscopy in neonates with perinatal cerebral hypoxic-ischemic injury: metabolite peak-area ratios, relaxation times, and absolute concentrations. *AJNR Am J Neuroradiol* 2006; **27**(7): 1546–54.
34. Cady E, D'Souza P, Penrice J, Lorek A. The estimation of local brain temperature by in vivo ^{1}H magnetic resonance spectroscopy. *Magn Reson Med* 1995; **33**(6): 862–7.
35. Vigneron DB, Barkovich AJ, Noworolski SM, *et al.* Three-dimensional proton MR spectroscopic imaging of premature and term neonates. *AJNR Am J Neuroradiol* 2001; **22**(7): 1424–33.
36. Scheurer E, Ith M, Dietrich D, *et al.* Statistical evaluation of time-dependent metabolite concentrations: estimation of post-mortem intervals based on in situ ^{1}H-MRS of the brain. *NMR Biomed* 2005; **18**(3): 163–72.
37. Brown MA, Semelka R. *MRI: Basic Principles and Applications*, 3rd edn. Chichester: JohnWiley, 2003.
38. de Certaines JD, Bovee WMMJ, Podo F. *Magnetic Resonance Spectroscopy in Biology and Medicine*. Oxford, UK: Pergamon Press, 1992.
39. Rabenstein DL, Nakashima TT. Spin-echo Fourier transform nuclear magnetic resonance spectroscopy. *Anal Chem* 1979; **51**: 1465A–1474 A.
40. Haase A, Odol F, von Kienlin M, *et al.* NMR probeheads for in vivo applications. *Concepts Magn Reson* 2000; **12**: 361–88.
41. Malamateniou C, Counsell S, Allsop J, *et al.* The effect of preterm birth on neonatal cerebral vasculature studied with magnetic resonance angiography at 3 Tesla. *Neuroimage* 2006; **32**(3): 1050–59.
42. Ment L, Bada H, Barnes P, *et al.* Practice parameter: neuroimaging of the neonate. Report of the Quality Standards Subcommittee of the American Academy of Neurology and the Practice Committee of the Child Neurology Society. *Neurology* 2002; **58**(12): 1726–38.
43. Tofts P. *Quantitative MRI of the Brain. Measuring Changes Caused by Disease*. England: John Wiley & Sons, 2003.
44. Almli CR, Rivkin MJ, McKinstry RC; Brain Development Cooperative Group. The NIH MRI study of normal brain development (Objective-2):

newborns, infants, toddlers, and preschoolers. *Neuroimage* 2007; **35(1)**: 308–25.

45. Conturo TE, McKinstry RC, Aronovitz JA, Neil JJ. Diffusion MRI: precision, accuracy and flow effects. *NMR Biomed* 1995; **8(7–8)**: 307–332.

46. Le Bihan D, Urayama S, Aso T, Hanakawa T, Fukuyama H. Direct and fast detection of neuronal activation in the human brain with diffusion MRI. *Proc Natl Acad Sci USA* 2006; **103(21)**: 8263–68.

47. Basser P, Mattiello J, LeBihan D. MR diffusion tensor spectroscopy and imaging. *Biophys J* 1994; **66(1)**: 259–67.

48. Basser P. Inferring microstructural features and the physiological state of tissues from diffusion-weighted images. *NMR Biomed* 1995; **8(7–8)**: 333–44.

49. Counsell S, Shen Y, Boardman J, *et al.* Axial and radial diffusivity in preterm infants who have diffuse white matter changes on magnetic resonance imaging at term-equivalent age. *Pediatrics* 2006; **117(2)**: 376–86.

50. Le Bihan D, Poupon C, Amadon A, Lethimonnier F. Artifacts and pitfalls in diffusion MRI. *J Magn Reson Imaging* 2006; **24(3)**: 478–88.

51. Mori S, Crain B, Chacko V, van Zijl P. Three-dimensional tracking of axonal projections in the brain by magnetic resonance imaging. *Ann Neurol* 1999; **45(2)**: 265–69.

52. Mori S, Zhang J. Principles of diffusion tensor imaging and its applications to basic neuroscience research. *Neuron* 2006; **51(5)**: 527–39.

53. Basser P, Pajevic S, Pierpaoli C, Duda J, Aldroubi A. In vivo fiber tractography using DT-MRI data. *Magn Reson Med* 2000; **44(4)**: 625–32.

54. Parker G, Alexander D. Probabilistic Monte Carlo based mapping of cerebral connections utilising whole-brain crossing fibre information. *Inf Process Med Imaging* 2003; **18**: 684–95.

55. Berman J, Mukherjee P, Partridge S, *et al.* Quantitative diffusion tensor MRI fiber tractography of sensorimotor white matter development in premature infants. *Neuroimage* 2005; **27(4)**: 862–71.

56. Dubois J, Hertz-Pannier L, Dehaene-Lambertz G, Cointepas Y, Le Bihan D. Assessment of the early organization and maturation of infants' cerebral white matter fiber bundles: a feasibility study using quantitative diffusion tensor imaging and tractography. *Neuroimage* 2006; **30(4)**: 1121–32.

57. Neema M, Stankiewicz J, Arora A, *et al.* T1- and T2-based MRI measures of diffuse gray matter and white matter damage in patients with multiple sclerosis. *J Neuroimaging* 2007; Suppl **1**(16S–21S).

58. Rugg-Gunn F, Boulby P, Symms M, Barker G, Duncan J. Whole-brain T2 mapping demonstrates occult abnormalities in focal epilepsy. *Neurology* 2005; **64(2)**: 318–25.

59. Fenrich F, Beaulieu C, Allen P. Relaxation times and microstructures. *NMR Biomed* 2001; **14(2)**: 133–9.

60. Thornton J, Amess P, Penrice J, Chong W, Wyatt J, Ordidge R. Cerebral tissue water spin-spin relaxation times in human neonates at 2.4 tesla: methodology and the effects of maturation. *Magn Reson Imaging* 1999; **17(9)**: 1289–1295.

61. Counsell S, Kennea N, Herlihy A, *et al.* T2 relaxation values in the developing preterm brain. *AJNR Am J Neuroradiol* 2003; **24(8)**: 1654–60.

62. Shanmugalingam S, Thornton J, Iwata O, *et al.* Comparative prognostic utilities of early quantitative magnetic resonance imaging spin-spin relaxometry and proton magnetic resonance spectroscopy in neonatal encephalopathy. *Pediatrics* 2006; **118(4)**: 1467–77.

63. Williams L, Gelman N, Picot P, *et al.* Neonatal brain: regional variability of in vivo MR imaging relaxation rates at 3.0 T – initial experience. *Radiology* 2005; **235(2)**: 595–603.

64. Kreis R, Hofmann L, Kuhlmann B, Boesch C, Bossi E, Huppi P. Brain metabolite composition during early human brain development as measured by quantitative in vivo ¹H magnetic resonance spectroscopy. *Magn Reson Med* 2002; **48(6)**: 949–58.

65. Govindaraju V, Young K, Maudsley A. Proton NMR chemical shifts and coupling constants for brain metabolites. *NMR Biomed* 2000; **13(3)**: 129–53.

66. Urenjak J, Williams S, Gadian D, Noble M. Specific expression of N-acetylaspartate in neurons, oligodendrocyte-type-2 astrocyte

progenitors, and immature oligodendrocytes in vitro. *J Neurochem* 1992; **59(1)**: 55–61.

67. Mandel P, Edel-Harth S. Free nucleotides in the rat brain during post-natal development. *J Neurochem* 1966; **13(7)**: 591–95.

68. Bachelard H. *Magnetic Resonance Spectroscopy and Imaging in Neurochemistry. Advances in Neurochemistry.* New York: Plenum, 1997.

69. Glonek T, Kopp S. Ex vivo P-31 NMR of lens, cornea, heart, and brain. *Magn Reson Imaging* 1985; **3(4)**: 359–76.

70. Bolinger L, Seeholzer S, Kofron J, Leigh JS. A guide to chemical shifts of 31-P, 1-H and 13-C. *News Metabol Res* 1984; **1**: 32–45.

71. Ernst T, Hennig J. Coupling effects in volume selective ¹H spectroscopy of major brain metabolites. *Magn Reson Med* 1991; **21(1)**: 82–96.

72. Connelly A, Van Paesschen W, Porter D, Johnson C, Duncan J, Gadian D. Proton magnetic resonance spectroscopy in MRI-negative temporal lobe epilepsy. *Neurology* 1998; **51(1)**: 61–6.

73. Rabenstein D, Nakashima T. Spin-echo Fourier transform nuclear magnetic resonance spectroscopy. *Anal Chem* 1979; **51**: 1465A–1474A.

74. Vanhamme L, van den Boogaart A, van Huffel S. Improved method for accurate and efficient quantification of MRS data with use of prior knowledge. *J Magn Reson Imaging* 1997; **129**: 35–43.

75. Naressi A, Couturier C, Devos J, *et al.* Java-based graphical user interface for the MRUI quantitation package. *Magn Reson Materials Physics Biol Med (MAGMA)* 2001; **12**: 141–52.

76. Corbett R, Laptook A, Nunnally R. The use of the chemical shift of the phosphomonoester P-31 magnetic resonance peak for the determination of intracellular pH in the brains of neonates. *Neurology* 1987; **37**: 1771–9.

77. Petroff O, Prichard J. Cerebral intracellular pH by ³¹P nuclear magnetic resonance spectroscopy. *Neurology* 1985; **35**: 781–8.

78. Williams G, Smith M. Application of the accurate assessment of intracellular magnesium and pH from the ³¹P shifts of ATP to cerebral hypoxia-ischemia in neonatal rat. *Magn Reson Med* 1995; **33**: 853–7.

79. De Vita E, Thomas D, Roberts S, *et al.* High resolution MRI of the brain at 4.7 Tesla using fast spin echo imaging. *Br J Radiol* 2003; **76**: 631–7.

80. De Vita E, Bainbridge A, Cheong J, *et al.* Magnetic resonance imaging of neonatal encephalopathy at 4.7 tesla: initial experiences. *Pediatrics* 2006; **118**: e1812–e1821.

81. Medicines and Healthcare Products Regulatory Agency UK. *Guidelines for Magnetic Resonance Equipment in Clinical Use.* 2002. www.mhra.gov.uk.

82. National Radiological Protection Board. Principles for the protection of patients and volunteers during clinical magnetic resonance diagnostic procedures. *Documents of the NRPB* 1991; **2(1)**.

83. International Non-Ionizing Radiation Committee of the International Radiation Protection Association. Protection of the patient undergoing a magnetic resonance examination (guidelines). *Health Phys* 1991; **61**: 923–8.

84. International Electrotechnical Commission. Medical electrical equipment – particular requirements for the safety of magnetic resonance equipment for medical diagnosis. *IEC* **2002**; 60601-2-33.

85. American Academy of Pediatrics, Committee on Environmental Health. Noise: a hazard for the fetus and newborn. *Pediatrics* 1997; **100**: 724–7.

86. National Radiological Protection Board. Restrictions on human exposure to static and time-varying electromagnetic fields and radiation. *Documents of the NRPB* 1993; **4(5)**.

87. International Commission on Non-Ionizing Radiation. Guidelines for limiting exposure to time-varying electric, magnetic and electromagnetic fields (up to 300 GHz). *Health Phys* 1998; **74**: 494–522.

88. Belliveau JW, Kwong KK, Kennedy DN, *et al.* Magnetic resonance imaging mapping of brain function. Human visual cortex. *Invest Radiol* **1992** [Suppl 2]: S59–S65.

89. Azzopardi D, Wyatt JS, Cady EB, *et al.* Prognosis of newborn infants with hypoxic-ischemic brain injury assessed by phosphorus magnetic resonance spectroscopy. *Pediatr Res* 1989; **25(5)**: 445–51.

JANET M. RENNIE,
CORNELIA F. HAGMANN, *and*
NICOLA J. ROBERTSON

Introduction

The anterior fontanelle provides a convenient acoustic window through which to image the neonatal brain. An infinite number of different images can be produced, but several views have become standard because they allow visualization of important structures such as the germinal matrix. The standard coronal sections are shown in Fig. 4.1 and the sagittal sections in Fig. 4.2. The pictures and diagrams in this chapter are designed to help the novice ultrasonographer find his or her way around the intracranial anatomical landmarks of these standard views. Once these have been learnt there is then no substitute for time spent trying to identify the same structures in many different subjects. Reviewing scans with others, and relating ultrasound imaging appearances to the anatomy, which is illustrated with MRI, are an invaluable part of the learning process. We have included a description of three axial sections because these are such a standard aspect of MRI although of course axial sections are difficult to produce with ultrasound (Fig. 4.3).

We have relied on several sources, including our neuroradiology colleagues, for neuroanatomical information, but we find the atlases by Bayer and Altman to be a particularly useful resource [1].

Performing a cranial ultrasound examination

Begin by placing the transducer on the fontanelle with the plane of the ultrasound passing from ear to ear to produce a coronal section. The convention is to display the image in the same way as an X-ray, with the left hand side of the patient on the right-hand side of the image as you look at it on the screen. Set the depth of the image to allow the bright base of the skull to appear at the bottom of the imaged arc, which should be as wide as possible. The depth will correspond to about 7 cm in a small baby. The transducer can then be angled as far forward as the fontanelle will allow, when it is usually possible to identify the orbital ridge of the skull. The transucer is then angled back from this position through at least six "stations"

(Fig. 4.1). When the coronal sections are complete, turn the transducer through 90°, which will place the plane of the image from front to back and produce sagittal and parasagittal sections. The convention now is to have the baby "looking" to the the left of the picture as shown in the images which follow. The transducer can now be angled to give a plane as near as possible to the surface of the brain, and if the size of the fontanelle allows an image can be produced which is almost like the external appearance of the whole brain. Several planes of section can be identified including a midline sagittal view (Fig. 4.2).

The whole examination can be recorded on videotape, but if hard copies are required pictures of the standard coronal sections with a midline sagittal and an angled parasagittal section obtained from both sides of the brain are usually made. A detailed examination can be completed in about 5 min with little disturbance to the baby. The examples used in the chapter are from mature infants. The appearance of the very immature brain will be discussed in Chapter 5.

Notes on the standard coronal sections

Coronal section 1: frontal lobes (Fig. 4.4a–e)

The most anterior coronal section contains mostly frontal lobe. The orbital ridge of the skull forms the boundary of this image with a lemon-shaped profile. The anterior cerebral arteries can often be seen pulsating as they lie close together in the interhemispheric fissure. The appearances should be symmetrical with the interhemispheric fissure in the midline; the pathological specimen is in fact slightly asymmetrical. Blood vessels provide useful landmarks throughout the examination but their small size mostly places them below the lower limit of resolution of ultrasound. The base of the skull is consistently the most echo-reflectant structure and provides a basis for comparison of other "bright" echogenic objects. The corresponding MRI is shown in Fig. 4.4e, and again consists mainly of frontal lobe. The surface of the brain is much more readily identified with MRI and detail of the sulci and gyri can

Neonatal Cerebral Investigation, eds. Janet M. Rennie, Cornelia F. Hagmann and Nicola J. Robertson. Published by Cambridge University Press. © Cambridge University Press 2008.

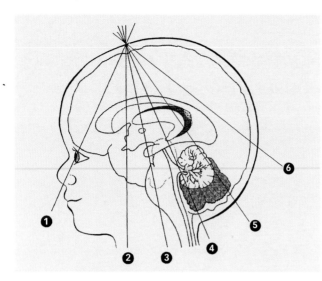

Fig. 4.1. **The six planes of section for coronal scans**

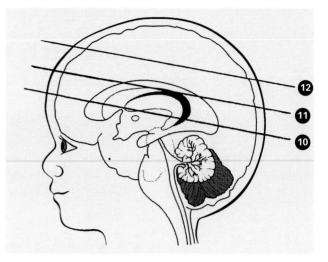

Fig. 4.3. **Planes of section for axial MRI scans.**

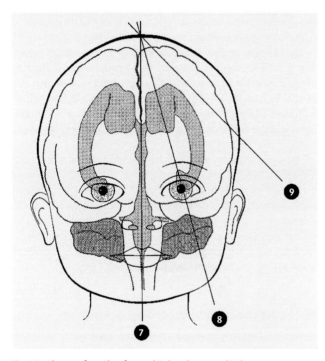

Fig. 4.2. **Planes of section for sagittal and parasagittal scans.**

be made out. An understanding of the anatomy and patterning of the main sulci is important when considering the maturity of the brain (Chapter 5), and when considering a diagnosis of lissencephaly (p. 262).

Coronal section 2: anterior frontal horns of the lateral ventricles (Fig. 4.5a–e)

As the transducer is moved in a coronal plane back from the most anterior position the frontal horns of the lateral ventricles appear as slitlike structures, placed either side of the midline. The cerebrospinal fluid (CSF) within the ventricles transmits ultrasound freely (it is echolucent) making the

cavity appear dark; occasionally the cavity of the ventricle is so small that the walls appear in apposition as bright lines. Mature infants have smaller ventricular cavities than premature infants. In the example the cavity of both lateral ventricles is almost obliterated; this is a normal finding for the first 24 h after birth and cannot be used to diagnose brain swelling (p. 146). There is often minor asymmetry between the ventricles and this is not abnormal. The cavum septum pellucidum is often very large in preterm babies and lies between the lateral ventricles and not below them, a feature which enables it to be distinguished from the third ventricle. The posterior portion is termed the cavum vergae and this can also be seen in neonatal cranial ultrasound scans. The tissue of the corpus callosum lies in the midline with the callosal sulcus appearing above it, forming a "tramline" appearance above the cavum septum pellucidum. The cingulate gyrus sits above the level of the corpus callosum with the cingulate sulcus easily seen traversing outwards from the midline.

The other major landmark in this plane during real-time examination comes from the pulsation of the middle cerebral artery arising from the bifurcation of the internal carotid artery. A long straight section of the course of the artery can often be seen as it travels in the Sylvian fissure. The middle cerebral artery gives off branches throughout its course, the lenticulostriate arteries, and occlusions of these (or the main trunk) are important causes of stroke (Fig. 7.5c and pp. 103–114). The basal ganglia at this level consist of the caudate nucleus in its position immediately inferior to the lateral ventricles, together with the putamina, and these can usually be made out as rather denser appearing gray matter.

Understanding the relationship of the deep gray matter structures is a crucial part of neonatal neuroradiology, because these structures are so vulnerable to damage. Figure 4.6 is redrawn from Netter [2], to give an idea of the spatial relationship of the thalamus, the lentiform nucleus, the caudate, and the amygdaloid body.

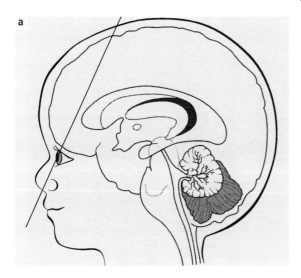

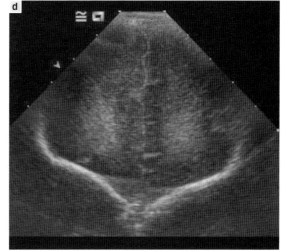

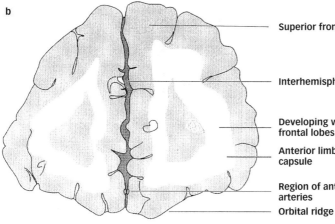

b

Superior frontal gyrus

Interhemispheric fissure

Developing white matter of frontal lobes

Anterior limb of internal capsule

Region of anterior cerebral arteries

Orbital ridge

Fig. 4.4a–e. **Coronal sections at the level of the frontal lobes. (a) Diagram of surface marking at this level. (b) Labeled line diagram to show the main anatomical landmarks. (c) Pathological specimen cut in the plane of section. (d) Ultrasound scan corresponding to the plane of section. (e) T$_1$-weighted MR image in this plane.**

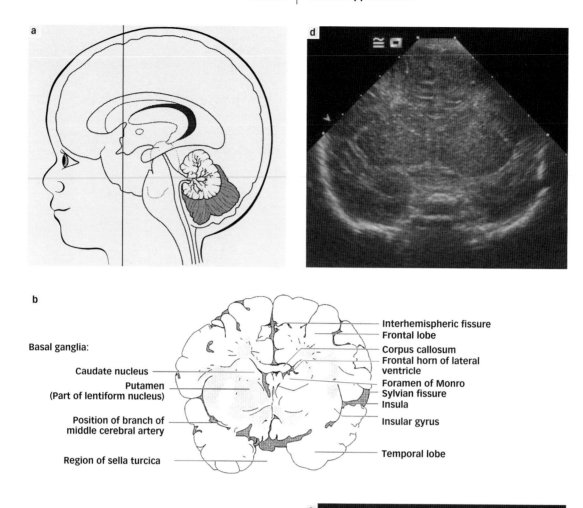

Basal ganglia:

Caudate nucleus

Putamen
(Part of lentiform nucleus)

Position of branch of
middle cerebral artery

Region of sella turcica

Interhemispheric fissure
Frontal lobe
Corpus callosum
Frontal horn of lateral
ventricle
Foramen of Monro
Sylvian fissure
Insula
Insular gyrus

Temporal lobe

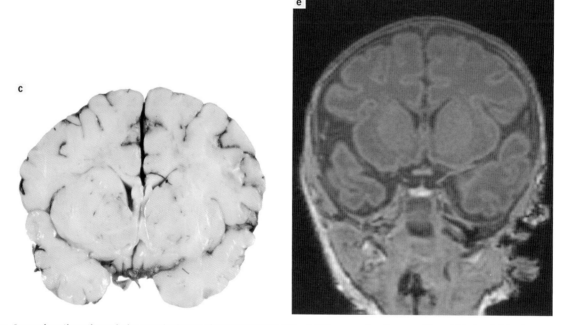

Fig. 4.5a–e. **Coronal sections through the anterior horns of the lateral ventricles.** (a) Diagram of surface marking at this level. (b) Labeled line diagram to show the main anatomical landmarks. (c) Pathological specimen cut in the plane of section. (d) Ultrasound scan corresponding to the plane of section. (e) T$_1$-weighted MR image in this plane.

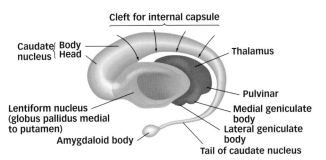

Fig. 4.6. **Diagram of the relationships of the deep gray matter structures (adapted from Netter [2] with permission). Interrelationship of thalamus, lentiform nucleus, caudate nucleus, and amygdaloid body (schema): left lateral view.**

Coronal section 3: level of the third ventricle (Fig. 4.7a–e)

The third ventricle varies considerably in width but can usually be made out as a small echo-free area appearing in the midline, below and between the lateral ventricles and the cavum septum pellucidi. The connections between the lateral and the third ventricle (the foramen of Monro) can usually be clearly seen in real time, by slight angulation of the transducer. The anatomy of the ventricular system is such an important basis for relating associated structures that a diagram of a cast of the system is shown in Fig. 4.8. Throughout these planes of section the Y shape of the Sylvian fissure provides a constant lateral landmark. This fissure becomes deeper and more convoluted with maturity, as explained in the next chapter. The position of the deep gray matter, which is prominent in this plane of section, is marked on the diagram so that when abnormalities are identified their anatomical location can be recognized (see Chapter 10). When the deep gray matter are abnormal, the region of the internal capsule can be identified as an echolucent line running through this area, in a "stripe" between the thalami and the lentiform nuclei. The appearance of the thalamus is usually uniform and relatively hypoechoic, but occasionally bright spots or a candelabra-like appearance can be identified within it, the latter being termed thalamo-striate vasculopathy (Chapter 10). As the plane of the section is moved backwards the deep gray matter structures are replaced by the more echodense appearance of the brainstem, which appears as a tree or star-like shape.

Coronal section 4: level of the cerebellum (Fig. 4.9a–e)

The plane of the transducer moves through the brainstem structures, which are echoreflectant and appear gray-white. The quadrigeminal cisterns also appear echoreflectant, like the interpeduncular cisterns, probably because of the presence of structures within them in spite of the fact that they contain CSF. This results in the characteristic overall appearance of this plane, that of a Christmas tree, or a three-pointed crown. The vermis of the cerebellum appears brighter than the cerebellar hemispheres, which are bounded by the tentorium cerebelli.

Coronal section 5: level of the trigone (Fig. 4.10a–e)

Scanning further posteriorly gives a tangential cut through the trigone of the lateral ventricles, which dominates this plane of posterior sections. The glomus of the choroid plexus often fills the cavity of the lateral ventricles in this position, and is particularly large in preterm babies. Choroid plexus hemorrhage can be difficult to diagnose and depends on asymmetry of the appearances. Choroid plexus cysts are a common finding during pregnancy and can sometimes be seen in newborns (Chapter 10). In this plane the white matter around the ventricles tends to appear quite echodense. This appearance has been termed the "peritrigonal blush" or "periventricular halo" [3,4]. The blush is thought to be due to the neurovascular bundles traveling at right angles to the ultrasound beam and thus acting as a good reflector as they are surrounded by a brain of high water content in premature babies. Myelin was not present in this region at postmortem in 28 preterm cases [3]. Normally the blush is less bright than the skull base or the choroid plexus and is symmetrical, and has the appearance of fine brush strokes within it. The normal range of appearance is of importance as there is a distinction to be made between blush and a "flare" in this region, which may represent subtle pre-white matter injury, perhaps due to inflammatory cell infiltrate. The cavum vergae can sometimes be seen between the lateral ventricles in this view.

Coronal section 6: level of the occiptal lobes (Fig. 4.11a–e)

By angling the transducer even further posteriorly the occipital cortex can be imaged, beyond the posterior horns of the lateral ventricles. This is a useful plane for confirming the presence of flare and for looking for the small occipital cysts of periventricular leucomalacia. In mature babies superficial sulci are well seen in this plane of section.

Midline sagittal (7) (Fig. 4.12a–e)

This useful image gives a great deal of information. In the midline the cerebellum vermis forms a highly echogenic landmark in the posterior fossa, with its anterior surface dented by a small cleft which is the fourth ventricle. Inferior to the cerebellum is the echo-free zone of the cisterna magna. The area which the cerebellar vermis occupies can be estimated. The anterior brainstem, in front of the narrow aqueduct, is not particularly echogenic in this plane; the pons is slightly more echoreflectant. Anterior to the brainstem is a more echoreflectant area which in fact marks a region of CSF, the interpeduncular cistern. Above the superior aspect of the brainstem is an echogenic structure, and this boundary is marked by a "figure of three" appearance formed in part by the superior colliculus. The massa intermedia can only usually be made out within the rhomboid-like space of the third ventricle when ventriculomegaly is present. The velum interpositum is located in the roof of the third ventricle, and sometimes a cavum velum interpositum can be seen as a CSF-containing space below the splenium of the corpus callosum.

The corpus callosum can be seen sweeping from the anterior to posterior direction in the midline view, bounded by

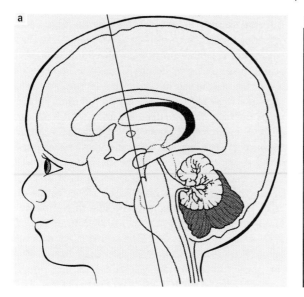

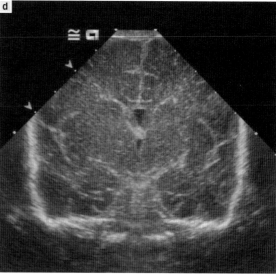

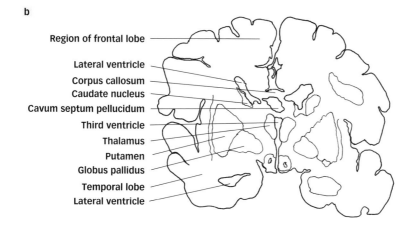

Region of frontal lobe

Lateral ventricle
Corpus callosum
Caudate nucleus
Cavum septum pellucidum
Third ventricle
Thalamus
Putamen
Globus pallidus
Temporal lobe
Lateral ventricle

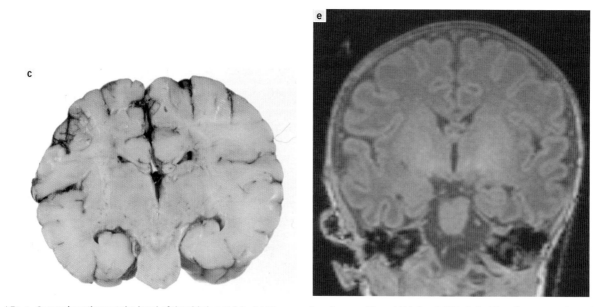

Fig. 4.7a–e. Coronal sections at the level of the third ventricle. (a) Diagram of surface marking at this level. (b) Labeled line diagram to show the main anatomical landmarks. (c) Pathological specimen cut in the plane of section. (d) Ultrasound scan corresponding to the plane of section. (e) T_1-weighted MR image in this plane.

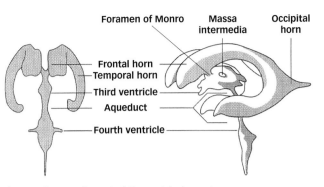

Fig. 4.8. **Diagram of a cast of the ventricular system.**

the callosal sulcus, which forms a clear echo boundary. The superior cingulate sulcus is above and roughly parallel to it, but is more convoluted due to secondary and tertiary gyri at term. The parieto-occipital sulcus forms another clear landmark above the posterior fossa, and the calcarine sulcus can often be made out. In mature infants the sulci are much more branched than in those who are immature, and the superior cingulate sulcus itself is more developed posteriorly (Chapter 5).

Angled parasagittal (8) (Fig. 4.13a–e)
This section is dominated by the C shape of the lateral ventricle. This is variable in size tending to be smaller in term infants. The lateral ventricle consists of a body (corpus), which forms the main part of the "C," which is seen in this plane, and three horns. The body lies within the frontal and parietal lobes and extends from the interventricular foramen to the splenium of the corpus callosum. There are three horns, which are anterior, posterior, and inferior. These are also sometimes termed the frontal, occipital, and temporal horns. The body of the lateral ventricle widens out at the point at which it becomes the posterior and inferior horns, and this part is called the trigone, or atrium.

The caudate nucleus lies below the floor of the frontal horn of the lateral ventricle with the thalamus behind and below it. The caudate nucleus is usually more echogenic than the thalamus. The glomus of the choroid plexus often fills the occipital horn of the lateral ventricle. The choroid plexus often extends anteriorly to tuck into the groove between the thalamus and the caudate nucleus, in the floor of the lateral ventricle, and often forms a bright spot, as in Fig. 4.13d. This is normal and should not be confused with a small hemorrhage into the germinal matrix capillary bed which is situated over the head of the caudate in a slightly more anterior position.

Tangential parasagittal (9) (Fig. 4.14a–e)
Further lateral angulation of the scanhead will produce a section that is tangential and superficial to the lateral ventricle. The Sylvian fissure is the landmark in this view. The number of sulci which can be identified increases with maturity. In less mature infants the insula can be glimpsed as the opercula have not yet fully enclosed it.

Axial section (10): level of the deep gray matter (Fig. 4.15a–e)
Axial sections can be made using ultrasound by placing the transducer on the posterior fontanelle, but we do not perform these as part of our standard imaging protocol. Axial sections are a standard part of MR imaging, and CT scans are of course only displayed in axial views, hence it is important to have an understanding of the structures that can be identified in these views. This plane contains the thalami, the lentiform nuclei (the putamina and the globi pallidi) and the head of the caudate nucleus; Fig. 4.6 shows the three dimensional interrelationship between these structures. The internal capsule runs between the caudate and the lentiform nucleus anteriorly, and between the thalamus and the lentiform nucleus posteriorly. At term, there is very little myelin in the brain. Some is present in the posterior limb of the internal capsule, and the characteristics of the appearances on MRI are discussed in the next chapter [5]. Usually the appearances are those of a spot of hypointensity in the generally hyperintense region on T_2-weighted images (Fig. 4.15e), with high signal intensity on T_1 inversion recovery images (Fig. 4.15d), but it is important to be certain of the range of normal appearances that are generated by the sequences in use in a particular institution (Chapter 2).

The genu and the splenium of the corpus callosum can be seen lying in between the anterior and posterior horns of the lateral ventricles respectively.

Axial section (11): level of the corona radiata (Fig. 4.16a–e)
The hemispheres should appear symmetrical and the pattern of sulci and gyri can be studied, together with the contrast between the gray and white matter of the brain. This axial slice shows the corona radiata. It is important to remember that the bodies of the caudate nuclei in fact extend this high up.

Axial section (12): level of the central sulcus (Fig. 4.17a–e)
This is the plane in which the pre- and postcentral gyri, lying either side of the central sulcus (sometimes termed the Rolandic sulcus), can be seen. The region in which the white matter of the corona radiata will develop can be seen in this plane. Further information about the anatomy of sulci and gyri is contained within the next chapter.

Normal variation

Cavum septi pellucidi and cavum vergae
The large size of the cavum septi pellucidi is often a striking feature in cranial ultrasound images of preterm babies (Fig. 4.18). The structure varies in size from a cavity much larger than that of the adjacent ventricles to a small slit. The cavum septi pellucidi has disappeared by 2 months of age in 85% of cases [6]. Closure of the cavum vergae begins at about 24 weeks of gestation. The cavum septi pellucidi can enlarge to a pathologic cyst, and hemorrhage can occur into it. The width of the cavum septi pellucidi varied from 2 mm to 10 mm in 102

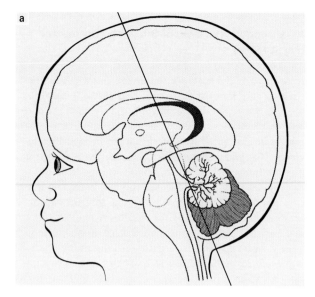

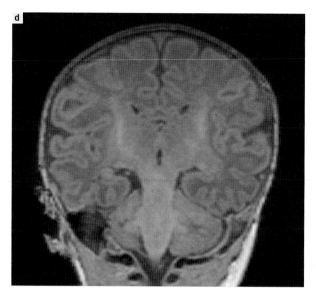

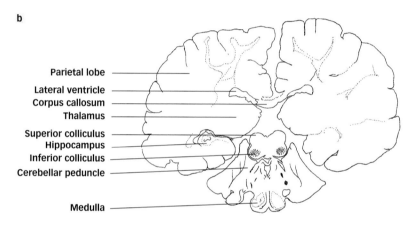

Parietal lobe
Lateral ventricle
Corpus callosum
Thalamus
Superior colliculus
Hippocampus
Inferior colliculus
Cerebellar peduncle

Medulla

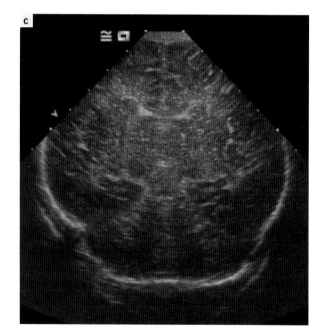

Fig. 4.9a–d. **Coronal sections at the level of the cerebellum. (a) Diagram of surface marking at this level. (b) Labeled line diagram to show the main anatomical landmarks. (c) Ultrasound scan corresponding to the plane of section. (d) T$_1$-weighted MR image in this plane.**

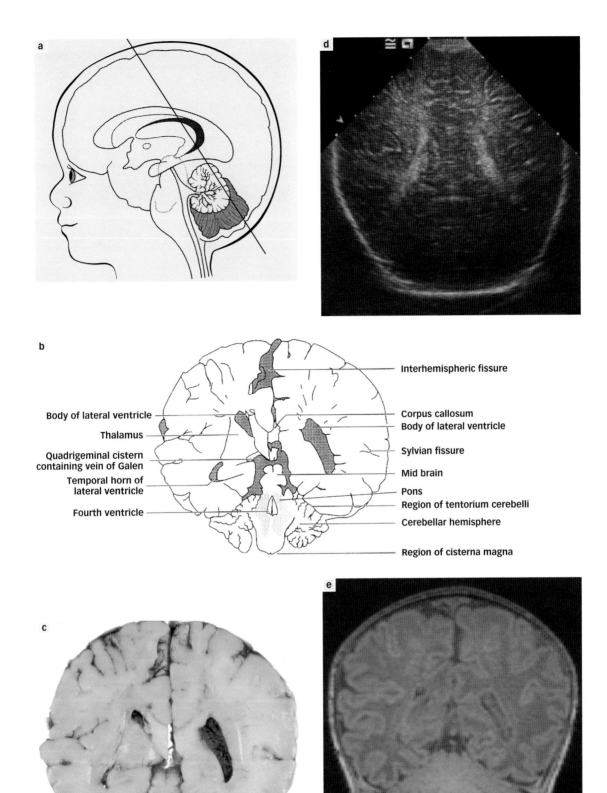

a

d

b

Body of lateral ventricle

Thalamus

Quadrigeminal cistern
containing vein of Galen

Temporal horn of
lateral ventricle

Fourth ventricle

Interhemispheric fissure

Corpus callosum
Body of lateral ventricle

Sylvian fissure

Mid brain

Pons

Region of tentorium cerebelli

Cerebellar hemisphere

Region of cisterna magna

c

e

Fig. 4.10.a–e. **Coronal section at the level of the trigone.** (a) Diagram of surface marking at this level. (b) Labeled line diagram to show the main anatomical landmarks. (c) Pathological specimen cut in the plane of section. (d) Ultrasound scan corresponding to the plane of section. (e) T_1-weighted MR image in this plane.

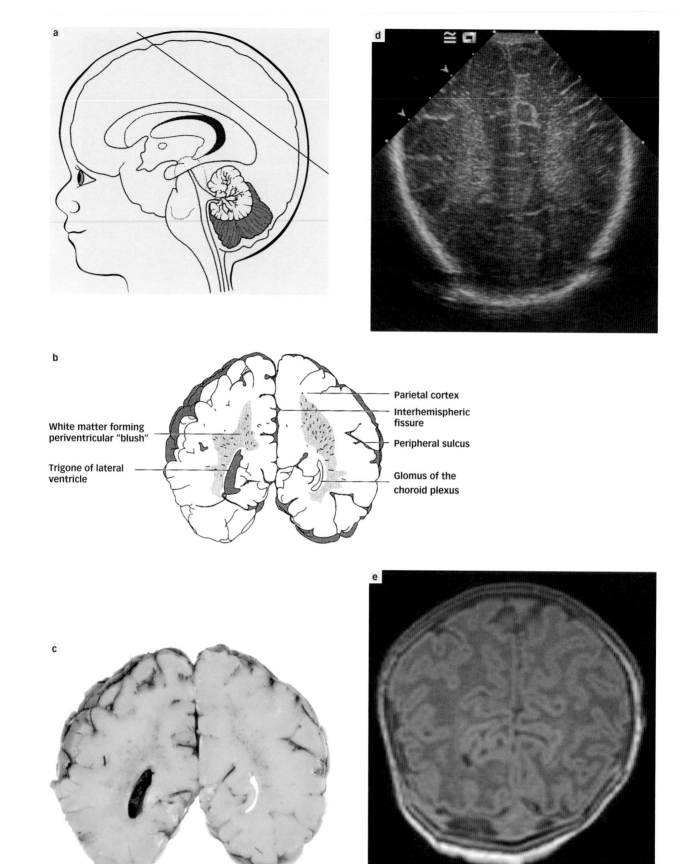

a

b

Parietal cortex

Interhemispheric
fissure

White matter forming
periventricular "blush"

Peripheral sulcus

Trigone of lateral
ventricle

Glomus of the
choroid plexus

c

d

e

Fig. 4.11a–e. Coronal section at the level of the occipital lobes. (a) Diagram of surface marking at this level. (b) Labeled line diagram to show the main anatomical landmarks. (c) Pathological specimen cut in the plane of section. (d) Ultrasound scan corresponding to the plane of section. (e) T$_1$-weighted MR image in this plane.

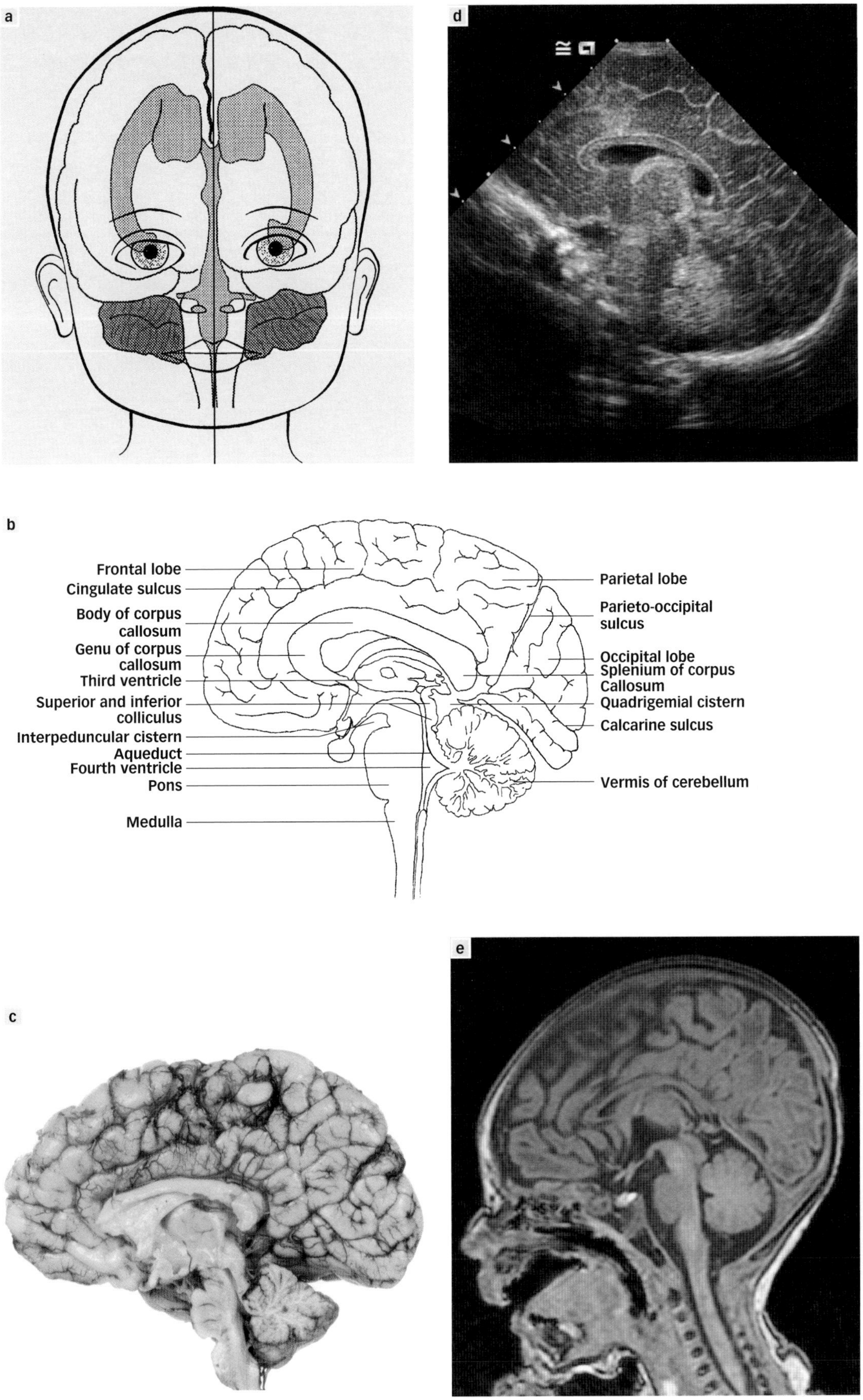
a
d
b
Frontal lobe
Cingulate sulcus
Body of corpus callosum
Genu of corpus callosum
Third ventricle
Superior and inferior colliculus
Interpeduncular cistern
Aqueduct
Fourth ventricle
Pons
Medulla
Parietal lobe
Parieto-occipital sulcus
Occipital lobe
Splenium of corpus Callosum
Quadrigemial cistern
Calcarine sulcus
Vermis of cerebellum
c
e

Fig. 4.12a–e. **Midline sagittal sections. (a) Diagram of surface marking at this level. (b) Labeled line diagram to show the main anatomical landmarks. (c) Pathological specimen cut in the plane of section. (d) Ultrasound scan corresponding to the plane of section. (e) T_1-weighted MR image in this plane.**

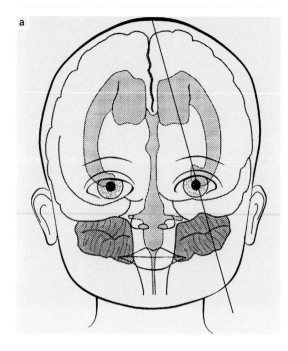

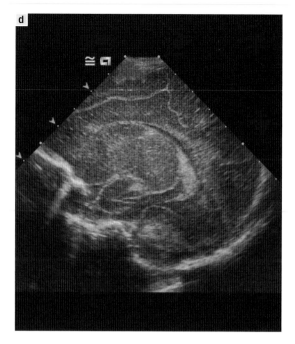

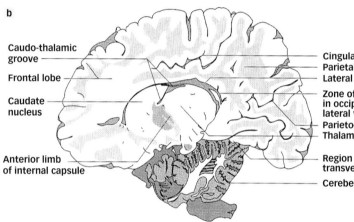

Caudo-thalamic groove

Frontal lobe

Caudate nucleus

Anterior limb of internal capsule

Cingulate sulcus
Parietal lobe
Lateral ventricle

Zone of choroid plexus in occipital horn of lateral ventricle
Parieto–occipital sulcus
Thalamus

Region of tentorium and transverse sinus

Cerebellum

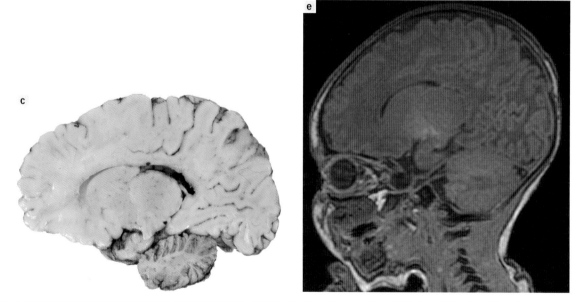

Fig. 4.13a–e. **Parasagittal sections through the lateral ventricles. (a) Diagram of surface marking at this level. (b) Labeled line diagram to show the main anatomical landmarks. (c) Pathological specimen cut in the plane of section. (d) Ultrasound scan corresponding to the plane of section. (e) T₁-weighted MR image in this plane.**

a

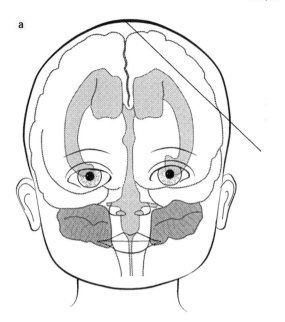

d

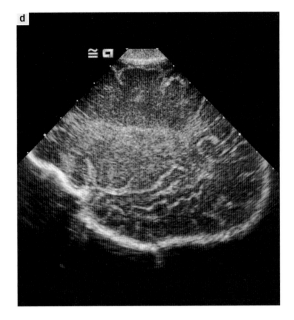

b

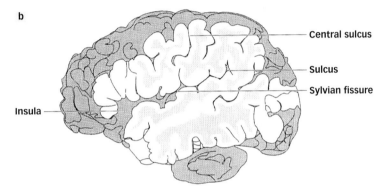

Central sulcus

Sulcus

Sylvian fissure

Insula

c

e

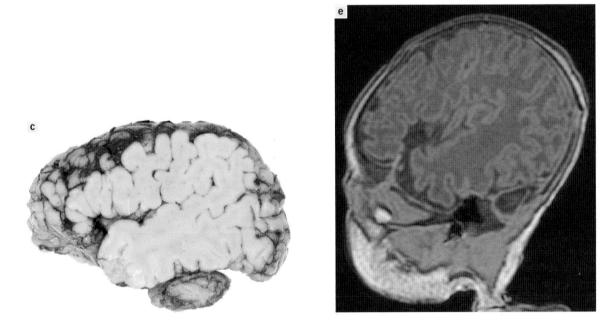

Fig. 4.14a–e. **Angled tangential parasagittal sections. (a)** Diagram of surface marking at this level. **(b)** Labeled line diagram to show the main anatomical landmarks. **(c)** Pathological specimen cut in the plane of section. **(d)** Ultrasound scan corresponding to the plane of section. **(e)** T$_1$-weighted MR image in this plane.

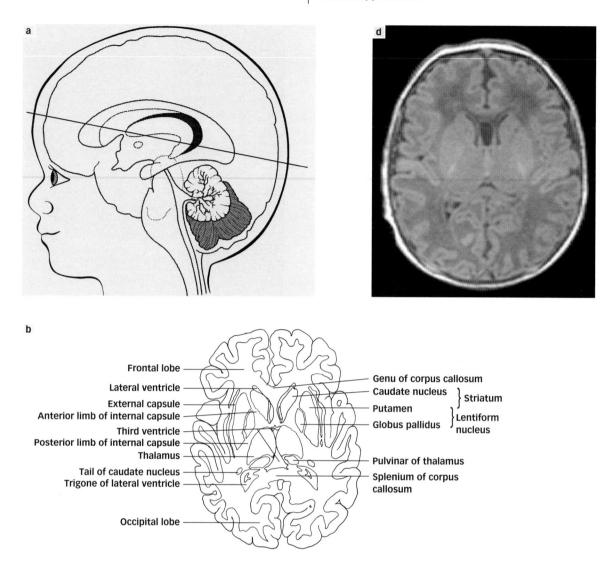

b

Frontal lobe

Lateral ventricle

External capsule
Anterior limb of internal capsule

Third ventricle
Posterior limb of internal capsule
Thalamus

Tail of caudate nucleus
Trigone of lateral ventricle

Occipital lobe

Genu of corpus callosum
Caudate nucleus $\Big\}$ Striatum
Putamen $\Big\}$ Lentiform
Globus pallidus $\Big\}$ nucleus

Pulvinar of thalamus

Splenium of corpus callosum

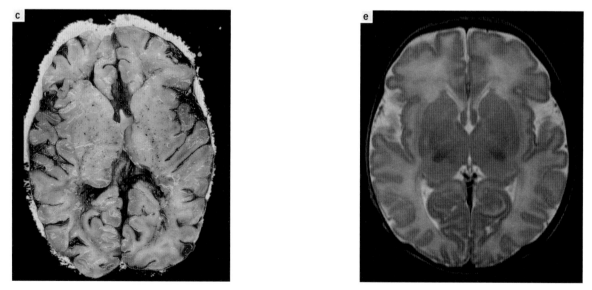

Fig. 4.15a–e. **Axial sections at level of the deep gray matter. (a) Diagram of surface marking at this level. (b) Labeled line diagram to show the main anatomical landmarks. (c) Pathological specimen cut in the plane of section. (d) T₁- and (e) T₂-weighted MR images from in this plane.**

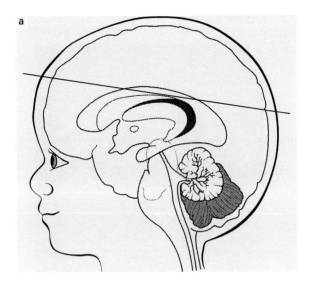

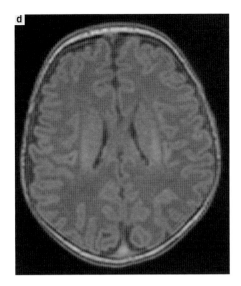

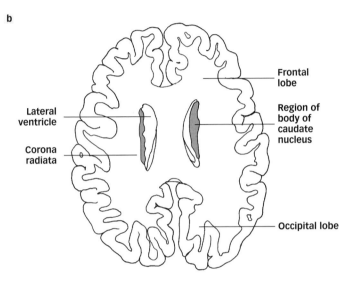

Frontal lobe

Lateral ventricle

Corona radiata

Region of body of caudate nucleus

Occipital lobe

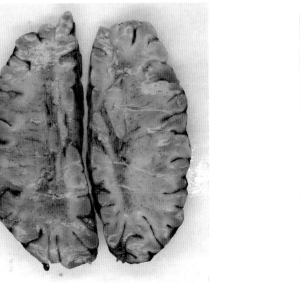

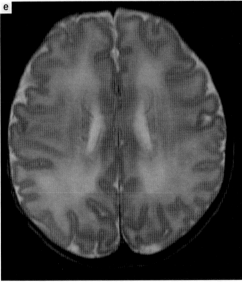

Fig. 4.16a–e. **Axial sections at level of the corona radiata. (a) Diagram of surface marking at this level. (b) Labeled line diagram to show the main anatomical landmarks. (c) Pathological specimen cut in the plane of section. (d) T₁- and (e) T₂-weighted MR images from in this plane.**

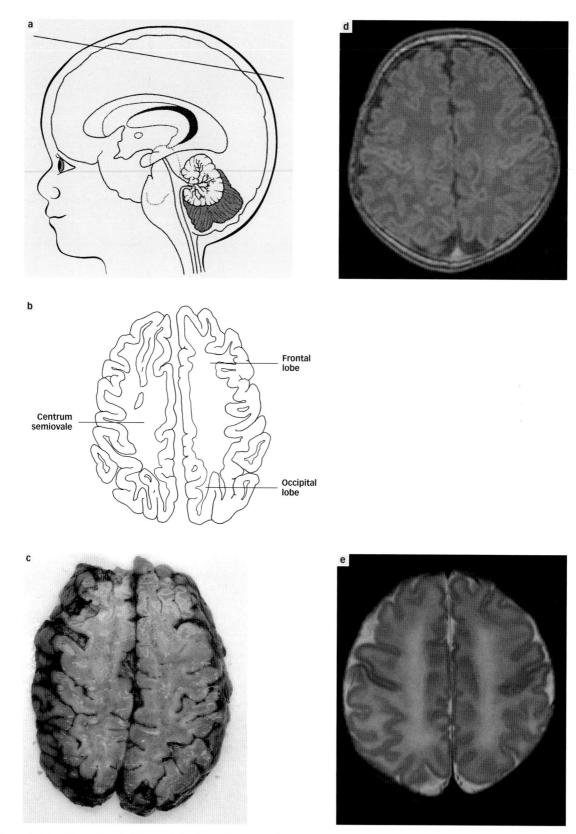

Fig. 4.17a–e. Axial sections at level of the central sulcus. (a) Diagram of surface marking at this level. **(b)** Labeled line diagram to show the main anatomical landmarks. **(c)** Pathological specimen cut in the plane of section. **(d)** T_1- and **(e)** T_2-weighted MR images from in this plane.

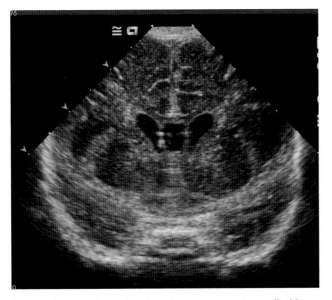

Fig. 4.18. **Ultrasound scan showing a large cavum septum pellucidum.**

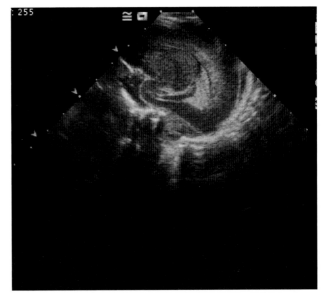

Fig. 4.20. **Poor choice of depth setting resulting in a minature image.**

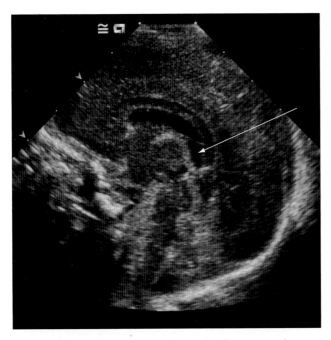

Fig. 4.19. **Midline sagittal ultrasound image showing cavum velum interpositum (arrow).**

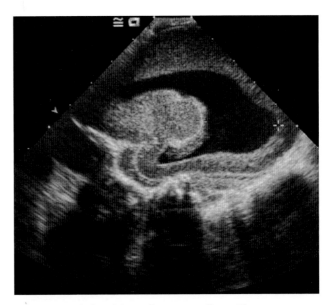

Fig. 4.21. **Poor choice of time-gain compensation setting.**

preterm infants studied by Ferrugia and Babcock [7]. The cavi are often in communication with each other but they do not communicate with the ventricular system.

Cerebrospinal fluid spaces

The lateral ventricles often differ considerably in volume, particularly in the occipital horns. For detail about the normal range of linear and area measurements see Chapter 9. The cisterna magna can be difficult to visualize and can also vary in height, the mean value being 4.5 mm [8]. Small size of the cisterna magna can be a clue to the presence of the Arnold–Chiari malformation. The subarachnoid spaces are more prominent in very preterm babies, with the appearance of separation of the Sylvian and interhemispheric fissures. Measurement of the subarachnoid space using a 10-MHz transducer was reported by Govaert *et al.* [9]. The results showed dimensions of less than 5 mm in normal newborns, similar to those obtained using MRI [10]. The subarachnoid space was often particularly wide over the parieto-occipital lobes. The isolated finding of a widened subarachnoid space (no measurements were given) was reported in 6 of a cohort of 75 preterm Canadian infants, all of whom developed normally [11]. As discussed, it is not unusual to be able to image the cavum velum interpositum in babies (Fig. 4.19).

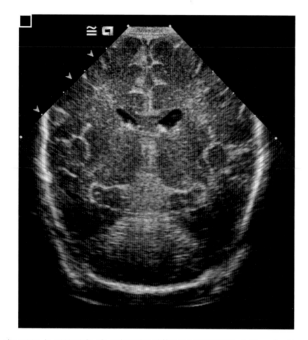

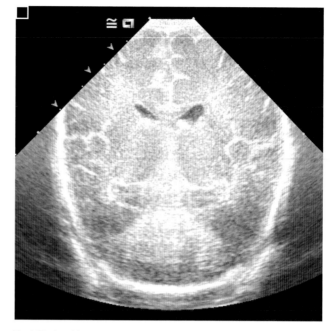

Fig. 4.22a, b. **Example showing the difference that the choice of gain setting makes. Images taken from the same baby at the same time, with different gain settings.**

Fig. 4.22. **(cont.)**

can also cause a series of "ripple"-like concentric rings to appear resulting from reverberation of ultrasound reflected between the transducer and the skin.

Incorrect setting of the time-gain compensation control

Time-gain compensation (TGC) is discussed in Chapter 1. Failure to optimize TGC can result in loss of detail from a large portion of the area of insonation (Fig. 4.21). Many modern machines have a setting which allows automatic optimization of TGC. Incorrect choice of setting on the TGC control (Chapter 1), or excessive "gain" (the amount of energy used to generate the ultrasound beam), can have a significant impact on the appearances of the image. It is essential to check the gain settings before making a diagnosis of "bright brain," which can be one feature of cerebral edema (pp. 146–147) (Fig. 4.22a, b). An incorrect diagnosis of cerebral edema, based only on increased echoreflectivity in an image with excessive gain settings, is the commonest error we see in scans made by inexperienced operators.

Acoustic shadow

Any structure that is highly echoreflectant allows little ultrasound to pass deeper and to be available to interrogate the structures lying below it (Fig. 4.23). Examples of structures that can cause acoustic shadowing are areas of calcification and ventricular catheters.

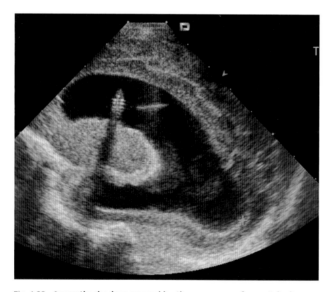

Fig. 4.23. **Acoustic shadow caused by the presence of a ventricular reservoir.**

Artifacts and common errors

Incorrect depth setting and/or not enough coupling gel

A poor choice of depth setting results in a minature image, which does not make the best use of the potential window for insonation (Fig. 4.20). There is nothing that can be done about a very small fontanelle, but it is important to use a generous quantity of coupling gel in order to avoid loss of information at the extremes of the angle of insonation. Lack of coupling agent

Normal neonatal neurological examination

Imaging the neonatal brain is a vital part of the assessment of the newborn, but it is important not to forget the importance of a detailed neurological examination. This is not as difficult

Table 4.1. System for neonatal neurological examination, from Rennie [12].

Neonatal CNS examination

Name: _____
DOB: _/_/_
GA: ___ weeks

Date of exam: _/_/_
Examiner: _____

States
0. Coma: no/little response to pain
1. Deep sleep, no movent, regular breathing
2. Light sleep, eyes shut, some movement
3. Dozing, eyes opening and closing
4. Awake, eyes open, minimal movement
5. Wide awake, vigorous movement
6. Crying

Orientation and behavior; note any adverse circumstances, e.g., excessive noise

	0	1 or 2	3 or 4	5 or 6
State at start	0	1 or 2	3 or 4	5 or 6
State at end of exam	0	1 or 2	3 or 4	5 or 6
Level of consciousness	Comatose	Lethargic	Hyperalert, stary	Normal, easily aroused
Consolability	High-pitched cry, continuous	Cries, difficult to console	Cries, easy to console	Not crying, consoling not needed
Irritability	Cries when not handled	Cries often and easily	Cries sometimes when handled, not irritable	Quiet all the time – too quiet
Visual orientation	Doesn't fix or follow, or roving eye movements	Fixes and follows but loses interest	Fixes and follows up to 90° horizontally	Fixes and follows reliably horizontally
Social interaction	Cannot engage at all	Tries to engage but does not succeed	Brief interest in stimuli or face of examiner	Easy to engage and makes eye contact

Posture and movement (normal and abnormal)

	0	1 or 2	3 or 4	5 or 6
Posture: draw here	Opistotonus, or flexed arms, extended legs	Arms + legs extended	Legs flexed, but not adducted	Normal, legs flexed, arms well flexed near abdomen
Spontaneous movements (observe quality and quantity)	No spontaneous movements	Paucity of movement, occasional random jerky movement, only stretching	Stereotyped or monotonous	Rich variety, smooth, fluent, good variability and range
Hand movements	Thumb fixed in palm, hand fisted all the time	No finger movements, intermittent fisting	Some occasional finger movements	Fine elegant finger movements, hands open
Tremors/startles	None, no reaction to loud noise or stimuli	Continuous tremors and startles	Frequent spontaneous startle and tremors when awake	Tremor after Moro, occasional spontaneous startle
Clinical seizures – describe	More than 6/day	3–6/day	<3/day	None

Trunk and limb tone

	0	1 or 2	3 or 4	5 or 6
Head control/head lag[a] draw here	No attempt to raise head, complete lag	Tries to lift head but effort better felt than seen, head drops back	Raises head very briefly, in line with body	Raises head – remains vertical and in front of body for brief time

Table 4.1. (cont.)

Ventral suspension[a] draw here	Back curved head and limbs hang straight	Back curved limbs slightly flexed	Back straight head in line limbs flexed	Back straight head above body
Leg recoil	No flexion	Incomplete	Complete, but slow	Complete and fast
Take both ankles with one hand, flex hips and knees, quickly extend, let go. Repeat × 3				
Truncal tone	Flaccid	Hyotonic	Hypertonic	Normal
Limb tone	Flaccid	Hyotonic	Hypertonic	Normal
Reflexes				
Tendon reflexes	Absent	Exaggerated	Clonus	Normal
Stepping[a]	No attempt to lift leg over the edge of the couch	Dorsiflexion of ankle	Flexes hip and knee and places sole on couch	Automatic walking easy to obtain
Moro[a]	Absent	Incomplete	Asymmetrical	Normal
Root[a]	Absent	Weak	Some head turn and mouth opening	Searches and localizes
Asymmetric tonic neck	Absent			Present
Sucking	Absent	Bites, clenches	Weak, irregular suck	Strong suck, strips
General observations				
Fontanelle/OFC	OFC: cm	Tense	Full	Normal
Skull	Caput	Subgaleal hematoma	Sutures overriding	Cephalohematoma
Respiration	IPPV for apnea	Brief apneas	Hyperventilation	Normal
Stability during exam	Unstable	Abnormal state throughout, no change	Little transition of state, slow transition	Rapid transition of state, well tolerated
Comments:				

Modified from Dubowitz 1981 [13] and other sources © JMR 2004.

[a] Do not examine in ventilated or very ill babies.

as many seem to think, and does not require the use of complex scoring systems to produce a sensible result. A semi-structured approach can help, particularly when there is a need for repeated assessment. Our current system, adapted from the work of Dubowitz and others by Rennie in 2005 [12], is reproduced in Table 4.1.

References

1. Bayer SA, Altman J. *The Human Brain During the Third Trimester*, 1st edn. Boca Raton, FL: CRC Press, 2004.

2. Rubin M, Safdieh JE. *Netter's Concise Neuroanatomy*. Philadelphia, PA: Sawnders.

3. Di Pietro MA, Brody BA, Teele RL. Peritrigonal echogenic "blush" on cranial sonography: pathologic correlates. *Am J Radiol* 1986; **146**: 1067-71.

4. Grant E, Schellinger D, Richardson J, Coffey M, Smirniotopoulous J. Echogenic periventricular halo: normal finding or neonatal cerebral haemorrhage. *Am J Neuroradiol* 1983; **4**: 43-6.

5. Cowan FM, de Vries LS. The internal capsule in neonatal imaging. *Semin Fetal Neonatal Med* 2005; **10**(5): 461-74.

6. Shaw CM, Alvord EC Jr. Cava septi pellucidi et vergae: their normal and pathological states. *Brain* 1969; **92**: 213-14.

7. Ferrugia S, Babcock DS. The cavum septi pellucidi: its appearance and incidence with cranial sonography in infancy. *Radiology* 1981; **139**: 147-50.

8. Goodwin L, Quisling R. The neonatal cisterna magna: ultrasononic evaluation. *Radiology* 1983; **149**: 691-5.

9. Govaert P, Pauwels W, Vanhaesebrouck P, De Praeter C, Afschrift M. Ultrasound measurement of the subarachnoid space in infants. *Eur J Pediatr* 1989; **148**: 412-13.

10. McArdle CB, Richardson CJ, Nicholas DA, Mirfakhraee M, Hayden CK, Amparo EG. Developmental features of the neonatal brain: MR imaging. *Radiology* 1987; **162**: 230-4.

11. Lui K, Boag G, Daneman A, Costello S, Kirplani H, Whyte H. Widened subarachnoid space in pre discharge cranial ultrasound: evidence of cerebral atrophy in immature infants? *Dev Med Child Neurol* 1990; **32**: 882-7.

12. Rennie JM. Examination of the central nervous system. Chapter 41, part 1, in Rennie JM (ed.) *Roberton's Textbook of Neonatology*, 4th edn. London, Churchill Livingstone, 2005; 1093-105.

13. Dubowitz L. *The Neurological Assessment of the Preterm and Full-Term Newborn Infant*, 1st edn. London, MacKeith Press, 1981.

Chapter 5 | The immature brain

JANET M. RENNIE,
CORNELIA F. HAGMANN, *and*
NICOLA J. ROBERTSON

Introduction

The stage of development of the cerebral fissures, sulci, and gyri can give an indication of the degree of maturity of the brain. A gyrus is bounded by two sulci or one sulcus and one fissure. The most important landmarks are the parieto-occipital sulcus (sometimes termed a fissure), the lateral sulcus (Sylvian fissure) and the cingulate sulcus, but there are many others. Chi made a detailed study of 507 brains between 10 and 44 weeks' gestation in order to document the appearance and development of the major sulci and gyri [1], and we have relied on the atlas of Feess-Higgins and Larroche [2], and the more recent book by Garel [3]. The ultrasound and magnetic resonance imaging (MRI) appearances lag behind the anatomical appearances [4]; the MRI appearances lag by at least a week, with the ultrasound appearances probably taking even longer [5]. There is thus a marked difference in the literature regarding the stage at which the major sulci have been reported to appear according to whether the features were identified with MRI, ultrasound imaging, or at autopsy. The effects of gender, twinning, and intrauterine growth restriction have yet to be evaluated in any detail. We have summarized the information available from various sources in the literature in Tables 5.1 and 5.2. In general, the sulci on the medial surfaces of the hemispheres (the parieto-occipital fissure, the calcarine and cingulate sulcus) appear earlier and are easier to recognize with ultrasound than the convexity sulci.

The appearances of the brain seen in very preterm babies born at around 22–23 weeks' gestation are those of a smooth brain surface with very few sulci and gyri. As a result, the diagnosis of lissencephaly (p. 262–263) cannot be entertained at this gestation. The parieto-occipital fissure forms a deep groove on the midline surface of the brain but the insula is wide open and the Island of Reil, part of the temporal lobe, is clearly visible from the lateral surface. On coronal section the Sylvian fissure (more correctly termed the circular sulcus at this stage) thus appears wide open. Scoring systems have been devised for the ultrasound appearances of immature brains in

standard sections [6], or comparison can be made with published photographs such as those in this chapter or in the literature (Fig. 5.1a, b) [7]. Some have measured the height of the frontal lobes with ultrasound as an index of brain growth and maturity

Table 5.1. Summary of the literature regarding the time of appearance of major cerebral sulci at autopsy, and on MRI. Information from [1,3,4,7,13,30]

	Gestational age (weeks)	
	Neuropathologic appearance	Present in more than 75% of brains on MRI
Sulci of the medial cerebral surface		
Interhemispheric fissure	10	22–23
Callosal sulcus	14	22–23
Parieto-occipital fissure	16	22–23
Cingulate sulcus (anterior part)	18	24–25
Cingulate sulcus (marginal part)	18–24	22–27
Calcarine fissure	16–18	23–25
Sulci of the lateral cerebral surface		
Sylvian fissure	14	16–18
Superior frontal sulcus	25	29
Inferior frontal sulcus	28	29
Superior temporal sulcus (posterior part)	23	27
Superior temporal sulcus (anterior part)		32
Insular sulci	34–35	34
Sulci of vertex		
Central sulcus	20	27
Precentral sulcus	24	27
Postcentral sulcus	25	28

Neonatal Cerebral Investigation, eds. Janet M. Rennie, Cornelia F. Hagmann and Nicola J. Robertson. Published by Cambridge University Press. © Cambridge University Press 2008.

Table 5.2. Timing of the appearance of major cerebral sulci seen with MRI. Information from [1,3,4,7,13,30].

Sulci as seen on MRI	Weeks of gestation							
	24	26	28	30	32	34	36	40
Sylvian fissure	+ (widely open)	+	+	+	+	+	+	+
Interhemispheric fissure	+	+	+	+	+	+	+	+
Callosal sulcus	+	+	+	+	+	+	+	+
Parieto-occipital fissure	+	+	+	+	+	+	+	+
Calcarine fissure	−/+	+	+	+	+	+	+	+
Cingulate sulcus (anterior part)	−/+	+	+	+	+	+	+	+
Central sulci	−	−	+	+	+	+	+	+
Superior temporal (posterior part)	−	−	+	+	+	+	+	+
Cingulate sulcus (marginal part)	−	−	−/+	+	+	+	+	+
Precentral sulci	−	−	−/+	+	+	+	+	+
Postcentral sulci	−	−	−/+	+	+	+	+	+
Superior frontal sulcus	−	−	−/+	+	+	+	+	+
Inferior frontal sulcus	−	−	−	+	+	+	+	+
Superior temporal (anterior part)	−	−	−	−	−	+	+	+
Insular sulci	−	−	−	−	−	−	+	+

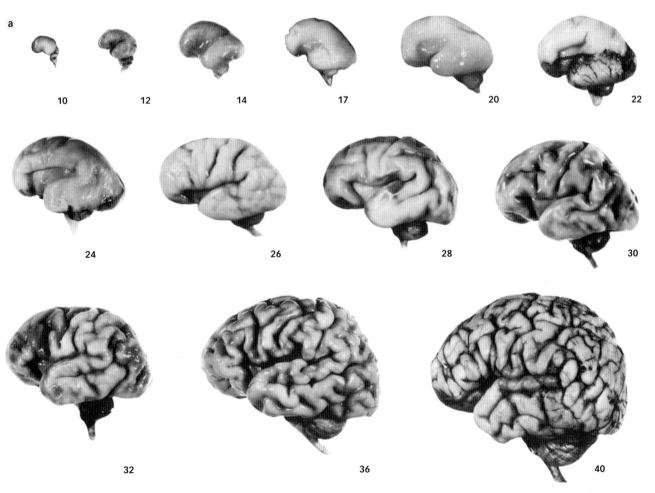

a

10   12   14   17   20   22

24   26   28   30

32   36   40

Fig. 5.1a,b. Characteristic configuration of fetal brain from 10 to 40 weeks of gestation at 2-week intervals. (a) External surface. (b) Midline sagittal. Reproduced with permission from Feess-Higgins and Larroche [2].

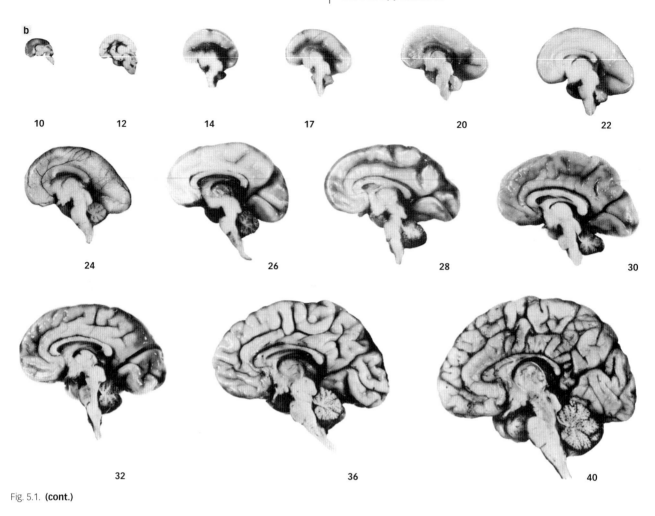

Fig. 5.1. **(cont.)**

but this was not more sensitive than head circumference [8]. The following description of the landmarks is summarized from many different published studies [6,9,10,11,12,13,14,15]. Maturation proceeds independently of gestational age at birth, although development can be retarded when there is brain injury [11].

Figure 5.2a–h shows the major sulci and gyri (Table 5.1) on the external surface (Fig. 5.2a, b), midline sagittal plane (Fig. 5.2c, d), coronal plane at the level of the third ventricle (Fig. 5.2e, f) and the axial plane at the level of the centrum semiovale (Fig. 5.2g, h). In the following section we discuss and show their appearance according to gestational age.

24 weeks (Fig. 5.3a–i)

The brain is virtually completely smooth with large cerebro-spinal fluid spaces between the interhemispheric fissure, easily seen in the coronal views. The tangential and midline views are dominated by the appearance of the parieto-occipital sulcus (Fig. 5.3b) which appears in virtually all fetuses and newborns at this gestation. The cingulate and calcarine sulci

are not yet always obvious on ultrasound but are usually visible on MRI [13]. The insula is prominent and is not yet overgrown and hence the Island of Reil is clearly visible in the lateral surface view (Fig. 5.3a). This is a striking feature of the immature brain which is also apparent on the coronal sections (Fig. 5.3c). By term, the insula will be almost completely buried. The corpus callosum has formed by 20 weeks and can be imaged by 24 weeks, but the structure will thicken and grow considerably over the coming months. The development of the corpus callosum is not finished when the pioneer axons have crossed the midline; more and more axons continue to cross until late in gestation. The full thickness is not reached until the tenth postnatal month. Myelination can been seen on MRI as T_1 hyperintensive signal at the level of the tegmentum, beginning at the cerebellar peduncle and vermis.

26 weeks (Fig. 5.4a–i)

The cingulate sulcus can usually be seen in the anterior portion in the parasagittal view by 26 weeks and on the anterior

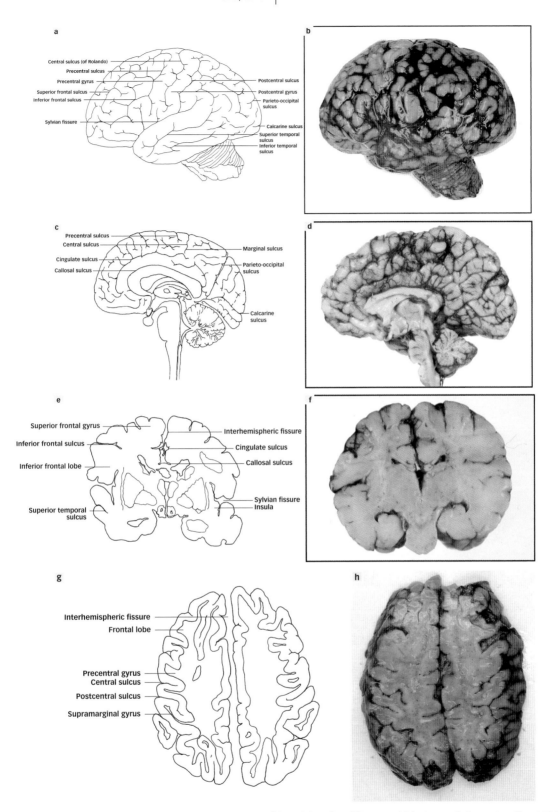

Fig. 5.2a–h. Line diagrams of the major landmarks showing the position of the sulci, gyri, and fissures which change during maturation. (a) Diagram of the external view of the brain with the major sulci, gyri, and fissures labeled. (b) Pathological specimen of the brain for comparison. (c) Diagram of the midline appearances of the brain with the major sulci, gyri, and fissures labeled. (d) Pathological midline specimen of the brain for comparison. (e) Line diagram of a coronal section of the brain with the major sulci, gyri, and fissures labeled. (f) Corresponding pathological specimen of the brain for comparison. (g) Diagram of an axial section of the brain at the level of the central sulcus with the major sulci, gyri, and fissures labeled. (h) Corresponding pathological specimen of the brain for comparison.

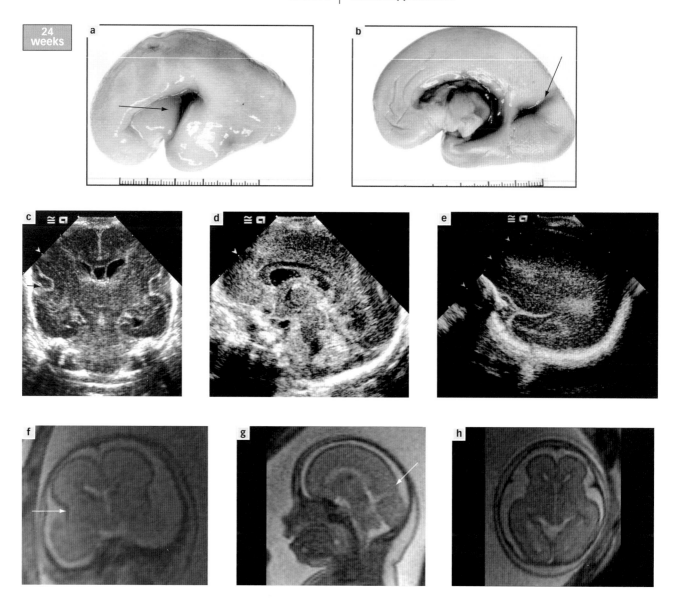

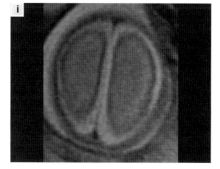

Fig. 5.3a–i. **Appearance of the brain at 24 weeks' gestation, and at postmortem with corresponding in vivo ultrasound and MRI images. (a) The superficial appearance of the brain on a pathological specimen. Arrow shows the insula. (b) The midline appearance of the brain on a pathological specimen. Arrow indicates the parieto-occipital sulcus. (c) Ultrasound appearances on a coronal scan sowing the open insula (arrow). (d) Ultrasound appearances on a midline sagittal scan. (e) Ultrasound appearances on a tangential parasagittal scan showing the open insula and smooth brain. (f) Coronal T$_2$-weighted MRI appearances at the level of the third ventricle, showing the open insula (arrow). (g) Sagittal T$_2$-weighted MRI appearances in the midline. The parieto-occipital sulcus can be seen (arrow). (h) Axial T$_2$-weighted MRI appearance at the level of the internal capsule and basal ganglia. (i) Axial T$_2$-weighted MRI appearance at the level of the centrum semiovale, showing how smooth the brain surface is at this gestation.**

coronal views, although it is not yet continuous or branched, and Fig. 5.4d is typical of the appearances at this gestation. The central sulcus can now be seen indenting the surface of the brain (Fig. 5.4a). The calcarine sulcus forms a Y shape at the junction with the parieto-occipital sulcus (Fig. 5.4b). Precentral and postcentral sulci may be seen on MRI (Fig. 5.4g, i). Other major sulci cannot be seen with ultrasound or MRI although they may appear as dimples on pathological specimens. The germinal matrix is extremely prominent at 24 and 26 weeks of gestation, and forms a band of high density on MR images all along the lateral margin of the lateral ventricles (Fig. 5.4h). The true extent of the germinal matrix can better be appreciated with MRI, and the appearances remind those used to imaging with ultrasound that the germinal matrix is not confined to a small volume of tissue at the head of the caudate nucleus.

28 weeks (Fig 5.5a–i)

The insula is still partly uncovered, but the formation of the Sylvian fissure can now be seen. The cingulate sulcus is now complete, stretching almost front to back, but there are no secondary branches yet. The cingulate sulcus can now usually be seen in the coronal plane of section on MR or ultrasound imaging, arising from the interhemispheric fissure. The parieto-occipital fissure is now very clearly seen and some occipital gyri have developed. The pre- and postcentral sulci are little more than mere dimples when the brain is examined at autopsy, and are still not very well defined with images in life. However, the central sulcus can usually be identified reliably with MRI and ultrasound, indenting the smooth surface of the brain particularly in the high axial slices (Fig. 5.5i) [13]. The superior temporal sulcus becomes visible on MRI, and myelin should be seen developing at the level of the vermis and cerebellar peduncles. Magnetic resonance imaging at this stage of gestation shows an appearance of "caps" around the lateral ventricles, which can be seen in Fig. 5.5h. This appearance is believed to represent a layer of migrating glial cells [16].

30 weeks (Fig. 5.6a–i)

The Sylvian fissure is now quite deep, and the insula is much more covered than earlier in development. The cingulate sulcus is now quite obvious even on the coronal section. The calcarine fissure shows a definite horizontal Y shape. The cingulate sulcus is now more tortuous than straight, and secondary branches can be seen. The marginal sulcus is now clearly visible, and can be seen on the ultrasound image in Fig. 5.6d (arrow). The parieto-occipital fissure is becoming slightly tortuous in the midline and tangential sections. The superior temporal sulcus appears by 30–31 weeks, and can probably be seen 2 weeks earlier with MRI [12]. It can sometimes be seen below the Y-shaped parieto-occipital and calcarine fissure on ultrasound scan and MR images. The cerebral white matter is still completely unmyelinated at this stage of

development. The nests of cells which previously formed the periventricular "caps" imaged with MRI can persist beyond 30 weeks, but are usually much less prominent by 30 weeks than earlier in gestation [12].

32 weeks (Fig. 5.7a–i)

Virtually all the primary sulci can be seen with MRI by 32 weeks (Table 5.2), and secondary sulci are now becoming apparent. They are easiest to see branching from the cingular sulcus, increasing the complexity of the imaging appearances. Insular sulci start to develop making the peripheral Y shape of the Sylvian fissure seen in the coronal sections a deeper and more complex structure. The superior temporal sulcus, anterior part, is present as is the inferior temporal sulcus. The superior frontal sulcus is usually well seen by 32 weeks [12].

34 weeks (Fig. 5.8a–h)

This period is characterized by a continuing increase in the complexity of sulci and gyri. Secondary sulci are now obvious in all the coronal and parasagittal sections, rendering the path of the insular, cingular, and occipital sulci more tortuous.

36 weeks (Fig. 5.9a–i)

Tertiary sulci are present making the superficial appearances resemble a bag of worms, very different to the featureless appearances of the 24-week-gestation infant. The cingulate sulcus is extensive and branched, with many minor gyri apparent. This appearance has been described as "cobblestone."

Term (Fig. 5.10a–i)

All the sulci and gyri seen in adult brains can be recognized at term, and after this time brain maturation is characterized by increasing complexity and development of myelination, rather than the formation of new sulci and gyri. On T_1-weighted MR images myelin in the posterior limb of the internal capsule appears hyperintense, with a characteristic spot of hypointensity in a more hyperintense band seen on the T_2 images (Fig. 5.10h) [17].

Figure 5.11 is a composite figure of a series of tangential parasagittal images showing just how much development can be seen between 24 and 38 weeks as the circular sulcus develops into the Sylvian fissure, with secondary branches. Figure 5.12 is a composite image showing the development of the precentral, central sulcus on axial T_2-weighted MR images between 24 and 38 weeks of gestation.

Myelination

The advent of MRI has allowed study of myelination during fetal and early neonatal life, and information is still accruing although the basic patterns are now fairly well defined [18,19,20].

26 weeks

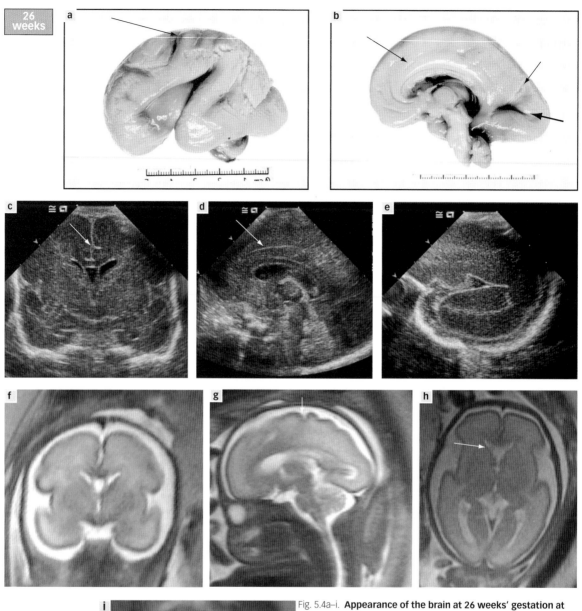

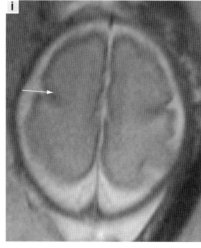

Fig. 5.4a–i. **Appearance of the brain at 26 weeks' gestation at postmortem with corresponding in vivo ultrasound and MRI images.** (a) The superficial appearance of the brain on a pathological specimen, arrow shows the central sulcus. (b) The midline appearance of the brain on a pathological specimen: the calcarine sulcus (thick arrow), parieto-occipital sulcus (short arrow) and the cingulate sulcus (long arrow) are now seen on ultrasound (c, d) and on MRI (f, g, and i). (c) Ultrasound appearances on a coronal scan showing the appearance of the cingulate sulcus (arrow). (d) Ultrasound appearances on a midline sagittal scan: arrow shows the cingulate sulcus. (e) Ultrasound appearances on a tangential parasagittal scan. (f) Coronal T$_2$-weighted MRI appearances at the level of the third ventricle, corresponding view to the ultrasound image in c. (g) Sagittal T$_2$-weighted MRI appearances in the midline. The central sulcus can be seen (arrow). (h) Axial T$_2$-weighted MRI appearance at the level of the internal capsule and basal ganglia. Arrow indicate the germinal matrix which forms a band of hypointensity along the lateral margin of the lateral ventricles (arrow). (i) Axial T$_2$-weighted MRI appearance at the level of the centrum semiovale. The central sulcus can be seen (arrow).

28 weeks

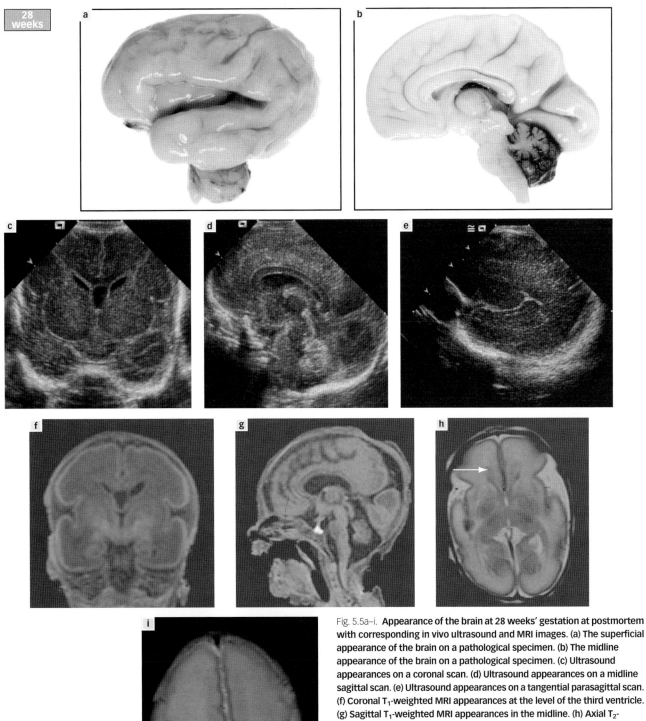

Fig. 5.5a–i. **Appearance of the brain at 28 weeks' gestation at postmortem with corresponding in vivo ultrasound and MRI images.** (a) The superficial appearance of the brain on a pathological specimen. (b) The midline appearance of the brain on a pathological specimen. (c) Ultrasound appearances on a coronal scan. (d) Ultrasound appearances on a midline sagittal scan. (e) Ultrasound appearances on a tangential parasagittal scan. (f) Coronal T_1-weighted MRI appearances at the level of the third ventricle. (g) Sagittal T_1-weighted MRI appearances in the midline. (h) Axial T_2-weighted MRI appearances at the level of the internal capsule and basal ganglia. This scan also shows a small right temporal lobe hemorrhage. Arrow shows periventricular "capping" white matter , also termed "crossroads." (i) Axial T_2-weighted MRI appearance at the level of the centrum semiovale. The postcentral sulcus can be seen (arrow).

Barkovich [20] has defined the ages at which the changes of myelination appear on T_1- and T_2-weighted images, and his work is summarized in Table 5.3. Myelination begins during the second trimester and proceeds long after birth in a caudal-rostral direction; hence (like sulcation) it is an index of the degree of maturity. In the brain myelination proceeds outwards from the center. Myelination is accompanied by an increase in the brain's lipid and protein content, whilst the water content is reduced. This results in a shortening of T_1 and T_2 relaxation times as the brain matures, and as white matter myelinates the signal generated by the area of brain involved changes from hypointense to hyperintense relative to gray matter on T_1-weighted images, and from hyperintense to hypointense relative to gray matter on T_2-weighted images [19].

Myelination in the internal capsule proceeds in a posterior to anterior fashion after birth, reaching the genu by 6 weeks post term, and the entire internal capsule is usually myelinated by 4–5 months post term, although the process continues for a year. The presence of a signal from myelin in the posterior limb of the internal capsule, as discussed above and shown in Fig. 5.10h, is a consistent finding at term. The absence of this normal signal has proved a useful sign in hypoxic-ischemia (Chapter 8) [17,21]. The corpus callosum is present from 20 weeks of gestation, but continues to grow throughout the rest of pregnancy and continues to thicken and develop during infancy, with a formed genu and splenium by 8–9 months of age.

In the following section we review some of the available normative data regarding ultrasound measurements of the fetal development of the corpus callosum, the septum pellucidum, the subarachnoid spaces, and the cerebellum. This information is helpful in the assessment of normal brain development and suspected brain malformations.

Normative ultrasound data of the fetal corpus callosum

Development of the corpus callosum is a late event in ontogenesis that takes place between 12 and 18 weeks. The rostral part of the corpus callosum, the genu, forms first and then grows caudally, forming the corpus and the splenium. Achiron and Achiron [22] demonstrated that ultrasound measurements of the three dimensions of the corpus callosum are feasible from 16 weeks of gestation and that the thickness and width of the corpus callosum increase three-fold during gestation, with approximately 50% of the thickness achieved between 16 and 20 weeks of gestation (Fig. 5.13). Further growth is apparent until 21–22 weeks of gestation and then remains stable throughout gestation.

Normative ultrasound data of the fetal cavum septum pellucidum

The septi pellucidi are two thin, translucent leaves that start to develop at 10–12 weeks of gestation and reach an adult form by 17 weeks of gestation. The cavum septum pellucidum is

Table 5.3. Time of the appearance of myelination in major parts of the brain when imaged with MRI; information largely obtained from the work of Barkovich [20].

Anatomic region	Ages when changes of myelination appear	
	T_1-weighted images	T_2-weighted image
Superior cerebellar peduncle	28 weeks of gestation	27 weeks of gestation
Median longitudinal fasciculus	25 weeks of gestation	29 weeks of gestation
Medial lemnisci	27 weeks of gestation	30 weeks of gestation
Lateral lemnisci	26 weeks of gestation	27 weeks of gestation
Middle cerebellar peduncle	Birth	Birth to 2 months
Cerebellar white matter	Birth to 4 months	3–5 months
Posterior limb of the internal capsule		
anterior part	First months	4–7 months
posterior part	36 weeks of gestation	40 weeks of gestation
Anterior limb of the internal capsule	2–3 months	7–11 months
Genu corpus callosum	4–6 months	5–8 months
Splenium of corpus callosum	3–4 months	4–6 months
Occipital white matter		
central	3–5 months	9–14 months
peripheral	4–7 months	11–15 months
Frontal white matter		
central	3–6 months	11–16 months
peripheral	7–11 months	14–18 months
Centrum semiovale	2–4 months	7–11 months

located in the midline between the two leaves of the septum pellucidum that separate the lateral ventricles. Jou et al. [23] provided normative fetal ultrasound measurements of the cavum septum pellucidum. They have shown that the width of this structure increases gradually with a rate of 0.37 mm per week between 19 and 27 weeks and then plateaus between 28 weeks of gestation and term [23] (Fig. 5.14). If the cavum septum pellucidum is larger than 10 mm at term and persistence of the cavum septum pellucidum beyond infancy occurs, further investigations are warranted (see Chapter 12).

Normative ultrasound data for subarachnoid spaces

In a prospective study by Lam et al. [24] subarachnoid spaces were measured in term infants and children (median 8 weeks,

30 weeks

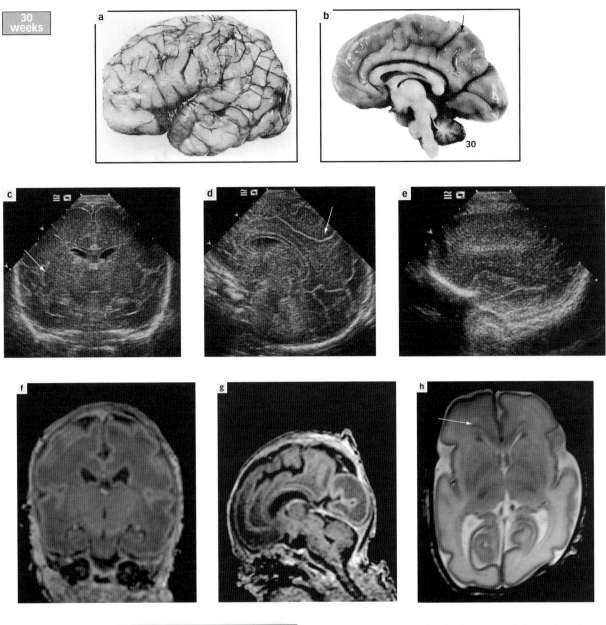

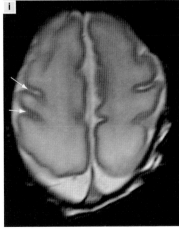

Fig. 5.6a–i. **Appearance of the brain at 30 weeks' gestation at postmortem with corresponding in vivo ultrasound and MRI images. (a) The superficial appearance of the brain on a pathological specimen. (b) The midline appearance of the brain on a pathological specimen. The marginal sulcus can be seen (arrow). (c) Ultrasound appearances on a coronal scan shows the ongoing operculization of the Sylvian fissure (arrow). (d) Ultrasound appearances on a midline sagittal scan. The parieto-occipital, calcarine and marginal sulcus (arrow) are seen. (e) Ultrasound appearances on a tangential parasagittal scan. (f) Coronal T$_1$-weighted MRI appearances at the level of the third ventricle. (g) Sagittal T$_1$-weighted MRI appearances in the midline. (h) Axial T$_2$-weighted MRI appearance at the level of the internal capsule and basal ganglia. The arrow shows the appearance of "caps" around the lateral ventricles. (i) Axial T$_2$-weighted MRI appearance at the level of the centrum semiovale showing the central and postcentral sulcus (arrow).**

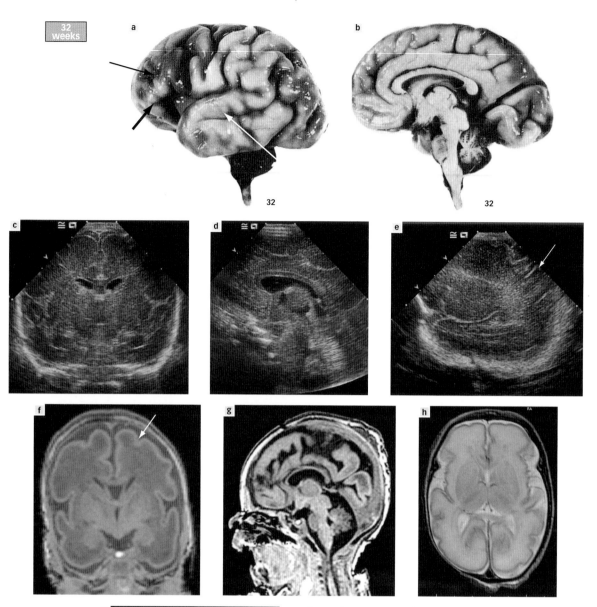

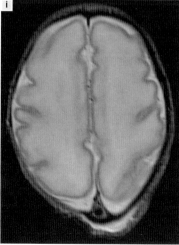

Fig. 5.7a–i. **Appearance of the brain at 32 weeks' gestation at postmortem with corresponding in vivo ultrasound and MRI images.** (a) The superficial appearance of the brain on a pathological specimen showing the superior (long black arrow) and inferior frontal sulcus (thick black arrow). The white arrow indicates the superior temporal sulcus; the inferior is not seen on this specimen. (b) The midline appearance of the brain on a pathological specimen. (c) Ultrasound appearances on a coronal scan showing more advanced opercularization. (d) Ultrasound appearances on a midline sagittal scan. (e) Ultrasound appearances on a tangential parasagittal scan, the central sulcus is seen in this view (arrow). (f) Coronal T_1-weighted MRI appearances at the level of the third ventricle; the superior frontal sulcus is seen (arrow). (g) Sagittal T_1-weighted MRI appearances in the midline. (h) Axial T_2-weighted MRI appearance at the level of the internal capsule and basal ganglia. (i) Axial T_2-weighted MRI appearance at the level of the centrum semiovale.

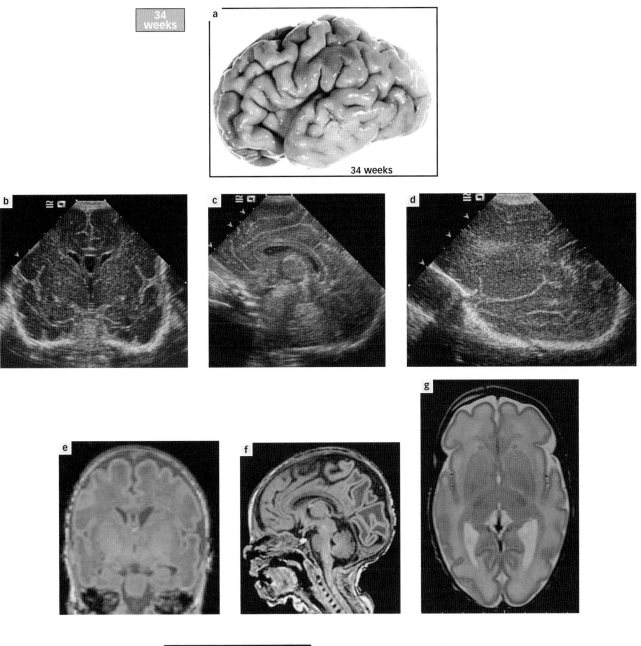

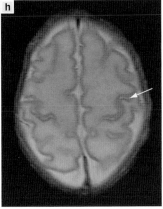

Fig. 5.8a–h. **Appearance of the brain at 34 weeks' gestation at postmortem with corresponding in vivo images on ultrasound and MRI. (a) The superficial appearance of the brain on a pathological specimen.** © Elsevier Ltd 2005, Standring: Gray's Anatomy 39e; www.graysanatomyonline.com. **(b) Ultrasound appearances on a coronal scan. (c) Ultrasound appearances on a midline sagittal scan. (d) Ultrasound appearances on a tangential parasagittal scan. (e) Coronal T$_1$-weighted MRI appearances at the level of the third ventricle. (f) Sagittal T$_1$-weighted MRI appearances in the midline. (g) Axial T$_2$-weighted MRI appearance at the level of the internal capsule and basal ganglia. (h) Axial T$_2$-weighted MRI appearance at the level of the centrum semiovale showing the central sulcus (arrow).**

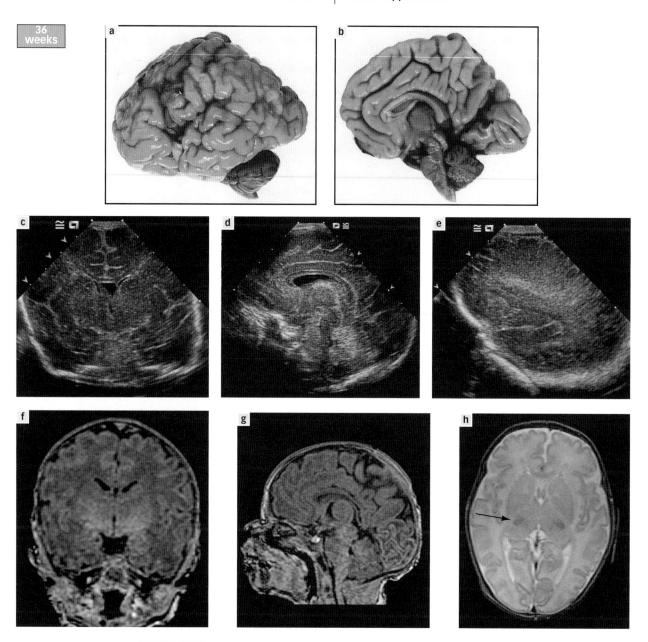

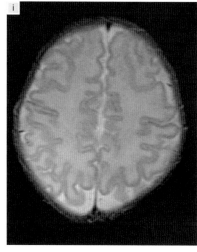

Fig. 5.9a–i. **Appearance of the brain at 36 weeks' gestation at postmortem with corresponding in vivo images on ultrasound and MRI. (a) The superficial appearance of the brain on a pathological specimen. (b) The midline appearance of the brain on a pathological specimen. (c) Ultrasound appearances on a coronal scan. (d) Ultrasound appearances on a midline sagittal scan. (e) Ultrasound appearances on a tangential parasagittal scan. (f) Coronal T_1-weighted MRI appearances at the level of the third ventricle. (g) Sagittal T_1-weighted MRI appearances in the midline. (h) Axial T_2-weighted MRI appearance at the level of the internal capsule and basal ganglia. Signal hypointensity within the posterior limb of the internal capsule starts to appear (arrow). (i) Axial T_2-weighted MRI appearance at the level of the centrum semiovale.**

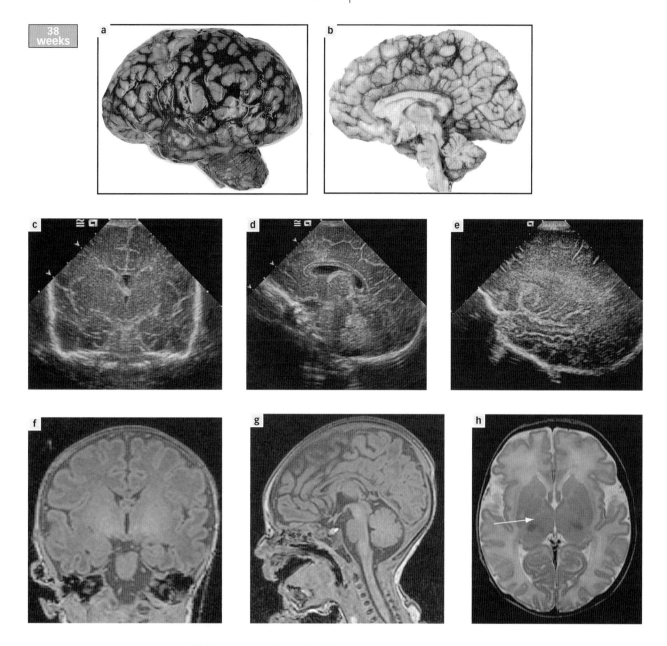

38 weeks

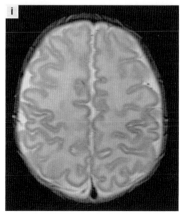

Fig. 5.10a–i. **Appearance of the brain at 38 weeks' gestation at postmortem with corresponding in vivo images on ultrasound and MRI. (a) The superficial appearance of the brain on a pathological specimen. (b) The midline appearance of the brain on a pathological specimen. (c) Ultrasound appearances on a coronal scan. (d) Ultrasound appearances on a midline sagittal scan. (e) Ultrasound appearances on a tangential parasagittal scan. (f) Coronal T_1-weighted MRI appearances at the level of the third ventricle. (g) Sagittal T_1-weighted MRI appearances in the midline. (h) Axial T_2-weighted MRI appearance at the level of the internal capsule and basal ganglia showing more myelin visible in the posterior limb of the internal capsule (arrow). (i) Axial T_2-weighted MRI appearance at the level of the centrum semiovale.**

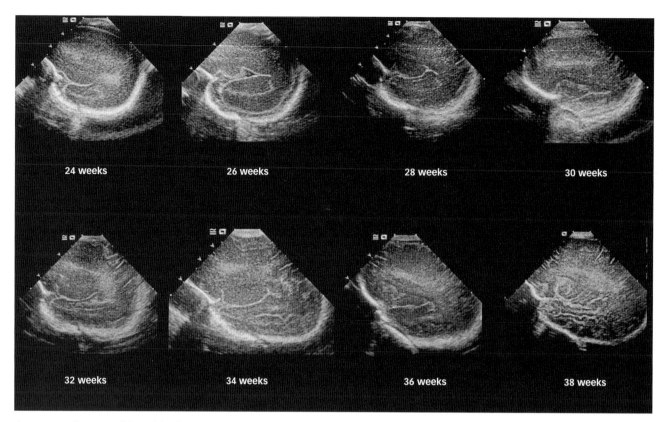

Fig. 5.11. **Development of the Sylvian fissure and insula seen on tangential parasagittal ultrasound images between 24 and 38 weeks of gestation.**

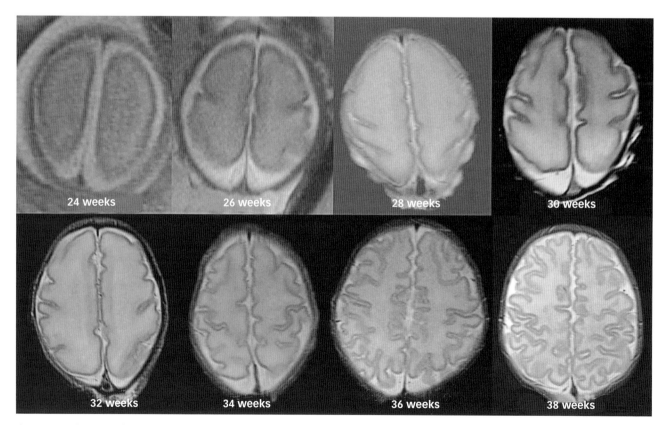

Fig. 5.12. **Development of the precentral, central and postcentral sulcus on axial T$_2$-weighted MR images between 24 and 38 weeks of gestation.**

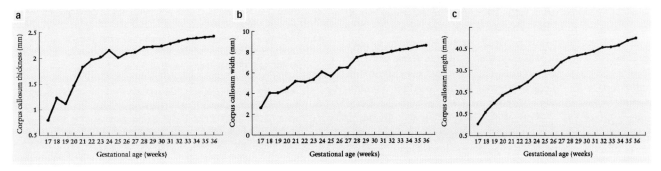

a

b

c

Fig. 5.13a–c. **Graph showing increase of corpus callosum thickness (a), width (b) and length (c) with gestational age. With permission from Achiron and Achiron [22].**

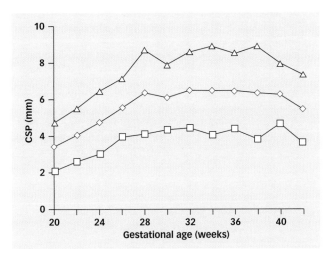

Fig. 5.14. **Mean width and two standard deviations of the fetal cavum septum pellucidum (CSP) at various gestational ages. With permission from Jou *et al*. [23].**

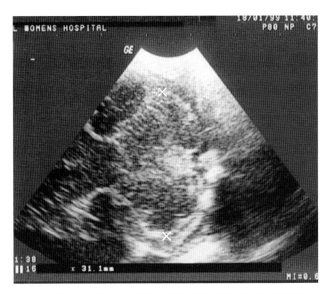

Fig. 5.16. **Ultrasound image of the posterior fossa demonstrating the measurement of the transverse cerebellar diameter. With permission from Davies *et al*. [29].**

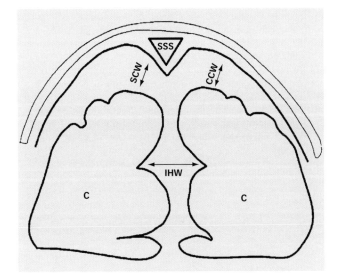

Fig. 5.15. **Anatomic landmarks and sonographic variables of the subarachnoid spaces in the coronal plane. C, cerebral hemisphere; CCW, craniocortical width; SCW, sinocortical width; IHW, interhemispheric width; SSS, superior sagittal sinus. With permission from Lam *et al*. [24].**

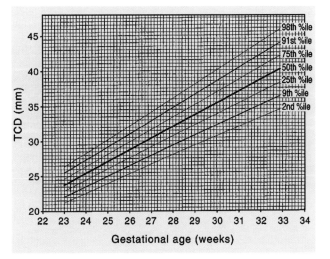

Fig. 5.17. **Percentile chart for transverse cerebellar diameter (TCD) by gestational age from 23 to 32 weeks and 6 days. With permission from Davies *et al*. [29].**

range 1 day to 1 year) (Fig. 5.15). They reported that there was an increasing width in the subarachnoid spaces with increasing age up to approximately 28 weeks of age (7 months of age), after which a decline was observed. However, these were not results of serial measurements. These data are consistent with older reports of "benign external hydrocephalus," an idiopathic condition in which infants are found to have a widened subarachnoid space with mild or no ventricular dilatation [25,26,27]. Usually the external hydrocephalus resolves after 18–24 months of age, and the prognosis is excellent [27]. One possible explanation for the widened subarachnoid spaces is thought to be that there is a differential rate of growth between the skull vault and cerebral hemisphere as the child grows.

Normative ultrasound data of the transverse cerebellar diameter

Fetal studies have shown a close relationship between the transcerebellar diameter (Fig. 5.16) and gestational age with linear growth during the second trimester [28]. Davies *et al.* [29] showed in preterm infants that the transverse cerebellar diameter increases linearly from 23 to 32^{+6} weeks of gestation and correlates closely with gestational age (Fig. 5.17). They have shown that this measurement is reproducible with minimal intra- and inter-observer differences. Transverse cerebellar diameter can be used to assess the gestational age or to assist in diagnosing cerebellar hypoplasia and abnormalities in cerebellar growth.

References

1. Chi JG. Gyral development of the human brain. *Ann Neurol* 1977; **1**: 86–93.
2. Feess-Higgins A, Larroche J-C. *Development of the Human Brain*, 1st edn. Paris, Inserm, 1987.
3. Garel C. *MRI of the Fetal Brain*, 1st edn. Berlin, Springer-Verlag, 2004.
4. Ghai S, Fong KW, Toi A, Chitayat D, Pantazi S, Blaser S. Prenatal US and MR imaging findings of lissencephaly: review of fetal cerebral sulcal development. *Radiographics* 2006; **26**: 289–405.
5. Toi A, Lister WS, Fong KW. How early are fetal cerebral sulci visible at prenatal ultrasound and what is the normal pattern of early fetal sulcal development? *Ultrasound Obstet Gynecol* 2004; **24**: 706–15.
6. Murphy NM, Rennie JM, Cooke RWI. Cranial ultrasound assessment of gestational age in VLBW infants. *Arch Dis Child* 1989; **64**: 569–72.
7. Dorovini-Zis K, Dolman CL. Gestational development of brain. *Arch Pathol Lab Med* 1977; **101**: 192–5.
8. Battisti O, Bach A, Gerard P. Brain growth in sick newborn infants: clinical and real time ultrasound analysis. *Early Hum Dev* 1986; **13**: 13–20.
9. Worthen NJ, Gilbertson V, Lau C. Cortical sulcal development seen on sonography: relationship to gestational parameters. *J Ultrasound Med* 1986; **5**: 153–6.
10. Huang C-C. Sonographic cerebral sulcal development in preterm newborn infants. *Brain Dev* 1991; **13**: 27–31.
11. Slagle TA, Oliphant M, Gross SJ. Cingulate sulcus development. *Pediatr Res* 1989; **26**: 598–602.
12. Fogliarini C, Chaumoitre K, Chapon F *et al.* Assessment of cortical maturation with prenatal MRI. Part 1 – normal cortical maturation. *Eur Radiol* 2005; **15**: 1671–85.
13. Cohen-Sacher B, Lerman-Sagie T, Lev D, Malinger G. Sonographic developmental milestones of the fetal cerebral cortex: a longitudinal study. *Ultrasound Obstet Gynecol* 2006; **27**: 494–502.
14. Garel C, Chantrel E, Brisse H *et al.* Fetal cerebral cortex: normal gestational landmarks identified using prenatal MR imaging. *Am J Neuroradiol* 2001; **22**: 184–9.
15. Garel C, Chantrel E, Elmaleh M, Brisser H, Sebgag G. Fetal MRI: normal gestational landmarks for cerebral biometry, gyration and myelination. *Childs Nerv Syst* 2003; **19**: 422–5.
16. Childs A-M, Ramenghi LA, Evans DJ *et al.* MR features of developing periventricular white matter in preterm infants: evidence of glial cell migration. *Am J Neuroradiol* 1998; **19**: 971–6.
17. Cowan FM, de Vries LS. The internal capsule in neonatal imaging. *Semin Fetal Neonatal Med* 2005; **10**(**5**): 461–74.
18. van der Knaap MS, Valk J. *Myelin and White Matter. Magnetic Resonance of Myelin, Myelination, and Myelin Disorders*, 2nd edn. Berlin, Springer, 1995; 4–51.
19. Barkovich AJ. Concepts of myelin and myelination in neuroradiology. *Am J Neuroradiol* 2000; **21**: 1099–109.
20. Barkovich AJ. Normal development of the neonatal and infant brain, skull and spine. In: Barkovich AJ, ed. *Paediatric Neuroimaging*, 4th edn. Philadelphia: Lippincott, Williams & Wilkins, 2005; 17–75.
21. Rutherford MA, Pennock JM, Counsell SJ *et al.* Abnormal magnetic resonance signal in the internal capsule predicts poor neurodevelopmental outcome in infants with hypoxic ischaemic encephalopathy. *Pediatrics* 1998; **102**: 323–8.
22. Achiron R, Achiron A. Development of the human fetal corpus callosum: a high-resolution, cross-sectional sonographic study. *Ultrasound Obstet Gynecol* 2001; **18**: 343–7.
23. Jou HJ, Shyu MK, Wu SC, Chen SM, Su CH, Hsieh FJ. Ultrasound measurement of the fetal cavum septi pellucidi. *Ultrasound Obstet Gynecol* 1998; **12**(**6**): 419–21.
24. Lam WW, Ai VH, Wong V, Leong LL. Ultrasonographic measurement of subarachnoid space in normal infants and children. *Pediatr Neurol* 2001; **25**(**5**): 380–4.
25. Ment LR, Duncan CC, Geehr R. Benign enlargement of the subarachnoid spaces in the infant. *J Neurosurg* 1981; **54**: 504–8.
26. Kendall B, Holland I. Benign communicating hydrocephalus in children. *Neuroradiology* 1981; **21**: 93–6.
27. Alvarez LA, Maytal J, Shinnar S. Idiopathic external hydrocephalus: natural history and relationship to benign familial macrocephaly. *Pediatrics* 1986; **77**: 901–7.
28. Goldstein I, Reece EA, Pilu G, Bovicelli L, Hobbins JC. Cerebellar measurements with ultrasonography in the evaluation of fetal growth and development. *Am J Obstet Gynaecol* 1987; **156**(**5**): 1065–9.
29. Davies MW, Swaminathan M, Betheras FR. Measurement of the transverse cerebellar diameter in preterm neonates and its use in assessment of gestational age. *Australas Radiol* 2001; **45**(**3**): 309–12.
30. Levine D, Barnes PD. Cortical maturation in normal and abnormal fetuses as assessed with prenatal MR imaging. *Radiology* 1999; **210**: 751–8.

Chapter 6 | The normal EEG and aEEG

GERALDINE B. BOYLAN,
DEIRDRE M. MURRAY, *and*
JANET M. RENNIE

Neonatal EEG: general features

The EEG of the newborn baby is unique. Patterns of electrical activity are seen that mirror the rapid maturational changes taking place in the brain. Waveforms appear that are not present at any other time of life. Sleep states are varied, change rapidly, and are very different from those seen in older children and adults.

The EEG of the neonate is best described in terms of the *background activity* or pattern. This is the baseline activity of the brain at rest, during wakefulness or sleep.

The EEG patterns of the full-term and of the preterm neonate are very different and it is best to consider them separately. However, the features used to describe the background activity are similar. The background activity of the neonatal EEG is generally described in terms of the following features: continuity, amplitude, frequency, synchrony and symmetry, maturational characteristics, state differentiation, and reactivity.

Continuity

The EEG of the normal full-term newborn shows continuous activity. This simply means that there is activity with a measurable voltage or amplitude present at all times (Fig. 6.1a). In contrast, preterm newborns exhibit a discontinuous EEG pattern (tracé discontinu) which is characterized by periods of continuous activity alternating with periods of little or no measurable voltage quiescence (Fig. 6.1b). In extremely preterm babies the EEG is very discontinuous and periods of quiescence can last up to 60 seconds. The EEG becomes progressively more continuous with increasing gestational age.

Amplitude or voltage

The amplitude of the normal neonatal EEG usually has a range of between 50 and 100 µV at term. In preterm neonates, particularly those less than 30 weeks, normal background amplitude is usually much higher; up 300 µV (Fig. 6.1a,b).

Frequency

In newborns, the predominant background activity is in the range 0.5–30 Hz (Fig. 2.8). This varies with sleep state. The frequency is lower in quiet compared to active sleep, whereas the voltage is higher. In other words, the EEG in quiet sleep tends to be high voltage low frequency, whereas in active sleep it is of lower voltage but higher frequency.

Synchrony and symmetry

Synchrony describes the degree with which activity appears simultaneously over both cerebral hemispheres. In the preterm infant (especially <32 weeks) the cerebral hemispheres may act independently and so EEG activity will appear asynchronous (Fig. 6.2). By term, both cerebral hemispheres should

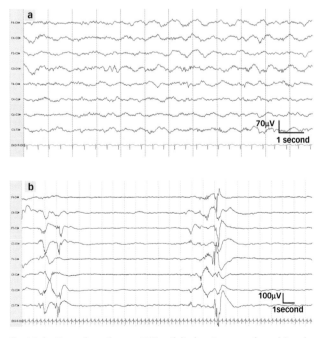

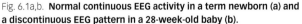

Fig. 6.1a,b. **Normal continuous EEG activity in a term newborn (a) and a discontinuous EEG pattern in a 28-week-old baby (b).**

Neonatal Cerebral Investigation, eds. Janet M. Rennie, Cornelia F. Hagmann and Nicola J. Robertson. Published by Cambridge University Press. © Cambridge University Press 2008.

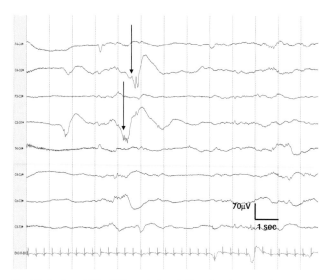

Fig. 6.2. **Preterm EEG at 28 weeks' gestation showing asynchrony between activity in the right and left hemispheres (arrows).**

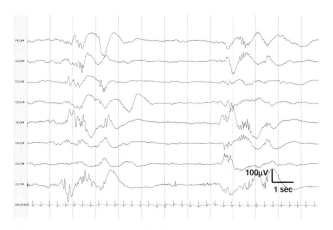

Fig. 6.4. **Preterm EEG at 28 weeks showing discontinuous EEG pattern and delta brushes (most prominent circled).**

show synchronous activity almost 100% of the time At all gestational ages, the amplitude on both sides should be the same. If one side consistently shows a lower amplitude (less than half that of the normal side), this indicates an abnormality on the side of the diminished amplitude (Fig. 6.3). In our experience, care must be taken when interpreting the EEG of a baby with a caput succedaneum or cephalohematoma, as an asymmetry may be seen, with amplitudes lower on the side of the swelling.

Maturational characteristics

Patterns such as delta brush activity, temporal saw-tooth activity, and frontal sharp transients appear in the neonatal EEG at specific gestational ages. Delta brush patterns appear at 28 weeks' gestation, are most prominent at 32 weeks, and then decrease so that they appear infrequently at term (Fig. 6.4). Gestation-specific features that may be present in the full-term EEG are anterior slow dysrhythmia (first appears from 35 weeks) and frontal sharp transients. These frontal sharp transients appear from 36 weeks' gestation and remain present until approximately 1 month post

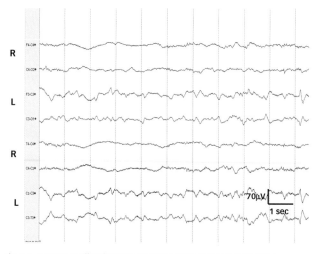

Fig. 6.3. **EEG recording in term neonate with hypoxic-ischemic encephalopathy and decreased amplitude evident in the right hemisphere (blue).**

term. Table 6.1 describes the EEG features that may be present at each gestational stage. It must be stressed that the presence of these features is an encouraging sign but their absence does not indicate an abnormality.

State differentiation

Sleep states are easily distinguishable from 36 weeks on the EEG. The normal term infant cycles through three behavioral states: quiet sleep, active sleep, and wakefulness. In our experience sleep state cycling can be seen in the normal term EEG immediately after birth and is an encouraging finding (Fig. 6.5). Information about the behavioral sleep state of the baby is essential before the neonatal EEG can be correctly interpreted. In addition to EEG analysis, behavioral staging can be determined by analyzing body movements, facial movements, and rapid eye movement. Newborns have a mean sleep cycle duration of 60 minutes with a range of 30–70 minutes. Hence, it is necessary to record the neonatal EEG for at least 1 hour. Sleep cycling may be absent in certain pathological conditions, and this may be the only abnormal finding in the neonatal EEG. The return of sleep cycling on an amplitude-integrated EEG (aEEG) has been linked to neurological outcome in babies who had sustained perinatal hypoxic ischemia [1].

Reactivity

A sensory stimulus, e.g., tactile or auditory, generally evokes changes in the background activity of the neonatal EEG, usually a generalized reduction in its amplitude (Fig. 6.6).

The EEG of the full-term newborn baby

The EEG of the normal full-term baby is continuous, synchronous, and symmetrical at all times. It contains moderate-voltage, mixed-frequency activity, shows fully developed sleep cycles, and is reactive to stimuli. However, accurate interpretation the neonatal EEG requires knowledge of the factors that can

Table 6.1. The normal features of the neonatal EEG at gestational intervals.* As, active sleep; IBI, interburst interval; QS, quiet sleep.

Gestational age (weeks)	Type of background activity	Max IBI (seconds)	SWC	Specific waveforms
22–23	Discontinuous	126–86 [23]	No	None reported
24–26	Discontinuous	10–60 [23,24,25]	No	STOPS
27–29	Discontinuous	10–40 [24,26,27]	No	PTθ, some delta brushes
30–32	Discontinuous generally but some semi-continuous periods during AS	3–20	AS emerges	PTθ, delta brushes abundant
33–34	Discontinuous in QS Continuous in AS and awake	≤10	Yes	Delta brushes, frontal sharp activity
35–37	Continuous AS and awake Semi-discontinuous in QS	< 10	Yes	Some encoche frontale; anterior slow waves; occipital delta brushes
Term	Continuous in all states	None	Yes	Sporadic temporal and rolandic sharp waves; encoche frontale; anterior slow waves

* Encoche frontale are sharp waves seen in the frontal regions of term newborns; a normal phenomenon.

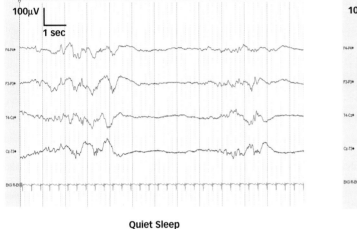

Quiet Sleep

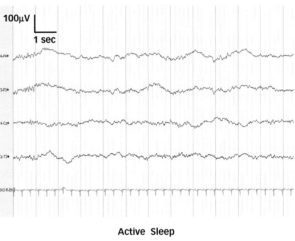

Active Sleep

Fig. 6.5. **Clear EEG sleep cycles seen in a normal term neonate soon after delivery.**

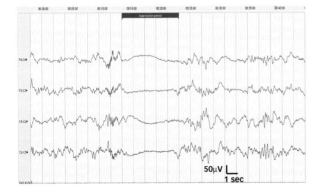

Fig. 6.6. **Normal full-term neonate in quiet sleep. Generalized attenuation lasting 5 seconds following auditory stimulation.**

influence its activity. The most important of these are behavioral state and the administration of neuroactive medications.

Sleep wake cycling

The first of the distinctive sleep states to develop is active (rapid eye movement or REM) sleep. Active sleep onset is characteristic of the neonatal period and the features of active sleep after a period of wakefulness are slightly different to those seen after a period of quiet sleep. Active sleep is characterized by continuous activity of mixed frequency, irregular respiration and rapid eye movements (Fig. 6.7a). "Active sleep onset" is sometimes called a mixed pattern of REM sleep as it contains diffuse mixed-frequency rhythmic activity with voltages of 40–100 µV. Active sleep that occurs after a period of quiet sleep is of lower amplitude (20–50 µV) and this pattern is sometimes referred to as a low-voltage irregular pattern (LVI). At 3 months of age REM onset of sleep disappears and active sleep shows less variability.

Quiet (non-rapid eye movement sleep) begins to appear at approximately 34 weeks' gestation. During quiet (non-rapid eye movement) sleep the EEG may show one of two distinctive patterns. The first consists of high-voltage slow wave sleep (HVSW) at 1–2 Hz. As sleep progresses, this can change to a pattern of bursts of activity alternating with periods of decreased amplitude, termed tracé alternant (TA) (Fig. 6.7b, c). In contrast to the discontinuous activity seen in the preterm or the encephalopathic neonate, the low amplitude periods of TA continue to show some activity, and are never completely suppressed. The frequency during TA alternates between periods of low-amplitude beta and theta activity and 3- to 5-second bursts of higher voltage (1–3 Hz) activity occurring at 3- to 10-second intervals.

In wakefulness the characteristic pattern is one of continuous mixed frequency irregular activity at 25–50 µV. This pattern is sometimes termed activité moyenne.

85

a Active sleep

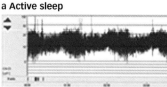

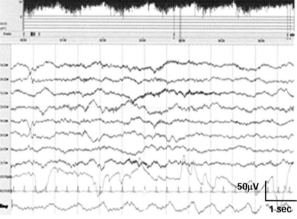

50μV

1 sec

b HVSW sleep

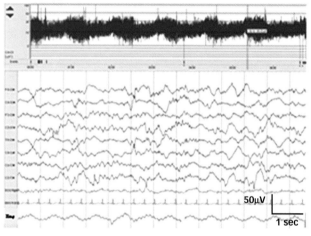

50μV

1 sec

c Tracé alternant

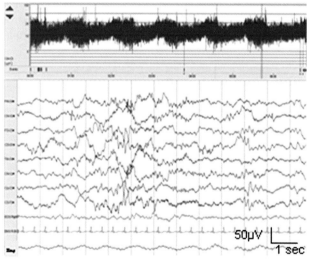

50μV

1 sec

Fig. 6.7a–c. **Active sleep and quiet sleep patterns in a normal term newborn. The aEEG trace shows sleep cycling over a 7-hour period. HVSW, High voltage slow wave.**

The EEG of the preterm baby

Rapid maturational changes take place in the brain of the human newborn during the last trimester of fetal life. These changes take place in an extrauterine environment in the prematurely born infant. The weight of the brain increases fourfold from 28 weeks' to 40 weeks' conceptional age and changes from a very smooth peanut-like structure at 26 weeks to a complex convoluted walnut-like structure at term (Fig. 5.1 Chapter 5). During this time, maturational changes also take place in neurons, synapses, and in the myelination of axons. This is reflected in the gradual maturation of the EEG as gestation progresses.

The EEG of the very premature baby is striking and reflects the immaturity of the fetal brain. The EEG can be recorded from babies born as early as 22 weeks' gestation, but the types of activity recorded would be considered extremely abnormal in adult life and in a term infant. The most striking features of the very preterm EEG are long periods of quiescence, containing little or no background activity. This is interrupted only by bursts of high-voltage, mixed-frequency waves (Fig. 6.1).

The lengths of quiescent periods are directly proportional to the degree of prematurity and this normal background pattern is referred to as "tracé discontinu" or discontinuous pattern. The intervals between bursts are referred to as "interburst intervals" (IBI). As the neonate matures, the EEG becomes progressively more continuous (Fig. 6.1), and the maximum accepted interburst interval decreases. The reported maximum accepted interburst intervals at earlier gestations vary. This may be because many previous studies included preterm infants who did not have normal neurological outcomes. A summary table (Table 6.1) illustrates the accepted guidelines for IBI durations at various gestational ages.

Prolonged IBIs in preterm infants have been associated with abnormal development at 3 years [2]. Holmes and Lambrusco found that at 33–36 weeks' gestation an IBI >20 seconds was associated with poor neurological prognosis [3].

Characteristic patterns consisting of sharp theta waves in the occipital regions (STOPs) and temporal areas (premature temporal theta PTθ) may be seen in extremely preterm infants (Table 6.2), but these should not be present at term.

Difficulty may arise when trying to decide whether a preterm infant is displaying characteristic periods of preterm discontinuity (tracé discontinu), or whether suppression and discontinuity of the EEG activity is occurring secondary to encephalopathy (often termed burst suppression). A useful point to remember is that during tracé discontinu, the activity will show variation, with IBIs of varying duration, the EEG will remain reactive to stimuli, and gestationally appropriate sleep cycles should be present. Encephalopathic burst suppression will lack these features (Fig. 2.10).

The effect of premature birth on EEG maturation

Early studies did not find any significant differences between the EEG patterns of premature babies at term (40 weeks post-conception) and term infants [4]. However, more recent studies have found different patterns in the ex-preterm infant. Longer

Table 6.2. Showing normal maturational features of the neonatal EEG.

Name	GA range recorded	Type of Activity
Delta brush activity	26–38	
STOPS Sharp theta on the occipitals of prematures	23–34	
PTθ Premature Temporal Theta	26–38	
(a) Encoches Frontale (Frontal sharp transients)	35–44	
(b) Anterior slow waves	34–44	

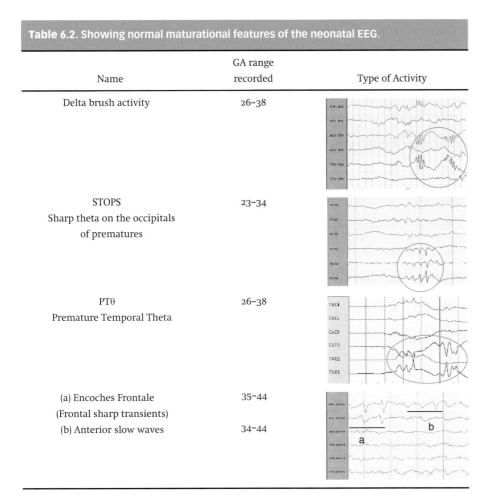

bursts during tracé alternant (TA) and more immature EEG patterns have been described [5]. More recently, differences in architectural, phase, continuity, spectral, and autonomic measures have been described, suggesting that functional brain maturation in the preterm neonate at term is not equivalent to that of gestational term babies [6].

Sleep–wake states in the preterm baby

As already stated, the term neonate alternates between three behavioral states: active sleep, quiet sleep, and wakefulness. In the preterm baby it is more difficult to determine behavioral state. Sleep states are difficult to distinguish prior to 30 weeks' gestation. At approximately 30 weeks, sleep states start to emerge and are clearly definable by 36–37 weeks.

In very preterm babies, state may need to be identified by behavioral and physiological characteristics rather than EEG patterns. At specific gestational stages different methods of determination are more appropriate [7]. For example, from 28 weeks, body movements predominate, with facial movements becoming increasingly common as the baby approaches term. At 32 weeks REM can be seen during active sleep. At 36 weeks, the

EEG can be used as a reliable predictor of sleep state. At term the electromyograph (EMG, chin) can also be analyzed. Although rhythmic movements of the chin appear in early prematurity, the EMG is not a reliable predictor of sleep state until 40 weeks.

A state that cannot be clearly identified as one of the three states is sometimes termed indeterminate or transitional sleep. The very premature baby is predominately in transitional sleep. By term however the baby spends just 3% of sleep time in this state. Active sleep occupies 60% of the sleep time of a baby at 34 weeks. This decreases to 50% at term and is less than 25% in adulthood.

The effect of medication on the background activity of the neonatal EEG

One of the major strengths of neonatal EEG is its ability to provide prognostic information based on the background activity. In particular, after hypoxic-ischemic injury, EEG background is often used to predict long-term neurological outcome [8]. Amplitude-integrated EEG has been used to recruit asphyxiated infants to large multicenter trials of therapeutic hypothermia [9]. However, the amplitude and continuity of the

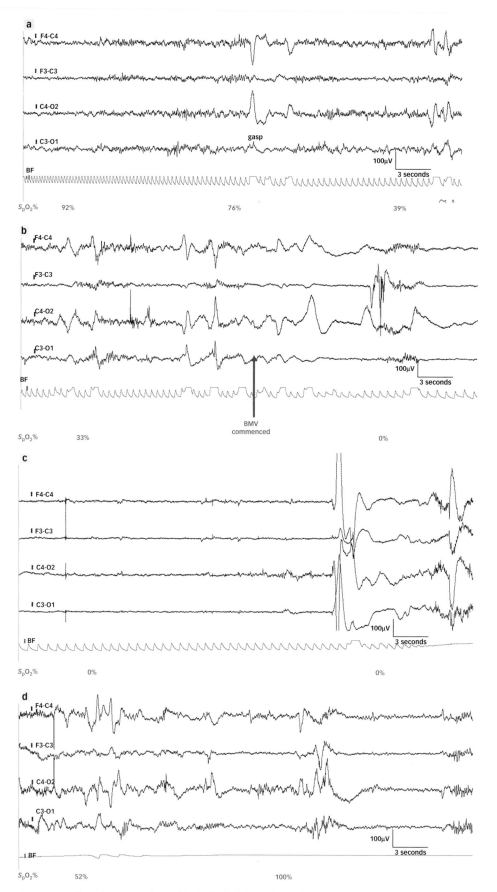

Fig. 6.8a–d. **Term newborn, saturations decreasing due to blocked tube (a). Continued from previous EEG, bag and mask ventilation (BMV) started, note loss of EEG activity (b). Continued from previous EEG, complete loss of all background EEG activity (c). Continued from previous EEG, return of EEG activity as oxygenation starts to improve (d).**

Table 6.3. Showing the normal background patterns of the aEEG with increasing gestational age. Adapted from reference [28]. (CNV, Continuous normal voltage; DNV, discontinuous normal voltage.)

Gestational age (weeks)	Background pattern	Sleep-wake cycles present	Minimum amplitude (µV)	Maximum amplitude (µV)
24–25	DNV	No	2–5	25–100
26–27	DNV	No	2–5	25–100
28–29	DNV/CNV	No	2–5	25–30
30–31	CNV/(DNV)	Yes	2–6	20–30
32–33	CNV/DNV in quiet sleep	Yes	2–6	20–30
34–35	CNV/DNV in quiet sleep	Yes	3–7	15–25
36–37	CNV/DNV in quiet sleep	Yes	4–8	17–35
38 +	CNV/DNV in quiet sleep	Yes	7–8	15–25

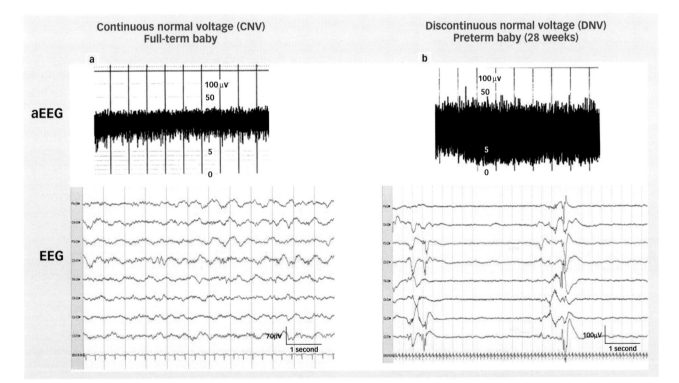

Fig. 6.9. **Continuous normal voltage (CNV) in a full-term baby. Discontinuous normal voltage (DNV) in a preterm baby (28 weeks).**

background EEG may be affected by a number of commonly used medications, in particular anticonvulsants and sedative agents. It is often the very babies who are receiving anticonvulsants and/or sedatives who stand to gain the most benefit from accurate interpretation of their EEG. Unfortunately, there is little information available on the exact effects of these drugs on the neonatal EEG.

Anticonvulsants and the neonatal EEG

Phenobarbitone is still the first-line treatment for neonatal seizures despite many studies demonstrating its lack of effect in suppressing electrographic seizures [10,11]. There are very few studies published on the effects of phenobarbitone on background EEG activity; those that have been reported consistently describe suppression of the background EEG activity, with increased discontinuity and increased IBIs. This effect seems to be greater with concurrent administration of diazepam. Even a single dose of diazepam given to a baby already treated with phenobarbitone is followed by a marked increase in the degree of EEG suppression, which prolongs the effect by 11–12 hours [12]. The degree of suppression seems to depend on the degree of underlying encephalopathy [13].

Box 6.1 Points to remember

- The normal full-term EEG should show continuity at all times, i.e., a measurable voltage throughout.
- EEG frequencies are mixed and do not have a regular pattern.
- Sporadic sharp waves are common and are a normal phenomenon.
- In term babies the EEG should have an average amplitude of at least 50 μV but in the preterm infant EEG voltages of up to 300 μV can be seen.
- The neonatal EEG should be recorded for a minimum period of 60 minutes to establish the presence or absence of sleep-wake cycling.
- Sleep-wake cycling should always be present in full-term neonates even immediately after delivery.
- The normal newborn EEG is reactive to stimuli such as touch and sound and shows a diffuse augmentation or attenuation.
- The normal newborn EEG is synchronous and symmetrical over both cerebral hemispheres at full term but can be asynchronous at preterm.
- The average interburst interval duration in extremely preterm neonates should be less than 1 minute.

The effects of other drugs on the neonatal EEG

Morphine and pethidine increase the interburst interval, depress the background activity, and alter sleep cycles in the same manner as phenobarbitone [12,14]. In addition, morphine has been reported to increase epileptogenic discharges. Young and da Silva [15] looked at the effect of morphine on the EEG of 20 normal newborns >26 weeks' gestation. They found that morphine produced prolonged periods of quiescence and excessive epileptiform activity in all infants [15]. These changes were largely reversible, although five of the babies continued to have excessive sharp waves when the morphine was discontinued.

Midazolam causes brief and moderate suppression of the aEEG, usually for short periods (approximately 2 hours) following administration. More profound, or prolonged suppression is seen with poor underlying background activity [16]. A burst-suppression pattern has also been described with very high serum levels of midazolam [17].

Lignocaine has also been shown to produce EEG suppression, with the development of a burst-suppression pattern in some cases [18,19]. However, many of these cases had been previously treated with phenobarbitone.

The effects of the neuromuscular blocking agent pancuronium on the neonatal EEG have been studied and found to produce no significant change [14,20].

It is apparent that anticonvulsants and other drugs routinely used in neonatal intensive care units do have an effect on the neonatal EEG. However, most studies have been small, retrospective, contain a mixed population, and are little more than observational. Therefore, it is often difficult to quantify exactly the degree of suppression attributable to the medications alone. This may affect the ability of the EEG to provide accurate prognostic information in some cases.

The effect of oxygenation on the neonatal EEG

The precise effect of hypoxia of varying duration on the neonatal EEG is not known. Animal work does suggest however that it may take as long as 30–40 minutes for the EEG to become suppressed [21,22]. This time may be shorter in the human neonate; anecdotally, we had the opportunity to examine the continuous EEG trace of a baby who developed a blocked ventilation tube whose oxygen saturation levels fell sharply. The EEG showed a rapid deterioration and loss of all background activities approximately 10–15 seconds after the oxygen saturation fell to 0% (Fig. 6.8). With bag and mask ventilation the saturations improved with rapid return of EEG activity, i.e., within 5–10 seconds.

The normal aEEG

Two normal patterns exist in aEEG monitoring of the newborn: a continuous normal voltage pattern (CNV), which is seen in term newborns; and a discontinuous normal voltage pattern (DNV), which is seen in preterm newborns. Figure 6.9 illustrates these two patterns and the associated EEG patterns from multi channel conventional EEG recordings. The aEEG matures, as does the EEG, with increasing gestational age, becoming more continuous. Table 6.3 illustrates the normal background patterns seen in the aEEG with increasing gestational age. It should be noted however that the amplitudes displayed on the cerebral function monitor are smoothed and rectified and are usually less than those displayed on the corresponding raw EEG tracing.

Conclusion

In summary, the neonatal EEG is complex and varied. Its patterns change with gestational age, sleep state, and the administration of medications. However, when these factors are accounted for, the accurate interpretation of the neonatal EEG may yield extremely valuable information about neonatal cerebral function. Information regarding the presence of encephalopathy, seizures, or structural abnormalities may be obtained, aiding long-term prognosis. The neonatal EEG is a non-invasive and safe investigation that provides real-time functional information that may not be provided by either structured neurological examination or detailed neuroimaging.

References

1. Osredkar D, Toet MC, van Rooij LG, van Huffelen AC, Groenendaal F, de Vries LS. Sleep-wake cycling on amplitude-integrated electroencephalography in term newborns with hypoxic-ischaemic encephalopathy. *Pediatrics* 2005; **115**(2): 327–32.
2. Hughes JR. *EEG in Clinical Practice*, 2nd edn. London, Butterworth-Heinemann, 1994.
3. Holmes GL, Lambrusco CT. Prognostic value of background patterns in the neonatal EEG. *J Clin Neurophysiol* 1993; **10**(3): 323–52.
4. Parmelee AH Jr, Schulte FJ, Akiyama Y, Werner WH, Schultz MA, Stern E. Maturation of EEG activity during sleep in premature infants. *Electroencephalogr Clin Neurophsyiol* 1968; **24**(4): 319–29.

5. Nunes ML, Da Costa JC, Moura-Ribeiro MV. Polysomnographic quantification of bioelectrical maturation in preterm and fullterm newborns at matched conceptional ages. *Electroencephalogr Clin Neurophsyiol* 1997; **102**(3): 186–91.

6. Scher MS, Bova JM, Dokianakis SG, Steppe DA. Positive temporal sharp waves on EEG recordings of healthy neonates: a benign pattern of dysmaturity in pre-term infants at post conceptional term ages. *Electroencephalogr Clin Neurophsyiol* 1994; **90**(3): 173–8.

7. Stern E, Parmelee AH, Harris MA. Sleep state periodicity in prematures and young infants. *Dev Psychobiol* 1973; **6**(4): 357–65.

8. van Lieshout HBM, Jacobs JWFM, Rotteveel JJ, Geven W, v't Hof M. The prognostic value of the EEG in asphyxiated newborns. *Acta Neurol Scand* 1995; **91**: 203–205.

9. Coolcap Study Group. Selective head cooling with mild systemic hypothermia after neonatal encephalopathy: multicentre randomised trial. *Lancet* 2005; **365**: 663–670.

10. Boylan GB, Rennie JM, Pressler RM, Wilson G, Morton M, Binnie CD. Phenobarbitone, neonatal seizures, and video-EEG. *Arch Dis Child Fetal Neonatal Ed* 2002; **86**(3): F165–F170.

11. Painter MJ, Scher MS, Stein AD et al. Phenobarbital compared with phenytoin for the treatment of neonatal seizures. *N Engl J Med* 1999; **341**(7): 485–489.

12. Bell AH, Greisen G, Pryds O. Comparison of the effects of phenobarbitone and morphine administration on EEG activity in preterm babies. *Acta Paediatr* 1993; **82**(1): 35–39.

13. Staudt F, Scholl ML, Coen RW, Bickford RB. Phenobarbital therapy in neonatal seizures and the prognostic value of the EEG. 1. *Neuropediatrics* 1982; **13**: 24–33.

14. Eaton DG, Wertheim D, Oozer R, Royston P, Dubowitz L, Dubowitz V. The effect of pethidine on the neonatal EEG. *Dev Med Child Neurol* 1992; **34**(2): 155–163.

15. Young GB, da Silva OP. Effects of morphine on the electroencephalograms of neonates: a prospective, observational study. *Clin Neurophysiol* 2000; **111**(11): 1955–1960.

16. van Leuven K, Groenendaal F, Toet MC et al. Midazolam and amplitude-integrated EEG in asphyxiated full-term infants. *Acta Paediatr* 2004; **93**(9): 153–154.

17. ter Horst HJ, Broswer OF, Bos AF. Burst suppression on amplitude-integrated electroencephalograph may be induced by midazolam: a report on three cases. *Acta Paediatr* 2004; **93**(4): 559–563.

18. Rey E, Radvanyi-Bouvet MF, Bodion C et al. Intravenous lidocaine in the treatment of convulsions in the neonatal period: monitoring plasma levels. *Ther Drug Monit* 2007; **12**(4): 316–320.

19. Hellstrom-Westa L, Westgren U, Rosen I, Svenningsen NW. Lidocaine for treatment of severe seizures in newborn infants. I. Clinical effects and cerebral electrical activity monitoring. *Acta Paediatr* 1988; **77**(1): 79–84.

20. Staudt F, Roth JG, Engel RC. The usefulness of electroencephalography in curarized newborns. *Electroencephalogr Clin Neurophsyiol* 1981; **51**(2): 205–208.

21. Williams CE, Gunn AJ, Synek B, Gluckman PD. Delayed seizures occurring with hypoxic-ischemic encephalopathy in the fetal sheep. *Pediatr Res* 1990; **27**(6): 561–565.

22. Gunn AJ, Parer JT, Mallard EC, Williams CE, Gluckman PD. Cerebral histologic and electrocorticographic changes after asphyxia in fetal sheep. *Pediatr Res* 1992; **31**(5): 486–491.

23. Hayakawa M, Okumura A, Hayakawa F et al. Background electroencephalographic (EEG) activities of very preterm infants born at less than 27 weeks gestation: a study on the degree of continuity. *Arch Dis Child Fetal Neonatal Ed* 2001; **84**(3): F163–F167.

24. Hahn JS, Monyer H, Tharp BR. Interburst interval measurements in the EEGs of premature infants with normal neurological outcome. *Electroencephalogr Clin Neurophysiol* 1989; **73**(5): 410–418.

25. Vecchierini MF, d'Allest AM, Verpillat P. EEG patterns in 10 extreme premature neonates with normal neurological outcome: qualitative and quantitative data. *Brain Dev* 2003; **25**(5): 330–337.

26. Selton D, Andre M, Hascoet JM. Normal EEG in very premature infants: reference criteria. *Clin Neurophysiol* 2000; **111**(12): 2116–2124.

27. Biagioni E, Bartalena L, Boldrini A, Cioni G, Giancola S, Ipata AE. Background EEG activity in preterm infants: correlation of outcome with selected maturational features. *Electroencephalogr Clin Neurophysiol* 1994; **91**(3): 154–162.

28. Hellstrom-Westas L, Rosen I, DeVries LS, Griesen G. Amplitude integrated EEG. Classification and interpretation in preterm and term infants. *Neoreviews* 2007; **7**: e76–e87.

Chapter 7

JANET M. RENNIE,
CORNELIA F. HAGMANN, *and*
NICOLA J. ROBERTSON

Clinical manifestations of neonatal seizure

All those involved in the care of babies need to maintain a high index of suspicion regarding the possibility of seizures. Not only are seizures common in the first few days of life, but they are also difficult to diagnose because the clinical manifestations are varied, subtle, and unlike those seen at other times of life. The diagnosis of seizure should be considered if a baby makes odd repetitive stereotyped movements of the limbs or face. Subtle seizures can manifest as repetitive blinking, chewing, eye-rolling or darting tongue movements. Seizures can also involve a stare without blinking, forced eye deviation, peculiar limb postures, apnea or a fixed smile. Ocular manifestations are common, and eye closure during a suspicious event makes the diagnosis of seizure less likely, although it does not exclude it completely [1]. Myoclonic jerks can be normal in sleep but myoclonic epilepsy does occasionally manifest in the neonatal period. Clinical seizures are often short-lived in babies; typically the baby becomes still, there is a change in breathing pattern (sometimes apnea), and a change in level of alertness followed by subtle repetitive movements involving the face or limbs. The whole episode may be over in less than a minute, but the same pattern does tend to recur, in which case it becomes more suspicious.

Babies with a history of fetal distress or difficult delivery are usually closely observed for signs of seizure, but it is important to remember that seizures can, and do, occur in any baby and are not confined to those with known risk factors. Seizures are diagnosed clinically in about 10% of very low birthweight babies (approximately 50 per 1000 low birthweight deliveries) and about 3 per 1000 of those born at term. Relying on clinical diagnosis vastly underestimates the seizure burden, and probably the prevalence, and there is poor inter-observer agreement [2,3]. In a study of 41 babies only 84/393 (21%) of the identified electrographic seizures were accompanied by any clinical manifestation [4]. A similar finding was reported in a video-EEG study of over 1000 seizures in 31 Australian babies [5]. Our experience with prolonged video-EEG supports these findings.

A neonatal seizure is an emergency, and should be the stimulus for detailed investigation and prompt treatment. Delayed diagnosis of a treatable cause such as hypoglycemia (pp. 215–217), meningitis (pp. 277–280), or an expanding posterior fossa subdural hematoma (p. 119) can have disastrous consequences for the long-term neurodevelopmental outcome of the child. Babies with a history of fetal distress and birth depression who seize do not necessarily have neonatal encephalopathy due to hypoxic ischemia (pp. 137–169) although that is clearly an important differential diagnosis. Early infantile encephalopathy or Ohtahara syndrome (p. 126) can present this way, and so can viral encephalitis, pyridoxine dependency (pp. 123–124), intracranial hemorrhage (pp. 115–122) and congenital myopathy. Babies with pre-existing cerebral malformations or stroke can seize in the neonatal period. Inadequate investigation at this crucial time can result in a "default" diagnosis of hypoxic ischemia, which can lead to inappropriate criticism of the obstetric management, with all that entails.

There have been some exciting advances in basic laboratory research that have uncovered important differences in the neurotransmitters and their receptors in the neonatal brain compared with the adult brain, and these advances should soon translate into more effective antiepileptic drug regimens [6,7,8]. Given the wealth of experimental evidence that seizures are harmful to the developing brain [9,10], better seizure control may also have a beneficial effect on outcome.

Incidence and epidemiology

Virtually all the published studies have relied on the clinical diagnosis of seizure for case identification, and many report the incidence from high-risk populations cared for in tertiary referral institutions. As discussed, clinical diagnosis of subtle seizure is fraught with difficulty and there is poor inter-observer agreement [2], hence the results are likely to represent an under-estimate of the true incidence. Nevertheless, they provide some important baseline information. A retrospective study of hospital records in Fayette County, Kentucky was carried out for births in the years 1985–89, yielding an incidence figure for clinically recognized neonatal seizures of

Neonatal Cerebral Investigation, eds. Janet M. Rennie, Cornelia F. Hagmann and Nicola J. Robertson. Published by Cambridge University Press. © Cambridge University Press 2008.

Table 7.1. Risk factors for neonatal seizures.

Abnormal CTG in labor

Depressed Apgar score (less than 5 at 5 min)

Need for resuscitation at birth

Low fetal scalp or cord pH

Prolonged membrane rupture

Maternal pyrexia in labor or post-partum

Maternal drug abuse

Instrumental delivery

Emergency caesarean section delivery during labor

Neonatal pyrexia

Abnormal neonatal neurological behavior; poor feeding

Family history of neonatal seizures

Prematurity

Small for gestational age

3.5 per 1000 live births [11]. The risk for babies of very low birthweight was 57.5 per 1000, significantly higher than the risk for heavier babies; for those of birthweight 2.5–4 kg the risk was 2.8 per 1000. The same authors went on to analyze US national hospital discharge survey information for the years 1980–91, producing a rather lower incidence figure of 2.84 per 1000 live births [12]. A prospective study was carried out in Newfoundland between 1990 and 1994; a nurse co-ordinator carried out training sessions using video clips before recruitment started and all suspected cases were transported to a single center [13]. The incidence was 2.6 per 1000 live births (1.9 for ≥38 weeks and 8.6 for <38 weeks). Finally, a population-based study in Harris County Texas between 1992 and 1994 estimated the incidence of seizure as 1.8 per 1000 live births, 19 per 1000 amongst those weighing less than 1500 g [14].

Seizures usually occur early in neonatal life; half of all cases were recognized by the third day, and 70% within the first week in one study [14]. Scher found that term babies were particularly likely to seize in the first 48 h, and 87% of his cases had developed seizures by then [15]. A high-risk group can be defined (Table 7.1), and when we monitored babies with risk factors prospectively with video-EEG seizures were found in at least 30%. Connell also monitored high-risk babies prospectively (with four channels of EEG) and found seizures in 25% of them [16].

Investigation of the baby with seizure

History taking in the baby with a suspected seizure

As elsewhere in this book, we make no excuse for continuing to stress the importance of basic clinical skills when assessing a baby with a suspected seizure. A detailed history should be taken regarding the pregnancy and the family whenever a diagnosis of seizure is made. Gentle questioning may uncover maternal drug abuse, or use of prescription drugs such as selective serotonin reuptake inhibitors (SSRIs) or benzodiazepines, which can produce a neonatal withdrawal syndrome [17,18]. The withdrawal syndrome of SSRIs is usually mild but

seizures have been reported [19]. There may be a family history of neonatal seizures, usually in the father, suggesting a diagnosis of benign familial neonatal seizures (p. 125). As ever, clues to sepsis include a history of maternal pyrexia, prolonged rupture of membranes and fetal tachycardia, and a history of vaginal herpes is always important. Details of the delivery, the condition of the baby at birth, the need for resuscitation, and the early feeding history are all essential. Given the importance of hematological disorders (both bleeding disorders and thrombophilia) a family history of thromboembolic disease may be relevant, and it is vital to know whether the baby received vitamin K (and if so, how much and by which route).

Clinical examination of the baby with a suspected seizure

The baby who is still making abnormal movements

When called to see a baby who is thought to be seizing, the first assessment of the baby may provide vital information. If the baby is in a crib next to his mother, move him to a resuscitaire in a good light, place him gently on his side and examine him; if he is still making abnormal movements take a moment or two to document them. Suck out any secretions if his color is poor, and consider whether he needs oxygen or respiratory support. Are the movements "marching" Jacksonian fashion through his body? Can you stop them by stilling a limb? What are the facial movements like? Check his heart rate and respiratory pattern; in a baby already receiving intensive care it should be possible to check the blood pressure and oxygen saturation.

The most urgent investigation is the blood glucose level, which must be checked immediately in any baby with suspicion of a seizure. Whilst this is being done, attempt to site an intravenous line and collect a small sample of blood from the cannula for a laboratory glucose level. If the glucose level is low give 3 ml/kg of 10% dextrose intravenously, and in any case arrange immediate admission to the nursery. In general, seizures are not sustained in babies (87% last less than 5 min, and 97% less than 9 min), but if the abnormal movements continue give 20 mg/kg of phenobarbitone slowly intravenously over 20 min once the baby has been admitted and is in an incubator with cardiovascular and respiratory monitoring in place. When the situation has stabilized take a careful history and examine the baby; measure his head as a baseline and feel the fontanelle. Explain gently to the parents that the baby has had a fit and will need investigation and treatment, but do not attempt to give a prognosis at this stage. Many of the causes of neonatal seizure (Table 7.2) have an excellent prognosis, although broadly speaking a third of term babies will have sequelae.

The baby in whom there is a history of possible seizure

In this situation it is important to take a careful history and examine the baby in a good light, and to have a low threshold for admitting him to the neonatal unit for observation and

Table 7.2. Causes of neonatal seizure.
Perinatal hypoxic ischemia
Cerebral arterial infarction (perinatal arterial stroke)
Cerebral venous sinus thrombosis
Intracranial hemorrhage
Subarachnoid hemorrhage
Subdural hemorrhage
Intraventricular hemorrhage
Parenchymal (lobar) hemorrhage
Thalamic hemorrhage
Cerebellar hemorrhage
Meningitis or encephalitis, bacterial, fungal or viral
Neonatal abstinence syndrome, other drug withdrawal (SSRIs) or drug intoxication
Structural cerebral malformations
Metabolic causes
Hypoglycemia
Hyponatremia
Hypernatremia
Hypocalcemia
Hypomagnesemia
Hyperbilirubinemia (kernicterus)
Inborn errors of metabolism
Pyridoxine dependency
Biotinidase deficiency
Glucose transporter type 1 deficiency (Glut-1 deficiency, De Vivo syndrome)
Amino acid, organic acid disorders
Syndromes
Benign familial neonatal convulsions
Benign non-familial neonatal convulsions
Early infantile epileptic encephalopathy (Ohtahara syndrome)
Early myoclonic encephalopathy (neonatal myoclonic encephalopathy)

SSRI, Selective serotonin reuptake inhibitor.

Table 7.3. Investigations in neonatal seizure.
EEG or aEEG
Glucose
Urea and electrolytes
Calcium and magnesium
Full blood count, differential white cell count, nucleated red cell count
Blood gas
Blood culture
Lumbar puncture (remember PCR for herpes virus)
Urine culture
Urine toxicology screen if there is a suspicion of maternal drug abuse
Cranial ultrasound scan
TORCH screen
MR imaging
Ammonia, lactate
Biotin
Prolonged EEG with pyridoxine administration
Urinary organic acids
Plasma and urinary amino acids

PCR, Polymerase chain reaction; TORCH toxoplasmosis, rubella, cytomegalovirus, herpes simplex and HIV.

investigation. If the baby remains on the postnatal ward with his mother, then an observation and feed chart should be set up, and glucose levels should be checked regularly until they are known to be normal and stable for at least 12 h.

Laboratory tests in the baby with a seizure

Investigations are aimed at establishing the diagnosis and finding the cause, particularly treatable causes such as meningitis and hypoglycemia. The first-line investigations are outlined in Table 7.3 and in our opinion lumbar puncture is a first-line investigation in seizure. Once these results are available it should be possible to place the baby into one of the broad diagnostic categories discussed later in this chapter.

Lumbar puncture

There has been an increasing reluctance to perform lumbar puncture in babies in recent years. In our view this is a pity

because meningitis is easily missed. The normal values are given in Table 13.1. If there is a high cerebrospinal fluid (CSF) white cell count with no organisms seen on microscopy in a baby who has not been treated with antibiotics, then herpes simplex encephalitis should be considered. The baby should be treated empirically with aciclovir until the result of polymerase chain reaction (PCR) for herpes can be obtained.

In the first instance, lumbar puncture is directed at excluding meningitis, but CSF may need to be examined specifically for glycine (high in non-ketotic hyperglycinemia, glycine encephalopathy) or lactate (high in mitochondrial disorders). One very rare syndrome, glucose transporter type 1 deficiency (GLUT-1 deficiency, De Vivo syndrome), is caused by a deficiency of the facilitative glucose transporter across the blood–brain barrier [20]. As a result, CSF glucose levels are low whereas blood glucose levels are normal, with low to normal CSF lactate levels.

The EEG in neonatal seizure

General points about the EEG confirmation of neonatal seizure

Even when the clinical diagnosis of seizure is unequivocal, the EEG can provide helpful information about the possible cause and prognosis, the type of seizure and the seizure burden as well as the background activity. When the diagnosis is uncertain, only EEG can settle the question. Electrographic seizures, like their clinical counterparts, are brief in the newborn. Most electrographic seizures in term babies last about 2–3 min, with 97% being over in less than 9 min [21,22,23]. Neonates do not sustain electrical or clinical seizure activity in the same way as

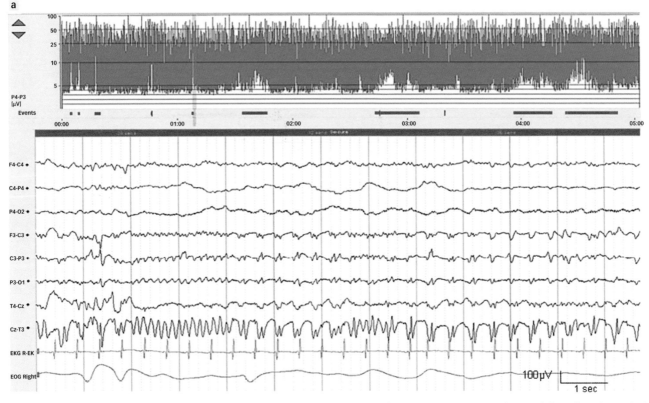

Fig. 7.1a–d. **EEG showing different types of neonatal seizure. In each panel the top trace is the aEEG; bottom channels show full EEG from the marked position on the aEEG. The bottom two channels on the EEG part of the trace show the electrocardiogram (ECG) (labeled EKG) and the electro-oculogram (EOG). (a) The evolving nature of a neonatal seizure; note frequency and morphology change. (b) A clear right-sided (blue channels) high-amplitude seizure, which is detected on aEEG. (c) High-amplitude seizure; note the frequency difference over right (blue) and left red sides within the same seizure. This detail is lost on aEEG. (d) Note how seizure discharge swaps from the right to the left side of the brain (blue to red channels).**

older children and adults, and hence the definitions that are used for status epilepticus (e.g., electrographic seizure that is sustained for more than 30 min) are not suitable for use in babies. Some groups have arbitrarily defined neonatal "status epilepticus" (better termed non-convulsive status epilepticus) as electrographic seizure activity for more than 50% of the recording time [22,24]. Others have used a definition of "serial seizures" over 20 min [25]. Our experience, based on continuous video-EEG monitoring of a large number of high-risk neonates, showed that if a definition of more than 30 min of electrographic seizure activity in an hour (not necessarily continuous, as required for the definition of status in older children) is adopted, about a third of monitored babies will meet this criterion [26].

Electrographic seizures are described in terms of location, duration, morphology, and amplitude. The location describes the site of seizure origin and spread, and the precision with which this can be determined is defined by the number and location of electrodes used to record the EEG. The morphology of neonatal seizures varies, but characteristically consists of monophasic repetitive discharges of sharp or slow waves or (more rarely) spike and wave activity (Fig. 7.1). Most neonatal seizures generalize from a unifocal discharge or from multifocal trains of abnormal waves, with the temporal lobe a

common site of origin. A primary generalized spike-wave discharge is extremely rare in a baby. Neonatal seizures can migrate, and have different morphology even within a single event. Babies can have seizures with different morphology in different parts of the brain at the same time, a remarkable feature that does not occur in adults or children, who have more mature synaptic connections (see Fig. 7.1).

The duration of a seizure can be more difficult to determine than would be expected, even on EEG: an electrographic seizure should have a clear onset and conclusion. Clancy and Ledigo [21] used an arbitrary cut-off of 10 s as a minimum duration; this definition was also adopted by Scher et al. [22] and is the one we adopt for clinical use and in our research studies. Others have used 5 s [27]. The International Federation of Clinical Neurophysiology recommend that the definition of a neonatal seizure should be an event of 5 s with a normal background EEG and 10 s when the background is abnormal. Abnormal discharges that are shorter than 5 or 10 s are sometimes called brief intermittent rhythmic discharges (BIRDS), but the significance of these remains to be established [28].

There is often asynchrony between the clinical and electrical diagnoses of neonatal seizures (electroclinical dissociation) [29], and this tends to increase after antiepileptic drugs have been given [30,31,32]. One explanation for the occurrence

b

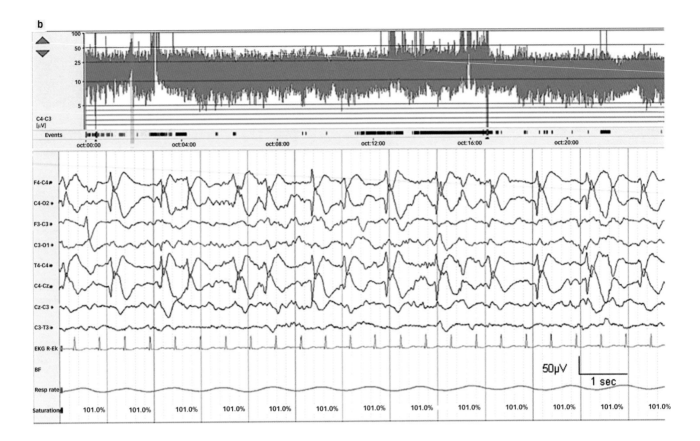

c

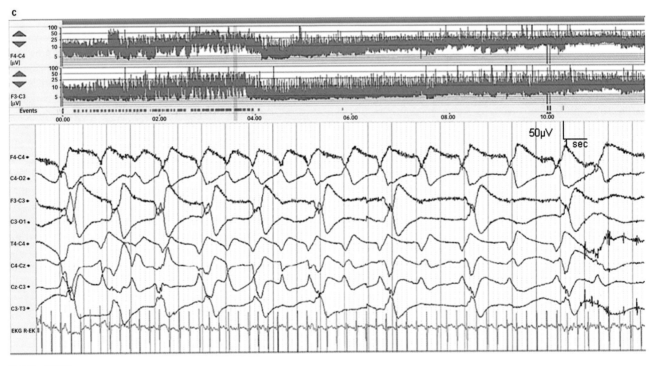

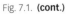

Fig. 7.1. **(cont.)**

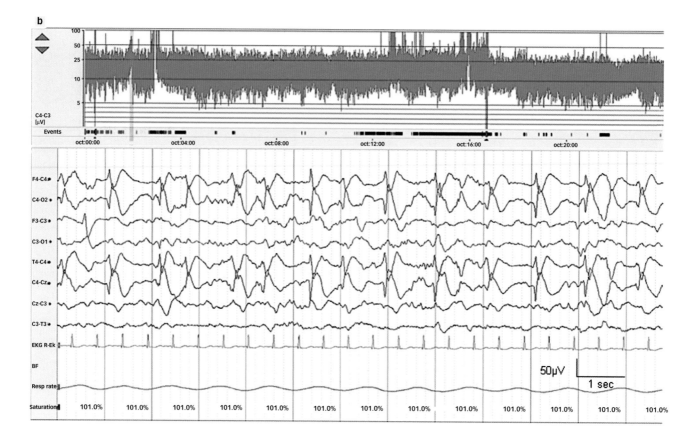

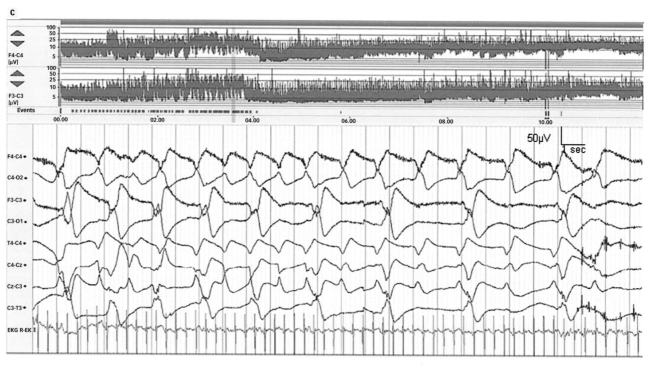

Fig. 7.1. **(cont.)**

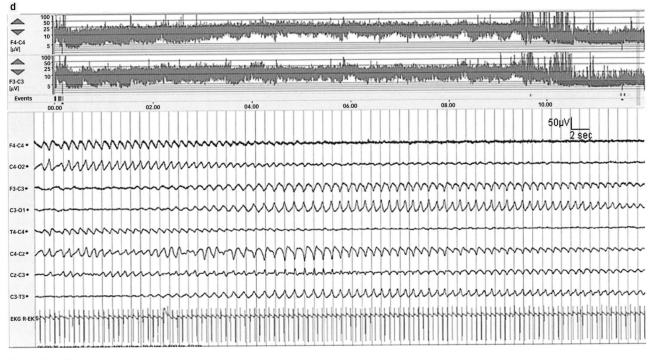

Fig. 7.1. **(cont.)**

of clinical seizures without electrographic discharge is that scalp electrodes are incapable of recording from every part of the brain; depth electrodes reveal an otherwise unsuspected electrical focus in 10% of adult patients. An alternative explanation proposed by Mizrahi's group is that the motor manifestations arise because of discharges from the brainstem and spinal cord, which are "released" because of lack of inhibition from higher centers [33]. In our experience, phenobarbitone treatment temporarily depresses the background EEG but this effect does not interfere with interpretation in the longer term, providing the plasma levels remain within the therapeutic range. Given the importance of the background EEG in the diagnosis and prognosis of neonatal encephalopathy (p. 143) more work needs to be done in this area.

Modern digital EEG systems allow prolonged recordings to be stored and manipulated with ease. These systems are much smaller and more compact than older paper-based analog EEG recorders. Digital files have the advantage that they can be transmitted electronically for interpretation at a remote site. In future, this technology should help to ensure that all babies have access to the limited expertise that is currently available to report neonatal EEG. Automated seizure detection using computerized analysis of EEG remains a "holy grail" in neonatal EEG research. Designing algorithms that can distinguish seizures of differing length and changing morphology from constantly varying background activity often clouded with movement artifact remains a formidable technical challenge. Nevertheless, advances in signal processing methods have also been impressive and there has been a welcome explosion of interest in the field over the last few years [34,35,36,37], which

may yield results, although no algorithm has as yet proved robust enough to be clinically useful.

The routine EEG in neonatal seizure

The duration of a standard EEG is 20–40 min, although 60 min is recommended for the newborn. Whilst there is no doubt that some seizures will be missed unless recording is prolonged beyond an hour, in many cases a standard EEG will show seizure activity [38]. Further, if abnormal background activity is recognized, it is worth continuing the recording because seizure is much more likely. If a limited montage is used, coverage should always include the temporal areas because so many neonatal seizures arise from this region in full-term babies.

Sheth has reported his 11-year experience in attempting confirmation of suspected neonatal seizures with routine 1-h EEG [39]. During this time 183 babies with suspected seizures were studied; 84 had epileptiform discharges on the first EEG and a further 29 on a repeat study. The EEG was normal in 39; this left 31, of whom 20 had electrical silence or a burst-suppression pattern, and 11 had dysmaturity. Sheth noted that confirmation was more likely in term babies (79%). This may have been because it is more difficult to distinguish between normal and abnormal motor activity in a preterm baby, or because of a longer interictal period in preterm babies. The seizure morphology cannot be used to determine the cause, and neither do focal seizures necessarily correlate with a lesion in the corresponding anatomical site [23].

aEEG monitoring in neonatal seizures

Whilst prolonged recording with video-EEG telemetry is the "gold standard" for seizure diagnosis, the equipment is

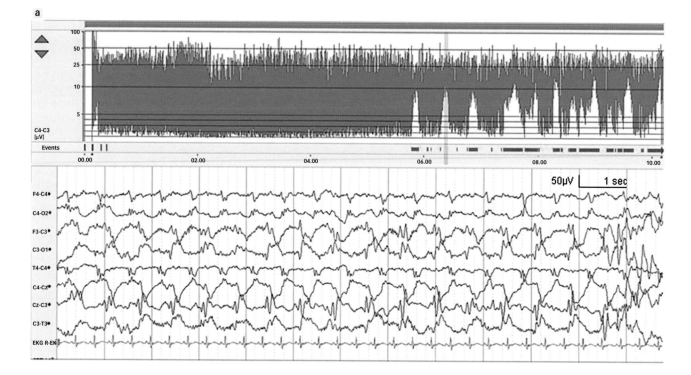

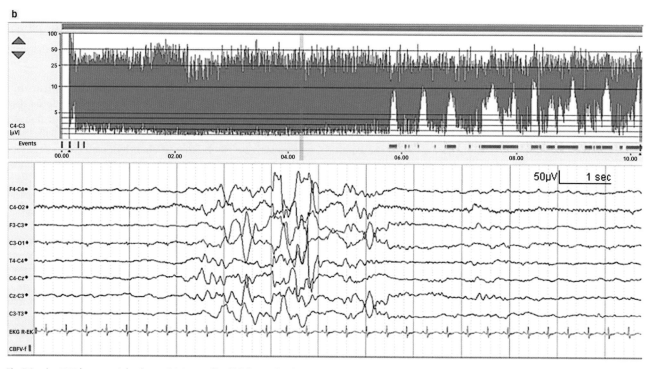

Fig. 7.2a–d. **aEEG in neonatal seizure. (a)** Generalized high-amplitude seizure which is easily seen on EEG. The baseline aEEG becomes saw-tooth. **(b)** Same baby as in (a) but showing background EEG. **(c)** Low-amplitude seizure that is not visible on the aEEG. **(d)** Term baby, very suppressed background EEG 4 h after delivery, seizures mainly not seen on aEEG.

not widely available. Most neonatal units rely on clinical diagnosis alone, supplemented by a routine EEG service. Others use aEEG monitoring. In our view, single-channel aEEG is not a suitable method with which to confirm or refute a diagnosis of neonatal seizure. This is because this method, which relies on a single channel of compressed and filtered EEG, cannot detect short seizures, or focal seizures, or distinguish low-votage seizures from a moderately abnormal

c

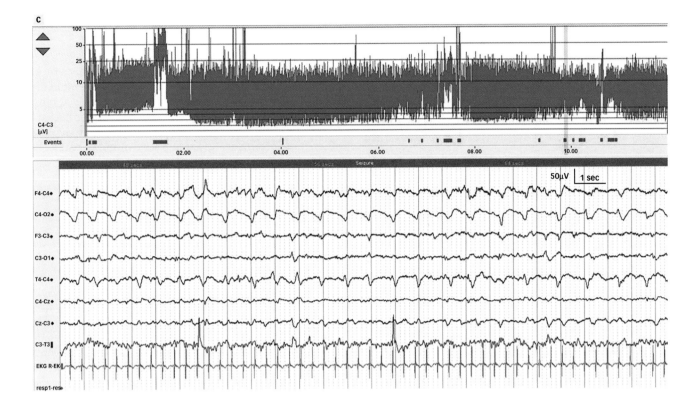

d

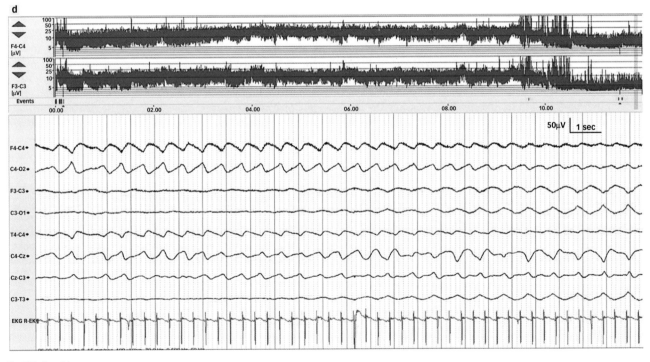

Fig. 7.2. (cont.)

background (Fig. 7.2). In a recent evaluation using four observers only 4/19 seizing babies were correctly identified by all observers, and there was poor intra-observer agreement [40]. Some seizures are easy to spot with aEEG and in these babies the method is ideal for monitoring the response to treatment (Fig. 7.2). We acknowledge that aEEG is better than clinical diagnosis alone, and the current generation of cotside aEEG monitors do offer the opportunity of multi channel recording and access to the raw EEG signal, which improves diagnostic accuracy.

Video-EEG monitoring

Capturing a period of stereotyped movement simultaneously with an electrographic paroxysm is the definitive method with which to diagnose neonatal seizure. Bye and Flanagan [5] used prolonged video-EEG recordings for the diagnosis of neonatal seizure, and reported that 13% of the 31 babies they studied had an interictal period of more than 60 min, implying that conventional EEG would have failed to detect their seizures [5]. However, most of their babies were outborn and had already been treated with antiepileptic drugs prior to the video-EEG study commencing. Our experience with video-EEG is that we confirm the diagnosis of seizure in about 65% of babies referred to us, and we agree with Seth's observations that confirmation is more likely in term babies (he found 79%), suggesting that clinical diagnosis is more reliable in this group. Digital technology has spread to video-EEG too, and the quality of the video recordings is now good enough to identify subtle facial movements. In future, cotside digital video-EEG telemetry will be the "gold standard" method for diagnosis and monitoring of neonatal seizures.

Cranial ultrasound imaging in neonatal seizure

Cranial ultrasound remains the first-line neuroimaging investigation in neonatal seizure. A cranial ultrasound scan should be performed at the first opportunity and repeated frequently thereafter. Sometimes abnormalities only appear after several days, and in other cases the appearances evolve over time.

The possible findings are listed below, and more detail can be found in this chapter regarding arterial and venous infarction, and all forms of intracranial hemorrhage at term. Further details regarding intracranial hemorrhage in preterm babies is given in Chapter 9 and for information regarding the focal abnormalities that can be seen in hypoxic ischemia see Chapter 8.

- Normal (pp. 45–60)
- Intracranial hemorrhage (p. 180–190)
- Focal cerebral infarction (p. 103–114)
- Cerebral edema (p. 146–147)
- Cerebral malformation (p. 251–267)
- Abnormalities of the deep gray matter or watershed areas (p. 154–163)
- Enlarged ventricles (p. 238–250)
- Strands within the ventricles suggesting infection (p. 274–281)

MRI in neonatal seizure

We are in no doubt that a baby with confirmed seizures should undergo magnetic resonance imaging (MRI). MRI provides valuable information regarding the precise nature of the abnormality even when ultrasound abnormalities are present, and this can assist in prognosis. Diffusion-weighted imaging is particularly useful in early stages, showing abnormalities at a time when conventional imaging may be normal. As with early neonatal encephalopathy, if a single MRI is planned the best time to perform the investigation is in the second week.

Diagnostic categories resulting from investigation of neonatal seizure

Neonatal encephalopathy (see Chapter 8)

Early neonatal encephalopathy is the most common cause of seizures in a term baby, and when the seizures present in the first 24 h of life in a baby who required resuscitation at birth and who had an early metabolic acidosis the cause is likely to be hypoxic ischemia, although it is very important to consider other causes of birth depression and early encephalopathy. For further information on the investigation, management, and prognosis of neonatal encephalopathy see Chapter 8.

Focal cerebral infarction or "perinatal arterial stroke"

Diagnosis, etiology, and prevalence

Clinical diagnosis of stroke

Focal arterial infarction, or "stroke" is by far the most likely diagnosis in a term baby whose antenatal course was unremarkable, who was born in a good or mildly depressed condition, and who remains alert between focal seizures which occur in the first few days of life. Stroke is the second most common cause of seizure at term, after hypoxic ischemia [41,42,43]. Neurological examination is usually normal and the baby often has preserved primitive reflexes. The seizures are typically focal, both clinically and on EEG, but they can generalize [44]. The background EEG is usually normal, and the babies are not usually encephalopathic, although they certainly can be [45,46,47]. Ultrasound cannot always detect small focal infarcts, and if the ultrasound scan is normal in this clinical situation then MR must be performed.

Stroke is a specific diagnosis, and should be clearly distinguished from hypoxic ischemia as a cause for neonatal encephalopathy or seizures in the minds of the treating clinicians and the parents. We agree with Karin Nelson, who observes that although early reports of perinatal stroke suggested an association with "birth asphyxia," these studies were done without the benefit of modern imaging techniques, and the association has not been confirmed in current series using a good standard of investigation [48]. Some of the confusion probably arose because some babies with stroke are encephalopathic, and others have a history of "difficult birth" with birth depression and/or a need for some resuscitation at birth. This does not prove that hypoxic ischemia was present or causal, and in a recent population-based case–control study there was no significant difference between cases and controls when a diagnosis of "birth asphyxia" was examined [49]. Perinatal arterial stroke is almost certainly under-diagnosed, because some babies have no abnormal signs in the neonatal period but present later in infancy with a hemiplegia, and hence are diagnosed only retrospectively [50]. Prenatal strokes are probably not as rare as was once thought, and cases have been detected with fetal ultrasonography [51] (Fig. 7.3). A few preterm cases also have been described [52]. The topic of perinatal arterial stroke has excited a great deal of interest in recent years, and has been the subject of several excellent reviews [48,53,54,55].

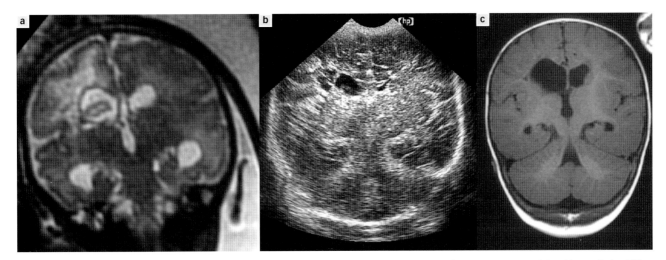

Fig. 7.3a–c. **Antenatal diagnosis of a right middle cerebral artery infarction. (a) A coronal single shot fast spin echo T$_2$-weighted image in fetal life shows intraventricular and ependymal hemorrhage, enlargement of the ventricle, and extensive white matter signal change. (b) Postnatal ultrasound in the baby, born at term, shows early echolucent cavities within the periventricular white matter. The baby was asymptomatic but developed a hemiplegia. (c) The coronal T$_1$-weighted MRI performed several weeks later shows dilatation of the right lateral ventricle and partial collapse of the white matter cavities.**

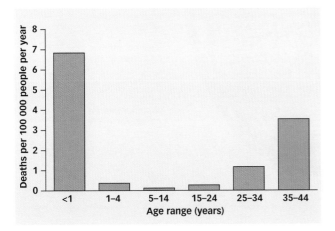

Fig. 7.4. **Mortality from arterial stroke related to age, from Nelson and Lynch with permission [48].**

Prevalence of perinatal arterial stroke

The disorder is not rare, and the frequency of perinatal stroke is estimated at around 1 in 4000–5000 births [42,56,57]. A recent Swiss population-based retrospective study revealed a higher prevalence of 1:2300 term babies, probably because of the liberal use of MRI [58]. This means that stroke is at least 17 times more common in the perinatal period than in later childhood, and the incidence does not rise as high as this again until much later in life (Fig. 7.4). The number of babies who have sustained a perinatal stroke but who do not develop clinical signs is of course impossible to estimate, but two cases were diagnosed with ultrasound in babies recruited to a term screening study at the Hammersmith Hospital in London, and the diagnosis was made in a further baby in a similar study of 2309 normal newborns in Taiwan [59,60]. Nelson and Lynch considered that about a third of all cases did not present in the neonatal period [48].

The most common arterial territory to be affected in cases of neonatal stroke is that of the middle cerebral artery (MCA), usually the left; estimates vary, but at least 75% of perinatal strokes involve the MCA. Infarction can be due to embolism or thrombosis. It is very helpful to have in mind the anatomy of the MCA and its branches, and to be aware of the territory supplied by the major arteries of the brain [52] (Figs. 7.5, 7.6). The territory that can be affected is very variable, but it is more common to see involvement of either the anterior or posterior trunk of the MCA rather than the whole of the main artery [56] (Fig. 7.6). More than one artery can be affected in the same baby, and strokes involving the posterior cerebral artery, the posterior inferior cerebellar artery, and the anterior cerebral artery have all been described. Govaert recently described 24 babies with strokes confined to the perforating branches of the MCA, none of which was a cause of seizures [62]. Neonatal stroke in the territory of the posterior cerebral artery territory is unusual, and in Govaert's series of 40 babies there were no cases although there were 3/47 in the Hammersmith series [56,59]. Bilateral changes are not uncommon: 25% of the cases in the Hammersmith series and 34% of the cases in Sreenan's series had changes on the contralateral side, with a smaller number having definite involvement of more than one arterial territory [59,63]. The full range of contralateral lesions is yet to be determined, because diffusion-weighted MRI can show small areas of abnormality which disappear after a week or so, and are never revealed with other imaging modalities. Rarely, babies have both focal arterial stroke and parasagittal watershed infarction [47].

Causes of perinatal arterial stroke

The etiology of perinatal stroke is not yet fully elucidated and no cause is ever identified in as many as 25%–47% of cases [56,64]. There are a large number of conditions which have been implicated; these are listed in Table 7.4 and discussed here.

One popular explanation for the observation that neonatal stroke is more common in the territory of the left MCA is that many cases are due to emboli from the placenta, which pass easily via the patent foramen ovale to the arterial side of the circulation during fetal life, when the pressure on both sides of the heart is high. Emboli leaving the left side of the heart via the aorta are more likely to pass into the left internal carotid artery and find their way into the left MCA. Histological examination of the placenta reveals "thrombotic vasculopathy" in a surprisingly high number of cases; in some this condition

a

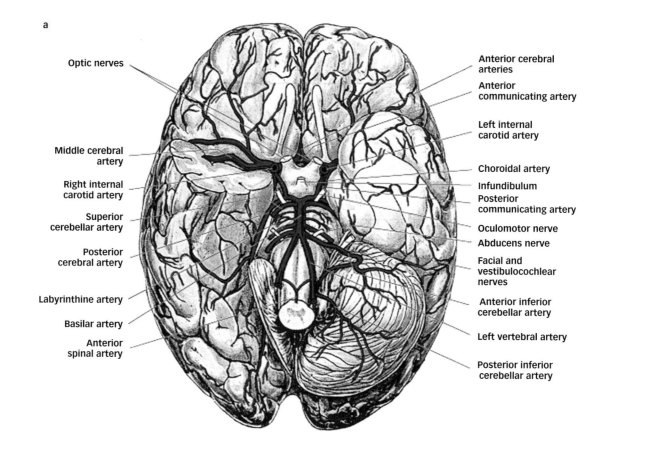

Optic nerves

Middle cerebral artery

Right internal carotid artery

Superior cerebellar artery

Posterior cerebral artery

Labyrinthine artery

Basilar artery

Anterior spinal artery

Anterior cerebral arteries

Anterior communicating artery

Left internal carotid artery

Choroidal artery

Infundibulum

Posterior communicating artery

Oculomotor nerve

Abducens nerve

Facial and vestibulocochlear nerves

Anterior inferior cerebellar artery

Left vertebral artery

Posterior inferior cerebellar artery

b

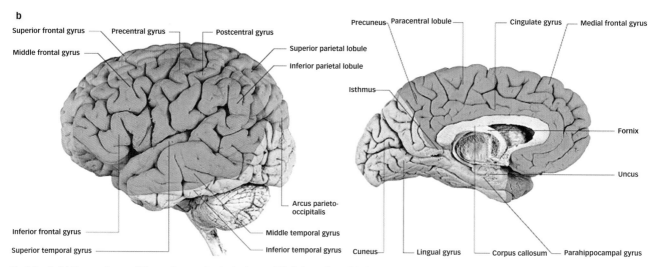

Superior frontal gyrus — Precentral gyrus — Postcentral gyrus

Middle frontal gyrus

Superior parietal lobule

Inferior parietal lobule

Precuneus Paracentral lobule — Cingulate gyrus — Medial frontal gyrus

Isthmus

Fornix

Uncus

Arcus parieto-occipitalis

Inferior frontal gyrus

Middle temporal gyrus

Superior temporal gyrus

Inferior temporal gyrus Cuneus — Lingual gyrus — Corpus callosum — Parahippocampal gyrus

Fig. 7.5a–d. **(a) The anatomy of the major cerebral arteries and their branches. (b) The territory of arterial supply of the major cerebral arteries. (c) Coronal view of the course of the middle cerebral artery and its branches. (d) Surface view of the course of the middle cerebral artery and its branches. (a), (b), (d) reproduced from** *Gray's Anatomy* **39e, www.graysanatomyonline.com, (c) Elsevier Ltd 2005, with permission; (c) reproduced from plate 134, Netter [61] with permission.**

c

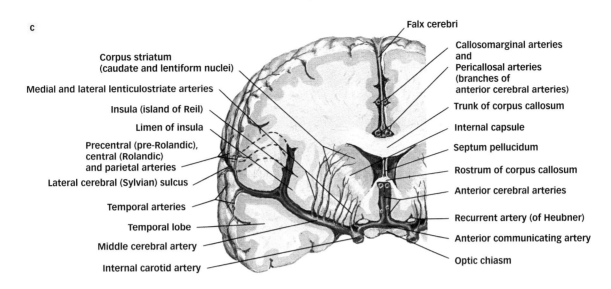

Falx cerebri

Corpus striatum
(caudate and lentiform nuclei)

Medial and lateral lenticulostriate arteries

Insula (island of Reil)

Limen of insula

Precentral (pre-Rolandic),
central (Rolandic)
and parietal arteries

Lateral cerebral (Sylvian) sulcus

Temporal arteries

Temporal lobe

Middle cerebral artery

Internal carotid artery

Callosomarginal arteries
and
Pericallosal arteries
(branches of
anterior cerebral arteries)

Trunk of corpus callosum

Internal capsule

Septum pellucidum

Rostrum of corpus callosum

Anterior cerebral arteries

Recurrent artery (of Heubner)

Anterior communicating artery

Optic chiasm

d

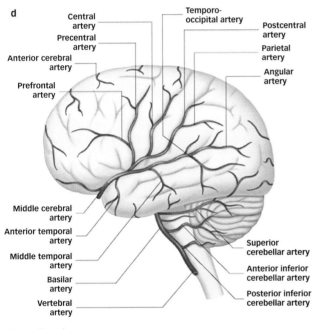

Central
artery

Precentral
artery

Anterior cerebral
artery

Prefrontal
artery

Temporo-
occipital artery

Postcentral
artery

Parietal
artery

Angular
artery

Middle cerebral
artery

Anterior temporal
artery

Middle temporal
artery

Basilar
artery

Vertebral
artery

Superior
cerebellar artery

Anterior inferior
cerebellar artery

Posterior inferior
cerebellar artery

Fig. 7.5. **(cont.)**

appears to be linked to maternal thrombotic disorder [65]. The sick newborn is also at risk of paradoxical emboli because of right-to-left shunting associated with respiratory or heart disease, and stroke has been linked to persistent pulmonary hypertension [56,66,67]. The reason for this may be that the persisting high pressure on the right side of the heart allows paradoxical embolization via the patent foramen ovale in early neonatal life, and because these ill newborns require vascular catheterization. Babies with pulmonary hypertension or meconium aspiration syndrome who require extracorporeal membrane oxygenation (ECMO) are at high risk of stroke [68,69]. Intracardiac thrombi and interventional procedures such as cardiac catheterization and exchange transfusion have long been identified as a cause of stroke. Emboli from umbilical vascular catheters are responsible for some cases [70].

Neonatal stroke does appear to be more common after "complicated" pregnancy and labor; factors such as primigravid mothers, chorioamnionitis, long labors, occipito posterior position, instrumental delivery, and a long second stage have all been implicated [57]. However, as discussed, there is little evidence for hypoxic ischemia as a cause, and there are many cases of stroke reported in babies born normally after uneventful labors, or delivered by elective caesarean section, or in whom the diagnosis clearly antedated the onset of labor. Preeclampsia has also been found to be associated with an increased risk of fetal or neonatal stroke [57]. The reason for these observations may be that these factors increase the risk of placental embolization, or that the babies are observed more carefully in the neonatal period and hence subtle signs of seizure (e.g., apnea) are detected and the diagnosis made.

Further work is needed with careful MR angiography of the neck vessels in neonatal stroke cases in order to elucidate whether carotid artery thrombi and carotid artery dissection are common causes of embolization to the cerebral circulation in the neonatal period: arterial dissection is certainly well recognized as a cause of stroke in older children [71,72]. Another lesson from adult practice which might be relevant is the observation that vasospasm is a complication of blood in the subarachnoid space and this can lead to arterial infarction [73]. Govaert has suggested that the presence of subdural blood, related to traumatic delivery, can cause vasospasm [74]. One old but highly cited case report describes a baby girl who died, in whom there was evidence of intracranial trauma at autopsy, with subarachnoid hemorrhage and widespread hemorrhagic necrosis. The findings included thrombus in the MCA, which was considered to have arisen as a result of a "stretch" injury to the artery itself during the high forceps delivery [75], but in retrospect might also have been due to vasospasm.

Some cases of neonatal stroke have been ascribed to direct trauma of the internal carotid artery in the neck causing dissection of the artery with formation of a thrombus, but the evidence remains largely anecdotal [76,77]. In some babies, carotid artery lesions have been found without a history of

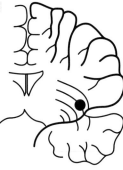
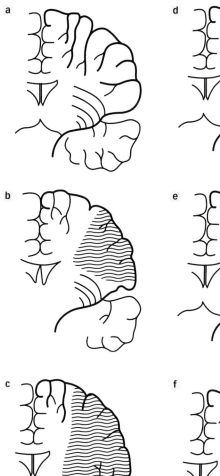
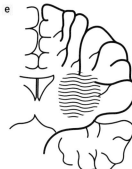
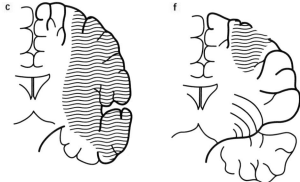

Fig. 7.6a–f. **Schematic drawing showing (a) the different branches of the middle cerebral artery with (b) involvement of a cortical branch, (c) involvement of the main branch, (d) involvement of one or (e) more lenticulostriate arteries and (f) the boundary zone between the anterior and middle cerebral artery. From De Vries *et al.* 1997 with permission [52].**

Table 7.4. Factors which have been identified as increasing the risk of perinatal arterial stroke.

Maternal disorders and maternal complications of pregnancy
　Anticardiolipin antibodies
　Pre-eclamptic toxemia
　Cocaine abuse
　Diabetes mellitus

Fetal complications of pregnancy
　Twin-twin transfusion syndrome

Placental disorders
　Chorioamnionitis
　Placental "thrombotic vasculopathy"

Hematological disorders
　Polycythemia
　Protein C deficiency
　Protein S deficiency
　Factor V Leiden mutation (factor V G1691A)
　Prothrombin G20210A
　MTHFR genotype 677TT or C677 T with high homocysteine levels

Cardiovascular disorders, disorders and manipulation of the blood vessels
　Congenital heart disease, particularly requiring surgery or cardiac catheterization
　Right-to-left shunts associated with pulmonary hypertension
　Internal carotid artery dissection, trauma to the internal carotid artery with thrombus formation
　Umbilical artery and vein catherization, exchange transfusion, ECMO
　Possibly vasospasm associated with significant amounts of blood in the basal cisterns (needs more confirmation, see text)

CNS infection
　Meningitis

Metabolic disorders
　Hyperhomocysteinemia

ECMO, Extra corporeal membrane oxygenation.

trauma [78]. One very interesting case report describes a 5-month-old child whose term delivery was normal, but was a 6-month fetus at the time of a maternal road traffic accident, who had a complete congenital Horner's syndrome, left hemiplegia, and microcephaly [79]. MRI showed a small left cerebral hemisphere with streak flow in the internal carotid artery, and the diagnosis was considered to be a "whiplash" injury to the carotid artery at the level of the neck during fetal life affecting the entire territory of the anterior and middle cerebral arteries.

Pregnancy is a prothrombotic state; there is a heightened maternal thrombotic response with activation of coagulant mechanisms at around the time of birth, probably acquired as a result of an evolutionary adaptation due to the high risk of hemorrhage during labor and the puerperium. The fetal and neonatal hematocrit is high. Recent studies have confirmed that there is a link between inherited thrombotic disorders and neonatal focal arterial infarction, and it may be that an inherited thrombophilic tendency and the procoagulant state of later pregnancy combine to "tip the balance" towards thrombosis at this time, explaining the high incidence of perinatal (and maternal) stroke in this group [80,81]. Hematological disorders associated with perinatal stroke include polycythemia, protein C deficiency, protein S deficiency, antithrombin III deficiency, prothrombin G20210A mutation, factor V Leiden mutation, and methylene tetrahydrofolate reductase variant (MTHFR) [50,80,82,83,84,85,86]. In one study 62 of 91 (68%) neonatal stroke cases had at least one prothrombotic risk factor compared to 24% of controls [80,87], and the risk was higher when more than one prothrombotic risk factor was present [64]. Only one recent study contradicts the wealth of evidence supporting the role of prothrombotic risk factors in neonatal stroke; a series of 59 neonates with arterial or venous stroke were not distinguishable from 437 normal babies in California when a range of gene polymorphisms was examined [88]. Debate continues about the role of the MTHFR variant. The heterozygous state, with C677 T MTHFR producing a "thermolabile" variant, is very common in Caucasian populations (about 44%). Some heterozygotes and those who are homozygous, with the MTHFR 677TT genotype, have hyperhomocystinemia (particularly if folate and vitamin B_{12} levels are low). High homocysteine levels do appear to be a risk factor for thrombosis [89], and Nowak-Gottl *et al.* [90] have suggested that MTHFR gene testing should be omitted from thrombophilia screens and replaced with estimation of homocysteine levels. Certainly it is the level of homocysteine which appears to be important, and affected individuals can reduce their levels with dietary manipulation and supplementation. Details of our current "thrombophilia" screen are given in Table 7.5, and it is important to carry out the tests 3–6 months after the acute episode and to use appropriate infant normal ranges when interpreting the results [90].

Maternal antiphospholipid antibodies (including lupus anticoagulant and anticardiolipin) can also predispose to perinatal arterial stroke, probably because phospholipids are involved in the activation of protein C and in the coagulation pathway [91,92,93]. On occasion, the diagnosis of perinatal arterial stroke has led to the diagnosis of antiphospholipid antibody syndrome in the mother [94]. Nelson and her colleagues found elevated levels of anticardiolipin antibodies and inflammatory mediators (interleukins and tumor necrosis factor) in neonatal blood samples from children with cerebral palsy compared to controls [95]. Other maternal diseases that have been implicated in neonatal thrombotic disorders with vascular occlusions (not just stroke) include diabetes mellitus [96].

Perinatal arterial stroke in the preterm infant
A recent hospital-based study by de Vries demonstrates that perinatal arterial stroke is not uncommon in preterm infants with a gestational age ≤34 weeks, with an incidence of 7/1000 [52,97]. This relatively high incidence may be explained by the use of routine cranial ultrasound in this population and possibly by their exposure to more invasive procedures during their stay in the neonatal intensive care unit. Interestingly, risk factors for perinatal arterial stroke in the preterm infant differ from those in the term infant: fetal heart rate abnormalities and the presence of twin-to-twin transfusion syndrome (see Chapter 10) were independent risk factors. Hypoglycemia was the only independent risk factor identified in the immediate neonatal period. As in the term population, the majority of strokes involved the MCA (81%); however, the involvement of different branches of the MCA changed with gestational age. Involvement of one or more lenticulostriate branches was most common among infants with a gestational age of 28–32 weeks (Fig. 7.7).

Table 7.5. Investigations to be performed in babies with focal aterial infarction ("perinatal arterial stroke"); tests are best carried out 3 months after the acute episode. Similar investigations should be considered in babies with venous thrombosis.

Blood tests
Blood cell count
Ratio of prothrombin time to partial thromboplastin time
Protein C activity
Protein S activity
Factor V111c
Von Willebrand factor
Antithrombin activity
Phospholipid antibodies
Cardiolipin antibodies
Homocysteine levels
Lipoprotein a
Plasminogen
Fibrinogen
Amino acids

Genetic tests
Factor V Leiden mutation
Prothrombin G20210A mutation
MTHFR mutation (see text, some suggest homocysteine levels are sufficient because the heterozygous MTHFR mutation is so common)

Urine tests
Organic and amino acids

Tests on parents who wish to undergo screening
Thrombophilia screen on mother and father as below:
Blood cell count
Ratio of prothrombin time to partial thromboplastin time
Protein C activity
Protein S activity
Antithrombin activity
Phospholipid antibodies
Cardiolipin antibodies
Lipoprotein a
Plasminogen
Fibrinogen
Factor V111c
Von Willebrand factor
Factor V Leiden mutation
Prothrombin G20210A mutation
MTHFR mutation

MTHFR, Methylene tetrahydrofolate reductase.

The EEG in neonatal stroke
Babies with stroke frequently have clinical seizures which are usually focal, although generalized seizures have been described [44,98]. A corresponding focus with spikes and/or

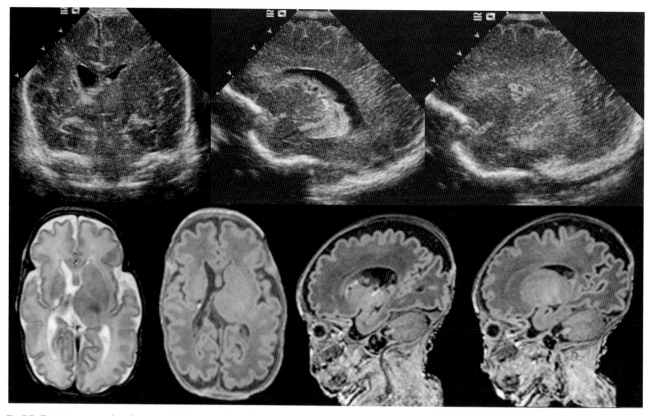

Fig. 7.7. **Top row: coronal and parasagittal images show the cystic changes within the basal ganglia of a preterm infant of 28 weeks of gestation at term-equivalent age. The lesion was first seen as a wedge-shaped increased echogenicity in the basal ganglia at 30 weeks of corrected gestational age. Bottom row: axial T₂- and T₁-weighted, and parasagittal T₁-weighted MR images at term-equivalent age show mature right thalamic caudate and white matter damage with cavitation and volume loss in keeping with infarction. The last parasagittal MR image shows normal left side.**

sharp waves on the EEG is also common [98,99], but the background EEG is usually normal [100]. Periodic lateralized epileptiform discharges (PLEDS) have been described as an early characteristic feature of neonatal stroke [101]. The location of electrographic seizures corresponded to the area of infarction in seven babies with pulmonary hypertension [67]. Prolonged EEG recording is undoubtedly useful in babies with definite cerebral pathology and clinical seizures. Babies with stroke and an abnormal background EEG in the neonatal period probably have a worse outlook than those whose background activity remains normal [46,100].

Imaging diagnosis of neonatal stroke

Ultrasound imaging is insensitive for the diagnosis of stroke, and the findings can be normal even when the diagnosis is confirmed with MRI and the ultrasound images are examined with the benefit of hindsight [102]. In the cases of neonatal stroke that can be diagnosed with ultrasound the usual appearance is initially an increased echogenicity and asymmetry in the region of the Sylvian fissure (Fig. 7.8a,b). Repeated ultrasound imaging is often required to demonstrate the abnormalities, which may only reveal changes after the third day [59]. There can be midline shift, and the ventricle on the affected side is often compressed. Sometimes extensive infarction of the territory of the MCA leaves an area that is paradoxically "bright" because it is supplied by the anterior cerebral artery

and hence is the only perfused area on that side of the brain (Fig. 7.9). Small wedge-shaped areas of infarction in the caudate nuclei, thalami or putamina can be seen which are due to involvement of a lenticulostriate or perforating branches of the MCA, but the lesions are not always of the classic triangular shape [62]. These small branches appear more likely to be affected in preterm babies [97]. The echodense lesions progress to cavity formation, or resolution.

Doppler ultrasound studies of the intracranial arteries have been of limited value in the diagnosis and assessment of neonatal stroke. Coker et al. found no significant difference in the cerebral blood flow velocity in the left and right MCAs in 15 cases of neonatal stroke [103], although others have found transient abnormalities of flow velocity in a few cases [104].

The MRI findings vary from tiny areas of infarction in the area of the internal capsule through an area supplied by a branch of the MCA to massive involvement of almost the whole hemisphere or both MCA territories (Fig. 7.10a–c). The internal capsule can only be identified with MRI, and because the prognosis is in part determined by whether there is involvement of the internal capsule (see below), MRI is helpful for prognostic purposes even when the diagnosis of stroke has been made with confidence using ultrasound.

Diffusion-weighted (DW) MRI can show ischemic change within hours of onset, and is the most sensitive technique for

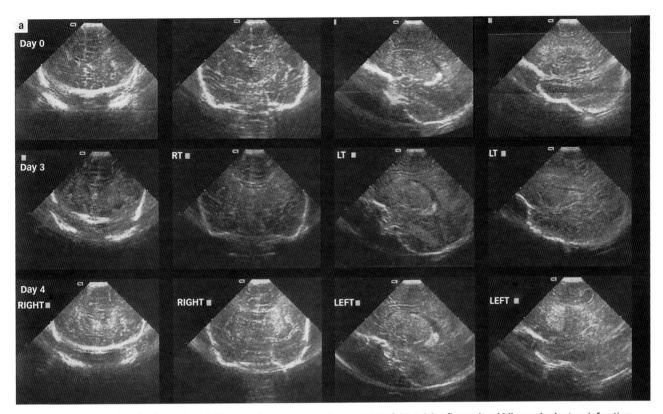

Fig. 7.8a,b. **Ultrasound** imaging in stroke. (a) Ultrasound appearances of asymmetry of the Sylvian fissure in middle cerebral artery infarction. This term infant presented with seizures on day 2 of life. The top row shows the images obtained on admission with normal appearances. On day 4 an area of increased echogenicity was seen in the territory of the middle cerebral artery resulting in an asymmetry of the Sylvian fissure (corresponding MR images in Fig. 7.10c). (b) This term infant presented with focal seizures of the right arm at 6 h of age. The top row shows the images obtained on day 2; the bottom row, day 11. The scan on admission was normal. There are subtle abnormalities in the region of the left Sylvian fissure, more prominent on day 11. The MRI from the same case is shown in Fig. 7.10a.

the early diagnosis of stroke [105,106,107,108]. Serial imaging demonstrates that, as expected, the changes seen with DW MRI are transient, and "pseudonormalization" occurs in the first week (earlier than in adult cases) [108,109] (Fig. 7.10b). Diffusion-weighted imaging with apparent diffusion coefficient (ADC) mapping at the level of the cerebral peduncles has been used to identify abnormality in this region, and in the posterior limb of the internal capsule, early in acute arterial stroke, and was predictive of outcome [110]. Conventional MRI, in contrast, can be normal in the early stages and show abnormalities only on follow-up scans, although after the first week diagnosis has to rest mainly on T_2-weighted MRI [108]. The thalamus on the side of the lesion can shrink in the months following the stroke, a finding thought to be due to retrograde neuronal degeneration [111]. Wallerian degeneration can also occur, manifesting as abnormal signal intensity and reduced volume in the brainstem (Fig. 7.11).

Special investigations in babies with stroke

Once the diagnosis of a neonatal stroke has been confirmed, the baby (and his parents, if they wish) should undergo thrombophilia screening although testing is best delayed for at least 6 weeks to allow low neonatal levels to recover. Our current thrombophilia screen is given in Table 7.5.

Treatment and prognosis of neonatal stroke

There is no specific treatment for stroke. Seizures should be controlled. As yet, no treatment for inherited thrombophilic tendencies is recommended, with the exception of folate and B_{12} supplementation for babies with high homocysteine levels related to their MTHFR status. Thrombolytic therapy is probably not an option in the acute phase because of the risk of hemorrhage, and there are few reports of its use (or the use of aspirin) in neonatal stroke. All four of the cases studied carefully with MRI in Tubigen were heparinized (1.5 mg/kg per day), with no evidence of bleeding complications [108], but experience is limited and we do not currently advise anticoagulation in babies found to have an arterial stroke.

The recurrence risk for stroke appears to be very low, even in the presence of a thrombophilic disorder, although children with more than one inherited thrombophilic factor who had venous thrombosis in the neonatal period may be at increased risk of future thrombotic events [112,113]. The childhood stroke study group followed up 215 neonates with arterial ischemic stroke for a median time of 3.5 years, during which 7 children (3.3%) developed symptomatic thromboembolism – 5 of these children had a prothrombotic risk factor and the second event was often triggered by a specific underlying problem such as immobilization or mastoiditis [112].

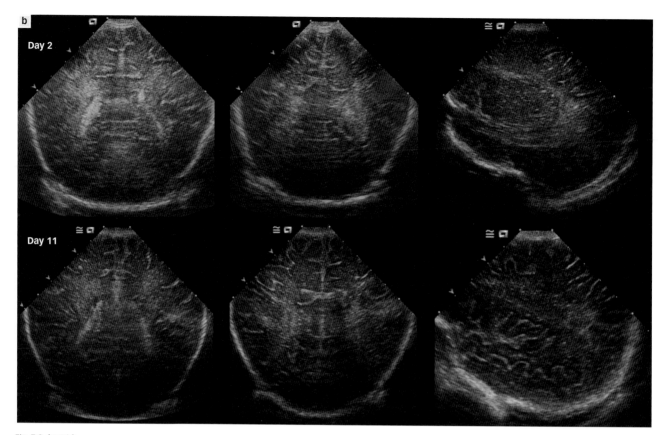

Fig. 7.8 **(cont.)**

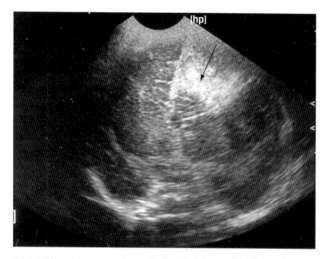

Fig. 7.9. **The appearance of paradoxical "brightness" in the territory of the anterior cerebral artery, which is the only remaining perfused part of the brain in extensive middle cerebral artery infarction. The normal brain, which appears bright, is arrowed.**

Adverse outcomes include hemiparesis, visual field defects, epilepsy, language delay, and behavioral problems, although many children escape without any deficit and most are mobile [42,114,115,116]. All of the outcome studies so far show that the outcome for babies with stroke is better than that for older children and adults [117,118,119]. This is probably due to the plasticity of the newborn brain, and babies with stroke are able to preserve and use some of the ipsilateral connecting pathways which would normally "drop out" during development. Estimates of the risk of disability vary, and many of children in older series were not imaged with MRI, hence only those who presented with neonatal seizures and could be detected with ultrasound or computed tomography (CT) were included. One large single center study from Toronto which enrolled babies born between 1992 and 1999 found that 11/33 (33%) of those who sustained a perinatal arterial stroke had no neurological deficit [117]. Lynch and Nelson [120] estimated that 40% of infants with perinatal stroke were later neurologically normal [120], and in another follow-up study, 15 of 46 (33%) children had a normal outcome; the others had cerebral palsy and/or cognitive impairment [63]. The size of the lesion alone is not always a good guide to prognosis, but in general small infarcts in the territory of the posterior cerebral or the posterior cortical branches of the MCA have a good prognosis [59], whereas large cortical infarcts involving Broca's area around the inferior frontal gyrus do worse [121]. Govaert speculated that involvement of the anterior trunk was more likely to produce upper limb hemiplegia whereas damage in the distribution of the posterior trunk tended to be associated with spatial and orientation disturbances [56]. Children with involvement of the internal capsule, even when the lesion is very small, are more likely to develop hemiplegia, and involvement of the internal capsule, hemisphere, and basal ganglia was a poor

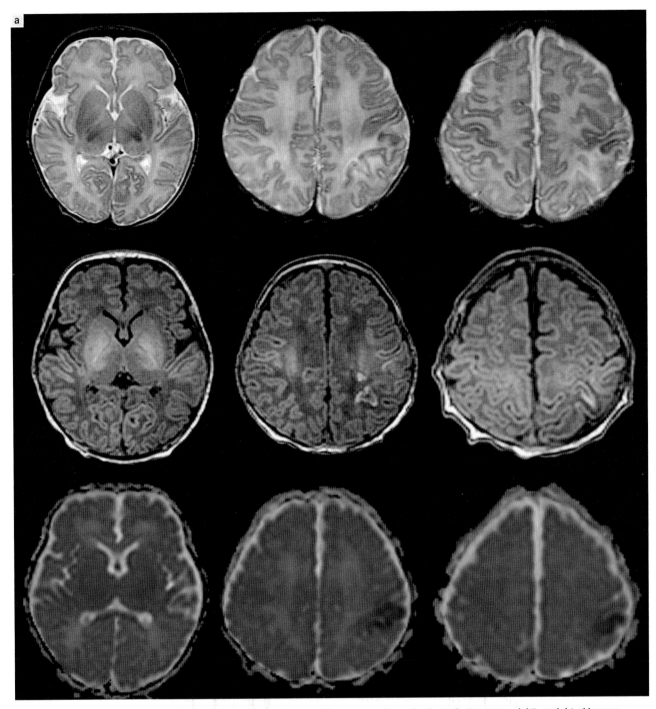

Fig. 7.10a–c. (a) MRI images done on day 7, of a baby whose ultrasound images are shown in Fig. 7.8b. Top row: axial T_2-weighted images show increased signal within the cortex and white matter, with loss of the cortical ribbon in keeping with edema, and hypointensity within the cortex in keeping with hemorrhagic products. Middle row: axial T_1-weighted images show cortical highlighting. Bottom row: apparent diffusion coefficient (ADC) maps show restricted diffusion in the same area shown as abnormal on the T_2-weighted scans. This is consistent with an infarct in the left middle cerebral artery (MCA). (b) Axial T_2-weighted scans show increased signal involving cortex and white matter in the right MCA territory in keeping with a subacute infarct in another case. The ADC map shows regions of normal and increased diffusion as pseudonormalization occurs. (c) Axial T_2-weighted image at 4.7 T shows an acute left MCA infarct with swelling and increased signal within the white matter and cortex, left head of caudate nucleus and lateral lentiform nucleus.

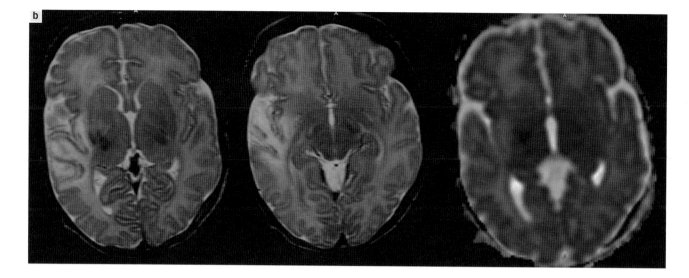

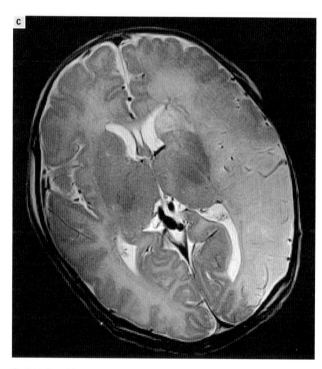

Fig. 7.10 **(cont.)**

and we do not currently amend our counseling regarding the prognosis when a diagnosis of factor V Leiden deficiency is made. Visual field defects, delay in visual maturation, and abnormal results on tests of cortical visual processing were found in 6/16 (38%) of one group of children with stroke [122].

Children with hemiplegia have always been noted to have a high risk of learning disability (especially with language) and neuropsychiatric problems [123], and these difficulties were noted in as many as 25% in one large follow-up study [121]. Many children with hemiplegic cerebral palsy have fidgety behavior, poor concentration, and distractibility which affects their education and their lives, although of course these problems are not confined to such children. Some have attention deficit hyperactivity disorders and a small number have autistic features, with intense and peculiar preoccupations with objects such as washing machines, toy cars, or long bits of string, and impoverished and repetitive imaginative play. Unsurprisingly, the risk of epilepsy increases over time, and after a seizure-free interval of between 1 and 8 years 3 out of 14 children with stroke required antiepileptic medication in one study [115]; more than half of 29 children required AEDs at some point in childhood in another, and 39% of the Toronto group had postnatal seizures [121,124].

Extracranial hemorrhage

Subgaleal (subaponeurotic) hemorrhage

The subgaleal space is a large potential space which lies in the loose connective tissue below the skin of the scalp; to be precise it lies between the epicranial aponeurosis of the scalp and the periosteum of the bone (Fig. 7.12). Bleeding into this space is a serious and potentially life-threatening complication of delivery, and there is a very strong association with delivery using a vacuum cup [125,126,127,128]. The incidence of subgaleal hematoma has been estimated as 7 per 1000 vacuum deliveries compared to around 1 per 1000 normal births [129,130]. Hospitals with active surveillance programs have estimated the incidence to be much higher than this, reporting

prognostic combination in two series (probably overlapping) of 19 and 28 neonatal cases [100,118]. Early demonstration of involvement of the internal capsule has been achieved with ADC mapping using DWI MRI [110]. The motor disability is usually spastic hemiplegic cerebral palsy and there were no cases of dystonia in the neonates who were followed up at the Hammersmith. These workers also found that babies who were heterozygous for factor V Leiden had a worse prognosis than those without this thrombophilic risk factor, and all the children with this genetic mutation and stroke developed a hemiplegia. These results have not been confirmed, however,

figures of 19.7 and 210 per 1000 vacuum deliveries [131,132]. The risk appears to be increased with increased cup application time, number of pulls, cup pop-offs, and a deflexed (occipito-posterior) cup position [133]. Current guidelines generally suggest using no more than four pulls and a maximum cup

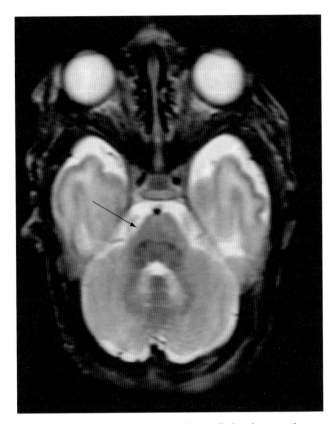

Fig. 7.11. **Axial T$_2$-weighted image showing Wallerian degeneration (arrow); this image is of the same infant as in Fig. 7.7.**

application time of 20 min with a negative suction pressure of no more than 0.8 kg/m^2 [132]. The type of cup may be important; soft cups such as the Kiwi or Mighty-Vac are associated with less scalp trauma but a higher failure rate, which may reach 50% in babies with occipito-posterior presentations.

The diagnosis should be suspected if there is a fluctuant swelling which crosses suture lines, and suspicion should be heightened if a baby who was delivered with the Ventouse fails to respond to resuscitation, or collapses in the hours following delivery [132,134]. The head circumference may enlarge by several centimeters, and the amount of blood contained can be considerable (Fig. 7.13) [135]. The only effective treatment is intensive care support with replacement of blood and blood products, and massive volumes may be required. Neurosurgical drainage has nothing to offer. There is a significant mortality associated with subgaleal hematoma, around 20% in most series [130,131]. If effective volume replacement is achieved and there is no associated intracranial lesion the prognosis is good [131]. The lowest mortality ever reported (2.8%) was from the prospective series collected in Kuala Lumpur, which supports the observation that some cases are diagnosed too late for intensive care support to reverse the spiral of acidosis and hypoxic ischemia (including myocardial ischemia, renal failure, and disseminated intravascular coagulation) which the hypovolemic shock has triggered [132].

Intracranial hemorrhage

Etiology and prevalence

Diagnosis and management of this life-threatening and potentially disabling condition remains a challenging problem. Hanigan estimated the incidence of intracranial bleeding as 5:10 000 at term; the condition is much more common in preterm babies [136]. Suspicion of intracranial hemorrhage should

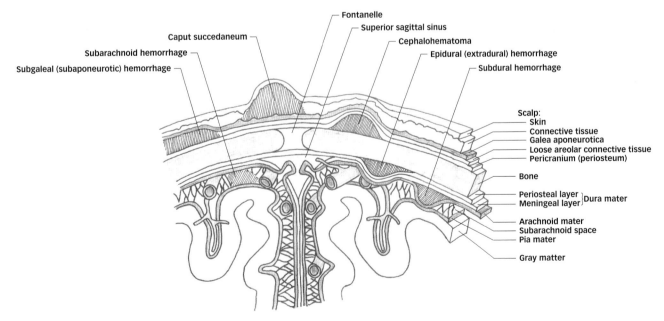

Fig. 7.12. **A diagram showing the layers of the scalp and coverings of the brain.**

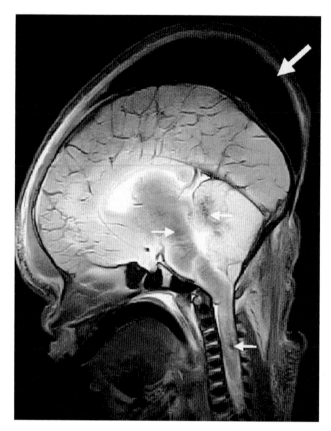

Fig. 7.13. **Large subgaleal collection: sagittal magnetic resonance scan at 4.7 T. The large arrow indicates subgaleal hemorrhage, the small arrows indicate signal intensity changes indicative of hemorrhagic infarction (from Cheong *et al*. with permission [135]).**

be raised if a baby is pale with a tense fontanelle and a moulded head after difficult delivery; heavily bloodstained CSF is obtained after an easy lumbar puncture; the baby has extensive petechiae and a low platelet count; there are seizures; or there is a family history of a bleeding diathesis. At the same time as arranging for investigation of the baby's neurological status, it is important to consider predisposing factors. Most important are underlying hematological disorders such as vitamin K deficiency bleeding, hemophilia A or B, or neonatal alloimmune thrombocytopenic purpura (NAITP). Sometimes bleeding arises from an arteriovenous malformation or a tumor. Neonatal liver disease often presents with vitamin K deficiency, and alpha-1-antitrypsin deficiency has presented with intracranial bleeding [137]. Cord abnormalities and thrombosis of the umbilical vein are rare causes of in utero intracranial hemorrhage [138].

Many conditions including NAITP can cause intracranial bleeding during intrauterine life [139]. Other cases are due to hemorrhagic venous infarction associated with cranial venous sinus thrombosis (sometimes termed a "venous stroke," see below) rather than a primary bleeding problem. Obstetric trauma remains an important cause of intracranial hemorrhage at term, particularly subdural hemorrhage [140,141]. A recent review reported that the outcome of fetal intracranial hemorrhage was poor, with 79 intracerebral, 10 infratentorial, and 20 subdural cases [142].

In a term baby with a low platelet count it is important to pursue investigation of the mother's platelet group and her platelet antibody status, because if the diagnosis is NAITP the condition is likely to recur in the next pregnancy and she will need advice from a specialist fetal medicine center. A male baby may be the first in his family with hemophilia, and if the diagnosis is missed his intracranial bleed will continue to enlarge and could prove fatal. If he dies without the diagnosis being made the opportunity to offer antenatal diagnosis in the next pregnancy will be lost. The risk of intracranial hemorrhage in a hemophiliac is greater in the newborn period than at any other time of life (about 1%–4%), and devastating bleeds have occurred even after caesarean section delivery. Some consider that this risk is sufficiently high to justify prophylaxis to a male baby who has had antenatal diagnosis or is at very high risk of having hemophilia [143]. Others suggest that prophylactic treatment increases the risk of later antibody formation against factor VIII rendering subsequent treatment more difficult, and is not indicated given the level of risk in the neonatal period.

Cerebral sino venous thrombosis
The increasing use of MR imaging has facilitated the diagnosis of sino venous thrombosis, and it has now become apparent that sino venous occlusion is a relatively common cause of intracranial hemorrhage (hemorrhagic venous infarction) in term babies, and later in life [144,145]. The Canadian registry study estimated the incidence as 0.67 per 100 000 children per year, with 43% of the cases being less than a month old at diagnosis [146]. The German thrombophilia registry reported a higher incidence, of 2.6/100 000 neonates per year [147]. As in adult patients, the sagittal and transverse sinuses are most commonly involved, with occasional involvement of the sigmoid or straight sinuses, the torcula, the internal cerebral veins or the vein of Galen (Fig. 7.14a,b) [145,146,148].

Sino venous thrombosis has been associated with all the thrombotic risk factors that have been implicated in perinatal arterial stroke, such as protein C or S deficiency, factor V Leiden mutation, antiphospholipid antibodies, infection, or polycythemia [147,148,150,151,152,153,154]. The list of implicated factors extends to include maternal diabetes mellitus, pre-eclamptic toxemia, neonatal congenital heart disease, ECMO and sepsis [148,154,155,156]. As with perinatal arterial stroke, it seems to be the combination of a prothrombotic risk factor with either another risk factor or an underlying condition that places the baby at most risk of sino venous thrombosis [147]. In general, it is now clear that the prothrombotic tendency associated with pregnancy is a risk factor for cerebral venous sinus thrombosis as well as stroke in both mother and baby [145], and no cause other than this generally increased risk is found in a relatively large number of cases. Hypernatremic dehydration was considered to be the cause of an extensive thrombosis of the sagittal and transverse sinusus in one baby with a 23% weight loss and a serum sodium of 171 mmol/l [157]. This baby was treated with heparin and urokinase. The clue to the diagnosis in

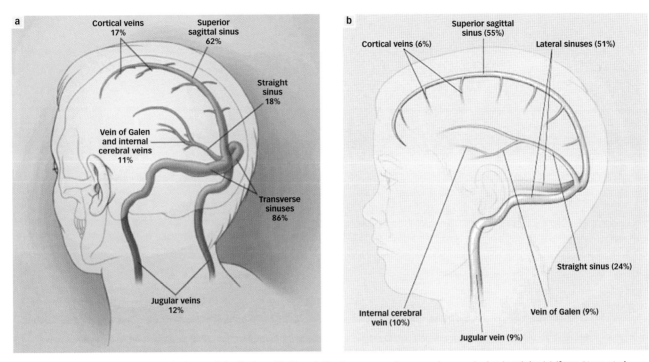

Fig. 7.14a–c. **Anatomy of the venous drainage of the brain, with the relative frequency of venous sinus occlusion in adults (a) (from Stam *et al*. with permission [146]) and in infants and children (b) (from De Veber *et al*. with permission [147]).**

this case was a high CSF protein and elevated D-dimers. Another case associated with hypernatremic dehydration has been described from Turkey [158]. In a further parallel with perinatal arterial stroke, there appears to be a link with "difficult" instrumental delivery [159], perhaps because of distortion or trauma to the vascular endothelium forming a nidus for clot formation at this time of generally heightened thrombotic response.

Cerebral venous sinus thrombosis characteristically presents with the sudden onset of seizures in the newborn [148,160], but (like arterial strokes) some cases are detected only with imaging carried out for another reason [159]. Some babies present with vomiting, hypotonia, lethargy, and poor feeding and a high index of suspicion is required in order to make the correct diagnosis in this situation [148,154,161]. Quite often the clinical signs are subtle in the presence of surprisingly extensive involvement of the deep venous sinuses (Fig. 7.14c). The most sensitive investigation for the diagnosis of suspected sino venous thrombosis is probably CT with venography, but the radiation dose is considerable. As in perinatal ischemic (arterial) stroke, the increasing availability of MRI has undoubtedly resulted in an increased awareness of sino venous thrombosis, which was previously under-diagnosed. Doppler ultrasound findings led to consideration of the diagnosis in a number of cases in Sydney [155]. It is possible that, like arterial stroke, venous sinus thrombosis can occur in fetal life and a few cases have been reported in which unilateral periventricular venous infarction was thought to have occurred in this way; the babies had focal gliosis at the site of the presumed infarct and the lateral ventricles had a normal contour [162].

As yet, it is not clear whether anticoagulation is indicated in babies found to have venous thrombosis, and discussions regarding possible randomized controlled trials in this area continue. The tendency for many of the associated venous infarctions to become hemorrhagic raises obvious concerns about the risk of anticoagulation. Endovascular thrombolysis is not usually an option for the affected neonate at present, and interventional neuroradiology is generally limited to treatment of vein of Galen aneurysms (p. 267); nevertheless, direct thrombolytic therapy has been tried [163]. If there is no associated venous infarction, the prognosis is generally good and the venous sinuses usually recanalize after a period of time, so that treatment may not be necessary; 77% of the children in the Canadian registry study had no sequelae at 2 years [117,146,161,164]. The outlook is understandably worse when there is associated infarction of the cortex, periventricular white matter, or deep gray matter [148].

An understanding of the epidemiology of sino venous thrombosis in neonates and children is necessary to develop interventional strategies. The Candian Pediatric Ischemic Stroke Registry was established in 1992 and aims to obtain comprehensive prospective epidemiologic data on stroke, including sino venous thrombosis. One important goal is to determine a global terminology for stroke and a working party has been set up with this objective.

Subarachnoid hemorrhage

Subarachnoid hemorrhage is common in babies who are born by normal vaginal delivery, and the incidence is higher

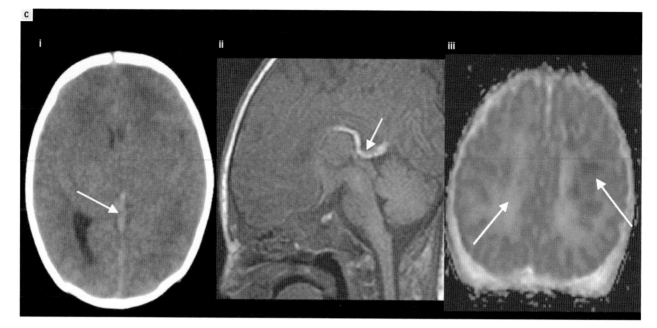

Fig. 7.14a–c. **(cont.) (c) Internal cerebral vein thrombosis (white arrow) and thalamic venous infarction (short white arrow). (i) A CT shows hyperdense thrombus within the internal cerebral veins (arrow). There is diffuse cerebral swelling in addition to marked bithalamic swelling and low density change in keeping with venous infarction. (ii) The sagittal T$_1$-weighted image shows hyperintense thrombus within internal cerebral vein and vein of Galen (arrow). (iii) The ADC map shows areas both of increased and restricted diffusion (arrow).**

following an instrumental birth [140,165]. Subarachnoid hemorrhage does not usually cause neonatal signs although some babies have seizures, but the condition is not a cause of long-term disability unless there is another intracranial lesion [166]. Further, many of the studies reporting seizures and adverse outcome after subarachnoid hemorrhage were done before MRI was widely available, meaning that associated intracerebral lesions were likely to have been missed [167].

Subdural hemorrhage

General points about subdural hemorrhage in babies
Massive subdural hemorrhage is fortunately now rare, although modern neuroimaging has revealed that small clinically unsuspected subdural collections are very common, particularly after vaginal delivery, with an increased risk after instrumental vaginal delivery in many studies [168,169,170,171,172,173]. Subdural hematomas in the neonatal period are often caused by tentorial tears, and small subdural collections around the falx cerebri or tentorium probably account for the frequent observation of high red cell counts in "normal" neonatal CSF [172]. Interestingly, one of the spin-offs of the MRI studies in babies with congenital heart disease before and after surgery has been the incidental finding that significant numbers have small subdural collections along the tentorium [174]. All the recent MRI studies showed that

the vast majority of neonatal subdural hematomas are peritentorial. As with arterial and venous stroke, better imaging with MRI has revealed more and more cases; Whitby and her colleagues described an incidence of 8% using 0.2-T MRI whereas Looney *et al.* [170,171] used 3-T MRI and found subdural hematomas in 26% of babies who had been born vaginally. Most of these smaller collections resolve within 4 weeks, do not cause any neonatal signs, and do not require treatment; it is as important to recognize this group in order to advise the parents accordingly and to avoid over-treatment as it is to identify the baby who is in need of urgent neurosurgical referral.

Subdural hemorrhage is associated with instrumental delivery, and in the large Californian series the risk was increased if the delivery was achieved by vacuum or forceps, and was particularly high if both these instruments failed and urgent operative delivery was required [140]. The risk is also high after a vaginal breech delivery [175], and breech babies can develop occipital osteodiastasis, which can give rise to posterior fossa subdural bleeding and damage to the cerebellum [176,177]. Subdural hematoma can develop in utero, either with or without apparent trauma [178,179]. Volpe discusses how the abnormal forces which are created during delivery with Ventouse or forceps can tear the tentorium or the bridging veins [180]. Tentorial tears from rupture of the straight sinus, the transverse sinus, or the vein of Galen can cause infratentorial bleeding, which can rapidly prove fatal. Bleeding that extends only supratentorially is usually less disastrous. Rupture of the superficial bridging veins results in a convexity subdural hemorrhage.

The clinical presentation includes that of a baby who is comatose from birth, with eye deviation, neck rigidity, and opisthotonos who rapidly develops fixed dilated pupils and dies, a baby who presents after a lucid interval of 12 h to several days after birth who then develops a tense fontanelle, irritability/seizures and perhaps a third nerve palsy, and a baby who presents late because of a slowly enlarging head [181]. As discussed above, many babies with small peritentorial subdural hematomas do not have neurological signs in the neonatal period.

Ultrasound is not reliable for the detection of subdural collections, particularly in the posterior fossa, but large collections over the convexity of the brain can be seen (Fig. 7.15). If subdural hemorrhage is suspected in the neonatal period the diagnosis must be confirmed with high-quality neuroimaging, at least CT and preferably MRI (Fig. 7.16a,b).

Convexity subdural hemorrhage

This type of subdural hemorrhage carries the best prognosis, and 80% of such cases in one Canadian study were normal at follow-up [182]. Large convexity subdural collections can be detected by ultrasound (Fig. 7.15) but the method is not reliable, and if there is a high index of suspicion CT or MRI must be arranged. Subdural tears associated with skull fractures can on occasion be the cause of a "growing fracture," a condition unique to infancy. In this condition subarachnoid fluid herniates through the dural tear and the fracture (or suture) line, keeping the bone edges apart and preventing healing of the

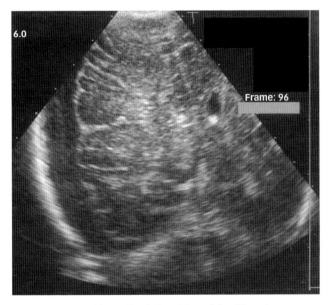

Fig. 7.15 **Ultrasound image in a baby with a subdural hematoma.**

skull fracture [183,184]. The condition presents with a scalp swelling which is pulsatile and increases in tension when the baby cries; the only effective treatment is neurosurgical repair of the dural tear, and the fracture will not heal until this is done.

Supratentorial subdural hemorrhage

Tentorial tearing can produce hemorrhage which extends both supratentorially and infratentorially. This type of hemorrhage, resulting from tearing at the falcotentorial junction leading to damage of the vein of Galen and internal cerebral vein, or both, was the most common type in one series [175]. In general, neonatal imaging studies suggest that most subdural hematomas form around the tentorium or the falx, and in the prospective 3-T MRI study in North Carolina all the lesions were peritentorial, with the hematoma forming infratentorially or low in the occipital or temporal areas [171]. In Hayashi et al.'s study the blood collected around the posterior hemispheric fissure, and if it did not reach the convexity or the posterior fossa subdural space the intracranial pressure did not rise above 200 mmHg, the babies did not require surgery, and they usually did well [175].

Infratentorial (posterior fossa) subdural hemorrhage

Posterior fossa subdural hematomas are associated with breech delivery or the use of forceps or vacuum extraction, and occipital osteodiastasis is an important risk factor for the condition after a vaginal breech delivery (now rarely performed) [185]. Signs of a posterior fossa subdural collection include a tense fontanelle, an increasing head circumference, apnea, bradycardia, loss of primitive reflexes or opisthotonos. This condition is potentially very serious because of the risk of brainstem compression, and neurosurgical intervention needs to be considered as a matter of urgency [186,187]. Surgical evacuation performed because of signs of brainstem compression in eight babies with posterior fossa subdural hematomas was followed by a normal outcome in all of them [188]. The babies with adverse outcomes in this series were those who had associated supratentorial injuries or hypoxic-ischemic damage. After a major tear of the tentorium with rupture of the vein of Galen, straight sinus, or transverse sinus (Fig 7.14a, b) the hemorrhage extends into the posterior fossa where it rapidly produces lethal brainstem compression. Less significant collections can present with neurological signs including irregular respiration, apnea, eye signs, irritability, and hypotonia. Figure 7.17 shows images from a baby born by Ventouse, who was well for a few days before presenting with irritability and a fixed dilated pupil on one side, but who rapidly deteriorated and died because of coning due to a posterior fossa subdural collection (Fig 7.17b). He was confirmed (after death) to have had hemophilia; there was no previous family history.

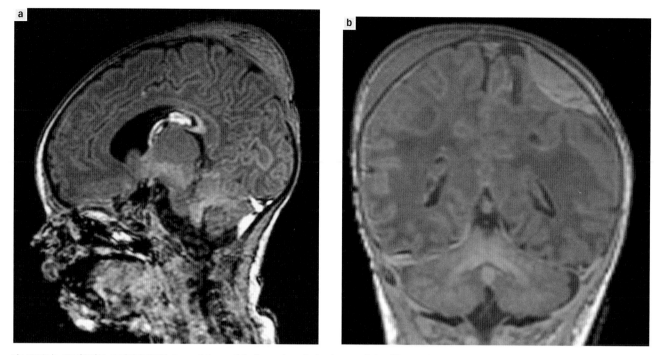

Fig. 7.16a,b. **Sagittal T₁-weighted MI shows intraventricular and posterior fossa subdural hemorrhage as well as a cephalohematoma (a). Coronal T₁-weighted MRI shows a left convexity extradural hematoma and extensive convexity subdural hematomas (b).**

Epidural hematoma

Bleeding into the epidural space can occur in the neonatal period. Spinal epidural hematomas can form after lumbar puncture, and the risk of this condition is the main reason why lumbar puncture is contraindicated in babies with thrombocytopenia or a coagulopathy. On occasion, babies can bleed into the intracranial epidural space. The imaging appearances are shown in Fig. 7.18.

Germinal matrix-intraventricular hemorrhage in the preterm baby

The diagnosis and investigation of this condition are dealt with in Chapter 9.

Intraventricular hemorrhage in the term baby

At term intraventricular hemorrhage (IVH) is more likely to arise from the choroid plexus than the germinal matrix [188,189], although remnants of the germinal matrix remain and can be a source of bleeding. Germinal matrix-intraventricular hemorrhage (GMH-IVH) is much less common at term than in preterm babies. Ultrasound is fairly reliable in the detection of GMH-IVH at all gestations, and is the first-line investigation (Fig. 7.19). Screening of asymptomatic cohorts of term babies has revealed an incidence of about 4% in some series [190]. There is an association with ECMO therapy (in part via retrograde thrombosis of the venous system associated with occlusion of the jugular vein, and in part due to changes in cerebral blood flow), coagulation defects, birth trauma, small-for-gestational-age babies, and vaginal delivery. Many cases of IVH at term represent secondary bleeding in association with thalamic hemorrhage, which in turn is often due to cerebral sino venous thrombosis (see above) [191]. We agree with Donna Ferriero's group, who recommend MRI in all cases of bleeding into the ventricles and deep gray matter which are recognized at term, because otherwise cases of sino venous thrombosis will be missed [154].

Lobar hemorrhage

Lobar cerebral hemorrhage at term (Fig. 7.20) is rare (estimates around 3 per 10 000 births), and is associated with perinatal hypoxia, coagulopathies (remember vitamin K deficiency), and low platelet counts especially due to NAITP [136,192,193]. As with IVH and thalamic hemorrhage, it is now appreciated that many lobar hemorrhages are hemorrhagic venous infarcts associated with venous sinus thrombosis, and MRI is usually required to demonstrate the venous occlusion, although some cases have been diagnosed with CT [154]. Rupture of arteriovenous malformations or bleeding into a tumor are other rare causes of lobar hemorrhage at term. Babies who had intrauterine growth retardation are more likely to have coagulation abnormalities, and we have seen a number with significant lobar hematomas. Nevertheless, there is still a substantial number of cases in whom no cause is identified [193].

Temporal lobe hemorrhage is not uncommon in babies, and growth-retarded babies seem particularly vulnerable, probably because many of them have a coagulopathy. Some consider that surgical evacuation of the hematoma is worthwhile; even if this is not done a careful watch needs to be kept on the baby

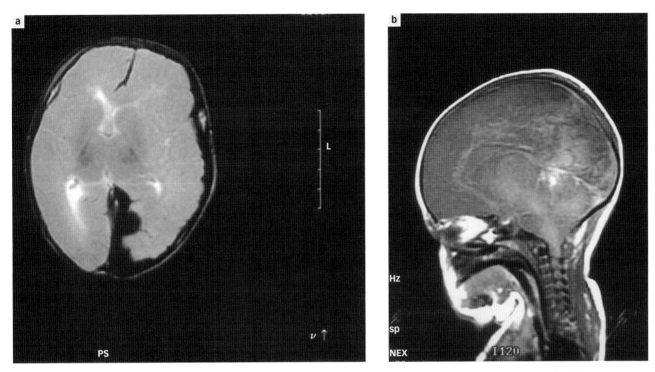

Fig. 7.17a,b. **Images from a baby delivered by Ventouse who developed a subdural hematoma. (a) The MR appearance soon after the CT was made. (b) The final appearance. There is coning. Bilateral tentorial tears were confirmed at autopsy, and postnatal investigation of abnormal coagulation confirmed hemophilia.**

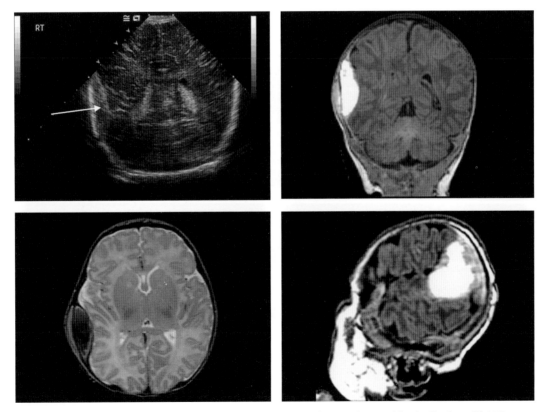

Fig. 7.18. **Coronal image with "dropout" in the parietal area (arrowed), which was shown to be an epidural collection with MRI.**

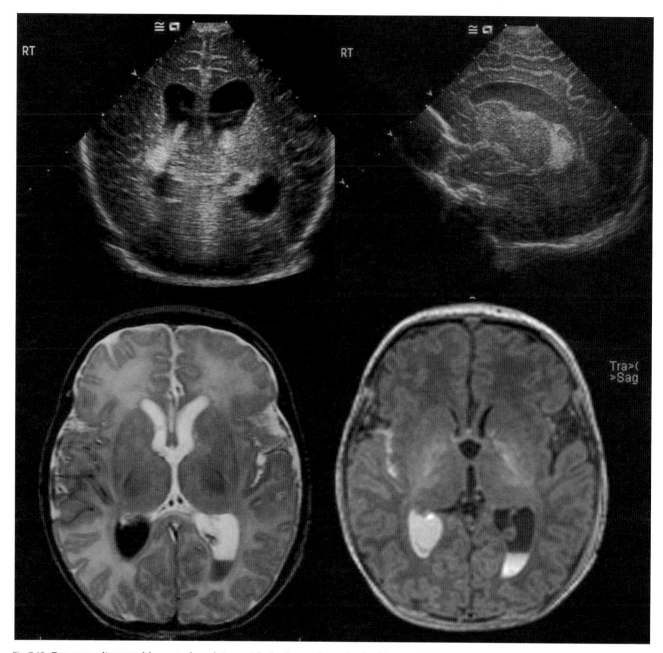

Fig. 7.19. **Top row: ultrasound images show intraventricular hemorrhage (IVH) with ventricular dilatation in a term infant. Bottom row shows axial T$_2$- and T$_1$-weighted images performed on the same day as the ultrasound images. At this stage of evolution of the hemorrhage, on T$_2$-weighted image the intraventricular blood appears hypointense whereas on the T$_1$-weighted image the blood appears hyperintense.**

because posthemorrhagic hydrocephalus is common [193]. Lobar hemorrhage, particularly into the frontal lobe, carries a high risk of sequelae and the parents should be counseled along these lines [182].

Thalamic hemorrhage

Thalamic hemorrhage should be clearly distinguished from bilateral thalamic abnormalities (bright thalami, hemorrhagic thalami) seen as a consequence of acute hypoxic ischemia

(p. 000). There are many reports of unilateral thalamic hemorrhage, usually with ipsilateral IVH, presenting in term babies who were previously well. Thrombosis of the internal cerebral vein (Figs. 7.14c, 7.21) resulting in hemorrhagic venous infarction is the cause in most cases [144,154,195]. The causes of sino venous thrombosis are discussed above, and as with a diagnosis of IVH it is essential to perform MRI in these babies (ideally with MR venography) in order to ascertain whether there is clot in the deep venous sinuses. One of Govaert's cases had

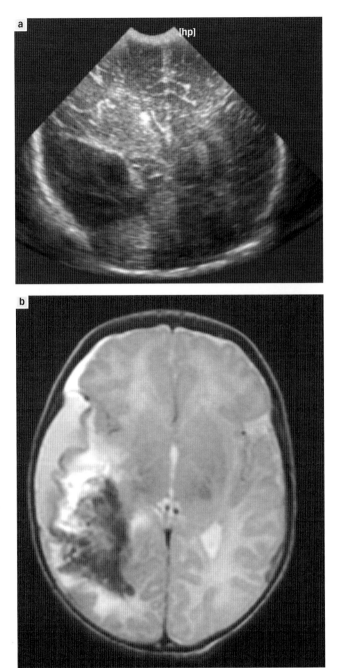

Fig. 7.20a,b. **Lobar hemorrhages. Ultrasound (a) and axial T$_2$-weighted MRI scan (b) show a large right temporo-parietal lobe hematoma.**

a 7-year period [197]. Babies with this condition usually present with seizures, often around a week old, and many have characteristic eye signs with sunsetting or forced eye deviation [198,199,200,201,202]. There is no specific treatment, and the majority of cases described have had neurologic sequelae, including posthemorrhagic hydrocephalus [144,148,164,197].

Cerebellar hemorrhage (see also Chapter 9)

Intracerebellar hemorrhage is more common in premature babies, but can accompany occipital osteodiastasis at term [203]. Ultrasound is not good at detecting posterior fossa lesions, including cerebellar hemorrhage, but cases have been diagnosed this way [204,205]. The prognosis may be better in term babies than their preterm counterparts, although not all would agree [206,207].

Brainstem hemorrhage

Brainstem hemorrhage is fortunately very rare, and affected babies usually die. We cared for one baby who remained ventilator dependent for several years because of the devastating effect on the respiratory center, a form of Ondine's curse.

Meningitis

The finding of an increased white cell count in the cerebrospinal fluid (CSF) suggests a diagnosis of meningitis; if organisms are not seen on Gram stain in a baby who has not received antibiotics viral meningitis should be suspected. Since aciclovir is the only effective treatment it should be offered until a result from polymerase chain reaction (PCR) of the CSF specifically looking for herpes is obtained. The EEG is of value in the prognosis of meningitis [208,209]. There are no specific imaging changes, but strands can be seen within the ventricle on occasion (pp. 274–279), and serial ultrasound scans should be carried out to exclude posthemorrhagic hydrocephalus (pp. 242–244).

Metabolic disease

Seizures can be a symptom of hypoglycemia, hypocalcemia or due to inborn errors of metabolism.

Pyridoxine dependency

The seizures in this rare autosomal-recessive disorder (about 1 in 100 000) usually begin between birth and 3 months of age [210,211]. An intravenous dose of pyridoxine (vitamin B$_6$) should be tried in all cases of resistant neonatal convulsions, administered under EEG control [212,213]. It has been said that the background EEG shows characteristic features [214], and background changes including burst suppression have been described (Fig. 7.23). Babies with pyridoxine dependency can present with birth depression, early-onset seizures and an encephalopathy, and their mothers may give a history of intrauterine "hammering" movement, suggesting fetal seizures. The usual dose of pyridoxine required for diagnosis is 50–100 mg, but some have suggested giving larger doses of up to 500 mg and waiting some time for a response. In classical

been ventilated in a negative pressure ventilator with a tight neck collar, and a case has been described after a central venous catheter entered the jugular vein. Thalamo-striate vasculopathy giving rise to a focal phlebitis in babies with central nervous system (CNS) infection accounts for a few cases [196]. Typical imaging findings include ventriculomegaly and are illustrated in Fig. 7.22.

The largest series is still that of Roland, who described 12 babies admitted to the neonatal unit in Vancouver over

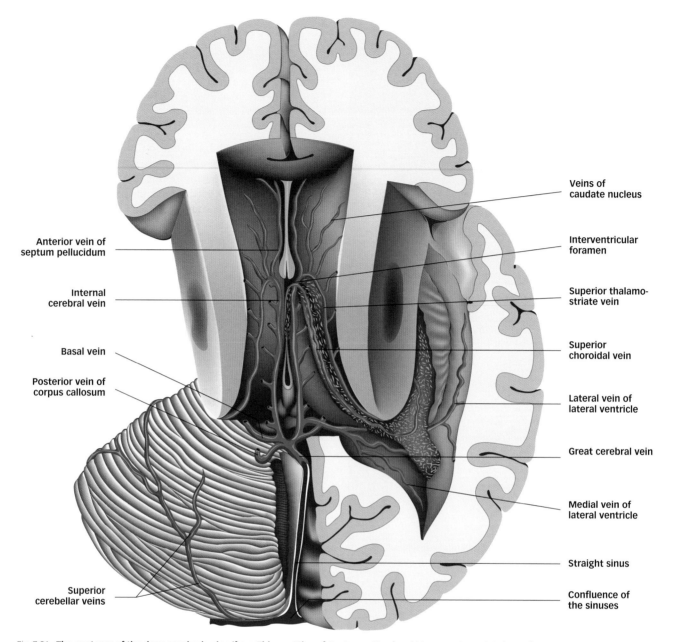

Fig. 7.21. **The anatomy of the deep cerebral veins (from Thieme Atlas of Anatomy: Head and Neuroanatomy [194], section 8.8 page 260 with permission).**

cases, this treatment stops the seizures within a short time; the occasional baby has developed transient but dramatic hypotonia after the first injection, presumed to be due to an effect on brain aminobutyric acid (GABA) levels [215]. Responders should be treated with at least 10 mg/kg per day pyridoxine, an amount far in excess of the daily requirements of 2 mg for an adult. Although the chromosome defect probably lies on chromosome 5 there is still no diagnostic test apart from monitoring the response to treatment and its withdrawal at about 4 years. Unfortunately children are often developmentally delayed even if the seizures are controlled.

GLUT-1 deficiency (De Vivo syndrome)

Glucose transport across the blood–brain barrier is mediated by the facilitative glucose transporter isoform 1 (GLUT-1). A deficiency of this transporter results in impaired energy supply to the brain, and was recognized by De Vivo in 1991 [20]. The diagnosis should be suspected if the CSF glucose is less than a third of the blood glucose level, and GLUT-1 deficiency can be confirmed with an assay that measures the uptake of [14C]-O-methyl-D-glucose in erythrocytes. Treatment is with a ketogenic diet, which is usually successful in controlling the seizures but does not always prevent the microcephaly, developmental delay,

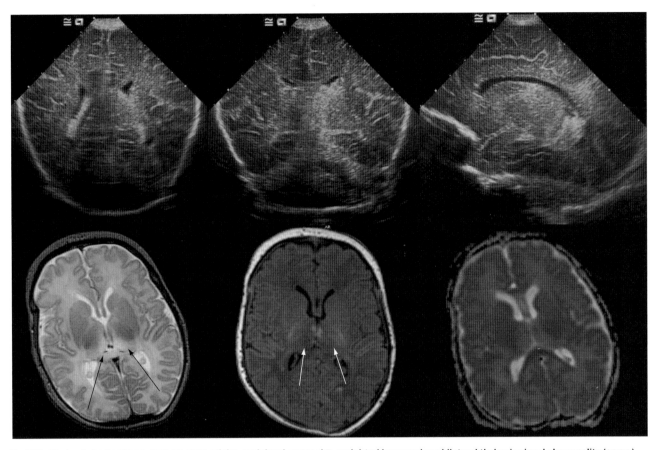

Fig. 7.22. **Thalamic hemorrhage. Bottom row: axial T$_2$-weighted, coronal T$_1$-weighted images show bilateral thalamic signal abnormality (arrow) in keeping with edema due to venous infarction and thrombus within the internal cerebral veins. The ADC map shows increased diffusion in the corresponding regions within the medial thalami. The appearances are most likely those of venous infarction due to internal cerebral vein thrombosis.**

and ataxia. Making the diagnosis is important because treatment with a ketogenic diet in some cases can lead to a normal outcome, and the disease is autosomal dominant [216,217].

Biotinidase deficiency

This is one of the few treatable causes of resistant neonatal seizures, hence the importance of considering this rare autosomal-recessive condition. There is usually a skin rash, similar in appearance to seborrheic dermatitis, and as the condition progresses there is ataxia and developmental delay. Screening using the neonatal blood spot is possible but is not currently carried out in the UK.

Cerebral malformations

Malformations such as schizencephaly and lissencephaly are often due to genetic defects, and are discussed in Chapter 12. Making a diagnosis of a neuronal migration disorder should not halt the search for an underlying metabolic disorder, because some are caused by peroxisomal disorders (e.g., Zellweger syndrome), mitochondrial disorders, disorders of cholesterol metabolism (e.g., Smith–Lemli–Opitz disease), or organic acidurias. Tuberous sclerosis has, very rarely, been recognized as causing seizures in the neonatal period (Fig. 7.24).

Neonatal epileptic syndromes

Benign familial seizures

Benign familial neonatal convulsions (BFNC) are linked to deletions of two potassium channel genes in most families [218]; the disorder is a "channelopathy." These are 20q13.3 (the voltage-gated potassium channel gene KNCQ2) and chromosome 8q24 (the potassium channel gene KCNQ3). The seizures in benign non-familial neonatal convulsions are usually partial with a normal interictal EEG, but we have recently seen one case with tonic-clonic seizures [219]. BFNC is one of three idiopathic epileptic syndromes caused by a single gene mutation. Seizures usually start between the second and fifth day of life, and cease before 6 weeks of age [220]. The prognosis of benign familial seizures, and neonatal non-familial seizures is excellent, although some children do continue having seizures into adult life.

Benign non-familial neonatal seizures (fifth day fits)

In some studies during the 1980s these seizures, of unknown etiology, were frequently reported. The disorder seems to have become much less common, although we still make the diagnosis occasionally. Like benign familial seizures, these dramatic clonic episodes usually begin around the second day and

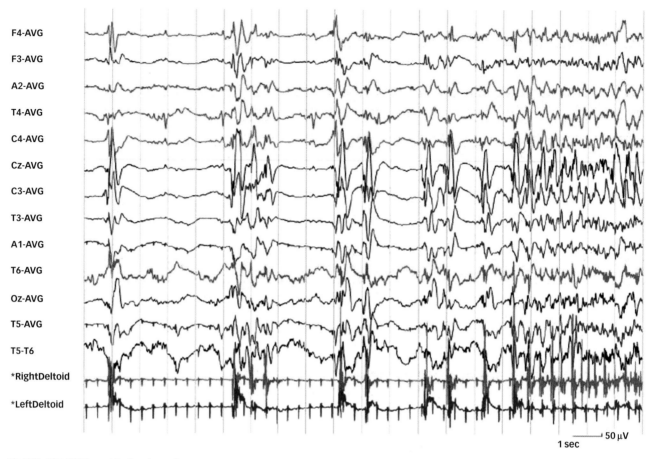

Fig. 7.23. **The EEG in pyridoxine dependency.**

continue for several days. Investigations are normal and the interictal background EEG is normal. The prognosis is excellent.

Benign neonatal sleep myoclonus

The myoclonus in this disorder, which may be quite dramatic, occurs *only* in sleep, and is most abundant during non-rapid-eye-movement sleep (quiet sleep). The EEG is entirely normal, as are the neurological examination and imaging. The prognosis is excellent and the myoclonus usually disappears over the first 6 months of life.

Early myoclonic encephalopathy

This rare disorder is characterized by erratic, fragmentary myoclonic jerks which begin in the first month of life. The EEG shows a characteristic suppression-burst pattern with spikes, sharp waves, and slow activity. Often no cause is found, although some babies with this presentation are discovered to have glycine encephalopathy or methylmalonic acidemia.

Early infantile epileptic encephalopathy (EIEE, Ohtahara syndrome)

Affected babies develop intractable tonic seizures in the early neonatal period, which do not improve (in contrast to the seizures of neonatal encephalopathy due to hypoxic ischemia).

Affected babies remain severely encephalopathic, and progression occurs. The disorder evolves into infantile spasms with hypsarrhythmia, and the uncontrollable seizures of Lennox-Gastaut syndrome. Many babies with Ohtahara syndrome have an underlying cerebral malformation, and Aicardi syndrome has also been associated with EIEE. Some have a focal cortical dysplasia and are helped by surgery. One case has been diagnosed to have cytochrome oxidase deficiency [221].

Treatment of neonatal seizure

There has always been controversy regarding the amount of damage seizures inflict on the immature brain, and this has previously driven a relaxed attitude to treatment. It is now clear that the neonatal brain is vulnerable to seizure damage, even though babies may be more resistant to damage from seizures than adults. Experimental work has shown that seizures impair neurogenesis, derange neuronal structure, function and connectivity, and can add to any primary insult by increasing the mismatch between energy supply and demand [222]. There is also evidence that seizures in early life may predispose ("sensitize") the brain to damage from seizures later on [223].

In the adult brain, glutamate is the primary excitatory neurotransmitter and GABA is the main inhibitory transmitter. GABA

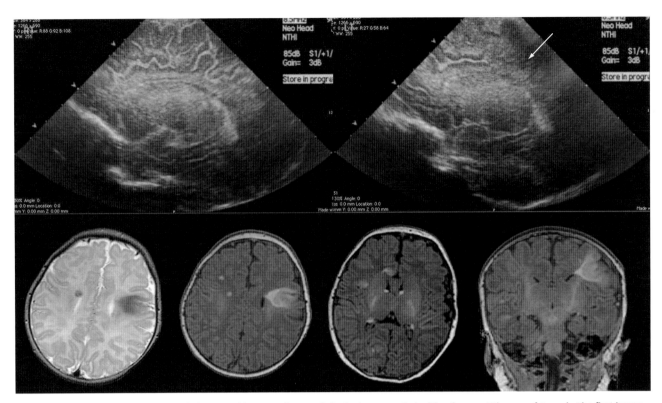

Fig. 7.24. **Top row show the parasagittal ultrasound images of a term infant who presented with seizures at the age of 1 week. The first image shows normal right parasagittal appearances, the second image shows a hypoechogenic lesion (arrow) which on MRI was identified as a tuber. Bottom row: axial T_2-, T_1-weighted pre- and T_1-weighted post contrast, and coronal T_1-weighted images in a neonate show multiple cortical tubers, some of which have signal characteristics suggestive of calcification and subependymal enhancing nodules including at the caudo-thalamic grooves. These are the typical features of tuberous sclerosis.**

receptors develop earlier than *N*-methyl-D-aspartate (NMDA) receptors, and in the neonatal brain GABA is probably excitatory [224] (Fig. 7.25). Further, there is an overabundance of excitatory glutaminergic receptors in the neonatal brain, and these are normally "pruned" later on. Seizures occurring during early life may interfere with pruning, permanently affecting connectivity: "neurons that fire together, wire together." Excess electrical activity can also disrupt developing circuits by altering the normal spontaneous activity, which is used to direct the formation of synapses. Seizures can also prompt genetic signaling, resulting in aberrant growth of granule cell axons or "mossy fibers" [225]. The brains of animals who suffered prolonged neonatal seizures are smaller than those who did not, with a particular reduction in dentate granule cells in the hippocampus [226,227]. The neonatal neuron has a high chloride content and consequently the developing brain has a different response to GABA (with an efflux of chloride rather than an influx), hence the response is excitatory rather than inhibitory. Recently, it has been discovered that the neonatal brain expresses a $Na^+K^+2Cl^-$ (NKCCl) co-transporter at birth and for some weeks after, explaining the high intracellular chloride levels compared to adult brain [228]. In addition to providing an elegant explanation for the observation that antiepileptic drugs which are effective in older children and adults do not work in babies, basic science research has also raised new questions about

the safety of currently used agents when used in babies with rapidly developing brains [229]. Recently, there has been the interesting and exciting observation that bumetanide, which is widely used as a diuretic and has a good safety profile, suppresses seizures in rat pups [228].

Phenobarbitone is still the first-line treatment of neonatal seizure, in spite of evidence that it is only effective in about a third of babies and the concern about apoptotic effects [230,231]. Experimental studies have shown that most commonly used antiepileptic drugs – phenytoin, phenobarbital, diazepam, clonazepam, vigabatrin, and valproate – cause apoptotic neurodegeneration in the developing rat brain at plasma concentrations relevant for seizure control in humans [229]. Interestingly, lamotrigine alone did not increase neuronal death when given up to doses of 50 mg/kg, but combination with phenytoin or phenobarbitone led to an attenuation of cell death [232]. More research is needed in this area as careful selection of drugs and doses may be needed to minimize neurotoxicity. Babies with a small seizure burden and a relatively normal background EEG are likely to respond to phenobarbitone. Phenobarbitone, for all its problems, has an established track record of safety, can be measured quickly in serum, and the neonatal pharmacokinetics are known. Consequently, until futher research is done, we suggest that phenobarbitone is retained as the first-line treatment, with phenytoin as second line.

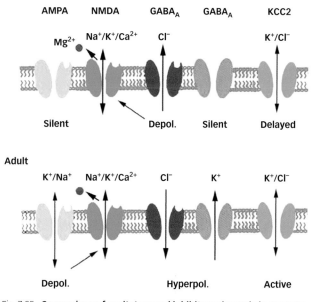

Fig. 7.25. Comparison of excitatory and inhibitory channels in neonate and adult. Depol, depolarization; Hyperpol, hyperpolarization. From [224] with permission.

Babies with an abnormal background EEG with a heavy seizure burden, or who are in neonatal status epilepticus, are unlikely to respond to any of the current antiepileptic drugs. Phenytoin controls some of them [231]. Lignocaine has proved popular in Europe, but the studies which showed that it was effective used cerebral function monitoring to assess the response [233] and our experience has been disappointing [234]. Paraldehyde is now difficult to obtain. There are anecdotal reports of success with sodium valproate, vigabatrin, lamotrigine, and carbemazepine. Finally, drugs of the benzodiazepine group (clonazepam, midazolam, diazepam) are frequently used [235], but our recent experience has been that no baby responded to clonazepam or midazolam when given as second line in an open study using video-EEG monitoring [234]. Surprisingly little has been published on the effectiveness of any neonatal anticonvulsant drug regimen measured using EEG.

Prognosis of neonatal seizure

Confirmation of the diagnosis of seizure considerably worsens the prognosis for any baby. Between 20% and 40% of term babies and 90% of preterm babies develop sequelae after neonatal seizures [15,236]. The prognosis does depend on the underlying lesion, and the combination of imaging findings, clinical and EEG data performed better than EEG alone in predicting outcome after neonatal seizure [237]. One group with a uniformly good prognosis is that with "clinical only" seizures and a normal background EEG, in whom all other investigations are also normal [238]. Babies whose neonatal neurological examination is normal do well [236].

Very many studies have confirmed the value of the background EEG in prediction of outcome in neonatal neurological illness. Even a single EEG can help in this respect, particularly if it is carried out in the first 3 days. A continuous EEG or aEEG is even better. A normal EEG at any time in the first few days conveys a good prognosis, and 42/47 (89%) of the babies in Tekgul's study who had a normal background EEG had a favorable outcome [236]. An EEG which shows persisting electrocortical inactivity (after the first 12–24 h), a continuous very low amplitude trace or burst suppression at term is an ominous finding (pp. 141–143). An EEG which is moderately abnormal should be repeated; persisting discontinuity indicates a poor prognosis.

In general the seizure burden alone does not help in prognosis, although not all would agree with this [24]. However, in association with an abnormal background EEG pattern a high electrographic seizure burden is predictive of a poor outlook. A heavy seizure burden increased the damage from hypoxia in neonatal rats, and the same may be true for babies [239,240].

The risk of seizure recurrence after neonatal seizures has remained unchanged at around 20% for many years [236,241]. In general, we only discharge a baby on phenobarbitone if he is continuing to seize, because of concerns about the effects of antiepileptic mediation on the developing brain [242]. However, practice varies, and in the US only 3% of neonatologists would stop antiepileptic drugs prior to discharge [244].

References

1. Bauder F, Wolhrab G, Schmitt B. Neonatal seizures: eyes open or closed? *Epilepsia* 2007; **48**(2): 394–6.
2. Malone A, Boylan G, Ryan CA, Connolly S. Ability of medical personnel to accurately differentiate neonatal seizures from non-seizure movements. *Clin Neurophysiol* 2006; **117**(S1): S1.
3. Murray DM, Boylan GB, Ali I, Ryan CA, Murphy BP, Connolly S. Defining the gap between electrographic seizure burden, clinical expression, and staff recognition of neonatal seizures. *Arch Dis Child* 2008; in press.
4. Clancy RR, Ledigo A, Lewis D. Occult neonatal seizures. *Epilepsia* 1988; **29**: 256–61.
5. Bye AME, Flanagan D. Spatial and temporal characteristics of neonatal seizures. *Epilepsia* 1995; **36**: 1009–16.
6. Holmes GL, Ben-Ari Y. The neurobiology and consequences of epilepsy in the developing brain. *Pediatr Res* 2001; **49**(3): 320–5.
7. Holmes GL. Effects of seizures on brain development: lessons from the laboratory. *Pediatr Neurol* 2005; **33**: 1–11.
8. Rennie JM, Boylan G. Treatment of neonatal seizures. *Arch Dis Child Fetal Neonatal Ed* 2007; **92**(2): 148–50.
9. Wasterlain CG. Recurrent seizures in the developing brain are harmful. *Epilepsia* 1997; **38**(6): 728–34.
10. Holmes GL. Seizure-induced neuronal injury. *Neurology* 2002; **59**: S3–S6.
11. Lanska MJ, Lanska DJ, Baumann RJ, Kryscio RJ. A population-based study of neonatal seizures in Fayette county, Kentucky. *Neurology* 1995; **45**: 724–32.
12. Lanska MJ, Lanska DJ. Neonatal seizures in the United States: results of the National Hospital Discharge Survey, 1980–1991. *Neuroepidemiology* 1996; **15**: 117–25.
13. Ronen GM, Penney S, Andrews W. The epidemiology of clinical neonatal seizures in Newfoundland: a population based study. *J Pediatr* 1999; **134**: 71–5.
14. Saliba RM, Annegers JF, Waller DK, Tyson JE, Mizrahi EM. Incidence of neonatal seizures in Harris County, Texas, 1992–1994. *Am J Epidemiol* 1999; **150**: 763–9.

15. Scher MS, Aso K, Beggarly ME, Hamid MY, Steppe DA, Painter MJ. Electrographic seizures in preterm and full-term neonates: clinical correlates, associated brain lesions, and risk for neurologic sequelae. *Pediatrics* 1993; **91**: 128–34.

16. Connell JA, Oozeer R, de Vries LS, Dubowitz LMS, Dubowitz V. Continuous EEG monitoring of neonatal seizures, diagnostic and prognostic considerations. *Arch Dis Child* 1989; **64**: 452–8.

17. Stiskal JA, Kulin N, Koren G, Ho T, Ito S. Neonatal paroxetine withdrawal syndrome. *Arch Dis Child* 2001; **84**: F134–F135.

18. Sanz EJ, de-las-Cuevas C, Kiuru A, Bate A, Edwards R. Selective serotonin reuptake inhibitors in pregnant women and neonatal withdrawal syndrome: a database analysis. *Lancet* 2005; **365**: 482–7.

19. Moses-Kolko EL, Bogen D, Perel J et al. Neonatal signs after late in utero exposure to serotonin reuptake inhibitors: literature review and implications for clinical applications. *J Am Med Assoc* 2005; **293**(19): 2372–83.

20. De Vivo D, Garcia-Alvarez M, Ronen G, Trifiletti R. Defective glucose transport across the blood-brain barrier as a cause of persistent hypoglycorrhachia, seizures and developmental delay. *New Engl J Med* 1991; **325**: 703–9.

21. Clancy RR, Ledigo A. The exact ictal and interictal duration of electroencephalographic neonatal seizures. *Epilepsia* 1987; **28**: 537–41.

22. Scher MS, Hamid MY, Steppe DA, Beggarly ME, Painter MJ. Ictal and interictal electrographic seizure durations in preterm and term neonates. *Epilepsia* 1993; **34**: 284–8.

23. Patrizi S, Holmes GL, Orzalesi M, Allemand F. Neonatal seizures: characteristics of EEG ictal activity in preterm and fullterm infants. *Brain Dev* 2003; **25**: 427–37.

24. McBride MC, Laroia N, Guillet R. Electrographic seizures in neonates correlate with poor neurodevelopmental outcome. *Neurology* 2000; **55**: 506–13.

25. de Alba GO, Mora EU, Valdez JM, Garcia DV, Crespo FV. Neonatal status epilepticus 11: electroencephalographic aspects. *Clin Electroencephalogr* 1984; **15**(4): 197–200.

26. Boylan GB, Murray DM, Greene BR, Ryan CA, MacNamara B, Connolly S. What is neonatal status epilepticus? *Clin Neurophysiol* 2006; **117**(S1): 1.

27. Shewmon DA. What is a neonatal seizure? Problems in definition and qualification for investigative and clinical purposes. *J Clin Neurophysiol* 1990; **7**: 315–68.

28. Oliveira AJ, Nunes ML, Haertel LM, Reis FM, Da Costa JC. Duration of rhythmic EEG patterns in neonates: new evidence for clinical and prognostic significance of brief rhythmic discharges. *Clin Neurophysiol* 2000; **111**: 1646–53.

29. Weiner SP, Painter MJ, Geva D, Guthrie RD, Scher MS. Neonatal seizures electroclinical dissociation. *Pediatr Neurol* 1991; **7**: 363–8.

30. Scher MS, Alvin J, Gaus L, Minnigh B, Painter MJ. Uncoupling of electrical and clinical expression of neonatal seizures after anti epileptic drugs. *Pediatr Neurol* 1994; **11**: 83.

31. Scher MS, Alvin J, Gaus L, Minnigh B, Painter MJ. Uncoupling of EEG-clinical neonatal seizures after antiepileptic drug use. *Pediatr Neurol* 2003; **28**: 277–80.

32. Boylan GB, Rennie JM, Pressler RM, Wilson G, Morton M, Binnie CD. Phenobarbitone, neonatal seizures and video-EEG. *Arch Dis Child* 2002; **86**: 165–170.

33. Mizrahi EM, Kellaway P. Characterization and classification of neonatal seizures. *Neurology* 1987; **37**: 1837–44.

34. Boylan GB, Rennie JM. Automated neonatal seizure detection. *Clin Neurophysiol* 2006; **117**: 1412–13.

35. Faul S, Boylan G, Connolly S, Marnane L, Lightbody G. An evaluation of automated neonatal seizure detection methods. *Clin Neurophysiol* 2005; **116**: 1533–41.

36. Greene BR, Boylan GB, Reilly RB, de Chazal P, Connolly S. Combination of EEG and ECG for improved automatic neonatal seizure detection. *Clin Neurophysiol* 2007; e pub ahead of print.

37. Greene BR, de Chazal P, Boylan GB, Connolly S, Reilly RB. Electrocardiogram based neonatal seizure detection. *IEEE Trans Biomed Eng* 2007; **54**(4): 673–82.

38. Glauser TA, Clancy RR. Adequacy of routine EEG examinations in neonates with clinically suspected seizures. *J Child Neurol* 1992; **7**: 215–20.

39. Sheth RD. Electroencephalogram confirmatory rate in neonatal seizures. *Pediatr Neurol* 1999; **20**: 27–30.

40. Rennie JM, Chorley G, Boylan GB, Pressler R, Nguyen Y, Hooper R. Non-expert use of the cerebral function monitor for neonatal seizure detection. *Arch Dis Child* 2004; **891**: 37–40.

41. Rennie JM. Seizures. In: Rennie JM, ed. *Roberton's Textbook of Neonatology*, 4th edn. Edinburgh, Elsevier, 2005; 1105–20.

42. Estan J, Hope PL. Unilateral neonatal cerebral infarction in full term infants. *Arch Dis Child* 1997; **76**: F88–F93.

43. Levy SR, Abroms IF, Marshall PC, Rosquete EE. Seizures and cerebral infarction in the full term newborn. *Ann Neurol* 1985; **17**: 366–70.

44. Clancy R, Malin S, Laraque D, Baumgart S, Younkin D. Focal motor seizures heralding stroke in full term neonates. *Am J Dis Child* 1985; **139**: 601–6.

45. Mercuri E, Cowan F, Rutherford M, Acolet D, Pennock J, Dubowitz LS. Ischaemic and haemorrhagic brain lesions in newborns with seizures and normal Apgar scores. *Arch Dis Child* 1995; **73**: F67–F75.

46. Mercuri E, Cowan F. Cerebral infarction in the newborn infant: review of the literature and personal experience. *Eur J Paediatr Neurol* 1999; **3**: 255–63.

47. Ramaswamy V, Miller SP, Barkovich AJ, Partridge JC, Ferriero DM. Perinatal stroke in term infants with neonatal encephalopathy. *Neurology* 2004; **62**: 2088–91.

48. Nelson KB, Lynch JK. Stroke in newborn infants. *Lancet Neurol* 2004; **3**: 150–8.

49. Wu YW, March WM, Croen LA, Grether JK, Escobar GJ, Newman TB. Perinatal stroke in children with motor impairment: a population-based study. *Pediatrics* 2004; **114**(3): 612–19.

50. Golomb MR, MacGregor DL, Domi T et al. Presumed pre- or perinatal arterial ischemic stroke: risk factors and outcomes. *Ann Neurol* 2001; **50**: 163–8.

51. Amato M, Herschkowitz N, Huber P. Prenatal stroke suggested by intrauterine ultrasound and confirmed by magnetic resonance imaging. *Neuropediatrics* 1991; **22**: 100–2.

52. de Vries LS, Groenendaal F, Eken P, van Haastert IC, Rademaker KJ, Meiners LC. Infarcts in the vascular distribution of the middle cerebral artery in preterm and fullterm infants. *Neuropediatrics* 1997; **28**: 88–96.

53. Miller V. Neonatal cerebral infarction. *Semin Pediatr Neurol* 2000; **7**(4): 278–88.

54. Chalmers EA. Perinatal stroke: risk factors and management. *Br J Haematol* 2005; **130**: 333–43.

55. Nelson K. Perinatal ischemic stroke. *Stroke* 2007; **38**: 742–5.

56. Govaert P, Mattys E, Zecic A, Roelens F, Oostra A, Vanzieleghem B. Perinatal cortical infarction within middle cerebral artery trunks. *Arch Dis Child* 2000; **82**: F59–F63.

57. Lee J, Croen LA, Backstrand KH et al. Maternal and infant characteristics associated with perinatal arterial stroke in the infant. *J Am Med Assoc* 2005; **293**(6): 723–9.

58. Schulzke S, Weber P, Luetsschg J, Fahnenstich H. Incidence and diagnosis of unilateral arterial cerebral infarction in newborn infants. *J Perinat Med* 2005; **33**: 170–5.

59. Cowan F, Mercuri E, Groenendaal F et al. Does cranial ultrasound imaging identify arterial cerebral infarction in term neonates? *Arch Dis Child* 2005; **90**(3): F252–F256.

60. Wang LW, Huang CC, Yeh TF. Major brain lesions detected on sonographic screening of apparently normal term neonates. *Neuroradiology* 2004; **46**: 368–73.

61. Netter FH. *Atlas of Human Anatomy*. London, Ciba Geigy Ltd.

62. Abels L, Lequin M, Govaert P. Sonographic templates of newborn perforator stroke. *Paediatr Radiol* 2006; **36**: 663-9.

63. Sreenan C, Bhargava R, Robertson CMT. Cerebral infarction in the term newborn: clinical presentation and long-term outcome. *J Pediatr* 2000; **137**: 351-5.

64. de Veber G, Monagle P, Chan A, et al. Prothrombotic disorders in infants and children with cerebral thromboembolism. *Arch Neurol* 1998; **55**: 1539-43.

65. Kraus FT, Acheen VI. Fetal thrombotic vasculopathy in the placenta: cerebral thrombi and infarcts, coagulopathies, and cerebral palsy. *Human Pathol* 1999; **30**: 759-69.

66. Klesh KW, Murphy TF, Scher MS, Buchanan DE, Maxwell EP, Guthrie RD. Cerebral infarction in persistent pulmonary hypertension of the newborn. *Am J Dis Child* 1987; **141**: 852-7.

67. Scher MS, Klesh KM, Murphy TE, Guthrie RD. Seizures and infarction in neonates with persistent pulmonary hypertension. *Paediatr Neurol* 1986; **2**: 332-9.

68. Lago P, Rebsamen S, Clancy R et al. MRI, MRA, and neurodevelopmental outcome following neonatal ECMO. *Pediatr Neurol* 1995; **12**: 294-304.

69. Jarjour IT, Ahdab-Barmada M. Cerebrovascular lesions in infants and children dying after extracorporeal membrane oxygenation. *Pediatr Neurol* 1994; **10**: 13-19.

70. Ruff RL, Shaw C-M, Beckwith JB, Iozzo RV. Cerebral infarction complicating umbilical vein catheterization. *Ann Neurol* 1979; **6(1)**: 85.

71. Fullerton HJ, Johnston SC, Smith WS. Arterial dissection and stroke in children. *Neurology* 2001; **57**: 1155-60.

72. Camacho A, Villarejo A, de Aragon AM, Simon R, Mateos F. Spontaneous carotid and vertebral artery dissection in children. *Pediatr Neurol* 2001; **25**: 250-3.

73. Topcuoglu MA, Pryor JC, Ogilvy CS, Kistler JP. Cerebral vasospasm following subarachnoid hemorrhage. *Curr Treat Options Cardiovasc Med* 2002; **4**: 373-84.

74. Govaert P, Vanhaesebrouck P, De Praeter C. Traumatic neonatal intracranial bleeding and stroke. *Arch Dis Child* 1992; **67**: 840-5.

75. Roessmann U, Tyler Miller R. Thrombosis of the middle cerebral artery associated with birth trauma. *Neurology* 1980; **30**: 889-92.

76. Alfonso I, Prieto G, Vasconcellos E, Aref K, Pacheco E, Yelin K. Internal carotid artery thrombus: an underdiagnosed source of brain emboli in neonates. *J Child Neurol* 2001; **16(6)**: 446-7.

77. Mann CI, Dietrich RB, Schrader MT, Peck WW, Demos DS, Bradley WG. Posttraumatic carotid artery dissection in children: evaluation with MR angiography. *AJR Am J Roentgenol* 1993; **160**: 134-6.

78. Lequin MH, Peeters EAJ, Holscher HC, de Krijger R, Govaert P. Arterial infarction caused by carotid artery dissection in the neonate. *Eur J Paediatr Neurol* 2004; **8**: 155-60.

79. Gupta M, Dinakaran S, Chan TK. Congenital Horner syndrome and hemiplegia secondary to carotid dissection. *J Pediatr Ophthalmol Strabismus* 2005; **42(2)**: 122-4.

80. Gunther G, Junker R, Strater R et al. Symptomatic ischemic stroke in full-term neonates role of acquired and genetic prothrombotic risk factors. *Stroke* 2000; **31**: 2437-11.

81. Golomb MR. The contribution of prothrombotic disorders to peri- and neonatal ischemic stroke. *Semin Thromb Hemost* 2003; **29(4)**: 415-24.

82. Kenet G, Sadetzki S, Murad H et al. Factor V Leiden and antiphospho-lipid antibodies are significant risk factors for ischemic stroke in children. *Stroke* 2001; **31**: 1283-8.

83. Zenz W, Bodo Z, Plotho J et al. Factor V Leiden and prothrombin gene G 20210. A variant in children with ischemic stroke. *Thromb Haemost* 1998; **80**: 763-6.

84. Lynch JK, Nelson KB, Curry CJ, Grether JK. Cerebrovascular disorders in children with the factor V Leiden mutation. *J Child Neurol* 2001; **16**: 735-44.

85. Lynch JK, Han CJ, Nee LE, Nelson KB. Prothrombotic factors in children with stroke or porencephaly. *Pediatrics* 2005; **116(2)**: 447-53.

86. Nowak-Gottl U, Strater R, Heinecke A et al. Lipoprotein (a) and genetic polymorphisms of clotting factor V, prothrombin, and methylene-tetrahydrofolate reductase are risk factors of spontaneous ischemic stroke in childhood. *Blood* 1999; **94(11)**: 3678-82.

87. Gunther G, Junker R, Strater R et al. Symptomatic ischemic stroke in full-term neonates: role of acquired and genetic prothrombotic risk factors. *Stroke* 2001; **31**: 2437-11.

88. Miller SP, Wu YW, Lee J et al. Candidate gene polymorphisms do not differ between newborns with stroke and normal controls. *Stroke* 2006; **37**: 2678-83.

89. Hogeveen M, Blom HJ, van Amerongen M, Boogmans M, van Beynum IM, Van de Bor M. Hyperhomocystinemia as risk factor for ischemic and hemorrhagic stroke in newborn infants. *J Paediatr* 2002; **141**: 429-31.

90. Nowak-Gottl U, Kosch A, Schlegel N. Thromboembolism in newborns, infants and children. *Thromb Haemost* 2001; **86**: 464-74.

91. Silver RK, MacGregor SN, Pasternak JF, Neely SE. Fetal stroke associated with elevated maternal anticardiolipin antibodies. *Obstet Gynecol* 1992; **80**: 497-9.

92. Akanli LF, Trasi SS, Thuraisamy K et al. Neonatal middle cerebral artery infarction: association with elevated maternal anticardiolipin antibodies. *Am J Perinatol* 1998; **15**: 399-402.

93. Chow G, Mellor D. Neonatal cerebral ischaemia with elevated maternal and infant anticardiolipin antibodies. *Dev Med Child Neurol* 2000; **42**: 412-13.

94. de Klerk OL, de Vries TW, Sinnige LGF. An unusual cause of neonatal seizures in a newborn infant. *Paediatrics* 1997; **100(4)**: e8.

95. Nelson KB, Dambrosia JM, Grether JK, Phillips TM. Neonatal cytokines and coagulation factors in children with cerebral palsy. *Ann Neurol* 1998; **44**: 665-75.

96. Moazzam A, Riaz M, Brennen MD. Neonatal gangrene in an extremity of an infant of a diabetic mother. *Br J Obstet Gynaecol* 2003; **110**: 75-6.

97. Benders MJNL, Groenendaal F, Uiterwaal CPM et al. Maternal and infant characteristics associated with perinatal arterial stroke. *Stroke* 2007; **38**: 1759-6.

98. Filipek PA, Krishnamoorthy KS, Davis KR, Kuehnle K. Focal cerebral infarction in the newborn: a distinct entity. *Pediatr Neurol* 1987; **3**: 141-7.

99. Koelfen W, Freund M, Varnholt V. Neonatal stroke involving middle cerebral artery in the term infants: clinical presentation, EEG and imaging study, and outcome. *Dev Med Child Neurol* 1995; **37**: 204-12.

100. Mercuri E, Rutherford M, Cowan F et al. Early prognostic indicators of outcome in infants with neonatal cerebral infarction: a clinical, electroencephalogram, and magnetic resonance imaging study. *Pediatrics* 1999; **103**: 39-46.

101. Rando T, Ricci D, Mercuri E et al. Periodic lateralized epileptiform discharges (PLEDs) as early indicators of stroke in full term newborns. *Neuropediatrics* 2000; **31**: 202-5.

102. Golomb MR, Dick PT, MacGregor DL, Armstrong DC, deVeber GA. Cranial ultrasonography has a low sensitivity for detecting arterial ischemic stroke in term neonates. *J Child Neurol* 2003; **18**: 98-103.

103. Coker SB, Beltran RS, Myers TF, Hmura L. Neonatal stroke: description of patients and investigation into pathogenesis. *Pediatr Neurol* 1988; **4**: 219-23.

104. Perlman JM, Rollins NK, Evans D. Neonatal stroke - clinical characteristics and cerebral blood flow velocity measurements. *Pediatr Neurol* 1994; **11**: 281-4.

105. Cowan FM, Pennock JM, Hanrahan J, Manji K, Edwards AD. Early detection of cerebral infarction and hypoxic ischaemic encephalopathy in neonates using diffusion weighted MRI. *Neuropediatrics* 1994; **25**: 172-5.

106. Venkataraman A, Kingsley PB, Kalina P et al. Newborn brain infarction: clinical aspects and magnetic resonance imaging. *CNS Spectrums* 2004; **9(6)**: 436-44.

107. Lovblad K, Ruoss K, Guzman R, Schroth G, Fusch C. Diffusion-weighted MRI of middle cerebral artery stroke in a newborn. *Pediatr Radiol* 2001; **31**: 374-6.

108. Kuker W, Mohrle S, Mader I, Schoning M. MRI for the management of neonatal cerebral infarctions: importance of timing. *Childs Nerv Syst* 2004; **20**: 742–8.

109. Mader I, Schoning M, Klose U, Kuker W. Neonatal cerebral infarction diagnosed by diffusion-weighted MRI. Pseudonormalization occurs early. *Stroke* 2002; **33**: 1142–5.

110. de Vries LS, van der Grond J, van Haastert IC, Groenendaal F. Prediction of outcome in newborn infants with arterial ischaemic stroke using diffusion weighted magnetic resonance imaging. *Neuropaediatrics* 2005; **36**: 12–20.

111. Giroud M, Fayolle H, Martin D *et al.* Late thalamic atrophy in infarction of the middle cerebral artery territory in neonates. *Child Nerv Syst* 1995; **11**: 133–6.

112. Kurnik K, Kosch A, Strater R, Schobess R, Heller C, Nowak-Gottl U. Recurrent thromboembolism in infants and children suffering from symptomatic neonatal arterial stroke. A prospective follow-up study. *Stroke* 2003; **34**: 2887–93.

113. Nowak-Gottl U, Junker R, Kreuz W *et al.* Risk of recurrent venous thrombosis in children with combined prothrombotic risk factors. *Blood* 2001; **97**: 858–62.

114. Wulfeck BB, Trauner DA, Tallal PA. Neurological, cognitive, and linguistic features of infants after early stroke. *Pediatr Neurol* 1991; **7**: 266–9.

115. Sran SK, Baumann RJ. Outcome of neonatal strokes. *Am J Dis Child* 1988; **142**: 1086–8.

116. Jan MMS, Camfield PR. Outcome of neonatal stroke in full-term infants without significant birth asphyxia. *Eur J Pediatr* 1998; **157**: 846–8.

117. de Veber GA, MacGregor D, Curtis R, Mayank S. Neurologic outcome in survivors of childhood arterial ischemic stroke and sinovenous thrombosis. *J Child Neurol* 2000; **15**: 316–24.

118. Boardman JP, Ganesan V, Rutherford MA, Saunders DE, Mercuri E, Cowan F. Magnetic resonance image correlates of hemiparesis after neonatal and childhood middle cerebral artery stroke. *Pediatrics* 2005; **115**(2): 321–6.

119. Lynch JK, Hirtz DG, deVeber G, Nelson KB. Report of the National Institute of neurological disorders and stroke workshop on perinatal and childhood stroke. *Pediatrics* 2002; **109**(1): 116–23.

120. Lynch JK, Nelson KB. Epidemiology of perinatal stroke. *Curr Opin Pediatr* 2001; **13**: 499–505.

121. Lee J, Croen LA, Lindan C *et al.* Predictors of outcome in perinatal arterial stroke: a population-based study. *Ann Neurol* 2005; **58**: 303–8.

122. Mercuri E, Anker S, Guzzetta A *et al.* Neonatal cerebral infarction and visual function at school age. *Arch Dis Child* 2003; **88**(6): 487–91.

123. Goodman R, Graham P. Psychiatric problems in children with hemiplegia: cross sectional epidemiological survey. *Br Med J* 1996; **312**: 1065–9.

124. Trauner DA, Chase C, Walker P, Wulfeck B. Neurologic profiles of infants and children after perinatal stroke. *Pediatric Neurol* 1993; **9**: 383–6.

125. Chadwick LM, Pemberton PJ, Kurinczuk JJ. Neonatal subgaleal haematoma: associated risk factors, complications and outcome. *J Paediatr* 1996; **32**: 228–31.

126. Vacca A. Birth by vacuum extraction: neonatal outcome. *J Pediatr Child Health* 1996; **32**: 204–6.

127. Vacca A. Risk factors associated with subaponeurotic haemorrhage in full-term infants exposed to vacuum extraction. *Br J Obstet Gynaecol* 2006; **113**(4): 491–9.

128. Cavlovich FE. Subgaleal hemorrhage in the neonate. *J Obstet Gynaecol Neonat Nursing* 1995; **24**: 397–404.

129. Govaert P, Vanhaesebrouck P, De Praeter C, Moens K, Leroy J. Vacuum extraction, bone injury and neonatal subgaleal bleeding. *Eur J Pediatr* 1992; **151**: 532–5.

130. Ng PC, Siu YK, Lewindon PJ. Subaponeurotic haemorrhage in the 1990's; a 3-year surveillance. *Acta Paediatr Scand* 1995; **84**: 1065–9.

131. Gebremariam A. Subgaleal haemorrhage: risk factors and neurological and developmental outcome in survivors. *Ann Trop Paediatr* 1999; **19**: 45–50.

132. Boo N-Y, Foong K-W, Mahdy ZA, Yong S-C, Jaafar R. Risk factors associated wtih subaponeurotic haemorrhage in full-term infants exposed to vacuum extraction. *Br J Obstet Gynaecol* 2005; **112**: 1516–21.

133. Plauche WC. Subgaleal haematoma: a complication of instrumental delivery. *J Am Med Assoc* 1980; **244**: 1597–8.

134. Benaron DA. Subgaleal hematoma causing hypovolemic shock during delivery after failed vacuum extraction: a case report. *J Perinatol* 1993; **13**: 228.

135. Cheong JL, Hagmann C, Rennie JM *et al.* Fatal newborn head enlargement: high resolution magnetic resonance imaging at 4.7 T. *Arch Dis Child* 2006; **91**: F202–F203.

136. Hanigan WC, Powell FC, Palagallo G, Miller TC. Lobar hemorrhages in full term neonates. *Child Nerv Syst* 1995; **11**: 276–80.

137. Hope PL, Hall MA, Millward-Sadler GH, Normand ICS. Alpha 1 antitrypsin deficiency presenting as a bleeding diathesis in the newborn. *Arch Dis Child* 1982; **57**: 68–79.

138. Fogarty K, Cohen HL, Haller JO. Sonography of fetal intracranial hemorrhage: unusual cases and a review of the literature. *J Clin Ultrasound* 1989; **17**: 366–70.

139. Sherer DM, Anyaegbunam A, Onyeije C. Antepartum fetal intracranial hemorrhage, predisposing factors and prenatal sonography: a review. *Am J Perinatol* 1998; **15**(7): 431–41.

140. Towner D, Castro MA, Evy-Wilkens E, Gilbert WM. Effect of mode of delivery in nulliparous women on neonatal intracranial injury. *N Engl J Med* 1999; **341**: 1709–14.

141. Govaert P. *Cranial Haemorrhage in the Term Newborn Infant*, 1st edn. London, Mac Keith Press; 1993.

142. Ghi T, Simonazzi G, Perolo A *et al.* Outcome of antenatally diagnosed intracranial hemorrhage: case series and review of the literature. *Ultrasound Obstet Gynaecol* 2003; **22**: 121–30.

143. Buchanan GR. Factor concentrate prophylaxis for neonatal haemophilia. *J Pediatr Haematol Oncol* 1999; **21**: 254–6.

144. Voutsinas L, Gorey MT, Goyuld R, Black KS, Scuderi DM, Hyman RA. Venous sinus thrombosis as a cause of parenchymal and intraventicular hemorrhage in the full-term neonate. *Clin Imaging* 1991; **15**: 273–5.

145. Stam J. Thrombosis of the cerebral veins and sinuses. *New Engl J Med* 2005; **352**: 1791–8.

146. de Veber G, Andrew M, Adams C *et al.* Cerebral sinovenous thrombosis in children. *N Engl J Med* 2001; **345**: 417–20.

147. Heller C, Heinecke A, Junker R *et al.* Cerebral venous thrombosis in children. A multifactorial origin. *Circulation* 2003; **108**: 1362–7.

148. Fitzgerald KC, Williams LS, Garg BP, Carvalho KS, Golomb MR. Cerebral sinovenous thrombosis in the neonate. *Arch Neurol* 2006; **63**: 405–9.

149. Carvalho KS, Bodensteiner JB, Connolly PJ, Garg BP. Cerebral venous thrombosis in children. *J Child Neurol* 2001; **16**: 574–80.

150. Sipahi T, Uner C, Yildiz YT, Akar N. Inherited protein-C deficiency, factor VG 1691 A and FV A 4070 G mutations in a child with internal cerebral venous thrombosis. *Pediatr Radiol* 2000; **30**: 420–3.

151. Vielhaber H, Ehrenforth S, Koch H, Scharrer I, van der Werf N, Nowak-Gottl U. Cerebral venous sinus thrombosis in infancy and childhood: role of genetic and acquired risk factors of thrombophilia. *Euro J Paediatr* 1998; **157**: 555–60.

152. Klein L, Bhardwaj V, Gebara B. Cerebral venous sinus thrombosis in a neonate with homozygous prothrombin G20210 A genotype. *J Perinatol* 2004; **24**: 797–9.

153. Pohl M, Zimmerhackl LB, Heinen F, Sutor AH, Schneppenheim R, Brandis M. Bilateral renal vein thrombosis and venous sinus thrombosis in a neonates with Factor V mutation (FV Leiden). *Paediatrics* 1998; **132**: 159–61.

154. Wu TW, Miller SP, Chin K *et al.* Multiple risk factors in neonatal sinovenous thrombosis. *Neurology* 2002; **59**: 438–40.

155. Hunt RW, Badawi N, Laing S, Lam A. Pre-eclampsia: a predisposing factor for neonatal venous sinus thrombosis? *Paediatr Neurol* 2001; **25**: 242–6.

156. Sebire G, Tabarki B, Saunders DE *et al.* Cerebral venous sinus thrombosis in children: risk factors, presentation, diagnosis and outcome. *Brain* 2005; **128**: 477–89.

157. Gebara BM, Everett KO. Dural sinus thrombosis complicating hypernatremic dehydration in a breastfed neonate. *Clin Pediatr* 2001; **40**: 45.

158. Korkmaz A, Yigit S, Firat M, Orran O. Cranial MRI in neonatal hypernatraemic dehydration. *Pediatr Radiol* 2000; **30**: 323-5.

159. Hanigan WC, Tracy PT, Tadros WS, Wright RM. Neonatal cerebral venous thrombosis. *Pediatri Neurosci* 1988; **14**: 177-83.

160. Konishi Y, Kuriyama M, Sudo M, Konishi K, Hayakawa K, Ishii Y. Superior sagittal sinus thrombosis in neonates. *Pediatr Neurol* 1987; **3**(4): 222-5.

161. Rivkin MJ, Anderson ML, Kaye EM. Neonatal idiopathic cerebral venous thrombosis: an unrecognised cause of transient seizures or lethargy. *Ann Neurol* 1992; **32**: 51-6.

162. Takanashi J, Barkovich AJ, Ferriero DM, Suzuki H, Kohno Y. Widening spectrum of congenital hemiplegia. Periventricular venous infarction in term neonates. *Neurology* 2003; **61**: 531-3.

163. Higashida RT, Helmer E, Halbach VV, Hieshima GB. Direct thrombolytic therapy for superior sagittal sinus thrombosis. *Am J Neuroradiol* 1989; **10**: S4-S6.

164. Barron TF, Gusnard DA, Zimmerman RA, Clancy RR. Cerebral venous thrombosis in neonates and children. *Pediatr Neurol* 1992; **8**(2): 112-16.

165. Huang AH, Robertson RL. Spontaneous superficial parenchymal and leptomeningeal hemorrhage in term neonates. *Am J Neuroradiol* 2004; **25**: 469-75.

166. Chaplin ER, Goldstein GW, Norman D. Neonatal seizures, intracerebral hematoma, and subarachnoid hemorrhage in full-term infants. *Pediatrics* 1979; **63**(5): 812-15.

167. Palmer TW, Donn SM. Symptomatic subarachnoid hemorrhage in the term newborn. *J Perinatol* 1991; **11**: 112-16.

168. Avrahami E, Frishman E, Minz M. CT demonstration of intracranial haemorrhage in term newborn following vaccuum extractor delivery. *Neuroradiology* 1993; **35**: 107-8.

169. Chamnanvanakij S, Rollins N, Perlman JM. Subdural hematoma in term infants. *Pediatr Neurol* 2002; **26**: 301-4.

170. Whitby EH, Griffiths PD, Rutter S *et al.* Frequency and natural history of subdural haemorrhages in babies and relation to obstetric factors. *Lancet* 2004; **363**: 846-51.

171. Looney CB, Smith JK, Merck LH *et al.* Intracranial hemorrhage in asymptomatic neonates: prevalence on MR images and relationship to obstetric and neonatal risk factors. *Radiology* 2007; **242**(2): 535-41.

172. Holden KR, Titus MO, von Tassel P. Cranial magnetic resonance imaging examination of normal term neonates: a pilot study. *J Child Neurol* 1999; **14**(11): 708-10.

173. Jhawar BS, Ranger A, Steven D, Del Maestro RF. Risk factors for intracranial hemorrhage among full-term infants: a case-control study. *Neurosurgery* 2003; **52**: 581-90.

174. Tavani F, Zimmerman RA, Clancy RR, Licht DJ, Mahle WT. Incidental intracranial hemorrhage after uncomplicated birth: MRI before and after neonatal heart surgery. *Neuroradiology* 2003; **45**: 253-8.

175. Hayashi T, Hashimoto T, Fukuda S, Ohshima Y, Moritaka K. Neonatal subdural hematoma secondary to birth injury. Clinical analysis of 48 survivors. *Child Nerv Syst* 1987; **3**: 23-9.

176. Currarino G. Occipital osteodiastasis: presentation of four cases and review of the literature. *Pediatr Radiol* 2000; **30**: 823-9.

177. Govaert P, Calliauw L, Vanhaesebrouck P, Martens F, Barrilari A. On the management of neonatal tentorial damage. Eight case reports and a review of the literature. *Acta Neurochir* 1990; **106**: 52-64.

178. Rotmensch S, Grannum PA, Nores JA, Hall C, Keller MS, McCarthy S. In utero diagnosis and management of fetal subdural haematoma. *Am J Obstet Gynecol* 1991; **164**: 1246-8.

179. Nogueira GJ. Chronic subdural hematoma in utero. *Child Nerv Syst* 1992; **8**: 462-4.

180. Volpe JJ. Intracranial haemorrhage: germinal matrix - intraventricular hemorrhage of the premature infant. In: Volpe JJ, ed. *Neurology of the Newborn*, 4th edn. 2000; 403-21.

181. Orrison WW, Robertson WC, Sackett JF. Computerized tomography in chronic subdural haematomas (effusions) of infancy. *Neuroradiology* 1978; **16**: 79-81.

182. Jhawar BS, Ranger A, Steven DA, Del Maestro RF. A follow-up study of infants with intracranial hemorrhage at full-term. *Can J Neurol Sci* 2005; **32**: 332-9.

183. King SJ, Boothroyd AE. Cranial trauma following birth in term infants. *Br J Radiol* 1998; **71**: 233-8.

184. Vas CJ. Growing skull fracture. *Dev Med Child Neurol* 1966; **8**: 734-40.

185. Menezes AH, Smith DE, Bell WE. Posterior fossa hemorrhage in the term neonate. *Neurosurgery* 1983; **13**(4): 452-6.

186. Scotti G, Flodmark O, Harwood-Nash DC, Humphries RP. Posterior fossa haemorrhages in the newborn. *J Comput Assist Tomogr* 1981; **5**: 68-72.

187. Perrin RG, Rutka JT, Drake JM *et al.* Management and outcomes of posterior fossa subdural hematomas in neonates. *Neurosurgery* 1997; **40**(6): 1190-200.

188. Donat JF, Okazaki H, Kleinberg F, Reagan TJ. Intraventricular hemorrhages in full term and premature infants. *Mayo Clin Proc* 1978; **53**: 437-41.

189. Lacey DJ, Terplan K. Intraventricular haemorrhage in the full term neonate. *Dev Med Child Neurol* 1982; **241**: 332-4.

190. Hayden CK, Shattuck KE, Richardson CJ, Ahrendt DK, House R, Swischuk LE. Subependymal germinal matrix hemorrhage in full-term neonates. *Pediatrics* 1985; **75**(4): 714-18.

191. Wu YW, Hamrick SEG, Miller SP *et al.* Intraventricular hemorrhage in term neonates caused by sinovenous thrombosis. *Ann Neurol* 2003; **54**: 123-6.

192. Hanigan WC, Powell FC, Miller TC, Wright RM. Symptomatic intracranial hemorrhage in full-term infants. *Child Nerv Syst* 1995; **11**(698): 707.

193. Sandberg DI, Lamberti-Pasculli M, Drake JM, Humphreys RP, Rutka JT. Spontaneous intraparenchymal hemorrhage in full term neonates. *Neurosurgery* 2001; **48**: 1042-1049.

194. Schuenke M, Schulte E, Schumacher U *et al. Thieme Atlas of Anatomy: Head and Neuroanatomy*. Stuttgart, Thieme Medical Publishers, 2007.

195. Govaert P, Achten E, Vanhaesebrouck P, De Praeter C, Van Damme J. Deep cerebral venous thrombosis in thalamo-ventricular haemorrhage of the term newborn. *Pediatr Radiol* 1992; **22**: 123-7.

196. de Vries LS, Smet M, Goemans N, Wilms G, Develiger H, Casaer P. Unilateral thalamic haemorrhage in the pre-term and full-term newborn. *Neuropediatrics* 1992; **23**: 153-6.

197. Roland EH, Flodmark O, Hill A. Thalamic haemorrhage with intraventricular haemorrhage in the full term newborn. *Pediatrics* 1990; **85**: 737-42.

198. Trounce JQ, Fawer C-L, Punt J, Dodd KL, Fielder AR, Levene MI. Primary thalamic haemorrhage in the newborn: a new clinical entity. *Lancet* 1985; **2**: 190-2.

199. Primhak RA, Smith MF. Primary thalamic haemorrhage in the first week of life. *Lancet* 1985; **1**: 635.

200. Montoya F, Couture A, Frerebeau PH, Bonnet H. Hemorragie intraventriculair chez le nouveau-ne a terme: origine thalamique. *Pediatrie* 1987; **42**: 205-9.

201. Adams C, Hochhauser L, Logan WJ. Primary thalamic and caudate hemorrhage in term neonates presenting with seizures. *Pediatr Neurol* 1988; **4**: 175-7.

202. Garg BP, DeMeyer WE. Ischemic thalamic infarction in children: clinical presentation, etiology, and outcome. *Pediatr Neurol* 1995; **13**: 46-9.

203. Grunnet ML, Shields WD. Cerebellar haemorrhage in preterm infants. *J Pediatr* 1975; **88**: 605-8.

204. Perlman JM, Nelson JS, McAlister WH, Volpe JJ. Intracerebellar haemorrhage in a premature newborn: diagnosis with real-time ultrasound and correlation with autopsy findings. *Pediatrics* 1983; **71**: 159-62.

205. Reeder JD, Setzer ES, Kaude JV. Ultrasonographic detection of perinatal intracerebellar haemorrhage. *Pediatrics* 1982; **70**: 385-6.

206. Martin R, Roessmann U, Fanaroff A. Massive intracerebellar haemorrhage in low birthweight infants. *J Pediatr* 1976; **89**: 290-3.

207. Chadduck WM, Duong DH, Kast JM, Donahue DJ. Pediatric cerebellar hemorrhages. *Child Nerv Syst* 1995; **11**: 579–83.

208. Chequer RS, Tuarp BR, Dreimane D, Hahn JS, Clancy RR, Coen RW. Prognostic value of EEG in neonatal meningitis: retrospective study of 29 infants. *Paediatr Neurol* 1992; **8**: 417–22.

209. Klinger G, Chin C-N, Otsubo H, Beyene J, Perlman M. Prognostic value of EEG in neonatal bacterial meningitis. *Pediatr Neurol* 2001; **24(1)**: 28–31.

210. Baxter P. Epidemiology of pyridoxine dependent and pyridoxine responsive seizures in the UK. *Arch Dis Child* 1999; **81**: 431–3.

211. Baxter P. Pyridoxine-dependent and pyridoxine-responsive seizures. *Dev Med Child Neurol* 2001; **43**: 416–20.

212. Gospe SM. Current perspectives on pyridoxine-dependent seizures. *J Pediatr* 1998; **132**: 919–23.

213. Gospe SM. Pyridoxine-dependent seizures: findings from recent studies pose new questions. *Pediatr Neurol* 2002; **26**: 181–5.

214. Nabbout R, Soufflet C, Plouin P, Dulac O. Pyridoxine dependent epilepsy: a suggestive electroclinical pattern. *Arch Dis Child* 1999; **81**: F125–F129.

215. Kroll J. Pyridoxine for neonatal seizures: an unexpected hazard. *Dev Med Child Neurol* 1985; **27**: 369–82.

216. Fishman RA. The glucose transporter protein and gluconeogenic brain injury. *N Engl J Med* 1991; **325**: 731–2.

217. Wang D, Pascual JM, Yang H *et al*. GLUT-1 deficiency syndrome: clinical, genetic and therapuetic aspects. *Ann Neurol* 2005; **57(1)**: 111–18.

218. Leppert M, Singh N. Benign familial neonatal epilepsy with mutations in two potassium channel genes. *Curr Opin Neurol* 1999; **12**: 143–7.

219. Guerra M, Rennie JM, Wilson G, Boylan G, Pressler RM. Tonic-clonic seizures in benign familial seizures. *Pediatr Neurol* 2002; **26**: 398–401.

220. Ronen G, Rosales TO, Connolly M, Anderson VE, Leppert M. Seizure characteristics in chromosome 20 benign familial neonatal convulsions. *Neurology* 1993; **43**: 1355–60.

221. Williams A, Gray RG, Poulton K, Ranami P, Whitehouse WP. A case of Ohtahara syndrome with cytochrome oxidase deficiency. *Dev Med Child Neurol* 1998; **40**: 568–70.

222. Kubova H, Druga R, Lukasiuk K *et al*. Status epilepticus causes necrotic damage in the mediodorsal nucleus of the thalamus in immature rats. *J Neurosci* 2001; **21(10)**: 3593–9.

223. Koh S, Storey TW, Santos TC, Mian AY, Cole AJ. Early-life seizures in rats increase susceptibility to seizure-induced brain injury in adulthood. *Neurology* 1999; **53**: 912–21.

224. Holmes GL, Khazipov R, Ben-Ari Y. New concepts in neonatal seizures. *Neuroreport* 2002; **13(1)**: A3–A8.

225. Holmes GL, Sarkisian M, Ben-Ari Y, Chevassus-Au-Louis N. Mossy fiber sprouting after recurrent seizures during early development in rats. *J Comp Neurol* 1999; **404**: 537–53.

226. Wasterlain CG. Effects of neonatal status epilepticus on rat brain development. *Neurology* 1976; **26**: 975–86.

227. McCabe BK, Silveira DC, Cilio MR *et al*. Reduced neurogenesis after neonatal seizures. *J Neurosci* 2001; **6**: 2094–103.

228. Dzhala VI, Talos DM, Sdrulla DA *et al*. NKCC1 transporter facilitates seizures in the developing brain. *Nature Med* 2005; **11**: 1205–13.

229. Bittigau P, Sifringer M, Genz K *et al*. Antiepileptic drugs and apoptotic neurodegeneration in the developing brain. *Proc Natl Acad Sci USA* 2002; **99**: 15089–94.

230. Boylan GB, Rennie JM, Pressler RM, Wilson G, Morton M, Binnie CD. Phenobarbitone, neonatal seizures, and video-EEG. *Arch Dis Child* 2002; **86(3)**: 165–70.

231. Painter MJ, Scher MS, Stein AD *et al*. Phenobarbital compared with phenytoin for the treatment of neonatal seizures. *N Engl J Med* 1999; **341**: 485–9.

232. Katz I, Kim J, Gale KN, Kondratyev AD. Effects of lamotrigine alone and in combination with MK-801, phenobarbital or phenytoin on call death in the neonatal rat brain. *J Pharmacol Exp Ther* 2007; e pub.

233. Hellstrom-Westas L, Westgren U, Rosen I, Svenningsen NW. Lidocaine for treatment of severe seizures in newborn infants. *Acta Paediatr Scand* 1988; **77**: 79–84.

234. Boylan G, Rennie JM, Chorley G *et al*. Second line anticonvulsant treatment of neonatal seizures: a video-EEG monitoring study. *Neurology* 2004; **62**: 486–8.

235. Andre M, Boutroy MJ, Dubruc C *et al*. Clonazepam pharmacokinetics and therapeutic efficacy in neonatal seizures. *Eur J Clin Pharmacol* 1986; **30**: 585–9.

236. Tekgul H, Gaubreau K, Soul J *et al*. The current etiologic profile and neurodevelopmental outcome of seizures in term newborn infants. *Pediatrics* 2006; **117(4)**: 1270–80.

237. Ortibus EL, Sum JM, Hahn JS. Predictive value of EEG for outcome and epilepsy following neonatal seizures. *Electroencephalogr Clin Neurophysiol* 1996; **98**: 175–85.

238. Boylan GB, Pressler RM, Rennie JM *et al*. Outcome of electroclinical, electrographic, and clinical seizures in the newborn infant. *Dev Med Child Neurol* 1999; **41**: 819–25.

239. Wirrell EC, Armstrong EA, Osman LD, Yager JY. Prolonged seizures exacerbate perinatal hypoxic-ischemic brain damage. *Pediatr Res* 2001; **50(4)**: 445–54.

240. Miller SP, Weiss J, Barnwell A *et al*. Seizure-associated brain injury in term newborns with perinatal asphyxia. *Neurology* 2002; **58**: 542–8.

241. Scher MS, Aso K, Beggarly ME, Hamid MY, Steppe DA, Painter MJ. Electrographic seizures in preterm and full-term neonates: clinical correlates, associated brain lesions, and risk for neurologic sequelae. *Pediatrics* 1993; **91**: 128–34.

242. Kaindl AM, Asimiadou S, Manthey D, Hagen MDH, Turski L, Ikonomidou C. Antiepileptic drugs and the developing brain. *Cell Mol Life Sci* 2006; **63**: 399–413.

243. Massingale TW, Boutross S. Survey of treatment practices for neonatal seizures. *J Perinatol* 1993; **13**: 107–10.

Chapter 8 | The baby who was depressed at birth

JANET M. RENNIE,
CORNELIA F. HAGMANN, *and*
NICOLA J. ROBERTSON

Clinical presentation of birth depression

When faced with the dire emergency of a baby who is white, floppy, not breathing and whose heart is beating very slowly, the attending neonatologist cannot spend time quizzing the mother about her family history, pregnancy and labor, and nor should she. Her first priority must be to resuscitate the baby along the usual lines, remembering that a baby who does not respond may have lost blood, be suffering from overwhelming sepsis, have endured a period of hypoxic ischemia, or have a myopathy or spinal cord damage. The one investigation that must be requested in the heat of the battle is a cord pH, preferably from both an umbilical artery and the vein. These results will be invaluable in a later analysis of the case, and in an emergency a double-clamped section of cord can be kept on one side and analyzed up to 60 min later without invalidating the result [1]. Normal scalp and cord blood pH values are given in Table 8.1. The most common cause of birth depression at term is hypoxic ischemia sustained during labor, and in preterm babies the most common cause is respiratory distress syndrome (RDS). Other causes are listed in Table 8.2, and sepsis is an important possibility.

Investigation of the baby with birth depression

Once the baby's condition is stable there will be time to gather more information. No baby is born in poor condition without a reason, and all babies have a medical history – which does not begin at the moment of birth. As in other branches of medicine, there is no substitute for a careful and detailed history, which should include a careful perusal of the mother's notes and a good family history. A few gentle but well-directed questions can pay dividends.

History

Family history, past obstetric history

Ask about any other relatives who have neurological disease, and about babies in the family who have died. Are the parents cousins? Previous male babies with bleeding problems suggest hemophilia; previous early neonatal deaths suggest metabolic disease or myopathy; the list could go on. A parent's occupation, a history of recent foreign travel and hobbies can all be relevant – the mother may be a farmer's wife or a veterinary surgeon.

Pregnancy

The pregnancy may have been troubled by bleeding; there may have been a lost twin. Prolonged rupture of membranes is obviously relevant, as is a history of pregnancy-associated hypertension or fetal growth retardation. There may have been an episode such as a road traffic accident or exposure to viral infection. Reduction of fetal movements is often reported in pregnancy, but a complete cessation of fetal movements is less common and can be ominous.

Labor and delivery

The cardiotocograph
The cardiotocograph (CTG) is a sensitive technique for the detection of intrapartum hypoxia but it is not very specific; unsurprisingly it is even less specific for the detection of neurological damage [5]. CTG has not lived up to the high expectations which were generated when it was introduced in the late 1960s [6]. Attempts to standardize interpretation continue (Table 8.3). In the meanwhile, for the neonatologist, a CTG that evolves from normal into a pattern of late decelerations with loss of variability strongly suggests intrapartum hypoxia as a cause for birth depression; so does a terminal bradycardia. A persistent unchanging loss of baseline variability is consistent with pre-existing central nervous system (CNS) damage [7,8], particularly when combined with a history of loss of fetal movements. A sinusoidal trace often accompanies fetal anemia.

Maternal pyrexia
A maternal intrapartum fever of more than 38 °C persisting for more than an hour is usually considered to be a clinical indicator of chorioamnionitis, and there is increasing realization

Neonatal Cerebral Investigation, eds. Janet M. Rennie, Cornelia F. Hagmann and Nicola J. Robertson. Published by Cambridge University Press. © Cambridge University Press 2008.

Table 8.1. Normal scalp and cord blood pH results (mean and standard deviation).

	Normal scalp pH results		
	Early first stage	Late first stage	Second stage
pH	7.33 ± 0.03	7.32 ± 0.02	7.29 ± 0.04
PCO_2 (mmHg)	44 ± 4.05	42 ± 5.1	46.3 ± 4.2
PO_2 (mmHg)	21.8 ± 2.6	21.3 ± 2.1	16.5 ± 1.4
Bicarbonate (mmol/l)	20.1 ± 1.2	19.1 ± 2.1	17 ± 2
Base deficit (mmol/l)	3.9 ± 1.0	4.1 ± 2.5	6.4 ± 1.8

	Normal cord blood pH results	
	Venous blood[a]	Arterial blood[b]
pH	7.35 ± 0.05	7.28 ± 0.05
PCO_2 (mmHg)	38 ± 5.6	49 ± 8.4
PO_2 (mmHg)	29 ± 5.9	18 ± 6.2
Base excess (mmol/l)	−4 ± 2	−4 ± 2
Bicarbonate (mmol/l)	20 ± 2.1	22 ± 2.5

	Venous blood[b]	Arterial blood[b]
pH	7.14–7.45	7.06–7.36
PCO_2		
(kPa)	3.2–7.5	3.7–9.1
(mmHg)	24–56	28–68
PO_2		
(kPa)	1.7–6	1.3–5.5
(mmHg)	12.3–45	9.8–41
Base excess (mmol/l)	−0.7 to −12	−0.05 to −15.3

[a] Data from [2].

[b] Data from [4]. Over 5000 samples analyzed within 75 min of delivery.

Source: Boylan PC. In: Creasy RK *et al.* (eds.) *Maternal-Fetal Medicine.* Philadelphia: Saunders, 1999. [3]

that perinatal infection is linked with low Apgar scores and later brain injury via inflammatory mediators [9,10]. Indeed, recent studies suggest that maternal intrapartum fever of more than 37.5 °C increases the risk of perinatal brain injury independent of infection [11]. Intrapartum fever, even when unlikely to be caused by infection, was associated with a four-fold increase in the risk of unexplained early-onset neonatal seizures at term [12]. The incidence of intrapartum fever (37.5 °C) was 6% in Dublin, and the risk of neonatal encephalopathy (NE) was increased in the babies born to pyrexial mothers, a risk that persisted when the results were corrected for the use of epidural analgesia, length of labor, and the use of oxytocin [13].

Experimental studies have shown that the combination of hypoxic ischemia and infection may be particularly damaging

Table 8.2. Causes of birth depression.

Hypoxic ischemia during labor or delivery

Intracranial trauma, especially massive infratentorial subdural hematoma

Extracranial trauma causing significant blood loss, e.g., a subgaleal (subapneurotic) hematoma

Sepsis, especially group B streptococcal septicemia

Muscle weakness – myopathy – e.g., X-linked myotubular mypopathy, nemaline myopathy, maternal myotonic dystrophy, Prader-Willi syndrome

Spinal cord trauma

Abnormal respiratory center (e.g., Ondine's curse)

Hypovolemia due to massive fetomaternal hemorrhage, vasa praevia or blood loss elsewhere into the fetal body or scalp (see extracranial trauma), or blood lost into an identical twin

Pre-existing central nervous system damage or malformation, including pre-labor hypoxic ischemia

Congenital airway problem, or blockage of the airway from blood, vernix, meconium or other matter

Congenital diaphragmatic hernia or other lung disorder, e.g., cystic adenomatoid malformation

Pneumothorax sustained during birth or early resuscitation

Maternal drug ingestion, including pethidine given during labor or the inadvertent administration of local anesthetic meant for the mother to the baby

to the neonatal brain [14], and that hyperthermia (40 °C) during hypoxic ischemia renders the immature brain unduly susceptible to damage. In other words, a mild hypoxic ischemic insult which would not usually be of sufficient severity to cause damage can do so when it occurs in combination with hyperthermia. Studies have shown that this is probably due to escalation of apoptotic cell death [15].

Cord and placenta

Unfortunately routine placental histology has gone out of fashion, but the placenta often contains important clues to the reason for birth depression. A placenta with a velamentous cord insertion, or one with a succenturiate lobe can be associated with vasa praevia, which can rupture and cause the baby to lose significant amounts of blood. Babies tolerate hypovolemia poorly and acute blood loss can cause circulatory collapse, before there is time for the anemia of hemodilution to develop. Examination of the placenta may show a hidden abruption, or chorioamnionitis, or areas of infarction. The cord may contain a true knot, although these do not usually cause cord compression and are often "red herrings" in the history [16]. Ideally the placenta should be subject to formal histology in all cases of birth depression. Placental microbiology can also be helpful, and even if histology is not available a small piece of placenta can be sent for culture.

Table 8.3. UK National Institute for Health and Clinical Excellence categorization[a] of fetal heart rate features.

Definition	Feature			
	Baseline (bpm)	Variability (bpm)	Decelerations	Accelerations[b]
Reassuring	110–160	≥5	None	Present
Non-reassuring	100–109 or 160–180	<5 for ≥40 but < 90 min	Early or variable, or 1 × prolonged (<3 min)	
Abnormal	<100 or >180 or sinusoidal (≥10 min)	<5 for ≥90 min	Atypical variable or late or 1 × prolonged (>3 min)	

[a] Categorization:

Normal   CTG where *all four* features (see above) fall into the reassuring category.

Suspicious   A CTG whose features fall into *one* of the non-reassuring categories, the remainder of the features being reassuring.

Pathological   A CTG whose features fall into *two or more* non-reassuring categories or *one or more* abnormal categories.

[b] The absence of accelerations in an otherwise normal CTG is of uncertain significance.

Examination

A baby who has been resuscitated from being half-dead or actually dead deserves a better quality neurological assessment than "fontanelle √".

Measure the head, check fontanelle tension, examine the eyes and the pupils, and assess tone, primitive reflexes, movement quality, and responsiveness to pain and touch. Is the baby adopting a normal flexed posture, moving fluently and elegantly with a good range of spontaneous movements, opening his hands and moving his fingers individually, rooting and sucking and opening his eyes to follow a bright toy? Is he consolable and "cuddly," nestling into the mother's shoulder or the crook of her arm, sleeping much of the time but waking for feeds? Or is he lying in an opisthotonic extended posture, stiff to handle, wide awake and startling in response to every little stimulus, with clenched fists, biting on the examiner's finger rather than sucking, and emitting only a high-pitched squeal? Worse still, is he comatose, ventilator-dependent, with fixed dilated pupils and unresponsive to pain? Much can be said about the baby in remarkably few words, and the neurological examination must be repeated frequently in the first few days. Whether the underlying cause of neonatal encephalopathy (NE) was a recent hypoxic ischemic insult, or a recent arterial infarction or intracranial hemorrhage then the clinical findings will evolve and change; if the NE remains static then another diagnosis becomes more likely. One way of documenting the findings and achieving some consistency between examiners is to use a simple form, and our current version (which owes much to the work of Dubowitz) is reproduced in Table 4.1. The findings on clinical examination can be used to form a score, which has been shown to be of diagnostic and prognostic value [17] (Table 8.4). A standardized neurological examination at 2–3 weeks is a simple but useful prognostic tool, and correlates well with magnetic resonance imaging (MRI) findings [18].

Laboratory tests

A basic set of tests in a baby with birth depression includes a blood gas, chest X-ray, glucose, electrolytes, creatinine, full blood count with nucleated red cell count, and coagulation studies. Other tests, such as ammonia and chromosome examination, may be indicated in certain situations; remember Prader–Willi syndrome and spinal muscular atrophy can now be identified quickly with genetic tests but the laboratory have to be asked the right question (Table 8.5). If the baby is hypovolemic or anemic a maternal Kleihauer test should be requested as soon as possible.

Lumbar puncture

There is increasing reluctance to perform neonatal lumbar puncture, which in our view is a pity. Meningitis is easily missed, particularly viral meningitis. Specific polymerase chain reaction (PCR) tests are available for herpes virus and should be considered, particularly if there are other clues to infection.

The electroencephalogram

An early electroencephalogram (EEG) can provide very helpful diagnostic information in babies with birth depression. Term babies who have suffered from significant intrapartum hypoxia often react in a similar way to experimental models [19]: their EEG becomes depressed and remains depressed for about 8 hours. Reactivity then returns, and seizures break through at about 8–12 hours, and often continue for several days [20,21]. A baby born in poor condition whose EEG in the first 12 hours remains entirely normal but who then develops seizures and abnormal imaging is very unlikely to have

Table 8.4. The Thompson encephalopathy score [17]. The score consists of clinical assessment of nine signs. Each sign is scored from 0 to 3 and the score for each day is totalled. The higher the score the more severely affected the infant. The maximum possible score on any day is 22.

Sign	Score			
	0	1	2	3
Tone	Normal	Hyper	Hypo	Flaccid
LOC	Normal	Hyperalert, stare	Lethargic	Comatose
Fits	Normal	Infrequent <3/day	Frequent >2/day	
Posture	Normal	Fisting, cycling	Strong distal flexion	Decerebrate
Moro	Normal	Partial	Absent	
Grasp	Normal	Poor	Absent	
Suck	Normal	Poor	Absent/bites	
Respiration	Normal	Hyperventilation	Brief apnea	Apneic
Fontanelle	Normal	Full, not tense	Tense	

LOC, Level of Consciousness.

Table 8.5. Laboratory investigations to consider in early neonatal encephalopathy.

Umbilical cord gas results

Full blood count with nucleated red blood cell count

Urea and electrolytes, glucose, creatinine

Blood culture

Lactate and ammonia

Early neonatal blood gas

Liver function tests

Coagulation screen

Thrombophilia screen

Toxicology screen

Plasma amino acids

Creatine kinase

Biotinidase

Acyl carnitine

Very long chain fatty acids and bile acids (Zellweger's, pseudo-Zellweger's)

Sulfate oxidase excretion

Chromosome studies – consider specific tests for Prader-Willi, spinal muscular atrophy and mitochondrial DNA mutations (Angelman syndrome has been reported as presenting in the newborn period with encephalopathy)

Plasma transferrin electrophoresis for carbohydrate-deficient glycoprotein syndrome

Urine amino and organic acids, urine reducing substances, toxicology

CSF lactate/pyruvate ratio and glycine for non-ketotic hyperglycinemia

Muscle biopsy for cytochrome oxidase deficiency and other respiratory chain disorders, e.g., pyruvate dehydrogenase deficiency

experienced an intrapartum hypoxic ischemic insult, whatever the CTG showed, even if the EEG subsequently changes to burst suppression. A baby who has electrographic status epilepticus at the age of 2 hours is likely to have sustained the hypoxic ischemic insult many hours earlier – possibly days earlier. An EEG pattern of burst suppression which persists, unvarying, for days or weeks suggests a diagnosis of metabolic encephalopathy or Ohtahara syndrome, not hypoxic ischemic encephalopathy. The EEG is often recorded after phenobarbitone, or other CNS-suppressing drugs, have been administered. Whilst EEG activity can show transient generalized suppression during the acute administration of phenobarbitone, we are in agreement with Staudt and colleagues in considering that a therapeutic level of phenobarbitone does not significantly alter the background EEG [22]. Massive doses of barbiturates can induce coma with an isoelectric EEG.

Cranial ultrasound

Like others, we believe that this imaging technique provides important information in babies with NE [23]. We image babies who have been depressed at birth as soon as possible after admission, and those who develop NE at 24 hours, 3–4 days, 7 and 14 days. The results of cranial ultrasound imaging do not usually allow a precise diagnosis or prognosis, but this investigation can identify pre-existing structural abnormalities or evidence of long-standing damage and assist in targeting other investigations and the timing of MRI. Occasionally the changes seen with ultrasound imaging are so clear cut that they are of prognostic value, for example obvious abnormality in the putamina and thalami or cystic breakdown of the white matter. Doppler ultrasound measurements of blood flow velocity in the anterior or middle cerebral arteries give useful information in babies with NE [24,25,26].

The following can be noted using cranial ultrasound in babies with NE, and will be described in more detail later in this chapter:

- The basic neuroanatomy; subtle abnormalities may be clues to metabolic, congenital or viral disease. For example, a hypoplastic corpus callosum (p. 254) may indicate a diagnosis of non-ketotic hyperglycinemia, and pseudocysts (pp. 229–231) can suggest mitochondrial, peroxisomal or viral disease.
- A persistence of small ventricular cavities beyond the 24 hours which is normal at term, associated with a loss of the definition of sulci and gyri and a "sparkly" appearance of the parenchyma – the "bright brain" of cerebral edema.
- Abnormal echogenicity in the parenchyma which can be present from the first scan, suggesting a long-standing insult, or develop over time.
- Abnormal echolucency or other evidence of cerebral atrophy.
- Increasing echogenicity in the basal ganglia and thalami; these changes are usually bilateral and support an acute hypoxic ischemic insult.
- Focal areas of hemorrhage or infarction (pp. 103–117); hemorrhage in the posterior fossa or the extracerebral space can be difficult to define with ultrasound.

Magnetic resonance imaging

Magnetic resonance imaging (MRI) has increased our understanding of the heterogeneity of brain injury associated with NE. The pattern of brain injury identified with MRI can help to distinguish between competing causes and can identify babies who are most at risk of adverse motor and cognitive outcomes [27]. Detailed descriptions of precise MR findings and their relation to later neurological outcome are available [28]. Magnetic resonance spectroscopy (MRS), in particular, assists in the identification of metabolic disorders, which can present with acute early NE. Magnetic resonance imaging has significant advantages over ultrasound in identification of abnormalities in the posterior fossa, and there are some useful signs (such as the absence of the normal signal from myelin in the posterior limb of the internal capsule) that are difficult or impossible to detect with ultrasound imaging.

In our opinion there is now sufficient evidence to recommend that MRI should be performed in all babies with moderate or severe NE, and similar recommendations have been made in the USA [29]. If resources allow only one image to be made, the optimal timing is in the second week of life; very early scans can give misleading results as they can appear almost normal even when there is severe brain injury.

The range of MR findings during the first few weeks in a baby with NE include:

- Normal
- Cerebral edema
- Abnormal signal from myelin in the posterior limb of the internal capsule
- Abnormal basal ganglia and thalami
- Cortical highlighting
- Cortical watershed abnormalities
- Focal white matter abnormalities
- Periventricular abnormalities
- Multicystic encephalomalacia
- Congenital malformation
- Intracranial hemorrhage

Broadly speaking, two main patterns of brain injury are detected with MRI in babies with NE that is due to hypoxic ischemia. These are, first, a watershed-predominant pattern, involving the white matter in the vascular watershed areas between the territory of the major cerebral arteries, and, second, a basal ganglia-thalamus predominant pattern which can involve the peri-Rolandic cortex when severe [30,31]. Scoring systems are available [27].

Diagnostic categories resulting from investigation of the baby with birth depression

Neonatal encephalopathy due to perinatal hypoxic ischemia

Terminology and prevalence

We have chosen to use the term "neonatal encephalopathy" (NE) in this chapter, and we have not used the terms "perinatal asphyxia," "birth asphyxia" or "hypoxic ischemic encephalopathy." We have done this in recognition of the variable timing, biological variability and the wide range of underlying causes and risk factors associated with this syndrome. Neonatal encephalopathy is often defined clinically as abnormal neurological behavior commencing in the first 24 hours of life, which consists of an altered conscious level with abnormalities of neuromuscular tone or sucking behavior. Seizures are the hallmark of NE, but the disorder manifests in other ways, including difficulty in initiating and maintaining respiration, abnormality of tone and reflexes, feeding problems, and alterations of state (hyper-alertness, abnormal sleep-wake cycling, or reduced responsiveness). There is a need for consensus regarding the definition of NE, not least because the lack of an agreed definition makes comparison between studies difficult and pooling of data impossible [32].

Recent UK data showed that the incidence of NE was 1.1 per 1 000 births in Trent [33]. The incidence of NE in a prospective study carried out in the Southwest Thames region of the UK between 1993 and 1995 was 2.62 per 1 000 births when an "over inclusive" definition (similar to that of Badawi [11]) was used, and 1.62 per 1 000 when the definition included at least one seizure [34]. Similar rates have been published for other countries including Scotland, France, and Australia, and these rates have remained largely unchanged for the past 20 years, although some claim to have seen a decline [35,36,37,38]. The incidence in developing countries is almost certainly much higher, and was estimated as 6 per 1 000 live births in the major maternity hospital in Kathmandu, Nepal [39]. This hospital delivers over 14 000 babies a year using only intermittent auscultation for fetal heart rate monitoring, does not use partograms, and has a caesarean section rate of 10%.

Using a broad definition of NE, studies in Western Australia uncovered a wide range of risk factors including many antepartum problems such as maternal hypothyroidism, preterm prolonged membrane rupture, and chorioamnionitis [11,40,41]. The contribution of intrapartum hypoxic ischemic events to later cerebral palsy (CP) was estimated as 10% of CP cases [42]. Other studies have found perinatal hypoxic ischemia to be the cause of CP in a larger proportion of cases, and it is notable that as the use of MRI has increased in the Swedish cohort studies the proportion of cases ascribed to "unknown" causes has fallen, whereas that attributed to perinatal hypoxic ischemia has tended to increase – reaching 35% in the 1995–98 birth cohort [43,44]. The Swedish data also show a rise in the subtype of dyskinetic CP, the type which is most likely to be caused by acute hypoxic ischemia at term – current estimates suggest that 80% of this type of CP is caused by intrapartum hypoxic ischemia [45]. When babies who had a syndromic diagnosis or a congenital defect were excluded, 90% of cases of NE in term-born babies cared for in London or Utrecht were considered to be have sustained intrapartum hypoxic ischemia [46]. This high figure may reflect the tertiary referral nature of the collaborating institutions; nevertheless, intrapartum monitoring that was limited to intermittent auscultation detected "evidence of hypoxia" (presumably fetal heart rate changes) in 43% of the encephalopathic babies in Kathmandu, and intrapartum complications were implicated in 60% [39].

Physiology of hypoxic ischemia in the term newborn brain

Knowledge of how babies react to hypoxic ischemia has been informed by a long sequence of experiments using animal models, dating back to Boyle's work in the seventeenth century with "kitlings" in bell jars, and continuing with the submersion experiments on baby rabbits in the eighteenth and nineteenth centuries. Since then the newborn of almost every available laboratory animal has been subject to hypoxic ischemia for research purposes, including the classic work on newborn primates [47], the more recent studies on lambs by the New Zealand group [48], piglets at University College London (UCL) [49] and baby rabbits in Illinois [50]. Of course human babies are different to animals, and there is more variation in prior vulnerability and the precise degree and duration of the hypoxic stresses to which human fetuses may be exposed. Animals have a smaller brain-to-body weight ratio than babies and are usually anesthetized throughout the hypoxic-ischemic insult, which itself is standardized and reproducible. Some anesthetics (e.g., ketamine) are now thought to be neuroprotective. For all these reasons, data from animal models of perinatal hypoxic ischemia have to be evaluated carefully but continue to provide invaluable insight into the human situation.

The animal models fall into two basic groups: prolonged partial (chronic partial) hypoxia and acute total hypoxia. Gluckman's group have recently added repeated acute insults, but there is still no animal model for the acute-on-chronic situation so often seen clinically [51]. A wide range of insults including maternal hypoxia, maternal hypotension, placental separation, prolonged complete umbilical cord occlusion,

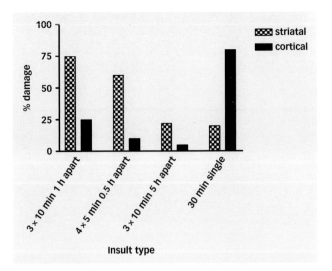

Fig. 8.1. **Pattern of brain damage sustained after different types of insult in the fetal lamb model. Data taken from the work of Mallard et al. [54,55].**

prolonged partial cord occlusion, repeated brief cord occlusions, and reversible occlusion of the common carotid arteries have been tried.

Acute near-total hypoxic ischemia

A sudden virtually complete obstruction to the fetal circulation produces a bradycardia within 90 seconds in animal models, with an initial rise in blood pressure followed by hypotension. There is no time for compensatory mechanisms to be called into play. A reduction in umbilical blood flow to 25% of normal produces a bradycardia of around 60 beats per minute in a lamb fetus. The pH falls rapidly in this situation, reaching levels as low as 6.8 in 12 minutes, with a base deficit of the order of 16 mmol/l. Animals resuscitated after more than 10 minutes of acute total asphyxia of this severity show damage to the nuclei of the basal ganglia and the thalami; those resuscitated after more than 25 minutes do not survive the neonatal period. The parts of the brain which show damage in this model are those with a high metabolic rate and glucose metabolism, and also those with a large number of excitatory glutaminergic inputs [52].

Gluckman's group have studied the result of brief repeated bilateral fetal carotid compression in lamb fetuses, which may be similar to the hypoxic ischemia experienced by the human fetus subjected to intermittent cord compression. Three 10-minute insults an hour apart caused damage in the striatum whereas a single 30-minute insult damaged the parasagittal cortex [53]. Four 5-minute occlusions of the umbilical cord 30 minutes apart also damaged the striatum [54]. Three 10-minute insults 5 hours apart did not damage the brain as much in this model, but there was some neuronal loss in the basal ganglia (Fig. 8.1).

The UCL group use a newborn piglet model of transient hypoxic ischemia induced by reversible occlusion of the common carotid arteries by remotely controlled vascular occluders

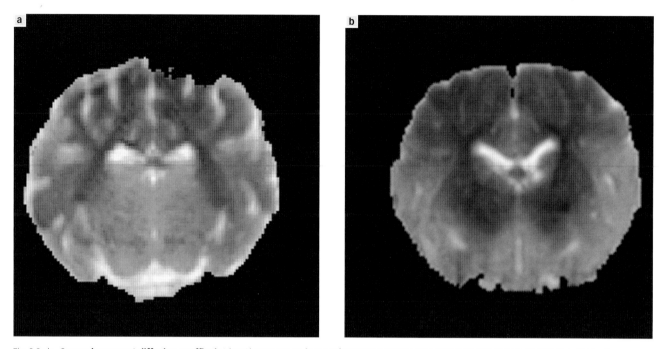

Fig. 8.2a,b. Coronal apparent diffusion coefficeint (ADC) maps at 15 hours after transient hypoxia ischemia (HI) in two piglets (a and b) who endured a moderate and severe hypoxic ischemia insult respectively. Darker areas indicate reduced ADC, which reflects energy depletion and cytotoxic edema limited to the parasagittal region in (a) and extending to involve the parasagittal region, cortex and thalamus in (b).

and simultaneous reduction in the inspired oxygen fraction to 0.08–0.12. An advantage of this model is that intensive care can be administered to the piglet and metabolic and physiological homeostasis maintained throughout the experiment, whilst monitoring cerebral energy metabolism continuously and non-invasively. The insult severity can be quantified using phosphorus-31 (^{31}P) MRS as the piglet remains in the bore of the magnet before, during, and after the insult, for up to 60 hours at a time [49]. A biphasic pattern of energy failure during and after hypoxic ischemia has been observed in this model; these data have contributed to the realization that neuroprotective strategies such as hypothermia may interrupt the cascade of irreversible injury if cooling is started in the "latent phase" when energy levels have "pseudo-normalized" after resuscitation [56]. Piglet studies have also shown that more severe insults are associated with shortening of the subsequent latent phase, worse secondary energy failure, and more severe cortical damage [57]. The brevity of the latent phase in severe insults may explain the lack of hypothermic neuroprotection seen in severe NE in the results of the clinical cooling trials [58]. Typical patterns of injury that are seen in this model are shown in Fig. 8.2a and Fig. 8.2b; it is remarkable that even in this model where the hypoxic ischemic insult can be quantified and standardized there is still a degree of biological variability, which may reflect previous pre-conditioning events or different pre-existing risk factors.

The selective vulnerability of the deep gray matter seen in the experimental models of acute hypoxic ischemia resembles that seen in the primate experiments conducted by Myers in the 1970s [47,59]. The "acute total" hypoxic-ischemic syndrome is now well recognized in babies, and classically occurs as a result of a catastrophe such as uterine rupture, cord prolapse or massive placental abruption [60,61]. Bradycardia can occur in the second stage (or even the first stage) of labor for no obvious reason, and persist long enough to cause acute total hypoxia of this kind [60,62]. Occasionally shoulder dystocia or a persisting vagal bradycardia associated with head compression during instrumental delivery is responsible. When the damaging acute hypoxic ischemia occurs in the immediate run-up to delivery, which is the usual situation, babies require cardiopulmonary resuscitation and usually have a 5-minute Apgar score of less than 5. Rarely, fetuses can recover after a severe in-utero insult and demonstrate all the features of an acute near-total hypoxic insult after birth without significant birth depression [63,64,65].

Prolonged partial hypoxic ischemia
Fetal animals show a consistent response to prolonged partial hypoxic ischemia whether it be induced by maternal hypoxemia, reduced uteroplacental blood flow or incomplete cord occlusion. At first the fetus increases its blood pressure and redistributes cardiac output away from the lungs, gut, and kidney towards the brain, heart, and adrenals; "centralization" of the circulation [66]. This compensatory phase can last some time, and has a parallel in human babies with uteroplacental insufficiency who can survive (albeit hypoxic and mildly acidotic) for weeks [67]. This adaptation is responsible for the "brainsparing" phenomenon seen in fetuses who have intrauterine growth retardation because of placental insufficiency.

Table 8.6. Sites of particular predilection for the diffuse form of selective neuronal injury seen after hypoxic ischemia in the term infant.

Brain region	Areas of particular vulnerability in the term infant with selective neuronal injury following hypoxia ischemia
Cerebral cortex	Somers sector of hippocampus – most vulnerable
	Calcarine and peri-Rolandic cortex affected in more severe injury
	Diffuse involvement of all cortex seen in very severe injury
	Neurons in deeper cortical layers and depths of sulci predominantly affected
Diencephalon	Thalamus consistently affected – may be combined with basal ganglia and brainstem injury
	Hypothalamus and lateral geniculate body also vulnerable
Basal ganglia	Caudate and putamen commonly affected in term infants – globus pallidus more often affected in preterm infants but not the rule. Putaminal-thalamic injury typical of hypoxic-ischemic injury in the term infant
Brainstem	Characteristic of hypoxic-ischemic injury in term infant
	Midbrain – inferior colliculus, trochlear, oculomotor, substantia nigra
	Pons – motor nuclei of 5th, 7th cranial facial nerves, dorsal cochlear nuclei
	Medulla – dorsal nuclei of vagus, 9th and 10th cranial nerves, inferior olivary nucleus, cuneate and gracile nuclei
Cerebellum	Purkinje cells
	Anterior lobe of the vermis commonly damaged in severe hypoxic ischemia

Hypoxic ischemia that is prolonged, repeated or very severe eventually causes the fetus to decompensate with a progressive acidosis and falling blood pressure. At this point brain damage becomes much more likely. The healthy fetus has a considerable reserve capacity because it is usually operating with a surplus of oxygen, meaning that a reduction of oxygen delivery of the order of 50% for at least an hour is usually required to produce acidosis, and even then not all acquire brain damage. Fetuses with reduced reserve probably acquire acidosis (and the possibility of brain damage) much sooner because they have reduced oxygen-carrying capacity, reduced glycogen stores, and blunted catecholamine responses. During a mild-to-moderate reduction in perfusion, the brain autoregulatory mechanisms preserve blood flow to the brainstem, cerebellum, and deep gray matter. This results in a reduction in perfusion of the cerebral watershed region, producing parasagittal lesions [68,69].

In fetal lambs uterine artery occlusion can be used to produce hypoxic ischemia; in one experiment it took over an hour before the fetal EEG was flattened, and in some animals it was necessary to put a bag over the ewe's head to produce additional hypoxia [70]. Of the 14 lambs who survived this insult, 8 had parasagittal cortical damage; the damaged lambs were those who had been hypotensive during the insult, and whose pH had fallen to around 7. The most useful postnatal predictor of damage was EEG suppression in the first 12 hours. Repeated occlusions of umbilical cords of fetal lambs (for 1 out of every 2.5 minutes for some hours) eventually led to acidosis, hypotension, and damage to the parasagittal cortex [71]. Reducing the ovine umbilical cord blood flow to 21% for 90 minutes led to a diversion of blood from the body to the brain, EEG suppression, and encephalopathy after recovery [72].

Neuropathology of hypoxic ischemia

The neuropathological changes seen after neonatal hypoxic ischemia vary with the gestational age of the infant, the nature of insult, type of interventions, and other factors that remain to be defined. Two main patterns are seen: (1) selective neuronal necrosis; and (2) parasagittal cerebral injury, although overlap between these groups is the rule rather than the exception.

Selective neuronal necrosis

Selective neuronal necrosis is the most common injury response observed after intrapartum hypoxic ischemia. The patterns include:

1. Diffuse neuronal injury. This typically occurs following a very severe, very prolonged insult. The major sites for predilection for diffuse neuronal necrosis in the term infant include the cerebral cortex, hippocampus, deep nuclear structures (in particular the caudate, putamen, and thalamus), and brainstem (Fig. 8.3a–c, Table 8.6).
2. Cerebral cortex – deep nuclear neuronal injury. This usually occurs following moderate to severe, prolonged insult and typically consists of injury to the peri-Rolandic cortex/putamen and thalamus (Fig. 8.3d).
3. Deep nuclear-brainstem neuronal injury. This typically follows a severe, abrupt insult. The typical topography of this pattern of injury is shown in Fig. 8.3e. The brainstem, thalamus, and basal ganglia have an active metabolism and the corresponding blood flow is abundant in these areas making them most vulnerable to acute anoxia.

Magnetic resonance imaging scans have revealed these patterns of injury with remarkable clarity. Another region of selective vulnerability after acute hypoxic ischemia is the anterior lobe of the cerebellar vermis [73,74] (Fig. 8.3f).

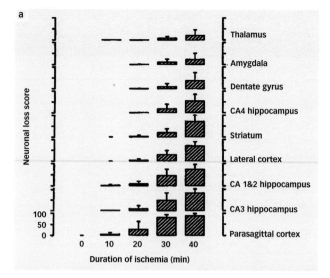

Fig. 8.3a–f. (a) Neuronal damage in nine brain regions following increasing durations of ischemia. These are ranked in inverse order of total damage scores: the parasagittal cortex was the most severely and easily damaged (bottom) whereas the thalamus (top) showed the least damage. The damage scores are on a linearized scale: 0 to 100, 0 no neuronal loss; 100, total necrosis. (Reproduced with permission from [19].)

Excitotoxicity is believed to be responsible for the neuronal damage caused by hypoxic ischemia in the developing brain [52]. Excitotoxicity can be regarded as the "Achilles heel" of neurons, which normally benefit from the trophic stimulation provided by well-modulated excitatory stimulation. There is evidence that the neuronal pattern of damage reflects the dysfunction of a set of excitatory neuronal circuits triggering selective neuronal death [75]. Brain injury after transient hypoxic ischemia is an evolving process: transient severe hypoxic ischemia and subsequent reperfusion/reoxygenation leads not only to immediate cell death but triggers complex biochemical events which result in further delayed neuronal death [52,76,77,78,79]. Although apoptotic cell death (cell suicide) is currently considered to be the main cause of delayed neuronal death after hypoxic ischemia in the developing brain, both apoptotic and necrotic cell death are observed after hypoxic ischemia in animal models and human infants who subsequently died. It is very important to understand the relative contribution of these different processes so that effective neuroprotective strategies can be developed, and much experimental work is currently directed towards this end.

Parasagittal cerebral injury
Parasagittal cerebral injury (also termed watershed or border-zone injury) is a lesion of the cerebral cortex and subcortical white matter with a characteristic distribution over the supero-medial aspects of the cerebral convexities (Fig. 8.4a). An excellent example of parasagittal injury was produced in the Myers primate model, in which the mother was rendered hypotensive for between 1 and 5 hours prior to the delivery of the fetus

(Fig. 8.4b). This pattern of injury is characterized by necrosis of the cortex and the immediately adjacent white matter, and usually affects the parieto-occipital regions (the posterior watershed) more than the anterior watershed [80]. The precuneus is an area of brain which lies at the junction of all three major cerebral arteries and is particularly vulnerable to damage in this pattern of injury. At the cellular level, laminar necrosis of cortical pyramidal neurons is typically seen.

Magnetic resonance imaging has greatly facilitated identification of these cases; in a recent study parasagittal injury was the commonest pattern (45% of cases) [30] (Fig. 8.5a–d). The depths of the sulci are less well supplied with blood than the tips, hence this relatively avascular area is especially vulnerable to a drop in perfusion pressure. This observation may explain why the cerebral injury in the parasagittal vascular border zones is more severe in the depths of the sulci and why the damaged gyri become mushroom shaped; this is called ulegyria. Ulegyria can be identified with late MRI (Fig. 8.5), when it remains specific for hypoxic ischemic damage at term; the immature or adult brain does not react this way.

The parasagittal pattern of injury has been seen in various experimental models: the monkey, sheep, rabbit, mouse, and piglet. In the near-term fetal lamb, there was greater vulnerability of the parasagittal regions, however with prolonged asphyxia many other regions became affected and the parasagittal predilection is less apparent [81]. This is similar to the findings in the piglet (see above).

Clinical course of neonatal encephalopathy
Neonatal encephalopathy due to hypoxic ischemia is an evolving clinical illness. Static NE suggests that the cause is not hypoxic ischemia, whereas babies who sustained an intrapartum hypoxic ischemic insult show clinical progression of their NE, with a worsening of neurological signs after the first 12–24 hours and a slow improvement after about 4–5 days. Encephalopathy scores usually demonstrate a peak on days 3–4 [17]. Most encephalopathy scores are based on the clinical criteria developed by Sarnat and Sarnat in 1976 and modified by Levene in 1986 [82,83]. Recent modifications have been directed at developing quantifiable scores with good reproducibility, and the Thompson score has a possible maximum of 22 (Table 8.4). Some scores claim prognostic value on the first day of life, whereas most of the earlier scoring systems were only of value when the worst grade was reached, or when considered over the first 7 days [84,85]. Whilst we wholly endorse the use of repeated careful neurological examination and find a structured system helpful (Table 4.1), we would not base a prognosis on the results of a neonatal neurological examination on the first day.

In general babies with Sarnat grade I encephalopathy, which includes a brief period of irritability and poor sucking but not seizures, do not develop any sequelae although Rosenbloom has described some who later developed dyskinetic cerebral palsy [86]. Babies with the basal ganglia/thalamus-predominant pattern of injury generally have the most intensive need for

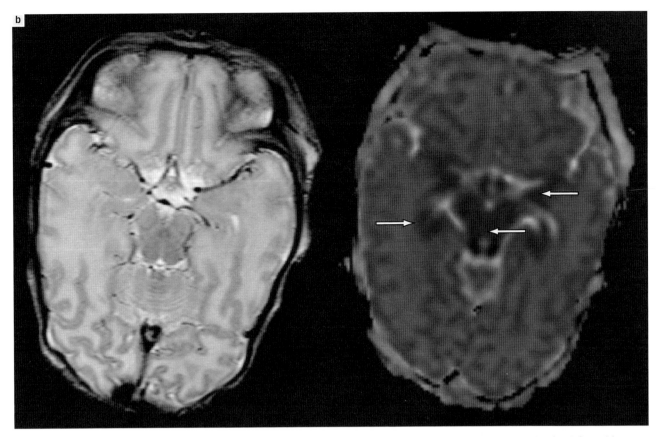

Fig. 8.3. (cont.) (b) Axial T$_2$-weighted images and apparent diffusion coefficient (ADC) trace map at the level of the mid brain of an infant with stage II Sarnat encephalopathy scanned on day 5. ADC trace map demonstrates restricted diffusion in the inferior mid brain, hippocampi, and amygdalae (arrows). This is not well demonstrated on the axial T$_2$-weighted image.

resuscitation at birth and the most severe clinical encephalopathy and seizures [30]. In general, babies who have sustained an intrapartum hypoxic insult of sufficient severity to cause brain damage have transient injury to other organ systems, including the kidney [87,88].

EEG in neonatal encephalopathy

The principles of EEG are discussed in Chapter 2 and the normal appearances described in Chapter 6. Both EEG and amplitude-integrated EEG (aEEG) are invaluable investigations in babies with NE, and can assist with diagnosis and prognosis, particularly when prolonged or repeated recordings are made. The EEG appearances, like the clinical syndrome and the neuroimaging appearances, evolve over time in NE due to hypoxic ischemia. EEG studies in asphyxiated fetal sheep showed that the EEG became isoelectric at the time of a 30-minute acute hypoxic ischemia insult and remained suppressed for about 8 hours afterwards [89]. During the recovery (reperfusion) phase EEG activity increased, with seizures breaking through at about 12 hours, but the background activity remained abnormal [19]. The electrographic seizures then

continued, coinciding with the phase of cerebral edema, and burnt out after about 48–72 hours [90,91].

In general, the seizure burden is not considered to be of prognostic importance [92], although McBride and her co-workers did find that babies with a large number of electrographic seizures had a worse outcome than those with fewer or no seizures [91]. In our experience, babies with NE due to hypoxic ischemia who are in electrographic status (defined as a seizure burden of 50% or more in a 1-hour period) fare badly. We have documented the emergence of seizures after a quiescent interval in several cases of NE, although the time to first seizure probably varies according to the type and duration of the insult, when it occurred, and whether or not antiepileptic medication has been given [20,93]. As discussed, the diagnosis of NE due to hypoxic ischemia should be reconsidered if the clinical and EEG signs remain static for several days, and further investigations are essential in this situation (Table 8.5). Repeated EEG testing from very early in life is more valuable than a single recording, but if resources are limited to a single EEG then it is best obtained between 24 and 48 hours. An EEG that is depressed in the first 12 hours can

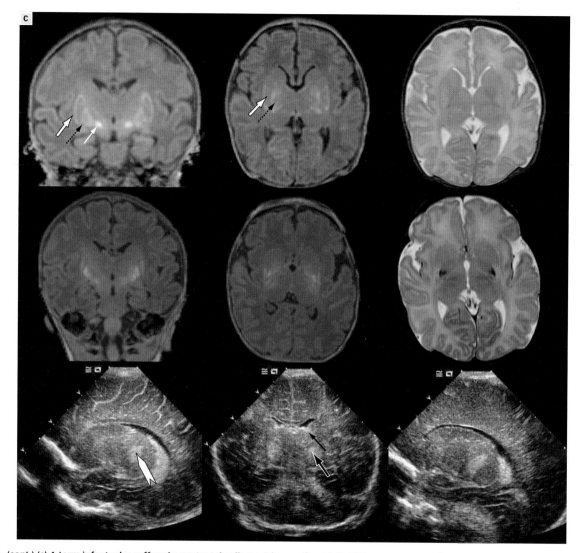

Fig. 8.3. **(cont.) (c) A term infant who suffered a postnatal collapse 3 hours after birth. MRI scans were preformed on day 6 and 16. Cranial ultrasound scans from day 16 are shown in the bottom row. Top row: the coronal-weighted image demonstrates (from medial to lateral) abnormal signal in the subthalamic nucleus (STN) (small white arrow), globus pallidus (dotted arrow), and putamen (large white arrow). The axial T$_1$-weighted image confirms the abnormal signal inthe globus pallidus (dotted arrow) and putamen (large white arrow). Middle row: these abnormalities persist on day 16. Bottom row: cranial ultrasound scans (right and left S2 and C4 views). The C4 view demonstrates echodense areas in the thalami (thin arrow) and globi pallidi (large arrow). On the right and left S2 views there are abnormal signals in the globi pallidi (large arrow). The dark stripe corresponding to an abnormal signal intensity in the posterior limb of the internal capsule (PLIC) can be seen on all views and is indicated on the first S2 view (white arrowhead).**

recover to a normal or mildly abnormal pattern and these babies generally do well [21,93,94].

The first attempt to combine EEG with clinical information for prognostic purposes was made in Oxford in 1960 [95]. At the time, they concluded that the striking EEG changes they observed were of no value, but the prognostic value of EEG between the second and seventh day of life in term babies with encephalopathy is now well established, and an EEG which is very depressed (less than 5 μV, now termed electro-cerebral inactivity), shows burst suppression or is markedly asymmetrical at this time presages a poor outcome [91,97,98,99,100] (Fig. 8.6). The vast majority of babies with persistent electro-cerebral inactivity will either die or have severe neurological sequelae [102,103]. The same is true for persisting burst suppression [104,105,106,107]. Babies with normal or mildly abnormal EEGs do well, as do those with moderate abnormalities which improve before 7 days of age [94,98,99]. Peliowski and Finer included some of these results in a meta-analysis in 1992; the risk of death or handicap with a severely abnormal EEG was 95%; with moderate abnormalities, 64%; and with mild or no abnormalities, 3% [108].

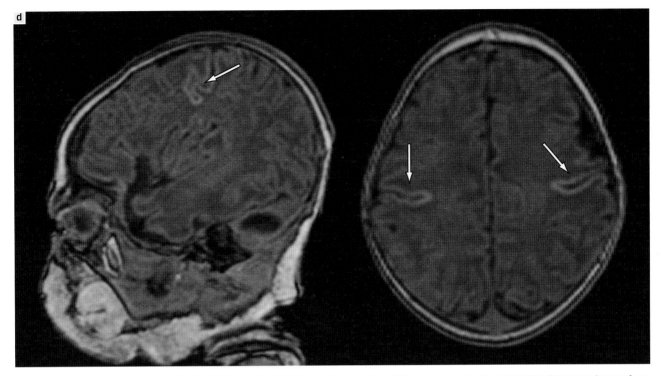

Fig. 8.3. (cont.) (d) T_1-weighted sagittal and axial images (level of the centrum semiovale) in a term infant with postnatal collapse at 3 hours of age. The abnormal SI in the lentiform nuclei and thalamus is clearly seen. The cortical highlighting in the peri-Rolandic cortex is clearly seen in both the sagittal and axial MR images.

The main drawback of an EEG obtained after 24 hours is that changes seen at this time can be secondary to hypoxic ischemia associated with sepsis, raised intracranial pressure due to an expanding subdural hematoma, or a metabolic disorder, and are not specific to an intrapartum hypoxic ischemia insult. In NE EEG abnormalities often persist for days, and occasionally weeks, but the background activity eventually normalizes. A normal EEG in the second week of life does not rule out a diagnosis of NE due to hypoxic ischemia; neither does it provide complete reassurance about the prognosis in this condition. The same is not true for a normal EEG in the first 24 hours, which excludes very recent (usually intrapartum) damaging hypoxic ischemia and indicates a much better chance of a normal neurological outcome (depending on the diagnosis). There has been a suggestion that the EEG should be performed when the baby's neurological signs were at their worst in order to obtain the reliable information for diagnosis and prognosis [109]. However, in our view the longer the time between a putative hypoxic ischemic insult and an abnormal EEG the worse the prognosis, but the more tenuous the diagnosis. The combination of repeated or continuous EEG from early in postnatal life, repeated clinical evaluation, appropriate laboratory evaluation with repeated ultrasound imaging, and a judiciously timed MRI can give very specific diagnostic and prognostic information when the results are correctly interpreted, and represents the current "gold standard" of investigation after birth depression [110]. Our aim is to encourage and facilitate this standard for all babies with NE.

Amplitude integrated (aEEG) in neonatal encephalopathy

The basis of the aEEG, a compressed filtered and rectified EEG signal, is described in Chapter 2 and the normal appearances and classification system in Chapter 6. In spite of the obvious limitations, the background EEG can be reliably assessed at term using this method [111,112]. Modern aEEG systems also have several advantages: they are compact, easy to use, and can store signals at the cotside over long periods of time. The method is not always reliable for the detection of seizures, but works well in many babies, and neonatal unit staff can be taught to interpret the results. aEEG shows the same basic patterns as EEG: normal, discontinuous, low voltage, burst suppression, and isoelectric (Chapter 6) (Fig. 8.6). The results obtained using aEEG to predict outcome are similar to those obtained using EEG; a very early trace showing burst suppression or electro-cerebral inactivity can normalize by 6 hours and the baby can do well, but persistent burst suppression, or persisting electro-cerebral inactivity carries a poor prognosis [21,26,111,113,114,115].

The aEEG background pattern has a good predictive value for neurodevelopmental outcome in NE by 12 hours (some say

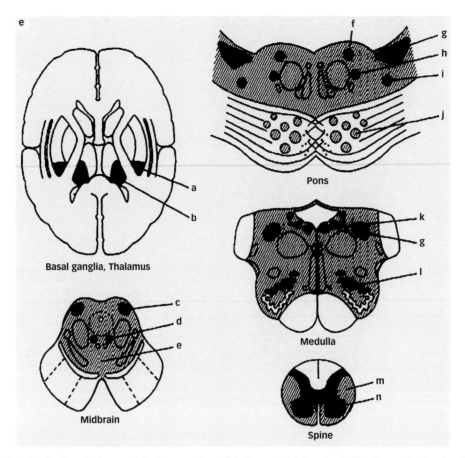

Fig. 8.3. **(cont.) (e) Typical distribution of microscopic lesions seen in a clinical case of total asphyxia [63]. The cerebral cortex did not exhibit any abnormality. The shaded area indicates nuclei with neuronal loss and the diagonally striped pattern indicates the area of marked gliosis. a, putamen; b, ventral posterolateral thalamic nuclei; c, inferior colliculus, d, trochlear nuclei; e, tegmentum; f, abducens nucleus; g, vestibular nucleus; h, facial motor nucleus; i, spinal tract of trigeminal nerve; j, longitudinal pontine bundles; k, hypoglossal nucelus; l, olivary nucleus; m, lateral funiculus; n, anterior horn. Reproduced with permission from [63].**

as early as 3 hours after birth) (Table 8.7) [26,111,113,114,116,117]. In a retrospective review of 160 babies with NE who had aEEG recordings which began within 6 hours of birth, 65 had traces that were initially of very low voltage (electro-cerebral inactivity) and 25 had burst suppression [21]. In only 6 of the 65 who had electro-cerebral inactivity did the trace normalize within 24 hours; 5 of these children were normal at follow-up and 1 had a major disability. In contrast, recovery was more likely in those with burst suppression (12 of 25) but the outcome was worse, with only 4 normal survivors. One of the children died, 5 had a moderate to severe disability and 2 had mild disability. This study is important because it highlights the need for early and continued aEEG monitoring of babies with NE, a view which we wholly endorse. It is recognized that drugs can affect the background pattern of the aEEG; the degree of the effect is dependent on the severity of the brain injury [101], but antiepileptic drugs did not affect the recovery of the aEEG in the Utrecht study, or in our own EEG study [93]. Burst suppression has been linked to treatment with midazolam [119]; hence, the prognostic value of aEEG may be limited when midazolam levels are high.

Sleep–wake cycling (SWC) is present in healthy term newborns and is a sign of brain integrity [120]. During wakefulness/active sleep the bandwidth of the aEEG tracing is narrower, whereas during quiet sleep the bandwidth is broader. Diagnosis of normal SWC rests on there being at least three consecutive cycles on aEEG tracing during a period of 5 hours [121]. The presence of normal SWC soon after birth was a valuable predictor of good neurodevelopmental outcome in NE [121]. In this study, an assessment 36 hours after birth proved to be the most valuable: a good neurodevelopmental outcome was predicted correctly by the onset of SWC before 36 hours in 82% of term newborns. The presence of seizures prolonged the time from birth to onset of SWC – it was not possible to determine whether this was due to the electrographic seizure activity or to the antiepileptic drugs. In our view, and that of others, aEEG is an essential tool in NE, and should be supplemented by formal EEG wherever possible [101]. Ideally, the aEEG recording should be continued long enough to allow the onset of SWC to be determined, but it is certainly important to continue recording for at least 48 hours.

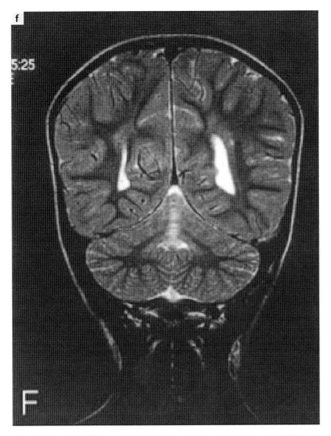

As explained in Chapter 2, the newer digital aEEG recorders simultaneously display and record EEG and aEEG, hence direct inspection of the raw EEG and comparison with the aEEG can be performed in real time and retrospectively. As experience with these new digital monitors grows, there is a realization that this facility is crucial for the correct interpretation of the aEEG. In particular we and others have recognized that EEG artifacts frequently occur despite the filtering process and can influence the interpretation of the aEEG recording [122] (Fig. 8.7a). For example, 200 hours of aEEG recordings from a representative sample of 20 infants with NE suggested that artifacts occurred in 12% of the recording time sampled (Fig. 8.7b); around 55% artifacts were derived from electrical interference and 45% from movement interference, and both could influence the voltage and width of the aEEG band [122].

The currently used aEEG classifications [123] rely heavily on the aEEG band voltage and background activity, thus artifacts may result in an erroneous classification. This is important especially if aEEG is used as a selection tool for neuroprotection intervention studies as, for example, elevation of the voltage band of activity from the baseline of <5 to >5 μV may suggest a more favorable prognosis and lead to exclusion from therapeutic hypothermic. The possibility of inspecting the raw EEG in the new digital aEEG systems facilitates the detection of artifacts and improves the accuracy of interpretation of the aEEG. However, although some artifacts may be easily recognized, for example the regular artifact caused by ECG interference, in many cases the recognition of an underlying artifact requires an ability to interpret the EEG [122].

Fig. 8.3. (cont.) (f) Abnormal high T_2 signal intensity in the central lobule of the anterior lobe of the cerebellar vermis secondary to profound hypoxia ischemia in the perinatal period is seen in this image from a 9-month-old girl with dyskinetic cerebral palsy. From [73].

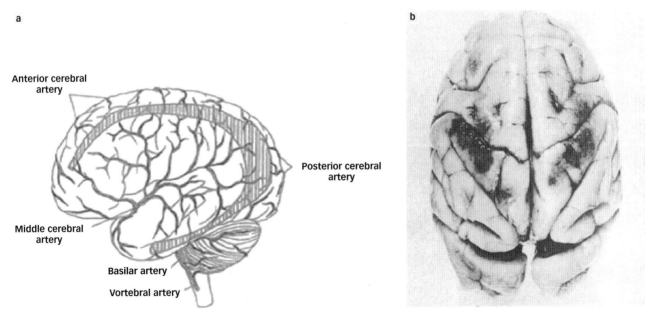

Fig. 8.4a,b. (a) Parasagittal cerebral injury. Schematic diagram of cerebral convexity, lateral view, showing distribution of major cerebral arteries. Distribution of injury, shown by shaded area, is in the border zones and end fields of these arteries. (b) Cerebral lesions in the term fetal rhesus monkey after severe partial asphyxia (intrauterine fetal asphyxia was produced by halothane-induced maternal hypotension for between 1 and 5 hours). At the end of the period of asphyxia, each fetus was surgically delivered and resuscitated. This is a superior view of the brain of a representative asphyxiated newborn monkey showing brain swelling combined with bilateral hemorrhagic infarcts of the middle paracentral regions of the cortex.

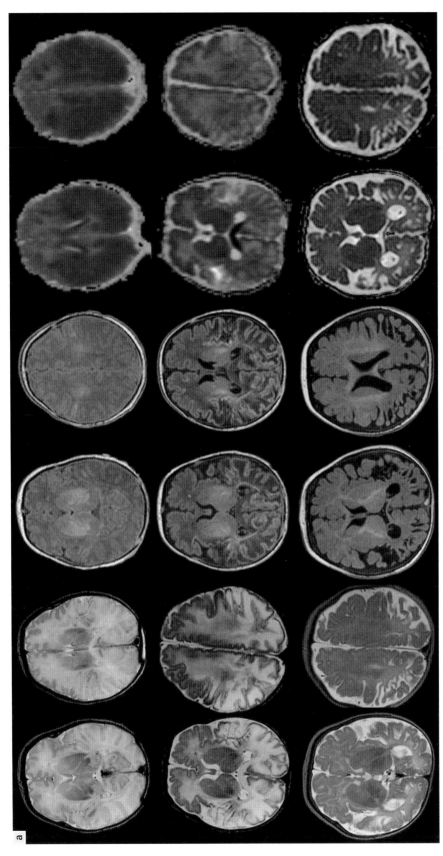

Fig. 8.5a–d. (a) Predominant parasagittal cerebral injury in a term infant who was born at 40 + 1 weeks' gestation with Apgar scores of 9 at 1 and 5 minutes, cord gas pH 7.3 and base deficit −8.1. There was some meconium at delivery and grunting developed at 30 minutes of age necessitating admission to the neonatal intensive care unit for continuous positive airways pressure (CPAP) and oxygen therapy. At 13 hours after birth the infant became apneic with neonatal seizures. MRI scans were acquired on day 5 (upper row), day 11 (middle row), and 4 months (bottom row). Upper row: T₂-weighted images show bilateral parasagittal cerebral hemispheric injury extending anteriorly. There is cerebral swelling and the cortex and white matter are involved, with loss of the cortical ribbon. T₁-weighted images show reduced gray-white matter differentiation. These areas show restricted diffusion on the ADC trace map. Middle row: the brain swelling is resolving on T₂-weighted images. ADC trace maps show a mixed pattern of restricted and increased diffusion. Bottom row: the cerebral infarction has matured and there is brain atrophy. The typical appearance of ulegyria due to more severe damage in the depths of the sulci is clearly seen in the posterior parasagittal watershed regions. ADC trace maps show predominantly increased signal in the posterior white matter.

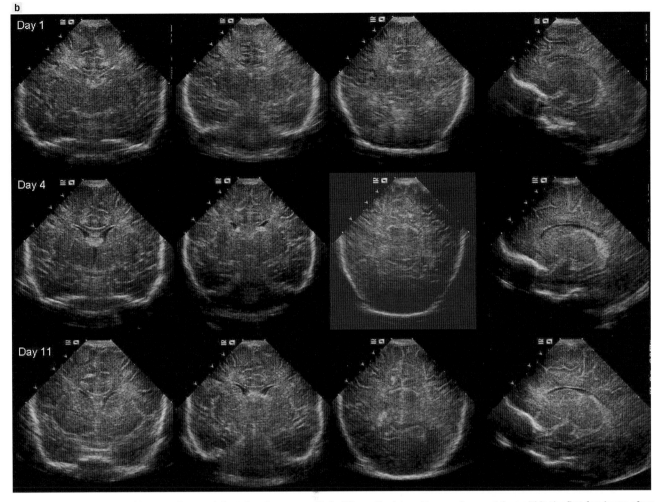

Fig. 8.5. **(cont.) (b)** Ultrasound images of a term infant showing parasagittal white matter injury. Top row: images taken within the first few hours after birth showing established clear area of abnormal echogenicity bilaterally in frontal and parieto-occipital regions. Middle row: the appearances on day 4; the ventricles are now normal size and the abnormal echogenicity is less obvious. Bottom row: the appearances on day 11 with little further evolution. The MRI and spectroscopy findings appear in (c) and (d). Taken together the findings confirm injury which was well established at the time of birth.

Cranial ultrasound in neonatal encephalopathy

Brain swelling and edema

Brain swelling is a non-specific cranial ultrasound finding which supports a diagnosis of hypoxic ischemia, but is not always present even in confirmed cases. The term "bright brain" has been applied to the ultrasound appearances of brain swelling since 1983 and has the merit of simplicity [124], but must be reserved for genuine cases. Given the importance which may be attached to a scribbled note reporting "bright brain" years later, long after the pictures have become detached from the records and destroyed by flooding in the hospital basement, great care needs to be taken before making this diagnosis using ultrasound. After the early phase of cytotoxic cerebral edema, edema is not a neuropathological feature of hypoxic ischemia until after 24 hours, and the swelling usually resolves before the end of the first week.

The ultrasound diagnosis of brain swelling requires more than a casual observation of "slit-like ventricles." Virtually all normal term babies have small lateral and third ventricular cavities, and a few hours spent imaging babies on postnatal wards will reveal the range of normal appearances at term. The ultrasound appearances of cerebral edema include loss of the normal anatomical detail with obscuration of the sulcal markings and closure of the interhemispheric and Sylvian fissures (Fig. 8.8a,b). The brain has a generally "sparkly" appearance, with increased echoreflectance, although care needs to be taken to check the gain settings (Fig. 4.22). The lateral ventricles are indeed small and may be completely obliterated, but the important feature is that the finding persists beyond the first day of life. Hence a diagnosis of cerebral edema can only reliably be made with ultrasound 24 hours after birth, although on occasion the associated

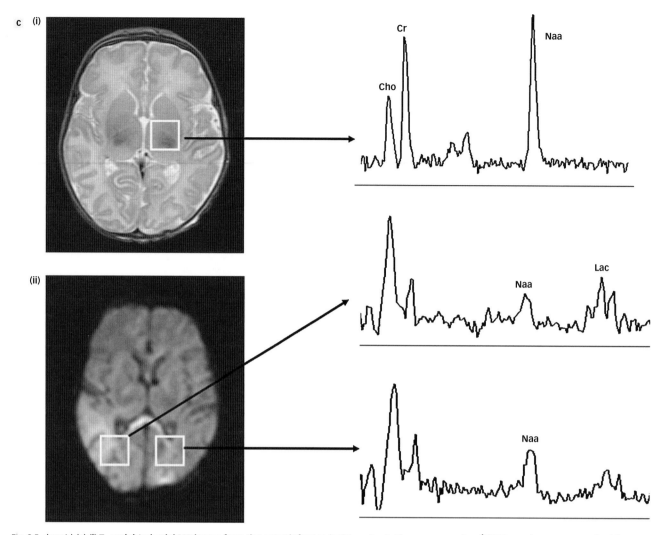

Fig. 8.5. **(cont.) (c) (i)** T_2-weighted axial MR image from the same infant as in (b) on day 5. The corresponding ¹H MR spectrum was acquired from an 8-cm³ voxel in the left basal ganglia and thalamus using a PRESS localization sequence (TE 288 ms). The Naa and Lac peak areas ratios appear normal; peak ratios were: Naa/Cr 1.19; Lac/Cr 0.26; Lac/Naa 0.24, which are within the normal range for control term infants. **(ii)** ADC trace map acquired on day 5 in the same infant showing restricted diffusion in the watershed or borderzone areas. The right side is more severely affected than the left. ¹H MR spectra were acquired from both right and left parieto-occipital lobes (8-cm³ voxels, PRESS localization, TE 288 ms). Consistent with the more widespread restricted diffusion on the right, the ¹H MR spectrum acquired from the right white matter shows higher lactate and reduced Naa, suggesting more severe injury. ¹H MRS peak area ratios from the left white matter were: Naa/Cr 2.27; Lac/Cr 1.46; Lac/Naa 0.64. ¹H MRS peak area ratios from the right white matter were: Naa/Cr 1.63; Lac/Cr 2.36; Lac/Naa 1.45.

parenchymal changes are so obvious that there is a high index of suspicion in the first 24 hours. A finding of cerebral edema is not useful for prognosis, nor is it a reliable indicator of the time of the insult. However, a "full house" of bright parenchyma, obliterated gyri, and tiny lateral ventricles seen in the first 24 hours would suggest that the hypoxic-ischemic insult had occurred well before birth, particularly if the changes rapidly resolved or evolved within a day or two into an established injury pattern. A Doppler cerebral blood flow velocity pattern which showed an increase in diastolic velocity at the same time (i.e., within 24 hours of birth) would support the conclusion that the hypoxic-ischemic insult was not recent.

Increased echogenicity in the basal ganglia and thalami
Following on from diffuse brain swelling, increased echogenicity of the deep gray matter can often be seen to emerge 2–4 days after an acute hypoxic ischemic injury. The published experience is now considerably greater than the single case reports and small series that were available when the first edition of this book was prepared [125,126,127]. If a clear and persistent bilateral abnormality of the basal ganglia and/or thalamic area is imaged with ultrasound then the prognosis is poor (Fig. 8.9 a,b) and there is a good correlation with MRI (Fig. 8.10a–e) [128]. Once seen, the appearances are unmistakable – the thalami, in particular, appear egg-shaped and

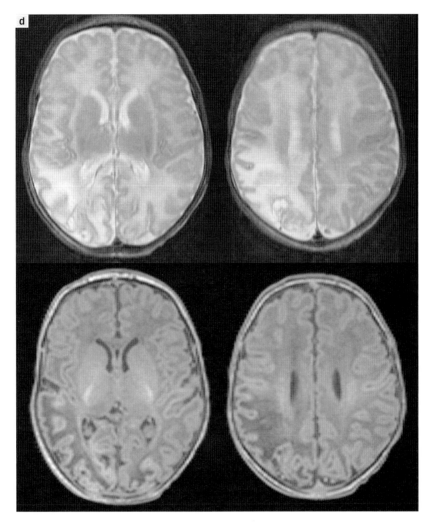

Fig. 8.5. (cont.) (d) These MR images (same baby as in (b) and (c)) were performed on day 13 after birth. Axial T$_1$- and T$_2$-weighted MR images show signal abnormality consistent with edema and early cavitations in the right parieto-occipital lobes, and some edema in the right thalamus. These are the typical appearances of watershed injury.

echoreflectant. In the coronal view, the internal capsule remains of normal echogenicity and gives rise to a "stripe" appearance as it sits between the thalami and lentiform nuclei, which are abnormally echoreflectant. This appearance, of a hypoechoic line running through the central gray matter, is probably a poor prognostic sign [129]. The imaging changes are probably due to areas of hemorrhagic infarction, and the accuracy of detection of thalamic neuronal necrosis using ultrasound appears to be good, with 100% sensitivity and 83% specificity in one autopsy study, in which there was only one false-positive result [130].

Cortical lesions

Areas of increased echogenicity in the superficial cortex, in the region immediately below the brain surface, can be detected with ultrasound in some babies with hypoxic-ischemic encephalopathy. A 10-MHz transducer improves the accuracy of detection of cortical lesions.

Extensive cortical change can be predicted from the "cotton-wool," patchily echodense appearance of the parenchyma in the early days (Fig. 8.11a). Figure 8.11b shows the evolving appearances as imaged with ultrasound over the first 7 days. The images show the development of extensive echogenicity in the subcortical and deep white matter. There is loss of the normal architectural detail. Over time there is often extensive cystic degeneration and loss of white matter, with the "swiss-cheese" appearance of multicystic encephalomalacia. Sometimes both the deep gray matter and the cortex are involved in a very destructive, almost total, brain injury leading to very poor head growth and a dismal outcome.

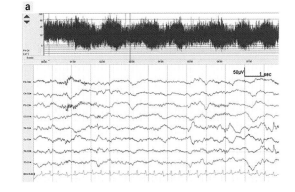

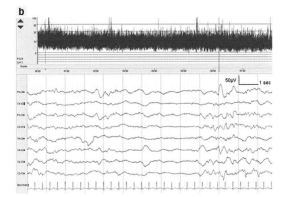

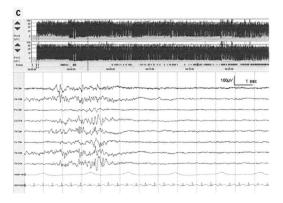

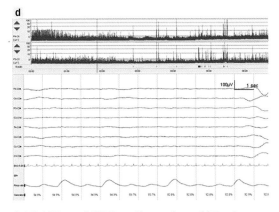

Fig. 8.6a–d. **EEG and aEEG traces seen in NE [101]. (a) Normal. (b) Discontinuous trace. (c) Burst suppression. (d) Very low amplitude, almost isoelectric trace.**

Periventricular lesions

Eken *et al.* found that ultrasound evidence of periventricular echodensity was surprisingly common in term babies with hypoxic-ischemic encephalopathy [130], and the same findings were reported in one of the first studies of ultrasound imaging in NE [131]. In Eken's study ten babies had areas of increased echogenicity in the periventricular white matter, which were confirmed at autopsy in eight. Two more had pathological lesions of antenatal origin which were missed. Interestingly, the periventricular lesions were imaged with ultrasound in the first 24 hours, in contrast to the other abnormalities which are usually detected in NE. This pattern of injury may reflect a watershed-predominant pattern affecting the posterior intervascular boundary zones of the brain [27]. Recent MR imaging studies have revealed a strikingly high incidence of white matter lesions in term babies with congenital heart disease who underwent complex surgery [31,132, 133].

Doppler cerebral blood flow studies in NE

Although the early reports of an increased diastolic flow velocity in babies with NE are now 20 years old the results have been confirmed many times, and the test has proved reliable and reproducible over the years [24,25,26,134]. The change can be detected from about 24 hours after the insult, and is usually assessed by the calculation of the Pourcelot Index (PI) [(peak systolic velocity – end-diastolic velocity)/peak systolic velocity]. There can be confusion with the Pulsatility Index, which is also often abbreviated to PI but is calculated from the formula (peak systolic velocity – end-diastolic velocity)/mean. Some manufacturers term the Pourcelot Index the Resistance Index, displaying the result as RI. More information on the physics of the Doppler effect is given in Chapter 1. The investigation of babies with NE remains the main clinical application of Doppler ultrasound in neonatal medicine, although the technique has been widely used for research into cerebral blood flow in the past [135,136] (Fig. 8.12a,b).

The change which is seen in babies with hypoxic ischemia is basically an increase in diastolic velocity (Fig. 8.12c). The effect is probably due to increasing resistance to blood flow associated with brain swelling, contributed to by the loss of autoregulation. The timing of the change coincides with the phase of "luxury perfusion" seen in animal models of hypoxic ischemia; in other words, the phase of overshoot in cerebral blood flow (CBF) which occurs after an early phase of low CBF (sometimes termed "no reflow"). As the diastolic velocity rises, the PI falls, and a PI of less than 0.55 is associated with a poor outcome. Before interpreting the result it is worth checking that the arterial carbon dioxide tension and blood pressure are within the normal range and that there is not a large patent ductus arteriosus (PDA). It does not appear to be critical which vessel is used; usually it is easiest to insonate the anterior cerebral artery via the anterior fontanelle, but good results can also be obtained using the temporal window to insonate the middle cerebral artery. The contrast between a normal CBF velocity pattern and that showing a low PI can be seen in Fig. 8.12c. In our

view, it is worthwhile performing Doppler estimation of CBF velocity in babies with hypoxic-ischemic encephalopathy because the information adds to the total picture and helps when assessing prognosis.

A reverberating CBF velocity pattern, with reversed diastolic flow, can be seen in "brain death" [137,138,139,140]. Caution is needed because a large left-to-right shunt can produce significant flow reversal in diastole, and because there is controversy regarding the definition of "brain death" in the newborn.

Conventional MRI in neonatal encephalopathy

Experience with MR imaging in newborn encephalopathy, particularly hypoxic-ischemic encephalopathy, has accrued quickly since the first descriptions in the early 1990s [46,141,142,143,144,145,146,147,148,149,150,151,152]. Centers in Zurich, London, and San Francisco have all imaged large cohorts of babies and followed them up. Specific patterns of abnormality that are characteristic of hypoxic-ischemic injury are now very well described [30,31,153,154]. Further, MRI can reliably identify signs of existing abnormality due to antenatal damage or a congenital malformation. There is better inter-observer agreement for MRI than for ultrasound [155]. Magnetic resonance imaging is increasingly seen as a standard first-line investigation in babies with NE [29,156]. Perinatally acquired brain lesions are most obvious on conventional MRI from day 5 onwards; indeed imaging within the first 2 days may show only subtle abnormalities even when there is significant brain injury. Neonatologists may wish to use MRI very early to aid clinical management, and early imaging should always include diffusion-weighted imaging (DWI) and if possible MR spectroscopy (see below), but even DWI can fail to discover the extent and severity of the lesions [152]. It is not yet known whether neuroprotective therapies such as hypothermia delay the evolution of changes seen with MRI.

Barkovich describes three main patterns of injury seen on conventional MRI in NE [27]: parasagittal injury, total cortical loss, and basal ganglia and thalamic lesions.

1. Parasagittal injury (also called borderzone or watershed injury)

   The classic "watershed" or "borderzone" damage described by Volpe and Pasternak [80] involves areas of white matter loss at the boundaries of the territories of the three major cerebral arteries (Fig. 8.5). This pattern of tissue loss is thought to result from prolonged hypotension associated with chronic partial hypoxia, producing an effect similar to dry patches on a lawn resulting from reduced water pressure to adjacent sprinklers. Babies can acquire a "mixed" pattern of damage with lesions in the borderzones and the deep gray matter, and a recent series of 173 cases described a mixed pattern in 31% of those with watershed injury; previously a mixed pattern had been thought to be rare [30]. The affected cortex on T_2-weighted imaging will appear hyperintense and on T_1-weighted images edematous cortex will appear as areas of low signal intensity in the cortex and adjacent white matter. The most obvious abnormality is loss of the gray–white matter distinction and interruption of the cortical ribbon. The parasagittal white matter has prolonged T_2. As the injury evolves, cortical thinning and loss of the underlying white matter are seen in the parasagittal vascular boundary zones.

2. Total cortical loss

   Cortical injury is diffuse, involving most of the cortex while sparing the underlying deep gray matter. This

pattern is much less common than the parasagittal injury or the basal ganglia–thalamus pattern [157]. The outcome is usually poor. In addition to the "bat's wing" of cortical highlighting seen in the peri-Rolandic cortex as part of the "acute total" asphyxia pattern, in some cases the entire cortex is abnormally highlighted on MR images made in the early weeks after the insult. This finding probably corresponds to the well-described neuropathological finding of laminar necrosis in the deep

Table 8.7. Predictive value of aEEG at 3, 6 and 12 hours of age in NE, from references cited in the text.

	Time (h)				
	3 (*n* = 68)	6 (*n* = 47)	6 (*n* = 68)	6 (*n* = 160)	12 (*n* = 24)
	Toet *et al.* [114]	Hellström-Westas *et al.* [113]	Toet *et al.* [114]	van Rooij *et al.* [118]	al Naqeeb *et al.* [111]
Sensitivity	85	95	91	93	100
Specificity	77	89	86	85	82
PPV	78	86	86	88	85
NPV	84	96	91	91	100

PPV, positive predictive value; NPV, negative predictive value.

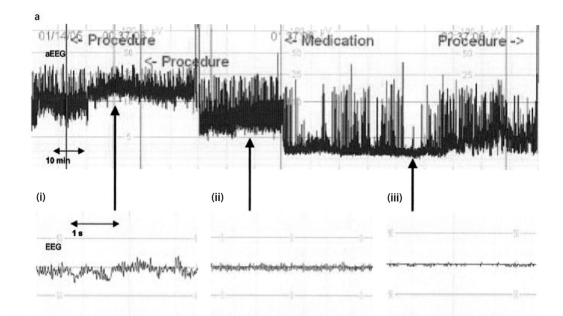

Fig. 8.7a,b. **(a) aEEG (normal impedance) and underlying single-channel raw EEG recordings from an infant with Sarnat Stage II encephalopathy at ~3 hours of age. The arrows define the points at which each underlying raw EEG was inspected. (i) High-frequency artifacts can be seen on the raw EEG. The basline is shifted upward >5 µV; (ii) The electrodes were moved closer to the vertex. The underlying raw EEG continued to show artifacts of lower amplitude and there was a slight shift of the aEEG baseline. (iii) After administration of pancuronium (medication marker) the underlying raw EEG showed fewer artifacts and was discontinuous. The aEEG background was classified as severely abnormal. ((a) and (b) reproduced with permission from [122].) (b) Frequency of observed artifacts observed during a random selection of 200 hours of aEEG recording in infants with NE.**

cortical layers. Extensive cortical abnormality usually presages the cystic breakdown of multicystic encephalomalacia (MCLE) (Fig. 8.11b, bottom row). We agree with the Dutch group, and with Rutherford [31,154], that babies who develop MCLE have often suffered a devastating encephalopathy characterized by marked cerebral

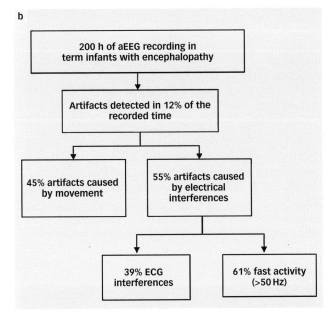

Fig. 8.7. **(cont.)**

edema after a surprisingly innocuous antenatal course; the CTG changes are often minor, the Apgar scores reasonable, and the long-term outcome and the amount of structural damage often seem disproportionate to the original insult. Others describe MCLE as occurring after "severe" hypoxia, but there is insufficient detail in the reports to determine whether the authors mean that the insult was severe, or they are describing the severity of the subsequent neonatal illness [149,158,159]. The condition is rare, so that even large series contain few cases. The percentage of babies with hypoxic ischemia who develop MCLE has been estimated as between 5% and 10% [149,153]. Perhaps future research will discover why some babies react to hypoxic ischemia this way – current ideas include the interaction of cytokine damage associated with infection and hypoxic ischemia, or "priming" of the apoptotic pathways by multiple asphyxial episodes.

3. Basal ganglia and thalamic lesions

More widespread use of MRI has revealed that the deep gray matter is extremely vulnerable to damage following acute near-total intrapartum hypoxic ischemia at term. The changes have been found remarkably frequently given the paucity of the previous autopsy descriptions. The basal ganglia consist of the globus pallidus and the putamen (which together form the lentiform nucleus), and the caudate nucleus. The normal appearances are shown in Chapter 4. Abnormalities can be seen in all parts of the basal ganglia and the thalami, and are often

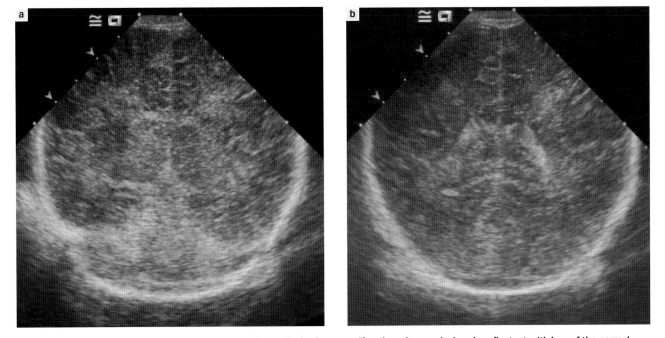

Fig. 8.8a,b. **Ultrasound scan images showing cerebral edema. The brains are uniformly and excessively echoreflectant with loss of the normal sulcal markings and small ventricles. The normal "Y" of the Sylvian fissure is obliterated.**

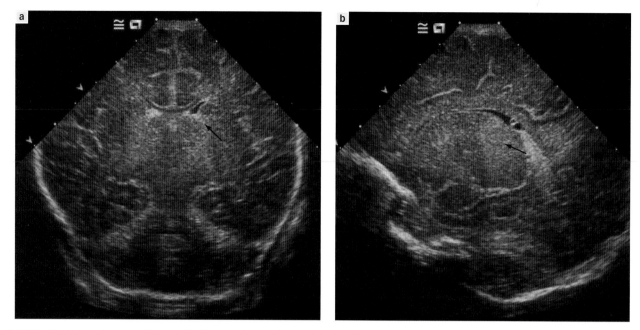

Fig. 8.9a,b. **Coronal and parasagittal cranial ultrasound scans from an infant with NE on day 3. The abnormal thalami appear as egg-shaped echoreflective lesions on the parasagittal views (thin black arrow), and can be located easily on the coronal image, medial to the similarly abnormally echoreflective lentiform nuclei. As a result the internal capsule appears as a "stripe" of darker tissue between the two.**

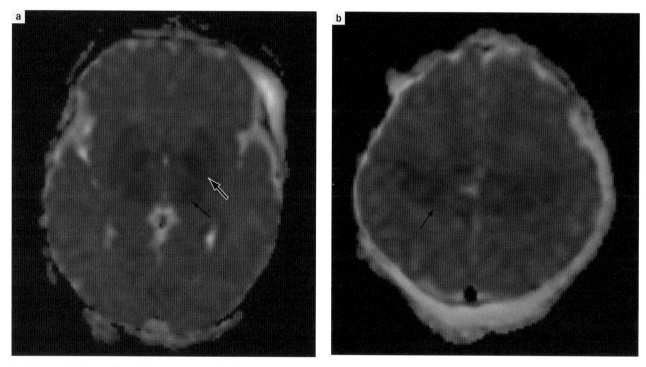

Fig. 8.10a–e. **ADC (day 4 after birth), conventional MR T$_1$-weighted and cranial ultrasound images (both day 10) from a term infant with Stage II Sarnat encephalopathy. The ADC trace maps in (a) show restricted diffusion within the thalami (thin arrow) and lentiform nuclei (globus pallidi and putamen) (large arrow) and in (b) in the peri-Rolandic cortex (thin arrow). These areas of ADC restriction have a similar pattern as the signal abnormality on the axial T$_1$-weighted images in (c) and (d) on conventional MRI on day 10 – abnormal signal intensities are present in the thalami (thin arrows) and lentiform nuclei (large arrows). A sagittal cranial ultrasound in the same infant is shown in (e). The posterior limb of the internal capsule appears as a stripe of darker tissue between the thalami and lentiform nuclei on the sagittal cranial ultrasound image (arrowhead).**

accompanied by damage to the corticospinal tracts around the central fissure (the peri-Rolandic cortex). However, the most vulnerable structures are the ventrolateral nuclei of the thalami and the posterior thirds of the putamina. The combination has been termed "central cortico-subcortical damage" [160]. The hippocampus can also be involved in this spectrum of damage, as can the lateral geniculate nucleus and the optic radiation. In severe total asphyxia the dorsal brainstem nuclei can be affected. Preterm babies can acquire damage in the deep gray matter, usually the thalamus, if they experience a near cardiac arrest [161].

There is a varying spectrum of damage, and several scoring systems have been devised [27,151]. The mildest changes include focal changes in the ventrolateral nuclei of the thalami, with normal signal in the posterior limb of the internal capsule (Fig. 8.13) (PLIC), but the spectrum evolves through more obvious changes in the putamina and thalami with accompanying change in the peri-Rolandic cortex and PLIC, into damage involving the whole of the lentiform nuclei, the thalami, and the caudate nuclei with or without cortical highlighting (Fig. 8.11). The deep gray matter can be totally destroyed and undergo cystic degeneration. There is a range of neurodevelopmental outcome corresponding to the different degrees of damage [28]; children with very small areas of focal change in the basal ganglia which can be imaged only with MR and not with ultrasound can be normal in the medium term, but the long-term outcome is not yet known. The thalamus is involved in executive functioning, which is the ability to hold ideas in the mind in order to plan and perform a complex sequence of events. Memory defects and defects of executive functioning were found in a group of children followed up after moderate or severe NE who did not have a motor

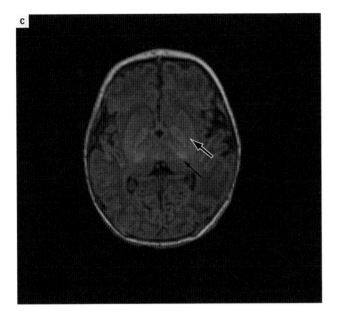

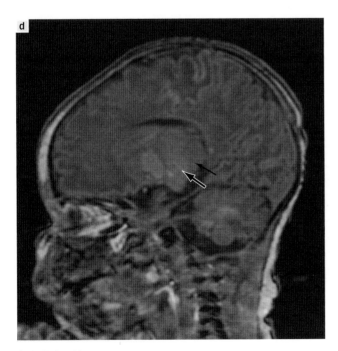

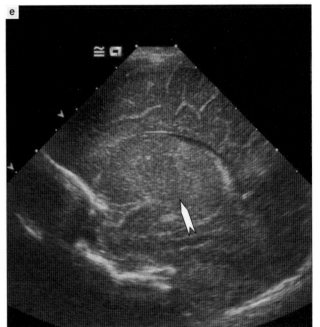

Fig. 8.10. **(cont.)**

disability, and more studies of this type are awaited [162]. Children who have damage in the posterior parts of the putamina usually have athetoid (dyskinetic) cerebral palsy at follow-up, often with preserved intelligence [163] although they can be very disabled by uncontrollable writhing movements, sometimes with a hemiballistic quality. Finally, children with widespread damage to the basal ganglia and thalami (in whom the PLIC signal is always abnormal) usually develop quadriplegic cerebral palsy with bulbar palsy and the associated feeding difficulties, often meaning that they have to be fed via a gastrostomy because their swallow is not safe.

Other observations on conventional MRI in the first 2 weeks include cerebral edema and focal and periventricular white matter abnormalities, as now discussed.

Cerebral edema

Early MRI, like ultrasound, shows brain swelling which usually develops 24 hours after a hypoxic-ischemic insult and persists for about 7 days. The imaging features which assist in making a correct diagnosis are the same as ultrasound; namely, small ventricles, loss of the normal anatomical detail with obscured sulcal markings and obliteration of the interhemispheric and Sylvian fissures. The prognostic implications are also the same – if cerebral edema resolves and the brain appears normal then the prognosis is good [145].

Focal and periventricular white matter abnormalities

Small punctate hemorrhagic lesions scattered in the white matter are occasionally seen with MRI in hypoxic-ischemic encephalopathy, and larger areas of focal hemorrhage occur

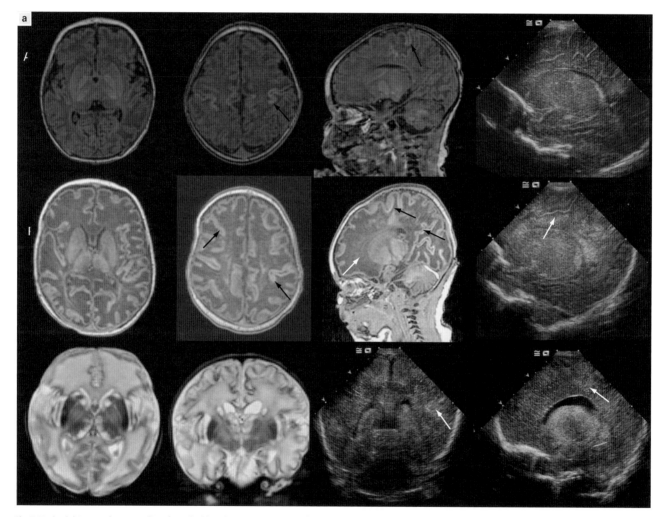

Fig. 8.11a,b. **(a) Increasing severity of cortical involvement in three infants with NE (1 infant per row). Top row: highlighting of the peri-Rolandic cortex (thin black arrow) is seen in addition to basal ganglia and thalamic injury in a term infant with Sarnat Stage II encephalopathy scanned on day 10. Middle row: more extensive cortical highlighting (black arrows) is observed as well as diffuse white matter signal abnormality (white arrow) in this infant with Stage III Sarnat encephalopathy scanned on day 10. A "cotton-wool" patchily echodense appearance of the parenchyma can be seen on the cranial ultrasound (white arrow). Bottom row: global extensive cerebral damage is seen in this term infant with Stage III encephalopathy scanned on day 14 affecting both hemispheres and deep gray matter with hemorrhagic change. On the cranial ultrasound, patchy parenchymal echodensities are seen (white arrows).**

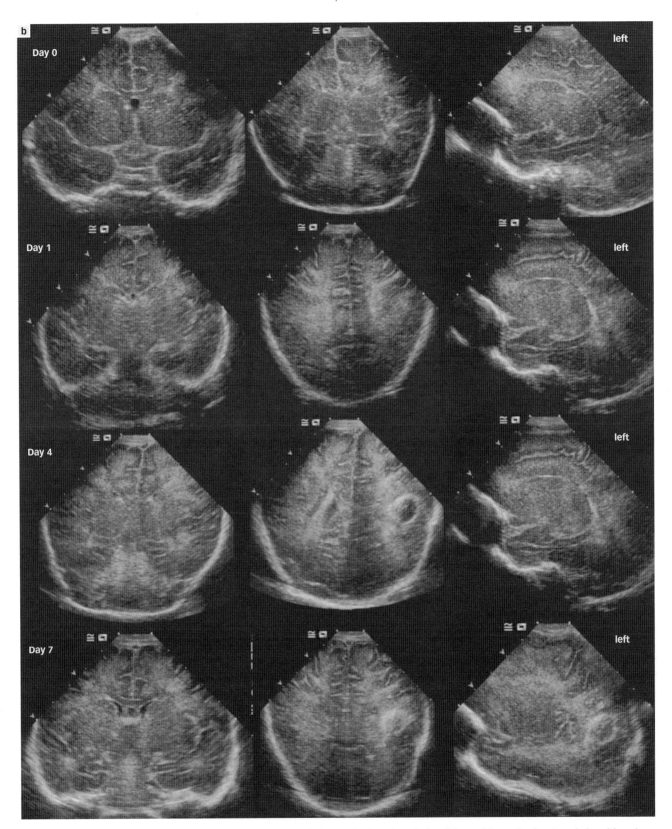

Fig. 8.11. (cont.) (b) Cranial ultrasound images showing evolution of changes in the subcortical and deep white matter in a term baby with early neonatal encephalopathy. Top row: day 0, almost normal appearances. Second row: day 1, patchy increased echogenicity in the white matter mainly seen in the frontal and periventricular white matter. By day 4 patchy, widespread "cotton-wool" echogenicity can be seen. Cortical highlighting is visible. In addition, there is a circumscribed cystic area in the left parietal lobe. Day 7, bottom row, widespread echogenicity of white matter, with cortical highlighting and slight interhemispheric fissure widening.

in around 5% of cases [153,164]. Baenziger is clearly of the view that periventricular leukomalacia-like lesions can be seen after hypoxic ischemia at term, with early periventricular high signal change which evolves into ventricular dilatation with a reduction in the periventricular white matter [144].

Rutherford has described the same sequence [154]. Others report periventricular high signal on MRI obtained between 4 and 12 months, but from these studies it is impossible to determine whether the abnormality originated in the perinatal period [165].

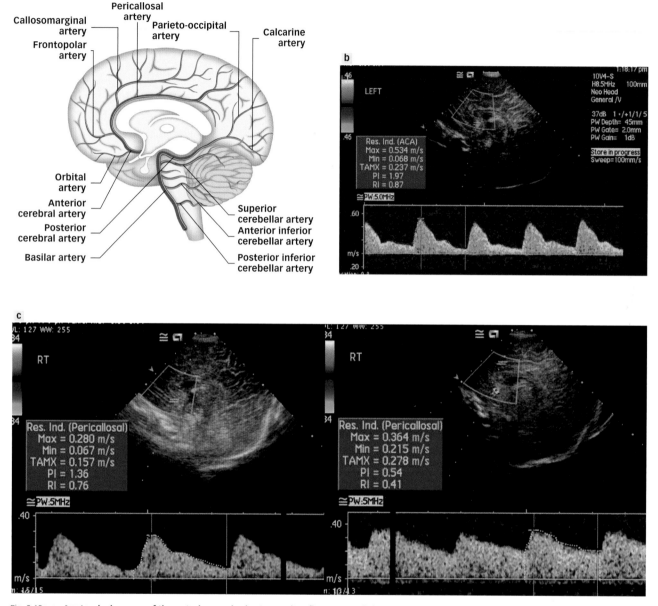

Fig. 8.12a–c. **Anatomical course of the anterior cerebral artery as it reflects around the corpus callosum and branches into the pericallosal and callosomarginal arteries. The easiest artery to insonate using Doppler ultrasound is the internal carotid artery just before it gives rise to the anterior carotid artery, because the angle of insonation is usually close to zero at this point reducing the errors. (b) Example of cerebral blood flow velocity using color Doppler in a normal infant. The results of the Doppler-shifted spectrum which has insonated the anterior cerebral artery are dispayed as a visual sonogram. The normal shape is pulsatile with a shoulder on the downstroke. The maximum velocity in systole and diastole can be assessed from the scale in the *y* axis. The resistance index of Pourcelot (PI) is: (peak systolic velocity – end-diastolic velocity)/peak systolic velocity. (c) Cerebral blood flow velocity of a term infant with Grade II NE at 2 and 4, days of age. The PI (labelled RI) is within the normal range on day 2 and has fallen to 0.41 on day 4, which is associated with a poor outcome.**

Quantitative MR techniques in NE

Diffusion-weighted imaging

Although DWI has revolutionized the diagnostic sensitivity of imaging in adult ischemic stroke [166], the value of DWI in NE has yet to be established [167]. Diffusion-weighted imaging can indicate the degree of free diffusion of water molecules, which is quantitated as the apparent diffusion coefficient (ADC), where ADC correlates with brain tissue energetics measured using ^{31}P MRS [168]. Primary and secondary energy failure associated with perinatal hypoxic ischemia results in intracellular (cytotoxic) edema, shrinkage of the extracellular compartment and consequently reduced ADC. The latter translates into a high DWI signal. The ADC values gradually return to normal 5–10 days after a hypoxic-ischemic insult and then increase in chronic lesions as vasogenic edema and cellular necrosis develop. Experimental adult stroke data suggest that the evolution of ADC varies with the severity of brain injury (Fig. 8.14a) [169]. There are interesting case reports of ADC mapping in individual babies in whom the exact time of the (postnatal) hypoxic ischemic insult was known [170]. We have experience of imaging cases in which the time of the insult was certain (Fig. 8.14b,c).

The neonatal brain (especially white matter) contains more water (with greater diffusion) than adult brain; furthermore, ADC decreases with brain maturation [171]. Although brain-water ADC is sensitive to injury in the first few days following perinatal hypoxic ischemia [172,173,174,175,176] it remains unclear whether DWI will be of early prognostic benefit: many groups report that DWI in the first week underestimates the injury revealed later by conventional MRI. New areas of reduced diffusion can appear during the first few days after hypoxic ischemia, whilst at the same time "pseudonormalization" is occurring in previously abnormal areas. This can result in confusion, with images which show an entirely different pattern of injury on diffusivity maps acquired at different times from the same baby [152].

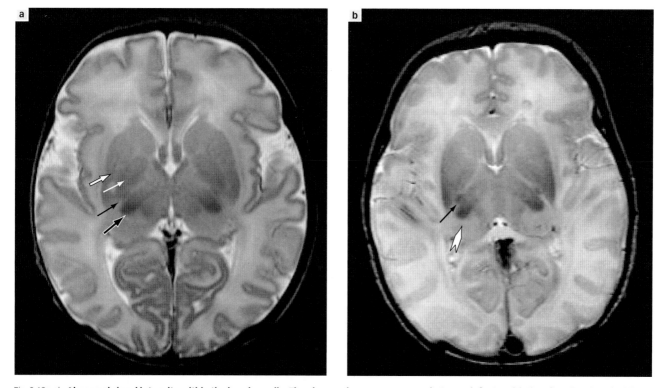

Fig. 8.13a–d. **Abnormal signal intensity within the basal ganglia.** The abnormal appearances vary between infants, with time from insult and with the windowing of the images but can be broadly divided into three groups of increasing severity. (a) T$_2$-weighted MRI from a normal term infant demonstrating normal signal hypointensity from myelin within the PLIC (small black arrow), ventrolateral thalamus (large black arrow), globus pallidus (small white arrow), and posterolateral putamen (large white arrow). (b) Mild abnormalities in the thalamus with increased signal suggestive of edema extending into the posterior part of the PLIC (white arrowhead). The low signal from myelin in the PLIC is still relatively preserved (small black arrow). (c) Severe involvement of lentiform nucleus and thalamus (double arrow) and abnormal SI within the PLIC with loss of normal low signal from myelin. As a result of increased contrast between the high signal of the lentiform nuclei and the low signal from the lenticulostriate vessels, the vessels appear more prominent (left arrow). (d) Extensive severe mature injury of all the basal ganglia including caudate nucleus (top arrow) and globus pallidus (middle arrow) with abnormal signal intensity in the PLIC (lower arrow).

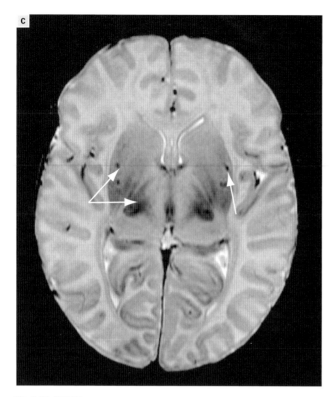

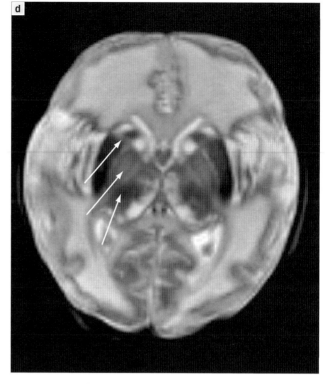

Fig. 8.13. **(cont.)**

The relationship between regional ADC and later neurodevelopmental outcome has been investigated: Zarifi *et al.* found no relationship between the ADC in the deep gray matter and outcome in term babies imaged 1–10 days after birth [172]. Others have found low ADC in the PLIC at a mean age of 5.6 days to be associated with an adverse outcome [176]. One of the largest studies is from the Hammersmith group, who studied the relationship between the contemporaneous DWI and conventional MRI in 63 infants with NE and 15 control infants [177]. The ADC values were significantly reduced in the first week after birth after severe injury to the basal ganglia-thalamus and white matter; values normalized at the end of the first week and then increased in week 2. The ADC values in infants with moderate injury were no different to controls, hence the additional information was not of great value in this group. These results show that the timing of the scan needs to be taken into account when interpreting the results.

Normal ADC values during the first week do not necessarily signify normal tissue. Apparant diffusion coefficient mapping may not detect moderate injury of the basal ganglia-thalamus or white matter, which can be associated with significant motor or cognitive impairment in the long term (Fig. 8.15). In severe injury, ADC is more helpful: ADC values $<1.1 \times 10^{-3}$ mm²/s are always associated with white matter infarction and values $<0.8 \times 10^{-3}$ mm²/s with thalamic infarction [177]. More sophisticated diffusion techniques, such as diffusion tensor imaging (DTI) may improve the ability to detect abnormal tissue as it brings in another parameter – anisotropy or directional diffusivity in a tissue [178]. In this study the fractional anisotropy (FA) was abnormal in both severe and moderate white matter and basal ganglia injury with no pseudonormalization at the end of the first week after birth.

T2 relaxometry

Quantitative MRI brain water T_2 (spin-spin relaxation time) measurements provide another method for early in vivo investigation of term infants with NE. T_2 is influenced by tissue properties including brain water content and its compartmental distribution, cerebral blood flow or volume, and tissue protein content. T_2 relaxometry utilizes multiple TEs to yield T_2 maps uncontaminated by other contrast mechanisms with absolute numerical values appropriate for intra- and inter-subject comparisons. T_2 relaxometry may reveal tissue abnormalities not apparent on conventional T_2-weighted imaging. A recent study at UCL demonstrated that deep gray matter T_2 was increased soon after birth (mean age 3.1 days, range 1–5) in infants with an adverse outcome. We found positive associations between basal ganglia and thalamic T_2 and lactate/Cr and lactate/Naa; there were negative correlations between basal ganglia and thalamic T_2 and Naa/Cr. Proton MRS peak area ratios were better predictors of adversity, however both ¹H MRS and T_2 were useful in assigning early prognosis (Fig. 8.16) [179].

The precise pathological cause of elevated T_2 in NE is unknown; histological studies in experimental models of both adult stroke and neonatal hypoxic ischemia have suggested that prolongation of T_2 reflects the onset of vasogenic edema associated with disruption of the blood–brain barrier and loss of tissue integrity. Given the considerable number of neurons and glial cells undergoing apoptotic death in the developing brain following hypoxic ischemia, the increased extracellular space due to cellular shrinkage may also contribute to T_2 prolongation. When the integrity of the plasma membrane is finally lost, T_2 may increase further due to the increased interstitial water content. Prolongation of T_2 may occur earlier and at a greater rate when necrosis is the dominant mode of cell death following hypoxic ischemia, as the disruption of the cellular architecture starts earlier compared to apoptosis [180].

MR spectroscopy

Over the last 25 years ^{31}P and ^{1}H MRS have advanced the understanding of pathophysiological changes in the developing brain. Interpretation of a MR spectrum can provide information about cellular energetics (phosphocreatine (PCr),

inorganic phosphate (Pi), adenosine triphosphate (ATP)), membrane turnover (phosphomonoesters (PME), phosphodiesters (PDE), choline (Cho)), neuronal function (N-acetyl aspartate (Naa), selected neurotransmitter activity (γ-aminobutyric acid (GABA), glutamate and glutamine) and the fate of anesthetic agents and certain drugs. The biochemical changes that occur in parallel with brain development are shown in Fig. 8.17. At a cellular level, processes such as neuronal organization, proliferation, differentiation of glial cells, and myelination occur in a highly ordered and stereotyped manner. Magnetic resonance spectroscopy has elucidated the biochemical mechanisms underlying these structural and cellular changes, and has demonstrated that metabolite concentrations vary in different regions of the brain [181]. An understanding of age-dependent and regional changes in metabolites is important to enable identification and recognition of metabolite abnormalities in pathological states.

Phosphorus-31 magnetic resonance spectroscopy (^{31}P MRS)

The first reported ^{31}P MR spectra were obtained in babies with NE at UCL in the early 1980s [182]. This technique has enormous

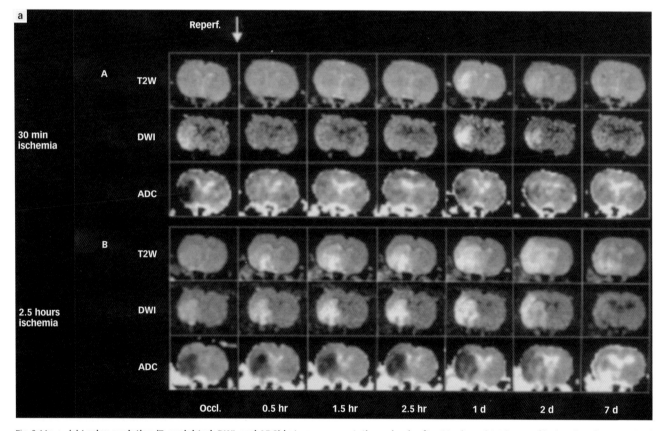

Fig. 8.14a–c. **(a)** Lesion evolution (T_2-weighted, DWI, and ADC) in two representative animals after 30 min and 2.5 hours of ischemia. After 30 min of ischemia, there is initially a complete reversal of DWI and ADC abnormalities during the first few hours of reperfusion, followed by the recurrence of the DWI lesion (and ADC abnormality) at 24 hours. After 2.5 hours of ischemia, the DWI abnormality does not reverse during early reperfusion. On the contrary, signal intensity increases rapidly in the previously ischemic region after recirculation due to the increase in the T_2 contribution to the DWI signal whereas ADC remains low until day 2. Reproduced with permission from [169].

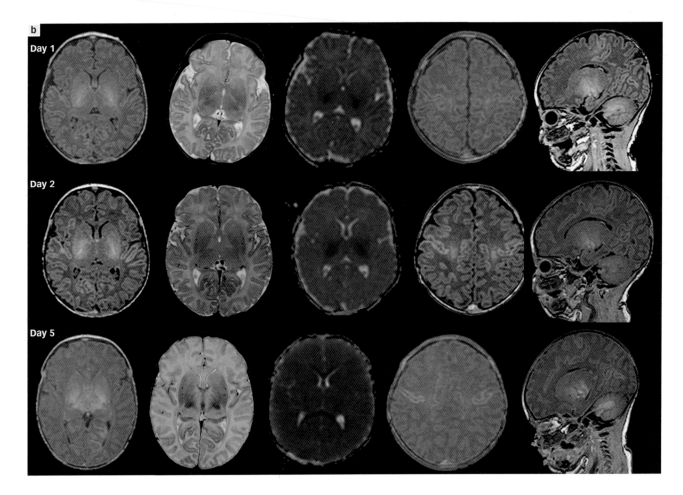

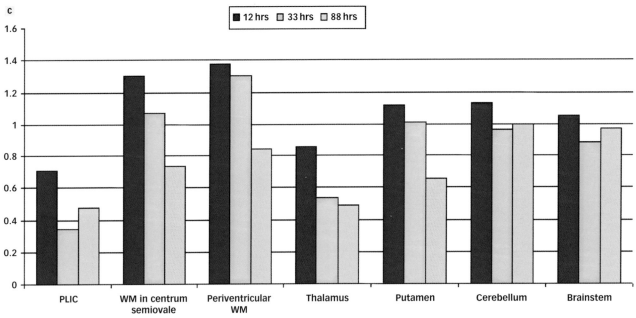

Fig. 8.14. (cont.) (b) Evolution of injury following a postnatal collapse in a term infant. The time of the insult was known; serial scans were performed at 12, 33, and 88 hours following the insult. On the first scan at 12 hours after insult (top row) the only definite abnormality seen is within the PLIC and ventrolateral thalamus on the ADC map. On the second scan at 33 hours after insult (middle row) signal abnormalities are seen in the thalami, PLIC, and putamen on the T_2-weighted images. The regions of restricted diffusion have extended to involve more of the thalamus. Peri-Rolandic cortical highlighting is seen. On the third scan at 88 hours there is more marked cerebral swelling. There is edema in cortex, white matter and deep gray matter matched by extensive diffusion changes. The deep gray matter, peripheral cortex, and white matter show slightly different temporal evolution in the development of diffusion changes. (c) Graph demonstrating evolution of regional ADC values with time (12, 33, and 88 hours following insult). The quantitative ADC values support the visual assessment of the ADC trace map and demonstrate that different regions develop restricted diffusion at different rates. For example the PLIC and the white matter in the centrum semiovale demonstrate early marked reductions in the ADC values, whereas areas such as the anterior white matter develop reductions in ADC at a later stage. WM, White Matter.

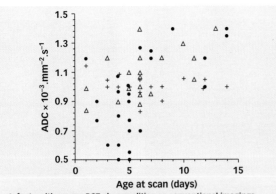

Fig. 8.15. **Apparent diffusion coefficient (ADC) values within the medial thalamus against age at scan in all infants divided into groups on the basis of their conventional MRI. In this study, a normal ADC value in the first week does not define normal tissue, as infants with moderately severe abnormalities on conventional MRI could have normal or increased ADC. BGT, Basal ganglia and thalamus. Reproduced with permission from [177].**

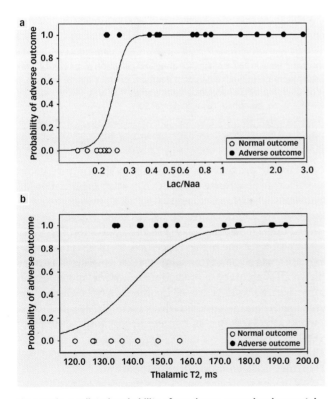

Fig. 8.16a,b. **Predicted probability of an adverse neurodevelopmental outcome versus cerebral Lac/Naa peak area ratios on thalamic ^{1}H MRS (a) and thalamic T_2 relaxometry (b) acquired within the first 3 days following birth in 21 infants with NE. Both techniques are useful for early prognosis when conventional MR imaging may appear normal. Reproduced with permission from [179].**

potential for studying brain energetics non-invasively, and the results obtained with ^{31}P MRS provided fundamental evidence, helping to elucidate the timing and pattern of primary and secondary energy failure in newborn babies. Studies from several groups [183,184,185,186] demonstrated that, following resuscitation after perinatal hypoxic ischemia, normal phosphorus MR spectra were seen, but 8–24 hours later there was a progressive decline in the PCr/Pi ratio despite adequate oxygenation and circulation. In the more severely affected babies there was also a decrease in ATP. The nadir of the energetic disturbance was seen after 12–24 hours [187] and the magnitude of the fall in the PCr/Pi ratio during secondary energy failure was seen to correlate with subsequent neurodevelopmental abnormality and reduced cranial growth 1 and 4 years later [188,189]. Sadly, today, few centers have the facilities to study infants using ^{31}P MRS.

The biphasic pattern of energy failure has been observed experimentally in the piglet [49], the rat pup [190] and, using different techniques, in the fetal sheep [90]. These studies provided a basis for the realization that rescue treatment after hypoxic ischemia might reverse or ameliorate secondary energy failure (Fig. 8.18). Experimental studies using moderate hypothermia as neuroprotection soon followed [56]. ^{31}P MRS continues to be used in the piglet model; recent work has demonstrated that hypothermia prolongs the latent phase, thus extending the therapeutic window for other pharamcological therapies [191] and that the duration of the latent phase shortens with increasingly severe hypoxic ischemia [57]. Although it is not feasible to perform ^{31}P MRS in infants with NE in the first 2 hours after birth, recent experimental data suggest that ^{31}P MRS provides an early robust marker of insult severity.

^{31}P MRS can also measure brain intracellular pH (pH$_i$) (Fig. 8.19a); see Chapter 3 on principles of MRI. Recent studies using ^{31}P MRS in infants with NE have demonstrated a remarkable phenomenon in the first 2 weeks after birth – a brain alkalosis, the extent of which was related to the severity of brain injury on MRI, neurodevelopmental outcome, and brain lactate peak areas ratios [192]. Brain pH$_i$ may be a marker of the severity of brain injury and it is likely that alkalosis itself is deleterious to brain cells (Fig. 8.19b). Amiloride is a drug which (amongst other actions) prevents the alkaline overshoot of pH$_i$ after hypoxic ischemia, and the investigation of its potential as a neuroprotective agent is an area of active research [193].

Proton magnetic resonance spectroscopy (^{1}H MRS)
The first ^{1}H MR spectrum from the neonatal brain was obtained in the early 1990s – almost a decade after the first neonatal ^{31}P MR spectrum. The information obtained from a ^{1}H MR spectrum is complementary to that obtained from a ^{31}P MR spectrum. Because of the greater sensitivity of the ^{1}H nucleus, data can be obtained from smaller regions of the brain. ^{1}H MRS has shown that cerebral lactate (Lac) rises during hypoxic ischemia but is rapidly cleared after successful resuscitation [194] only to be followed by a secondary increase after 12–24 hours [190,196]. This is thought to be due to renewed

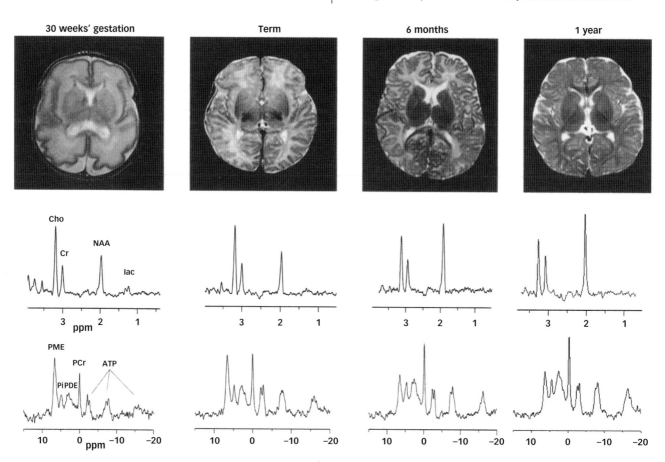

Fig. 8.17. Top row: representative T$_2$-weighted MR images; middle row: ^{1}H MR spectra; and bottom row: ^{31}P MR spectra from healthy newborn infants at 30 weeks' gestation, term, 6 months, and 1 year of age. The MR images show an increase in volume, surface area, and sulcation of cerebral cortex with development. Middle row: the series of ^{1}H MR spectra demonstrate a steady increase in brain NAA and a decrease in brain lactate with maturation. Bottom row: the series of ^{31}P MR spectra show changing rates of brain phospholipids and increasing energy reserves (PCr/Pi) with maturation. With permission from N. J. Robertson and J. S. Wyatt 2004; 89; 193–197, *Arch. Dis. Child. Fetal Neonatal Ed.*

production of lactate in brain tissue rather than entry via the circulation [197]. In the basal ganglia an increased Lac/total creatine (Cr; i.e., creatine plus PCr) peak-area ratio provides an early indication of the severity of brain injury in newborn infants following perinatal hypoxic ischemia, before changes are apparent on conventional longitudinal and transverse relaxation time (T$_1$ and T$_2$ respectively) weighted MRI. A number of groups have shown that the thalamic peak area ratios Lac/Cr, Lac/Naa, and or Lac/Cho provide accurate prognostic markers of the severity of brain injury and neurodevelopmental outcome [172,195,196,198,199,200,201]. Indeed such ratios may be more accurate than DWI and ADC of brain water in assessing injury severity [172]. In a recent UCL study we reported that the most accurate prognostic MR spectroscopy indices in NE are metabolite concentrations, in particular [NAA]. [NAA] was the only measure able to discriminate between all the outcome groups [202]. Representative ^{1}H MR spectra from a control infant and two infants with NE are shown in Fig. 8.20.

Metabolite peak-area ratios have been shown to be better predictors of an adverse outcome than other quantitative MR methods such as T$_2$ relaxometry [179]. Of all metabolite ratios Lac/NAA was the most useful. Lac/NAA and NAA/Cr demonstrated the highest sensitivity (84% and 85% respectively); Lac/NAA and Lac/Cr, the highest specificty (both 88%) for assigning cases to their actual outcome; and Lac/NAA demonstrated the greatest accuracy in predicting neurodevelopmental outcome. Further work is needed in order to assess whether the use of both basal ganglia and white matter ^{1}H MRS in the first 2 weeks after birth further refines the prognostic accuracy of ^{1}H MRS.

Treatment of neonatal encephalopathy

The year 2005 saw a landmark in the history of NE treatments, as the results of the first large multi center randomized trials of selective head and whole-body cooling were published [58,203]. The results of these trials suggest that 72 hours of mild hypothermia started within 6 hours of birth can

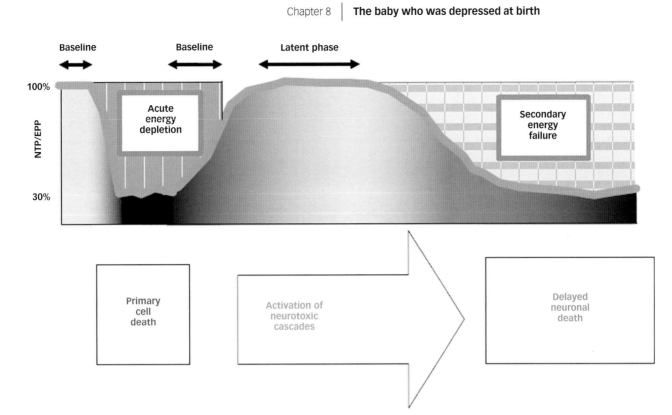

Fig. 8.18. **Schematic diagram illustrating the biphasic pattern of energy failure associated with a transient hypoxic ischemia (HI) insult visualized using serial ^{31}P MRS in the UCL newborn piglet model. The nucleotide triphosphate (NTP) concentration relative to the total high energy exchangeable phosphate pool (EPP = Pi + PCr + αNTP + βNTP + γNTP) is shown on the y axis (measure of cerebral oxidative metabolism). The change in NTP/EPP during transient hypoxic ischemia (HI), resuscitation, the latent phase (period between the recovery from acute HI and the evolution of secondary energy failure (SEF), and SEF itself are shown. During acute energy depletion, some cells undergo primary cell death, the magnitude of which will depend on the severity and duration of HI. Following reperfusion, the initial hypoxia-induced cytotoxic edema and accumulation of excitatory amino acids typically resolve over a period of 30–60 minutes, with apparent recovery of cerebral oxidative metabolism (latent phase). It is thought that the neurotoxic cascade is largely inhibited during the latent phase and that this period provides a "therapeutic window" for therapies such as hypothermia. Cerebral oxidative metabolism may then secondarily deteriorate 6–15 hours later (SEF). This phase is marked by the onset of seizures, secondary cytotoxic edema, accumulation of cytotoxins, and mitochondrial failure. Mitochondrial failure is a key step leading to delayed or programmed cell death.**

improve intact survival at 18 months of age. There are a number of possible mechanisms by which mild hypothermia may be neuroprotective following hypoxic ischemia in the developing brain. Hypothermia reduces the metabolic rate (4%-7% for a 1 °C drop); decreases the release of glutamate and other excitotoxic neurotransmitters; attenuates the activity of NMDA receptors; reduces the production of nitric oxide and oxygen radicals; and contributes to a reduction in intracranial pressure. Although mild to moderate hypothermia appears to be well tolerated in experimental models as well as in human studies [204], there are some potentially deleterious effects, which include cardiac suppression, reduced cerebral blood flow, increased thermogenesis, and increased blood viscosity.

Although the results of these trials are very exciting they raise important questions about the optimal modality and depth and duration of cooling that are needed to maximize neuroprotection. In addition, there is increasing evidence that

inter- and intra-subject variation (such as the size of the baby) can influence the neuroprotective potential of hypothermia [205]. Cooling may be less protective after very severe cerebral injuries [206,207] and the optimal temperature for neuroprotection may depend on the brain region that is affected. We have recently shown that cooling itself can prolong the latent phase [191]. Thus, if hypothermia delays the start of secondary energy failure, in addition to direct cerebroprotection, the therapeutic time window during which additional treatments may benefit may also be prolonged. The possible synergistic effects of cooling plus certain drugs and anesthetic agents is attracting attention and is currently the focus of many experimental studies [208].

At the time of writing the results of the MRC multicenter-based whole-body cooling (TOBY) trial are eagerly awaited. After considering the data available to them at the time recruitment ceased, the TOBY Data Monitoring Committee had no objection to infants being considered for treatment with

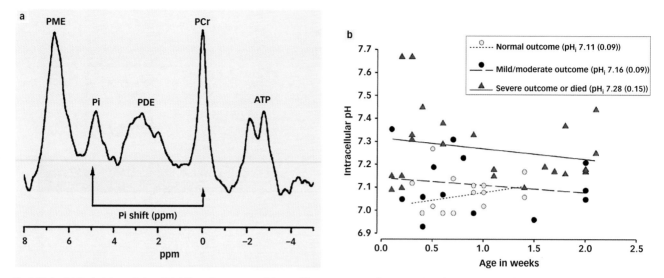

Fig. 8.19a,b. (a) Brain intracellular pH (pH$_i$) can be measured from a ^{31}P MR spectrum by measuring the chemical shift difference of the Pi resonance referenced to the PCr peak (δ). pH$_i$ can then be calculated using the Henderson–Hasselbalch equation:

$$pH = 6.75 + \log(\delta - 3.27)/(5.68 - \delta).$$

(b) Brain pH$_i$ in the first 2 weeks after birth in a cohort of term infants with NE according to neurodevelopmental outcome. Brain pH$_i$ was more alkaline in the severe/fatal outcome group ($p < 0.05$); this difference between groups was present during the first 2 weeks after birth and persisted for 20 weeks after birth; see [192].

cooling when recruitment to TOBY finishes, as long as treatment is according to a specified protocol. Many neonatologists will welcome the chance to offer a treatment that is already supported by some evidence, is economical to provide, and has the potential to minimize impairment following asphyxia, and we currently offer cooling according to the TOBY trial protocol. It is important that the use of cooling is audited and a cooling register has been set up in the UK by the National Perinatal Epidemiology Unit.

Magnetic resonance imaging studies of infants who have been cooled using whole-body or selective cooling demonstrate a decrease in basal ganglia and thalamic lesions in infants with a moderate aEEG abnormality but not in those with severe aEEG changes. A decrease in the incidence of severe cortical lesions was seen only in the infants treated with selective head cooling [209], unlike an Australian study which showed differential protection of the cortex with whole-body cooling [210].

It is important to provide optimal supportive care for babies with NE (with or without cooling), by controlling seizures, using ventilatory support if necessary, and to support blood pressure and fluid balance in the usual way. It is critical to avoid hyperthermia, especially in the period immediately after a hypoxic-ischemic insult, as fever of even moderate degree may markedly exacerbate brain injury [211]. There is still hope that the secondary wave of damage which occurs during the reperfusion phase can be reduced, and trials of hypothermia

protection are well under way. Seizure control is also an active area of research, because of the evidence that ongoing and uncontrolled seizures are detrimental to the developing brain. Management should include counseling the parents about the prognosis for their baby, and it is reasonable to offer to withdraw intensive care if there is near-certainty that the outlook is dismal. The prognosis cannot reliably be determined in the first 24 hours, except in the unusual circumstances of a completely unreactive EEG persisting beyond 12 hours in a comatose and unresponsive baby.

Prognosis of NE
As is generally the case in clinical medicine, no single test is available which can provide a consistently reliable prognosis when applied once in a baby with NE, even when the cause has been identified as hypoxic ischemia [212]. This is hardly surprising given the difference in prior state of the fetus, the degree and duration of the hypoxic ischemia, the wide differential diagnosis of NE, the rapidly evolving neurology, and the plasticity of the brain. To this has to be added the inevitable variation in test results due to inter-observer and laboratory error. In spite of the pressure, the neonatologist must resist the temptation to prognosticate too early; as Paneth once memorably put it, "don't hang crepe in the nursery too soon." Irreparable damage to the clinician's reputation and the family dynamics can be wreaked by an incorrect gloomy prognosis given in haste and regretted at leisure, based only on low

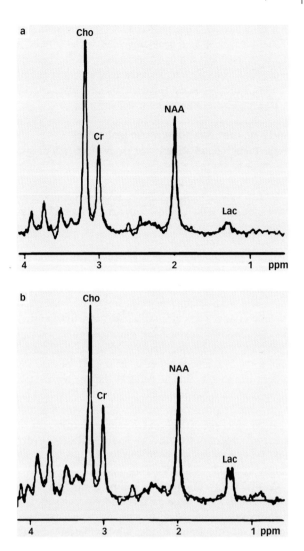

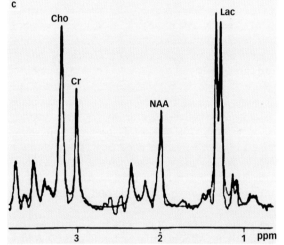

Fig. 8.20. **Representative brain ¹H MR spectra from a control infant and two infants with neonatal encephalopathy obtained from an 8-ml voxel centered on the thalami by using PRESS (TE 270 ms, TR 2 s). Lactate is visible at a low concentration in the control infant (a); the methyl doublet from lactate is very prominent in the severely affected infant (c). Increased brain lactate represents impaired oxidative phosphorylation. Note also the decreased NAA (representing neuronal loss/integrity) in the severely affected infant. We find the thalamic Lac/NAA peak area ratio particularly useful for prognosis from day 2 to 2 weeks after birth in term infants with NE. The dashed lines are the spectrum analysis Lorentzian profiles fitted to the peaks. (a) control; (b) mild/moderate outcome; (c) severe/fatal outcome. Cho, choline; Cr, creatine plus phosphocreatine; NAA, N-acetyl aspartate; Lac, lactate. Reproduced with permission from [202].**

Apgar scores, a cord blood acidosis, and a need for neonatal resuscitation. As we have pointed out, babies with "prolonged partial" hypoxic ischemia which can be followed by devastating parasagittal watershed damage are often born with only moderate birth depression, and are considered well enough to accompany their mothers to the postnatal ward, whereas those with a near-total acute profound hypoxic ischemia are usually significantly depressed and acidotic at birth, but can recover rapidly and survive without disability. Anyone who is feeling complacent about their ability to prognosticate would do well to reflect on their own clinical experience, and to read Shevell's account of the vastly different prophesies he obtained after presenting two sample cases to 40 "expert" neonatologists and pediatric neurologists [212]. Our experience has taught us to temper enthusiasm with caution, hence our advice is to be patient, assess the baby carefully and personally, and watch the NE evolve before jumping to conclusions.

Serial clinical assessments, review of the history, and the results of as many of the appropriate tests as it is possible to obtain will give the most accurate prognosis. Gathering all this information together can take a week or more. This is not to say that parents should not be kept informed during that time, but our advice is certainly to avoid making a hasty prediction of outcome in the first 12–24 hours because this is likely to be proved wrong later on. It is far better to take longer in order to give as accurate a prognosis as possible given the constraints of current technology, than to rush into discontinuing care inappropriately or to give false reassurance. Far more work needs to be done using discriminant analysis to weight the currently available prognostic indicators – one or two attempts have been made, but only with very small numbers of cases, and without information from MRI [213]. We have recently reviewed the range of outcomes which can be seen after hypoxic ischemia at term [214].

The following general points can be made about prognostication in early NE:

- Babies who have normal ultrasound scans, normal background EEG pattern within the first week, and normal MRI are not likely to develop a disability (providing the diagnosis of perinatal hypoxic ischemia at term is correct). The return of sleep-wake cycling (monitored with EEG) within 36 hours of birth after a hypoxic ischemia insult is a good prognostic sign.
- The importance of a careful, structured, neurological examination should not be forgotten [18].
- The most difficult group in which to prognosticate is that in which the EEG and the encephalopathy are moderately abnormal and the early ultrasound scans show cerebral edema; this is a group in which MRI should be performed for diagnosis and prognosis.
- The pattern of injury as defined with MRI conveys important prognostic information.
- Severe bilateral basal ganglia and thalamic injury is virtually always followed by severe spastic quadriplegic cerebral palsy with feeding difficulties, often with visual impairment and epilepsy, but even in this group the severity of the outcome can vary widely.
- Less severe damage in the basal ganglia and thalami usually requires MRI for diagnosis and most often results in athetoid (dyskinetic) cerebral palsy, with varying degrees of severity. Intelligence is preserved in some, and visual function is usually good [163]. Many children can walk although uncontrollable dystonic movements caused by damage to the deep gray matter can be very disabling, speech is often dysarthric and feeding can be problematic.
- Survivors of NE are at risk of developing cognitive deficits even in the absence of functional motor deficits. Cognitive problems occur in survivors of moderate and severe NE, particularly in the parasagittal pattern of injury involving the frontal white matter [162,215]. The cognitive outcome depends to some extent on the child's postnatal environment, socioeconomic conditions, and access to rehabilitation services.
- Extensive white matter involvement usually predicts cognitive difficulties, often (but not always) with accompanying motor disability. Repeated imaging may be required to discover the true extent of the damage in many of these babies. The recognition of cognitive deficits in the absence of motor disability may be delayed beyond the first year of life; in one cohort cognitive deficits associated with the parasagittal pattern of injury were detected at 30 months but were largely overlooked at a year [201].
- During the course of the first year of life a slowing of head growth velocity is usually an ominous sign, and is seen in association with both basal ganglia-thalamic and cortical damage [216].
- The hippocampus can be damaged by perinatal hypoxic ischemia (typically not in isolation), and damage in this region has been implicated as a cause of memory impairment [217,218]. The problems were with episodic memory (context-rich memory) rather than semantic memory (memory for facts) meaning that the true extent of the disability often only becomes apparent in later life, because early learning is often based on rote learning.

Early NE (not due to hypoxic ischemia)

In the French-population-based study of NE, 18% of cases of NE were due to antenatal causes or "birth defects" – biochemical, structural or genetic causes [38].

Inborn errors of metabolism, although individually rare, have considerable clinical impact and pose a diagnostic challenge to neonatologists. Accurate diagnosis is important for prenatal counseling and for antenatal diagnosis in subsequent pregnancies. The severity of the acute metabolic encephalopathy may fluctuate and is often precipitated by a metabolic stress such as an infection, fasting or surgery. The mechanisms of acute metabolic encephalopathy include changes to cerebral blood flow, fluid shifts, disturbances in neurotransmitters, deranged energy status of the brain and blood–brain barrier, free radical damage, and apoptosis. The age of onset is an important diagnostic and prognostic factor and in general the earlier the onset the more profound the metabolic disorder. Bilirubin encephalopathy has reduced in incidence but still presents with opisthotonic posturing and seizures despite the development of screening for glucose-6-phosphatase dehydrogenase deficiency in some parts of the world and the ready availability of anti-Rhesus immunoglobulin.

Cranial ultrasound may be helpful in detecting markers of metabolic disease, such as germinolytic cysts (p. 229), lenticulostriate vasculopathy (p. 226) or more extensive basal ganglia calcification, subtle white matter abnormalities and cortical and other structural abnormalities. Magnetic resonance imaging is extremely valuable in the imaging assessment of metabolic encephalopathy and inborn errors of metabolism, particularly in evaluating disorders of myelination [219]. Conventional MRI in neonatal metabolic disorders usually shows non-specific abnormalities (brain swelling, atrophy, delayed or hypomyelination). The MRI pattern may be classified by the predominant site of lesions. Disorders primarily affecting white matter include maple syrup urine disease (MSUD), non-ketotic hyperglycinemia, methylmalonic and propionic acidemia. Disorders primarily affecting gray matter include kernicterus – postero-medial border of globus pallidus. Combined lesions include mitochondrial encephalopathies [219]. In some of the diseases, imaging studies may reveal malformations of the brain, e.g., cortical dysplasia in Zellweger syndrome or callosal hypoplasia in non-ketotic hyperglycinemia. Diffusion-weighted imaging has been useful in newborns with MSUD [220] and non-ketotic hyperglycinemia [221].

^{1}H MRS may help to increase the specificity of diagnosis, although in most of the neurometabolic diseases with newborn onset ^{1}H MRS findings are non-specific. Nevertheless, they can provide useful additional information on the basic pathological processes occurring within the brain parenchyma. Disease-specific metabolites may occasionally be observed in metabolic diseases of neonatal onset: branched-chain amino acids in MSUD and glycine (3.56 ppm) at long TEs in nonketotic hyperglycinemia. The presence of a prominent lactate peak in mitochondrial encephalopathies may be helpful diagnostically.

Babies with early infantile encephalopathy can present with generalized seizures during the first day of life, and their EEG shows burst suppression. Babies with holoprosencephaly, polymicrogyria, schizencephaly, and other CNS malformations can also present with seizures and abnormal neurological behavior early in life (Chapter 12). They can be distinguished from babies with NE due to hypoxic ischemia by history, examination and investigation: there is no history consistent with intrapartum hypoxia, there is no damage to other organ systems, and the evolution of the illness is not characteristic. It is vital to consider further investigations, and to involve a specialist with experience in metabolic disease at an early stage.

Intracranial hemorrhage

See pp. 115–122.

Sepsis

See Chapter 13.

References

1. Armstrong L, Stenson B. Effect of delayed sampling on umbilical cord arterial and venous lactate and blood gases in clamped and unclamped vessels. *Arch Dis Child Fetal Neonatal Ed* 2006; **91(5)**: 342–5.

2. Yeomans ER, Hauth JC, Gilstrap LC, Strickland DM. Umbilical cord pH, PCO_2, and bicarbonate following uncomplicated term vaginal deliveries. *Am J Obstet Gynecol* 1985; **151**: 798–800.

3. Boylan PC. In Creasy RK *et al.* (eds) *Maternal–Fetal Medicine*. Philadelphia, Saunders, 1999.

4. Eskes TKAB, Jongsma HW, Houx PCW. Percentiles for gas values in human umbilical cord blood. *European J Obstet Gynaecol Reprod Med* 1983; **14**: 341–6.

5. Nelson KB, Dambrosia JM, Ting TY, Grether JK. Uncertain value of electronic fetal monitoring in predicting cerebral palsy. *N Engl J Med* 1996; **334**: 613–18.

6. Parer JT, King T. Fetal heart rate monitoring: is it salvageable? *Am J Obstet Gynecol* 2000; **182**: 982–7.

7. Phelan JP, Ahn MO. Perinatal observations in forty-eight neurologically impaired term infants. *Am J Obstet Gynecol* 1994; **171**: 424–31.

8. Schifrin BS. The CTG and the timing and mechanism of fetal neurological injuries. *Best Pract Res Clin Obstet Gynaecol* 2004; **18(3)**: 437–56.

9. Grether JK, Nelson KB. Maternal infection and cerebral palsy in infants of normal birth weight. *J Am Med Assoc* 1997; **278**: 207–11.

10. Nelson KB, Dambrosia JM, Grether JK, Phillips TM. Neonatal cytokines and coagulation factors in children with cerebral palsy. *Ann Neurol* 1998; **44**: 665–75.

11. Badawi N, Kurinczuk JJ, Keogh JM, Alessandri LM, O'Sullivan F, Burton PR. Intrapartum risk factors for newborn encephalopathy: the Western Australian case-control study. *Br Med J* 1998; **317**: 1554–8.

12. Lieberman E, Eichenwald E, Mathur G, Richardson D, Heffner L, Cohen A. Intrapartum fever and unexplained seizures in term infants. *Pediatrics* 2000; **106**: 983–8.

13. Impey L, Greenwood C, MacQuillan K, Reynolds M, Sheiel O. Fever in labour and neonatal encephalopathy: a prospective cohort study. *Br J Obstet Gynaecol* 2001; **108**: 594–7.

14. Eklind S, Mallard C, Leverin A-L *et al.* Bacterial endotoxin sensitizes the imature brain to hypoxic-ischaemic injury. *Eur J Neurosci* 2001; **13**: 1101–6.

15. Tomimatsu T, Fukuda H, Kanagawa T, Mu J, Kanzaki T, Murata Y. Effects of hyperthermia on hypoxic ischaemic brain damage in the immature rat: its influence on caspase-3-like protease. *Am J Obstet Gynaecol* 2003; **188(3)**: 768–73.

16. Spellacy WN, Gravem H, Fisch RO. The umbical cord complications of true knots, nuchal coils, and cords around the body. *Am J Obstet Gynecol* 1966; **94**: 1136–42.

17. Thompson CM, Puterman AS, Linley LL *et al.* The value of a scoring system for hypoxic ischemic encephalopathy in predicting neurodevelopmental outcome. *Acta Paediatr Scand* 1997; **86**: 757–61.

18. Mercuri E, Guzzetta A, Haataja L *et al.* Neonatal neurological examination in infants with hypoxic ischaemic encephalopathy: correlation with MRI findings. *Neuropediatrics* 1999; **30**: 83–9.

19. Williams CE, Gunn AJ, Mallard C, Gluckman PD. Outcome after ischemia in the developing sheep brain: an electroencephalographic and histological study. *Ann Neurol* 1992; **31**: 14–21.

20. Filan P, Boylan GB, Chorley G *et al.* The relationship between the onset of electrographic seizure activity after birth and the time of cerebral injury in utero. *Br J Obstet Gynaecol* 2005; **112**: 504–7.

21. van Rooij LGM, Toet MC, Osredkar D, van Huffelen AC, Groenendaal F, de Vries LS. Recovery of amplitude integrated electroencephalographic background patterns within 24 hours of perinatal asphyxia. *Arch Dis Child* 2005; **90(3)**: F245–F251.

22. Staudt F, Scholl ML, Coen RW, Bickford RB. Phenobarbital therapy in neonatal seizures and the prognostic value of the EEG. *Neuropediatrics* 1982; **13**: 24–33.

23. Leijser LM, de Vries LS, Cowan FM. Using cerebral ultrasound effectively in the newborn infant. *Early Hum Dev* 2006; **82(12)**: 827–35.

24. Archer N, Levene MI, Evans DH. Cerebral artery doppler ultrasound for prediction of outcome after perinatal asphyxia. *Lancet* 1986; **ii**: 1116–18.

25. Levene MI, Fenton A, Evans DH, Archer N, Shortland D, Gibson NA. Severe birth asphyxia and abnormal cerebral blood flow velocity. *Dev Med Child Neurol* 1989; **31**: 427–34.

26. Eken P, Toet MC, Groenendaal F, de Vries LS. Predictive value of early neuroimaging, pulsed doppler and neurophysiology in full term infants with hypoxic ischaemic encephalopathy. *Arch Dis Child* 1995; **73**: F75–F81.

27. Barkovich AJ, Hajnal BL, Vigneron D *et al.* Prediction of neuromotor outcome in perinatal asphyxia: evaluation of MR scoring systems. *Am J Neuroradiol* 1998; **19**: 143–9.

28. Cowan F. Outcome after intrapartum asphyxia in term infants. *Semin Neonatol* 2000; **5(2)**: 127–40.

29. Ment LR, Bada HS, Barnes P *et al.* Practice parameter: neuroimaging of the neonate. Report of the quality standards subcommittee of the American Academy of Neurology and the Practice Committee of the Child Neurology Society. *Neurology* 2002; **58**: 1726–38.

30. Miller SP, Ramaswamy V, Michelson D *et al.* Patterns of brain injury in term neonatal encephalopathy. *J Paediatr* 2005; **146**: 453–60.

31. Sie LTL, van der Knaap MS, Oosting J, de Vries LS, Lafeber HN, Valk J. MR patterns of hypoxic-ischemic brain damage after prenatal, perinatal or postnatal asphyxia. *Neuropediatrics* 2000; **31**: 128-36.

32. Leviton A, Nelson KB. Problems with definitions and classifications of newborn encephalopathy. *Pediatr Neurol* 1992; **8**: 85-90.

33. Marlow N, Budge H. Prevalence, causes, and outcome at 2 years of age of newborn encephalopathy. *Arch Dis Child* 2005; **90(3)**: 193-4.

34. Evans K, Rigby AS, Hamilton P, Titchiner N, Hall DMB. The relationships between neonatal encephalopathy and cerebral palsy: a cohort study. *J Obstet Gynaecol* 2001; **21(2)**: 114-20.

35. Levene MI, Kornberg J, Williams THC. The incidence and severity of post-asphyxial encephalopathy in full term infants. *Early Hum Dev* 1985; **11**: 21-6.

36. Adamson SJ, Alessandri LM, Badawi N, Burton PR, Pemburton PJ, Stanley F. Predictors of neonatal encephalopathy in full term infants. *Br Med J* 1995; **311**: 598-602.

37. Hull J, Dodd KL. Falling incidence of hypoxic ischaemic encephalopathy in term infants. *Br J Obstet Gynaecol* 1992; **99**: 386-91.

38. Pierrat V, Haouari N, Liska A, Thomas D, Subtil D, Truffert P. Prevalence, causes, and outcome at 2 years of age of newborn encephalopathy: population based study. *Arch Dis Child* 2005; **90(3)**: 257-61.

39. Ellis M, Manandhar N, Manandhar DS, de L Costello AM. Risk factors for neonatal encephalopathy in Kathmandu, Nepal, a developing country: unmatched case-control study. *Br Med J* 2000; **320**: 1229-36.

40. Badawi N, Kurinczuk JJ, Keogh JM et al. Antepartum risk factors for newborn encephalopathy: the Western Australian case-control study. *Br Med J* 1998; **317**: 1549-53.

41. Badawi N, Kurinczuk JJ, Mackenzie CL et al. Maternal thyroid disease: a risk factor for newborn encephalopathy in term infants. *Br J Obstet Gynaecol* 2000; **107**: 798-801.

42. Stanley F, Blair E. *Cerebral Palsy – Epidemiology and Causal Pathways*, 1st edn. Cambridge: MacKeith Press; 2000.

43. Himmelmann K, Hagberg G, Beckung E, Hagberg B, Uvebrant P. The changing panorama of cerebral palsy in Sweden. ix. Prevalence and origin in the birth-year period 1995-1998. *Acta Paediatr* 2005; **94**: 287-94.

44. Hagberg B, Hagberg G, Beckung E, Uvebrant P. Changing panorama of cerebral palsy in Sweden. viii. Prevalence and origin in the birth year period 1991-1994. *Acta Paediatr* 2001; **90**: 271-7.

45. Himmelmann K, Hagberg G, Wiklund LM, Eek MN, Uvebrant P. Dyskinetic cerebral palsy: a population-based study of children born between 1993 and 1998. *Dev Med Child Neurol* 2007; **49**: 246-51.

46. Cowan F, Rutherford M, Groenendaal F et al. Origin and timing of brain lesions in term infants with neonatal encephalopathy. *Lancet* 2003; **361**: 736-42.

47. Myers RE. Two patterns of perinatal brain damage and their conditions of occurrence. *Am J Obstet Gynecol* 1972; **112**: 246-76.

48. Gluckman PD. When and why do brain cells die? *Dev Med Child Neurol* 1992; **34**: 1010-21.

49. Lorek A, Takei Y, Cady EB et al. Delayed ('secondary') cerebral energy failure after acute hypoxia-ischaemia in the newborn piglet: continuous 48-hour studies by phosphorus magnetic resonance spectroscopy. *Pediatr Res* 1994; **36**: 699-706.

50. Derrick M, Drobyshevsky A, Ji X, Tan S. A model of cerebral palsy from fetal hypoxia-ischemia. *Stroke* 2007; **38**: 731-5.

51. Westgate JA, Bennet L, Gunn AJ. Intrapartum hypoxic-ischaemic brain injury. In: Donn SM, Sinha SK, Chiswick ML, eds. *Birth Asphyxia and the Brain: Basic Science and Clinical Implications*. New York, Futura, 2002; 243-79.

52. Johnston MV, Trescher WH, Ishida A, Nakajima W. Neurobiology of hypoxic-ischaemic injury in the developing brain. *Pediatr Res* 2001; **49**: 735-41.

53. Mallard EC, Williams CE, Gunn AJ, Gunning MI, Gluckman PD. Frequent episodes of brief ischemia sensitize the fetal sheep brain to neuronal loss and induce striatal injury. *Pediatr Res* 1993; **33**: 61-5.

54. Mallard EC, Williams CE, Johnston BM, Gunning MI, Davis S, Gluckman PD. Repeated episodes of umbilical cord occlusion in fetal sheep lead to preferential damage to the striatum and sensitize the heart to further insults. *Pediatr Res* 1995; **37**: 707-13.

55. Mallard EC, Waldvogel HJ, Williams CE, Faull RLM, Gluckman PD. Repeated asphyxia causes loss of striatal projection neurons in the fetal sheep brain. *Neuroscience* 1995; **65**: 827-36.

56. Thoresen M, Wyatt J. Keeping a cool head, post-hypoxic hypothermia – an old idea revisited. *Acta Paediatr* 1997; **86**: 1029-33.

57. Iwata O, Iwata S, Thornton JS et al. "Therapeutic time window" duration decreases with increasing severity of cerebral hypoxia-ischaemia under normothermia and delayed hypothermia in newborn piglets. *Brain Res* 2007; **1154**: 173-80.

58. Gluckman PD, Wyatt JS, Azzopardi D et al. Selective head cooling with mild systemic hypothermia after neonatal encephalopathy: multicentre randomised trial. *Lancet* 2005; **365**: 663-70.

59. Myers RE. Four patterns of perinatal brain damage and their occurrence in primates. *Adv Neurol* 1975; **10**: 223-4.

60. Roland EH, Poskitt K, Rodriguez E, Lupton BA, Hill A. Perinatal hypoxic-ischemic thalamic injury: clinical features and neuroimaging. *Ann Neurol* 1998; **44**: 161-6.

61. Pasternak JF, Gorey MT. The syndrome of acute near-total intrauterine asphyxia in the term infant. *Pediatr Neurol* 1998; **18**: 391-8.

62. Okumura A, Hayakawa F, Kato T, Kuno K, Watanabe K. Bilateral basal ganglia-thalamic lesions subsequent to prolonged fetal bradycardia. *Early Hum Dev* 2000; **58**: 111-18.

63. Natsume J, Watanabe K, Kuno K, Hayakawa F, Hashizume Y. Clinical, neurophysiologic, and neuropathological features of an infant with brain damage of total asphyxia type (Myers). *Pediatr Neurol* 1995; **13**: 61-4.

64. Krageloh-Mann I, Helber A, Mader I et al. Bilateral lesions of thalamus and basal ganglia: origin and outcome. *Dev Med Child Neurol* 2002; **44**: 477-84.

65. Naeye RL, Lin H-M. Determination of the timing of fetal brain damage from hypoxemia-ischaemia. *Am J Obstet Gynecol* 2001; **184**: 217-24.

66. Bennet L, Westgate JA, Gluckman PD, Gunn AJ. Pathophysiology of asphyxia. In: Levene MI, Chervenak FA, Whittle M, eds. *Fetal and Neonatal Neurology and Neurosurgery*, 3rd edn. London, Churchill Livingstone, 2001; 407-26.

67. Bobrow CS, Soothill P. Causes and consequences of fetal acidosis. *Arch Dis Child* 1999; **80**: F246-F249.

68. Brann AW, Myers RE. Central nervous system findings in the newborn monkey following severe in utero partial asphyxia. *Neurology* 1975; **25**: 327-38.

69. Ikeda T, Murata Y, Quilligan EJ et al. Physiologic and histologic changes in near-term fetal lambs exposed to asphyxia by partial umbilical cord occlusion. *Am J Obstet Gynecol* 1998; **178**: 24-32.

70. Gunn AJ, Parer JT, Mallard EC, Williams CE, Gluckman PD. Cerebral histologic and electrophysiologic changes after asphyxia in fetal sheep. *Pediatr Res* 1992; **31**: 486-91.

71. De Haan HH, Gunn AJ, Williams CE, Gluckman PD. Brief repeated umbilical cord occlusions cause sustained cytotoxic cerebral edema and focal infarcts in near-term fetal lambs. *Pediatr Res* 1997; **41**: 96-104.

72. Ball RH, Parer JT, Caldwell LE, Johnson J. Regional blood flow and metabolism in ovine fetuses during severe cord occlusion. *Am J Obstet Gynecol* 1994; **171**: 1549-55.

73. Connolly DJA, Widjaja E, Griffiths PD. Involvement of the anterior lobe of the cerebellar vermis in perinatal profound hypoxia. *Am J Neuroradiol* 2007; **28(1)**: 16-19.

74. Sargent MA, Poskitt KJ, Roland EH, Hill A, Hendson G. Cerebellar vermian atrophy after neonatal hypoxic ischaemic encephalopathy. *Am J Neuroradiol* 2004; **25**: 1008-15.

75. McDonald JW, Johnston MV. Physiological and pathophysiological roles of excitatory amino acids during CNS development. *Brain Res* 1990; **15**: 41-70.

76. Brown GC, Bal-Price A. Inflammatory neurodegeneration mediated by nitric oxide, glutamate, and mitochondria. *Mol Neurobiol* 2003; **27**: 325-55.

77. Northington FJ, Ferriero DM, Graham EM, Traystman RJ, Martin LJ. Early neurodegeneration after hypoxic ischemia in neonatal rat is necrosis while delayed neuronal death is apoptosis. *Neurobiol Dis* 2001; **8(2)**: 201-19.

78. Orrenius S, Zhivotovsky B, Nicotera P. Regulation of cell death: the calcium-apoptosis link. *Nature Rev Mol Cell Biol* 2003; **4(7)**: 552-65.

79. Taylor DL, Edwards AD, Mehmet H. Oxidative metabolism, apoptosis and perinatal brain injury. *Brain Pathol* 1999; **9(1)**: 93-117.

80. Volpe JJ, Pasternak JF. Parasagittal cerebral injury in neonatal hypoxic-ischaemic encephalopathy. *J Pediatr* 1977; **91**: 472-6.

81. Williams CE, Gunn AJ, Mallard C, Gluckman PD. Outcome after ischemia in the developing sheep brain: an electroencephalographic and histological study. *Ann Neurol* 1992; **31(1)**: 14-21.

82. Sarnat HB, Sarnat MS. Neonatal encephalopathy following fetal distress. *Arch Neurol* 1976; **33**: 696-705.

83. Levene MI, Sands C, Grindulis H, Moore JR. Comparison of two methods of predicting outcome in perinatal asphyxia. *Lancet* 1986; **i**: 67-8.

84. Miller SP, Latal B, Clark H et al. Clinical signs predict 30-month neurodevelopmental outcome after neonatal encephalopathy. *Am J Obstet Gynaecol* 2004; **190**: 93-9.

85. Robertson CMT, Finer NN. Long term follow up of term neonates with birth asphyxia. *Clin Perinatol* 1993; **20**: 483-500.

86. Rosenbloom L. Dyskinetic cerebral palsy and birth asphyxia. *Dev Med Child Neurol* 1994; **36**: 285-9.

87. Perlman JM, Tack ED. Renal injury in the asphyxiated newborn: relationship to neurologic outcome. *J Pediatr* 1988; **113**: 875-9.

88. Shah P, Riphagen S, Beyene J, Perlman M. Multiorgan dysfunction in infants with post-asphyxial hypoxic-ischaemic encephalopathy. *Arch Dis Child Fetal Neonatol Ed* 2004; **89**: F152-F155.

89. Williams CE, Gunn AJ, Synek B, Gluckman PD. Delayed seizures occurring with hypoxic-ischemic encephalopathy in the fetal sheep. *Pediatr Res* 1990; **27(6)**: 561-5.

90. Williams CE, Gunn A, Gluckman PD. Time course of intracellular oedema and epileptiform activity following prenatal cerebral ischaemia in sheep. *Stroke* 1991; **22**: 516-21.

91. McBride MC, Laroia N, Guillet R. Electrographic seizures in neonates correlate with poor neurodevelopmental outcome. *Neurology* 2000; **55**: 506-13.

92. Bye AME, Cunningham CA, Chee KY, Flanagan D. Outcome of neonates with electro-graphically identified seizures, or at risk of seizures. *Pediatr Neurol* 1997; **16**: 225-31.

93. Pressler RM, Boylan GB, Morton M, Binnie CD, Rennie JM. Early serial EEG in hypoxic ischaemic encephalopathy. *Clin Neurophysiol* 2001; **112**: 31-7.

94. Selton D, Andre M. Prognosis of hypoxic-ischaemic encephalopathy in full-term newborns - value of neonatal electroencephalography. *Neuropediatrics* 1997; **28**: 276-80.

95. Harris R, Tizard JPM. EEG in neonatal convulsions. *J Pediatr* 1960; **57**: 510-14.

96. Rose A, Lombroso CT. Neonatal seizure states: a study of clinical, pathological, and electroencephalographic features in 137 full-term babies with a long-term follow-up. *Pediatrics* 1970; **45**: 404-25.

97. van Lieshout HBM, Jacobs JFM, Rotteveel JJ, Geven W, von dort Hoeffmann M. The prognostic value of the EEG in asphyxiated newborns. *Acta Neurol Scand* 1995; **91**: 203-7.

98. Takeuchi T, Watanabe K. The EEG evolution and neurological prognosis of perinatal hypoxia neonates. *Brain Dev* 1989; **11**: 115-20.

99. Watanabe K, Miyazaki S, Hara K, Hakamanda A. Behavioral state cycles, background EEGs and prognosis of newborn with perinatal hypoxia. *Electroencephalogr Clin Neurophysiol* 1980; **49**: 618-25.

100. Wertheim D, Mercuri E, Faundez JC, Rutherford M, Acolet D, Dubowitz L. Prognostic value of continuous electroencephalographic recording in full term infants with hypoxic ischaemic encephalopathy. *Arch Dis Child* 1994; **71**: F97-F102.

101. de Vries LS, Hellstrom-Westas L. Role of cerebral function monitoring in the newborn. *Arch Dis Child* 2005; **90(3)**: 201-7.

102. Holmes GL, Lombroso CT. Prognostic value of background patterns in the neonatal EEG. *J Clin Neurophysiol* 1993; **10(3)**: 323-52.

103. Aso K, Scher MS, Barmada MA. Neonatal electroencephalography and neuropathology. *J Clin Neurophysiol* 1989; **6**: 103-23.

104. Monod N, Pajot N, Guidasci S. The neonatal EEG: statistical studies and prognostic value in full term and preterm babies. *Electroencephalogr Clin Neurophysiol* 1972; **32**: 529-44.

105. Holmes G, Rowe J, Schmidt R, Testa M, Zimmerman A. Prognostic value of the electroencephalogram in neonatal seizures. *Electroencephalogr Clin Neurophysiol* 1982; **53**: 60-72.

106. Pezzani C, Radvani-Bouvet MF, Relier JP, Monod N. Neonatal electroencephalography during the first 24 hours of life in full term newborn infants. *Neuropediatrics* 1986; **17**: 11-18.

107. Grigg-Damberger MM, Coker SB, Halsey CL, Anderson CL. Neonatal burst supression: its developmental significance. *Pediatr Neurol* 1989; **5**: 84-92.

108. Peliowski A, Finer NN. Asphyxia in the term infant. In: Sinclair JC, Bracken MB, eds. *Effective Care of the Newborn Infant* 1st edn. Oxford, Oxford University Press, 1992; 249-79.

109. Tharp BR. Neonatal seizures and syndromes. *Epilepsia* 2002; **43(3)**: 2-10.

110. Biagioni E, Mercuri E, Rutherford M et al. Combined use of electroencephalogram and magnetic resonance imaging in full-term neonates with acute encephalopathy. *Pediatrics* 2001; **107**: 461-8.

111. al Naqeeb N, Edwards AD, Cowan F, Azzopardi D. Assessment of neonatal encephalopathy by amplitude-integrated electroencephalography. *Pediatrics* 1999; **103**: 1263-71.

112. Toet MC, van der Meij W, de Vries LS, Uiterwaal CPM, van Huffelen KC. Comparison between simultaneously recorded amplitude integrated electroencephalogram (cerebral function monitor) and standard electrocephalogram in neonates. *Pediatrics* 2002; **109**: 772-9.

113. Hellström-Westas L, Rosen I, Svenningsen NW. Predictive value of early continuous amplitude integrated EEG recordings on outcome after severe birth asphyxia in full term infants. *Arch Dis Child* 1995; **72**: F34-F38.

114. Toet MG, Hellstrom-Westas L, Groenendaal F, Eken P, de Vries LS. Amplitude integrated EEG 3 and 6 hours after birth in full term neonates with hypoxic-ischaemic encephalopathy. *Arch Dis Child* 1999; **81**: F19-F23.

115. Thornberg E, Ekstrom-Jodal B. Cerebral function monitoring: a method of predicting outcome in term neonates after severe perinatal asphyxia. *Acta Paediatr Scand* 1994; **83**: 596-601.

116. Ter Horst HJ, Sommer C, Bergman KA, Fock JM, Van Weerden TW, Bos AF. Prognostic significance of amplitude-integrated EEG during

the first 72 hours after birth in severely asphyxiated neonates. *Pediatr Res* 2004; **55**: 1026-33.

117. Toet MC, Lemmers PMA, van Schelven LJ, Van Bel F. Cerebral oxygenation and electrical activity after birth asphyxia: their relation to outcome. *Pediatrics* 2006; **17(2)**: 333-9.

118. van Rooij LG, Toet MC, Osredkar D, Van Heffelen AC, Groenendaal F, de Vries LS. Recovery of amplitude integrated electroencephalo-graphic background patterns within 24 hours of perinatal asphyxia. *Arch Dis Child Fetal Neonatal Ed* 2005; **90(3)**: F245-51.

119. Ter Horst HJ, Brouwer OF, Bos AF. Burst suppression on amplitude-integrated electroencephalogram may be induced by midazolam: a report on three cases. *Actra Paediatr Scand* 2004; **93**: 559-64.

120. Verma UL, Archbald F, Tejani NA, Handwerker SM. Cerebral function monitor in the neonate. I: normal patterns. *Dev Med Child Neurol* 1984; **26**: 154-61.

121. Osredkar D, Toet MC, van Rooji LGM, van Huffelen AC, Groenendaal F, de Vries L. Sleep-wake cycling on amplitude-integrated electroencephalography in term newborns with hypoxic-ischemic encephalopathy. *Pediatrics* 2005; **115(2)**: 327-32.

122. Hagmann CF, Robertson NJ, Azzopardi D. Artifacts on electroencephalograms may influence the amplitude-integrated EEG classification: a qualitiative analysis in neonatal encephalopathy. *Pediatr Experience Reason* 2006; **118(6)**: 2552-4.

123. Hellström-Westas L, Rosen I, de Vries LS, Greisen G. Amplitude-integrated EEG classification and interpretation in preterm and term infants. *Neoreviews* 2006; **7(2)**: E76-E87.

124. Sheehy-Skeffington F, Pearce RG. The "bright brain". *Arch Dis Child* 1983; **58**: 509-11.

125. Shen E-Y, Hunag CC, Chyou SC, Hung HY, Hsu CH, Hunag FY. Sonographic findings of the bright thalamus. *Arch Dis Child* 1986; **61**: 1096-9.

126. Voit T, Lemburg P, Neve E, Lumenta C, Stork W. Damage of thalamus and basal ganglia in asphyxiated full term neonates. *Neuropediatrics* 1987; **18**: 176-81.

127. Connolly B, Kelehan P, O'Brien NO *et al.* The echogenic thalamus in hypoxic-ischaemic encephalopathy. *Pediatr Radiol* 1994; **24**: 268-71.

128. Rutherford MA, Pennock JM, Dubowitz LMS. Cranial ultrasound and magnetic resonance imaging in hypoxic ischaemic encephalopathy: a comparison with outcome. *Dev Med Child Neurol* 1994; **36**: 813-25.

129. Leijser LM, Cowan FM. State-of-the-art neonatal cranial ultrasound. *Ultrasound* 2007; **15(1)**: 6-17.

130. Eken P, Jansen GH, Groenendaal F, Rademaker KJ, de Vries LS. Intracranial lesions in the fullterm infant with hypoxic ischaemic encephalopathy: ultrasound and autopsy correlation. *Neuropediatrics* 1994; **25**: 301-7.

131. Siegel MJ, Shackleford GD, Perlman JM, Fulling KH. Hypoxic ischaemic encephalopathy in term infants: diagnosis and prognosis evaluated by ultrasound. *Radiology* 1984; **152**: 395-9.

132. Galli KK, Zimmerman RA, Jarvik GP *et al.* Periventricular leukomalacia is common after neonatal cardiac surgery. *J Thorac Cardiovasc Surg* 2004; **127**: 692-704.

133. McQuillen PS, Barkovich AJ, Hamrick SEG *et al.* Temporal and anatomic risk profile of brain injury with neonatal repair of congenital heart defects. *Stroke* 2007; **38**: 736-41.

134. Van Bel F, Van de Bor M, Stijnen T, Baan J, Ruys JH. Cerebral blood flow velocity patterns in healthy and asphyxiated newborns: a controlled study. *Eur J Pediatr* 1987; **146**: 461-57.

135. Rennie JM, South M, Morley CJ. Cerebral blood flow velocity variability in infants receiving assisted ventilation. *Arch Dis Child* 1987; **62**: 1247-51.

136. Boylan G, Young K, Panerai RB, Rennie JM, Evans DH. Dynamic cerebral autoregulation in sick newborn infants. *Pediatr Res* 2000; **48**: 12-17.

137. McMenamin JB, Volpe JJ. Doppler ultrasonography in the determination of neonatal brain death. *Arch Neurol* 1983; **14**: 302-6.

138. Glasier CM, Seibert JJ, Chadduck WM, Williamson SL, Leithiser RE. Brain death in infants: evaluation with Doppler US. *Radiology* 1989; **172**: 377-80.

139. Hassler W, Steinmetz H, Gawlowski J. Transcranial doppler ultrasonography in raised ICP and in intracranial circulatory arrest. *J Neurosurg* 1988; **68**: 745-51.

140. Kirkham FJ, Levin SD, Padayachee TS, Kyme MC, Neville BGR, Gosling RG. Transcranial pulsed Doppler findings in brain stem death. *J Neurol Neurosurg Psychiatry* 1987; **50**: 1504-13.

141. Barkovich AJ, Truwit CL. Brain damage from perinatal asphyxia: correlation of MR findings with gestational age. *Am J Neuroradiol* 1990; **11**: 1087-96.

142. Barkovich AJ. MR and CT evaluation of profound neonatal and infantile asphyxia. *Am J Neuroradiol* 1992; **13**: 959-72.

143. Barkovich AJ, Westmark K, Partridge A, Sola A, Ferriero DM. Perinatal asphyxia: MR findings in the first 10 days. *Am J Neuroradiol* 1995; **16**: 427-38.

144. Baenziger O, Martin E, Steinlin M *et al.* Early pattern recognition in severe perinatal asphyxia; a prospective MR study. *Neuroradiology* 1993; **35**: 437-42.

145. Kuenzle CL, Baenziger O, Martin E *et al.* Prognostic value of early MR imaging in term infants with severe perinatal asphyxia. *Neuropediatrics* 1994; **25**: 191-200.

146. Byrne P, Welch R, Johnson MA, Darrah J, Piper M. Serial magnetic resonance imaging in neonatal hypoxic ischaemic encephalopathy. *J Pediatr* 1990; **117**: 694-700.

147. Truwit CL, Barkovich AJ, Koch TK, Ferriero DM. Cerebral palsy: MRI findings. *Am J Neuroradiol* 1992; **13**: 67-78.

148. Steinlin M, Dirr R, Martin E *et al.* MRI following severe perinatal asphyxia: preliminary experience. *Pediatr Neurol* 1991; **7**: 164-70.

149. Keeney SE, Adcock EW, McArdle CB. Prospective observations of 100 high-risk neonates in high field (1.5 tesla) magnetic resonance imaging of the central nervous system. II. Lesions associated with hypoxic-ischemic encephalopathy. *Pediatrics* 1991; **87**: 431-8.

150. Rutherford MA, Pennock JM, Schweiso JE, Cowan FM, Dubowitz LMS. Hypoxic ischaemic encephalopathy: early magnetic resonance image findings and their evolution. *Neuropediatrics* 1995; **26**: 183-91.

151. Rutherford M, Pennock J, Schwieso J, Cowan F, Dubowitz L. Hypoxic-ischaemic encephalopathy: early and late magnetic resonance imaging findings in relation to outcome. *Arch Dis Child* 1996; **75**: F145-F151.

152. Barkovich AJ, Miller SP, Bartha A *et al.* MR imaging, MR spectroscopy, and diffusion tensor imaging of sequential studies in neonates with encephalopathy. *Am J Neuroradiol* 2006; **27**: 533-47.

153. Rutherford M. Neuroimaging of hypoxic-ischaemic encephalopathy. In: Donn SM, Sinha SK, Chiswick ML, eds. *Birth Asphyxia and the Brain: Basic Science and Clinical Implications.* New York, Futura, 2002; 315-54.

154. Rutherford MA. The asphyxiated term infant. In: Rutherford MA, ed. *MRI of the Neonatal Brain,* 1st edn. London, W.B.Saunders, 2002; 99-128.

155. Jouvet P, Cowan FM, Cox P *et al.* Reproducibility and accuracy of MR imaging of the brain after severe birth asphyxia. *Ame J Neuroradiol* 1999; **20**: 1343-8.

156. Robertson NJ, Wyatt JS. The magnetic resonance revolution in brain imaging: impact on neonatal intensive care. *Arch Dis Child* 2004; **89(3)**: 193-7.

157. Barkovich AJ. MR imaging of the neonatal brain. *Neuroimag Clin North Am* 2006; **16**: 117–35.

158. Frigieri G, Guidi B, Zaccarelli SC et al. Multicystic encephalomalacia in term infants. *Child Nerv Syst* 1996; **12**: 759–64.

159. Weidenheim KM, Bodhireddy SR, Nuovo GJ, Nelson SJ, Dickson DW. Multicystic encephalopathy: review of eight cases with etiologic considerations. *J Neuropathol Exp Neurol* 1995; **54**: 268–75.

160. Rademakers RP, van der Knaap MS, Verbeeten B, Barth PG, Valk J. Central cortico-subcortical involvement. a distinct pattern of brain damage caused by perinatal and postnatal asphyxia in term infants. *J Comput Assist Tomogr* 1995; **19**: 256–63.

161. Barkovich AJ, Sargent SK. Profound asphyxia in the premature infant: imaging findings. *Am J Neuroradiol* 1995; **16**: 1837–46.

162. Marlow N, Rose AS, Rands CE, Draper ES. Neuropsychological and educational problems at school age associated with neonatal encephalopathy. *Arch Dis Child* 2005; **90(5)**: 380–7.

163. Barnett A, Mercuri E, Rutherford M et al. Neurological and perceptual-motor outcomes at 5–6 years of age in children wtih neonatal encephalopathy: relationship with neonatal MRI. *Neuropaediatrics* 2002; **33**: 242–8.

164. Childs A-M, Cornette L, Ramenghi LA et al. Magnetic resonance and cranial ultrasound characteristics of periventricular white matter abnormalities in newborn infants. *Clin Radiol* 2001; **56**: 647–55.

165. Konishi Y, Kuriyama M, Hayakawa K et al. Periventricular hyperintensity detected by magnetic resonance imaging in Infancy. *Pediatr Neurol* 1990; **6**: 229–32.

166. Muir KW, Buchan A, von Kummer R, Rother J, Baron JC. Imaging of acute stroke. *Lancet Neurol* 2006; **5(9)**: 755–68.

167. Barkovich AJ, Westmark KD, Bedi HS, Partridge JC, Ferriero DM, Vigneron DB. Proton spectroscopy and diffusion imaging on the first day of life after perinatal asphyxia: preliminary report. *Am J Neuroradiol* 2001; **22**: 1786–94.

168. Thornton JS, Ordridge RJ, Penrice J et al. Temporal and anatomical variations of brain water apparent diffusion coefficient in perinatal cerebral hypoxic-ischemic injury: relationships to cerebral energy metabolism. *Magn Reson Med* 1998; **39(6)**: 920–7.

169. Neumann-Haefelin T, Kastrup A, de Crespigny MA, Yenari T, Ringer GH. Serial MRI after transient focal cerebral ischemia in rats: dynamics of tissue injury, blood-brain barrier damage, and edema formation. *Stroke* 2000; **31**: 1311–17.

170. Soul JS, Robertson RL, Tzika AA, du Plessis AJ, Volpe JJ. Time course of changes in diffusion-weighted magnetic resonance imaging in a case of neonatal encephalopathy with defined onset and duration of hypoxic-ischemic insult. *Paediatrics* 2001; **108**: 1211–14.

171. Neil JJ, Shiran SI, McKinstry RC et al. Normal brain in human newborns: apparent diffusion coefficient and diffusion anisotropy measured by using diffusion tensor MR imaging. *Radiology* 1998; **209(1)**: 57–66.

172. Zarifi MK, Astrakas LG, Poussaint TY, Plessis AA, Zurakowski D, Tzika AA. Prediction of adverse outcome with cerebral lactate level and apparent diffusion coefficient in infants with perinatal asphyxia. *Radiology* 2002; **225(3)**: 859–70.

173. McKinstry RC, Miller JH, Snyder AZ et al. A prospective, longitudinal diffusion tensor imaging study of brain injury in newborns. *Neurology* 2002; **59**: 824–33.

174. Robertson RL, Ben-Sira L, Barnes PD et al. MR line-scan diffusion-weighted imaging of term neonates with perinatal brain ischemia. *Am J Neuroradiol* 1999; **20**: 1658–70.

175. Forbes KPN, Pipe JG, Bird R. Neonatal hypoxic-ischemic encephalopathy: detection with diffusion-weighted MR imaging. *Am J Neuroradiol* 2000; **21**: 1490–6.

176. Hunt RW, Neil JJ, Coleman LT, Kean MJ, Inder TE. Apparent diffusion coefficient in the posterior limb of the internal capsule predicts outcome after perinatal asphyxia. *Pediatrics* 2004; **114(4)**: 999–1003.

177. Rutherford M, Counsell S, Allsop J et al. Diffusion-weighted magnetic resonance imaging in term perinatal brain injury: a comparison with site of lesion and time from birth. *Pediatrics* 2004; **114(4)**: 1004–14.

178. Ward P, Counsell S, Allsop J et al. Reduced fractional anisotropy on diffusion tensor magnetic resonance imaging after hypoxic-ischemic encephalopathy. *Pediatrics* 2006; **117(4)**: E619–E630.

179. Shanmugalingam S, Thornton JS, Iwata O et al. Comparative prognostic utilities of early quantitative magnetic resonance imaging spin-spin relaxometry and proton magnetic resonance spectroscopy in neonatal encephalopathy. *Pediatrics* 2006; **118(4)**: 1467–77.

180. Martin LJ, Al-Abdulla NA, Brambrink AM, Kirsch JR, Sieber FE, Portera-Cailliau C. Neurodegeneration in excitotoxicity, global cerebral ischemia, and target deprivation: a perspective on the contributions of apoptosis and necrosis. *Brain Res Bull* 1998; **46(4)**: 281–309.

181. Pouwels PJ, Brockmann K, Kruse B et al. Regional age dependence of human brain metabolites from infancy to adulthood as detected by quantitative localized proton MRS. *Pediatr Res* 1999; **46(4)**: 474–85.

182. Cady EB, Costello A, Dawson MJ et al. Non-invasive investigation of cerebral metabolism in newborn infants by phosphorus nuclear magnetic resonance spectroscopy. *Lancet* 1983; **1**: 1059–62.

183. Hope PL, Costello AMDL, Cady EB et al. Cerebral energy metabolism studied with phosphorus NMR spectroscopy in normal and birth-asphxiated infants. *Lancet* 1984; **ii**: 366–9.

184. Younkin D, Delivoria-Papadopoulos M. Unique aspects of human cerebral metabolism evaluated with P31-NMR. *Ann Neurol* 1984; **16**: 581–6.

185. Laptook AR, Corbett RJ, Uauy R, Mize C, Mendelsohn D, Nunally RL. Use of 31-P NMRS to characterise existing brain damage after neonatal asphyxia. *Neurology* 1989; **39**: 709–12.

186. Martin E, Buchli R, Ritter S et al. Diagnostic and prognostic value of cerebral 31P magnetic resonance spectroscopy in neonates with perinatal asphyxia. *Pediatr Res* 1996; **40**: 749–58.

187. Azzopardi D, Wyatt JS, Reynolds EOR. Prognosis of newborn infants with hypoxic-ischaemic brain injury assessed by P-NIRS. *Pediatr Res* 1989; **25**: 445–51.

188. Roth SC, Edwards D, Cady EB et al. Relation between cerebral oxidative metabolism following birth asphyxia and neurodevelopmental outcome. *Dev Med Child Neurol* 1992; **34(4)**: 285–95.

189. Roth SC, Baudin J, Cady EB et al. Relation of deranged neonatal cerebral oxidative metabolism with neurodevelopmental outcome and head circumference at 4 years. *Dev Med Child Neurol* 1997; **39**: 718–25.

190. Blumberg RM, Cady EB, Wigglesworth JS, McKenzie JE, Edwards AD. Relation between delayed impairment of cerebral energy metabolism and infarction following transient focal hypoxia-ischaemia in the developing brain. *Exp Brain Res* 1997; **113(1)**: 130–7.

191. O'Brien FE, Iwata O, Thornton JS et al. Delayed whole-body cooling to 33 or 35 degrees C and the development of impaired energy generation consequential to transient cerebral hypoxia-ischemia in the newborn piglet. *Pediatrics* 2006; **117(5)**: 1549–59.

192. Robertson NJ, Cowan F, Cox IJ, Edwards AD. Brain alkaline intracellular pH after neonatal encephalopathy. *Ann Neurol* 2002; **52**: 732–42.

193. Kendall GS, Robertson NJ, Iwata O, Peebles D, Raivich G. *N*-Methyl-isobutyl-amiloride ameliorates brain injury when commenced before hypoxia ischemia in neonatal mice. *Pediatr Res* 2006; **59(2)**: 227–31.

194. Lei H, Peeling J. Effect of temperature on the kinetics of lactate production and clearance in a rat model of forebrain ischemia. *Biochem Cell Biol* 1998; **76**: 503–9.

195. Penrice J, Cady EB, Wylezinska M et al. Proton magnetic resonance spectroscopy of the brain in normal preterm and term infants, and early changes after perinatal hypoxia-ischaemia. *Pediatr Res* 1996; **40**: 6–14.

196. Amess PN, Wylezinska M, Lorek A et al. Early brain proton magnetic resonance spectroscopy and neonatal neurology related to neurodevelopmental outcome at 1 year in term infants after presumed hypoxic-ischaemic brain injury. *Dev Med Child Neurol* 1999; **41**: 436–45.

197. Rothman DL, Sibson NR, Hyder F, Shen J, Behar KL, Shulman RG. In vivo nuclear magnetic resonance spectroscopy studies of the relationship between the glutamate-glutamine neurotransmitter cycle and functional neuroenergetics. *Philos Trans R Soc London Biol Sci* 1991; **354**: 1165–77.

198. Groenendaal F, Veenhoven R, van der Grond J, Jansen GH, Witkamp TD, de Vries LS. Cerebral lactate and *N*-acetyl aspartate: choline ratios in asphyxiated full term neonates demonstrated in vivo using proton MRS. *Pediatr Res* 1994; **35**: 148–51.

199. Barkovich AJ, Baranski K, Vigneron D et al. Proton MR spectroscopy for the evaluation of brain injury in asphyxiated, term neonates. *Am J Neuroradiol* 1999; **20**: 1399–405.

200. Robertson NJ, Cox IJ, Cowan FM, Counsell SJ, Azzopardi D, Edwards AD. Cerebral intracellular lactic alkalosis persisting months after neonatal encephalopathy measured by magnetic resonance spectroscopy. *Pediatr Res* 1999; **46**: 287–96.

201. Miller SP, Newton N, Ferriero DM et al. Predictors of 30-month outcome after perinatal depression: role of proton MRS and socioeconomic factors. *Pediatr Res* 2002; **52(1)**: 71–7.

202. Cheong JL, Cady EB, Penrice J, Wyatt JS, Cox IJ, Robertson NJ. Proton MR spectroscopy in neonates with perinatal cerebral hypoxic-ischemic injury: metabolite peak-area ratios, relaxation times, and absolute concentrations. *Am J Neuroradiol* 2006; **27**: 1546–54.

203. Shankaran S, Laptook AR, Ehrenkranz RA et al. Whole-body hypothermia for neonates with hypoxic-ischemic encephalopathy. *N Engl J Med* 2005; **353(15)**: 1574–84.

204. Azzopardi D, Robertson NJ, Cowan FM, Rutherford MA, Rampling M, Edwards AD. Pilot study of treatment with whole body hypothermia for neonatal encephalopathy. *Pediatrics* 2000; **106(4)**: 684–94.

205. Iwata S, Iwata O, Thornton JS et al. Superficial brain is cooler in small piglets: neonatal hypothermia implications. *Ann Neurol* 2006; **60**: 578–85.

206. Haaland K, Loberg EM, Steen PA, Satas S, Thoresen M. The effect of mild post-hypoxic hypothermia on organ pathology in a piglet survival model of global hypoxia. *Prenat Neonat* 1997; **2**: 329–37.

207. Nedelcu J, Klein MA, Aguzzi A, Martin E. Resuscitative hypothermia protects the neonatal rat brain from hypoxic-ischemic injury. *Brain Pathol* 2000; **10(1)**: 61–71.

208. Ma D, Hossain M, Chow A et al. Xenon and hypothermia combine to provide neuroprotection from neonatal asphyxia. *Ann Neurol* 2005; **58(2)**: 182–93.

209. Rutherford MA, Azzopardi D, Whitelaw A et al. Mild hypothermia and the distribution of cerebral lesions in neonates with hypoxic-ischemic encephalopathy. *Pediatrics* 2005; **116(4)**: 1001–6.

210. Inder TE, Hunt RW, Morley CJ et al. Randomized trial of systemic hypothermia selectively protects the cortex on MRI in term hypoxic-ischemic encephalopathy. *J Paediatr* 2004; **145**: 835–7.

211. Kim Y, Busto R, Dietrich WD, Kraydieh S, Ginsberg MD. Delayed postischemic hyperthermia in awake rats worsens the histopathological outcome of transient focal cerebral ischemia. *Stroke* 1996; **27(12)**: 2274–3380.

212. Shevell MI, Majnemer A, Miller SP. Neonatal neurological prognostication: the asphyxiated term newborn. *Pediatr Neurol* 1999; **21**: 776–84.

213. Gray PH, Tudehope DI, Masel JP et al. Perinatal hypoxic ischaemic brain injury: prediction of outcome. *Dev Med Child Neurol* 1993; **35**: 965–73.

214. Rennie JM, Hagmann CF, Robertson NJ. Outcome after intrapartum hypoxic ischaemia at term. *Semin Fetal Neonatal Med* 2007; **12(5)**: 398–407.

215. Gonzalez FF, Miller SP. Does perinatal asphyxia impair cognitive function without cerebral palsy? *Arch Dis Child Fetal Neonat Ed* 2006; **91**: 454–9.

216. Mercuri E, Ricci D, Cowan FM et al. Head growth in infants with hypoxic-ischaemic encephalopathy: correlation with neonatal magnetic resonance imaging. *Pediatrics* 2000; **106**: 235–44.

217. De Haan M, Wyatt JS, Roth S, Vargha-Khadem F, Gadian D, Mishkin M. Brain and cognitive-behavioural development after asphyxia at term birth. *Dev Sci* 2006; **9**: 350–8.

218. Gadian DG, Aicardi J, Watkins KE, Porter DA, Mishkin M, Vargha-Khadem F. Developmental amnesia associated with early hypoxic-ischaemic injury. *Brain* 2000; **123**: 499–507.

219. Khong PL, Lam BCC, Tung HKS, Wong V, Chan FL, Ooi GC. MRI of neonatal encephalopathy. *Clin Radiol* 2003; **58**: 833–44.

220. Cavalleri F, Berardi A, Burlina AB, Ferrari F, Mavilla L. Diffusion-weighted MRI of maple syrup urine disease encephalopathy. *Neuroradiology* 2002; **44(6)**: 499–502.

221. Khong PL, Lam BC, Chung BH, Wong KY, Ooi GC. Diffusion-weighted MR imaging in neonatal nonketotic hyperglycinemia. *Am J Neuroradiol* 2003; **24(6)**: 1181–3.

Chapter 9 | The baby who had an ultrasound as part of a preterm screening protocol

JANET M. RENNIE,
CORNELIA F. HAGMANN, *and*
NICOLA J. ROBERTSON

Clinical presentation of preterm brain injury

Preterm babies who are found to have abnormal brain scans are usually asymptomatic, hence the importance of screening in this vulnerable group. Occasionally a baby develops a bulging fontanelle, shock, and seizures due to a massive intracranial hemorrhage. Encephalopathy is difficult to diagnose in a small ill baby who is ventilated and sedated. The current practice of routine screening was prompted by the high incidence of intracranial bleeding (around 50%) which was first revealed by systematic studies of neuroimaging in preterm babies using computerized tomography (CT) [1,2]. Once ultrasound became widely available cohort studies began in earnest, and continued to show a very high incidence of all grades of intracranial hemorrhage in this group throughout the 1980s (Fig. 9.1). Recently, the incidence has fallen to about 25% overall, with very few significant parenchymal lesions, but the prevalence of disability in affected survivors remains high. The most common lesions requiring assessment in preterm babies now are cerebral atrophy, ventriculomegaly, and delayed cortical development or diffuse white matter injury diagnosed with magnetic resonance imaging (MRI). It is important to remember that brain imaging screening meets very few of the criteria for screening set many years ago by the World Health Organization (WHO) (Table 9.1). In the absence of any effective treatment and no recognizable early stage of disease the aim of cohort screening studies is limited to audit, research, and to provide information for parents. In general, parents are keen to obtain as much information as possible about their preterm baby, but currently they are not routinely asked to consent for their baby to undergo brain imaging. In spite of the drawbacks, the American Academy of Neurology has stated that routine ultrasound screening should be the standard of care for all babies born at less than 30 weeks' gestation [8]. If the practice of screening is to continue, parents deserve to receive information based only on high-quality carefully interpreted serial imaging supported by information from detailed clinical assessment and the results of other appropriate investigations. Prognosis is the most difficult aspect of neonatal imaging, and must not be hasty or unrealistic. Our ability to predict motor impairment still far outstrips the accuracy of predicting neurodevelopmental delay or neuropsychiatric disorders. Experience has taught us not to be too dogmatic when giving a prognosis, and always to discuss the likely range of severity.

Investigative screening methods

Ultrasound is the only method which is currently suitable for routine screening in the nursery. In many hands this technique fails to detect any abnormality in about half of preterm babies who later develop cerebral palsy (CP) [9,10,11,12]. Some centers, notably Utrecht, claim far better results, albeit in a tertiary unit setting with expert observers using high-resolution sequential weekly cranial ultrasound repeated frequently until term-equivalent age. The results of this Utrecht study showed that 79% of children in whom CP was evident by 2 years had a major abnormality diagnosed with cranial ultrasound imaging in the neonatal period [13,14]. Ultrasound was not useful for the prediction of learning difficulties or sensorineural deficits. This group stresses the importance of repeated imaging, extending beyond the first 4 weeks after birth, in order not to miss the detection of transient cysts. These workers also stress the need to scan preterm infants of all gestational ages admitted to the neonatal unit, a practice we endorse.

Magnetic resonance imaging (MRI), with its multi-slice coverage of the whole brain and array of sequences, has, at term-equivalent age, been shown to have better sensitivity and specificity than ultrasound for the prediction of CP [15]. Although both ultrasound and MRI demonstrated high specificity in this study, in contrast to the Utrecht study very few late ultrasound images were made; repeat imaging was only done in babies with ultrasound abnormalities detected in the first

Neonatal Cerebral Investigation, eds. Janet M. Rennie, Cornelia F. Hagmann and Nicola J. Robertson. Published by Cambridge University Press. © Cambridge University Press 2008.

Table 9.1. Principles of screening formulated by Wilson and Junger for the World Health Organization in 1968.

1. The condition should pose an important health problem
2. The natural history of the disease should be well understood
3. There should be a recognizable early stage
4. Treatment of the disease at an early stage should be of more benefit than treatment started at a later stage
5. There should be a suitable test
6. The test should be acceptable to the population
7. There should be adequate facilities for the diagnosis and treatment of abnormalities detected
8. The chance of physical or psychological harm to those screened should be less than the chance of benefit

Table 9.2. UCLH scanning protocol (for preterm babies who remain as in-patients).

	< 30 weeks	31–35 weeks
As soon as possible after admission to intensive care	√	√
Day 1	√	
Day 2	√	
Day 3	√	
Day 4	√	
Day 7	√	√
Weekly to 32 weeks	√	
35 weeks	√	√
Term corrected	√	√
Discharge	√	

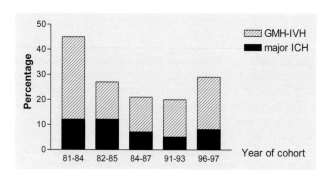

Fig. 9.1. **Incidence of intracranial hemorrhage detected with ultrasound screening over time. Data in colum 1 are from [3]; column 2, [4]; column 3, [5]; column 4, [6]; column 5, [7]. GMH-IVH, germinal matrix-intraventricular hemorrhage; ICH, intracranial hemorrhage.**

2 weeks. More comparative studies are needed, particularly studies which compare the prognostic abilities of ultrasound and MRI and in which a similar amount of time and expertise is devoted to image acquisition and expert analysis in both modalities. Neurological investigation of any sort cannot and should not be used to replace clinical examination, which assists considerably in detection of brain injury and in prognosis [12,16].

Ultrasound screening

Who?

Repeated ultrasound imaging can be used to examine the brain of preterm infants to identify abnormalities, and to time the onset and evolution. Cut-offs for screening vary between units, many screening all babies below 32 weeks' gestation at birth (the American Academy of Neurology suggests 30 weeks). Intraparenchymal hemorrhage is now virtually confined to the group less than 28 weeks' gestation, but babies of up to 32 weeks and beyond remain at risk of developing periventricular leukomalacia. Some have proposed limiting screening to babies born at less than 29 weeks' gestation plus those of 30-2 weeks who develop neurological signs, but this strategy would only be effective if the aim of screening did not include detection of white matter injury [17,18]. In our view, and in the view of the Hammersmith, Leeds, and Utrecht groups, cranial

ultrasound imaging is justified in all preterm babies admitted to neonatal units [14].

When?

In order not to miss abnormalities which may be of prognostic value, screening protocols should aim to include at least four or five scans (Table 9.2). The first scan should be made as early as possible, in order to detect any long standing intrauterine damage or congenital malformations. It is important to ascertain whether the scan looks normal at this time, whether the anatomy looks normal for the gestational age (Chapter 6), that there are no features to suggest congenital infection or metabolic disease, and to establish a baseline for the assessment of problems that may evolve later such as hemorrhage or white matter echogenicity.

The scan at around day 4 is essential, and is timed to detect intracranial hemorrhage, most of which has occurred by this stage. In very immature (<26 weeks) or sick babies scans should be done daily for the first 4–7 days for the same reason. Ideally, further images should be obtained at weekly intervals from day 7–10 onwards as long as the baby remains on the neonatal unit (certainly until 36 weeks' gestational age equivalent is reached) with a final scan at term-equivalent age (or discharge) to detect signs of brain atrophy and to see how any early lesions have resolved in the medium term. Repeated imaging can be very helpful when trying to distinguish between the potentially adverse effects of, say, a hostile intrauterine environment and a period of postnatal collapse or sepsis. Periventricular leukomalacia (PVL) often develops late (in de Vries's study cystic PVL was detected after 28 days in almost one-third of infants at <32 weeks' gestational age [13]), whereas intracranial hemorrhage rarely does [19,20]. As a result, repeat weekly imaging is the ideal if the aim is to identify all cases with small periventricular cysts, which may be transient. Our scanning protocol for preterm infants is given in Table 9.2.

Manpower or cost constraints may require reducing the screening protocol to a minimum, in which case a single early scan, with a second at 10 days and one at term would be our recommendation, with further scans in babies with neurological signs. This is similar to the US recommendation of one scan between 7 and 14 days and one between 36 and 40 weeks' gestational age equivalent, with the addition of our strong recommendation for a scan as early as possible [8]. We disagree strongly with the view that two normal scans are enough [21,22].

Why?

There is an urgent need for a bedside method to assess the effectiveness of neonatal therapies designed to improve cerebral development in low birthweight infants. It is unlikely that ultrasound imaging will be able to detect all the subtle white matter injury that may be responsible for school failure, the hippocampal damage that can affect memory, cerebellar damage, or a failure of gyral development [23,24]. However, this is an active area of research; a recent paper by Anderson *et al.* measuring the growth rate of the corpus callosum and cerebellar vermis between 2 and 6 weeks after birth suggested that early changes in the rate of growth of these structures are associated with CP at age 2 [25]. Such early quantitative information may be important for monitoring interventions. There is increasing evidence that signs of brain atrophy (enlarged subarachnoid space, widened interhemispheric fissure, reduced complexity of cortical folding) on sequential cranial ultrasound are associated with poor neurocognitive outcomes [26]; more studies with large numbers and precise quantitation with MRI correlations are required.

Parents are not usually consulted about their views on screening even if they refused antenatal testing. Further discussion and debate about the practice of screening for brain injury without informed consent are essential, particularly if MR imaging is to be used, because of the high probability of finding a subtle abnormality such as diffuse excessive high signal intensity (DEHSI), which carries an uncertain prognosis (see later). In the meanwhile, most neonatal units continue to image the brains of high-risk preterm babies with ultrasound in order to examine the effect of changes in practice over time, to compare their results to those of other units, and to inform parents about the prognosis for their baby. In the past, information from ultrasound imaging has proved invaluable in evaluating potential risk factors of preterm brain injury, and the results of such studies have contributed to the reduction in the prevalence of major ultrasound abnormalities (hyper- and hypocarbia are good examples, but there are others).

Useful information regarding the effects of different intensive care practices may yet be gained from comparative audits such as the one from Canada, where the incidence of intracranial hemorrhage varied between institutions from 14% to 57% [7]. Even after adjusting for factors such as illness severity and outborn status, three of the hospitals had a incidence which was significantly higher than the median value of 20%. Striking inter-unit variation has also been reported from Australia [27] and Japan [28]. Routine ultrasound scanning drew attention to an unusual pattern of brain injury emerging in some units [29]. The damage may have been due to vigorous chest physiotherapy although the debate about the mechanism continues [30]. High-frequency oscillatory ventilation used in a certain way was a further innovation which was found to be associated with a higher incidence of intracranial hemorrhage by screening [31].

MRI screening

To date, very few cohorts of preterm babies have been screened with MRI in the UK or USA, although 93% of Japanese neonatal units routinely perform CT or MRI [28]. From a sequential cohort of 41 babies born in London at less than 30 weeks' gestation, 28 had abnormalities diagnosed with MRI, a result remarkably reminiscent of that of the ground-breaking CT study conducted 20 years earlier [1,32]. The nature of the findings, though, has changed over time with germinal matrix-intraventricular hemorrhage (GMH-IVH) becoming much less common (9/41 babies). The most frequent finding (80% of infants) was DEHSI in the white matter, the nature and importance of which are not yet fully understood. The presence and severity of DEHSI were related to lower developmental quotients (DQ) at 18 months of age [33] which suggests that DEHSI represents an abnormality of white matter, although it is still unclear whether this is a maturational delay or secondary to injury due to vasogenic edema, oligodendrocyte damage or a reduced axonal diameter [34]. A cohort was imaged in Leeds, where 151/238 consecutive admissions were subjected to MRI in 1998–99 [35]. In this study 105 preterm babies were imaged with MRI, and, in contrast to the London series, 55% had normal MR brain scans; 26 had punctate white matter abnormalities thought to be micro-hemorrhagic change. Another cohort of 100 consecutive preterm infants underwent MRI at term equivalent age; these MRIs were assessed qualitatively [36] and quantitatively [37]. There was a high incidence of cerebral abnormality, particularly in the cerebral white matter at term-equivalent age. In keeping with the previous studies mentioned here, non-cystic diffuse white matter injury was more common than cystic white matter injury.

The extremely immature infant of <26 weeks' gestation may show a unique pattern of cerebral white matter abnormality characterized by ventriculomegaly and a marked reduction in white matter volume without cystic white matter abnormality or apparent signal abnormality and abnormal gray matter characterized by a delay in gyral development [36,37]. Interestingly, abnormalities in gray matter development were associated with the presence of white matter abnormalities. The quantitative volumetric MRI studies defined the abnormalities further: compared to term infants, preterm infants at term demonstrate prominent reductions in cortical gray matter and deep gray matter volumes and an increase in CSF volume [37]. In another cohort study of 89 consecutive babies less than 34 weeks' gestation scanned twice, at a median age of 32 weeks and before discharge, the severity of white matter abnormalities remained the same in both studies in 87%, increased in 9%, and resolved in 4% of the babies [38]. Non-cystic white matter abnormalities were reported in 52% of the babies with 23% having mild and 29% having moderate to severe abnormalities. The location and laterality were similar in the second study compared to the first.

Magnetic resonance imaging has several significant advantages for screening; the inter-observer agreement is much better than for ultrasound, and the method appears to be more sensitive for the detection of white matter lesions. The

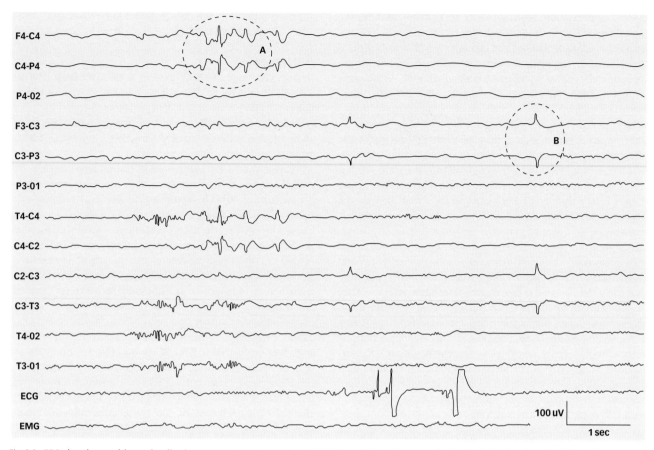

Fig. 9.2. **EEG showing positive Rolandic sharp waves. This example is from a term baby who was a twin who later developed multicystic encephalomalacia. The background is discontinuous. Surface positive sharp waves localized at C4 are shown (A). Positive broad-based sharp wave with a phase reversal in C3 is shown (B).**

disadvantages are cost, availability, and the fact that MRI (like ultrasound) does not meet stringent criteria for a screening test and may be overly sensitive. At the moment the cohort MR studies are at the same stage of research as the ultrasound studies were 20 years ago, and there is no doubt that much exciting progress will be made in the next decade.

EEG screening

Like ultrasound, EEG offers the potential for early cotside recognition of white matter injury, and can be repeated easily and safely. Electroencephalography has not often been used as a screening tool in preterm babies, but when it has the presence of a persistently normal background has proved a reliable indicator of a good outcome. Some claim that EEG is a more reliable predictor than clinical examination or cranial ultrasound in preterm babies [39]. In the early days of ultrasound, EEG was able to improve the reliability of diagnosis of suspected white matter lesions, and assist with prognosis [40,41]. Whether EEG could detect diffuse white matter injury, which is increasingly described in MR studies of preterm cohorts, is unknown. In research studies, EEG has great potential because detection of acute and chronic injury patterns offers the prospect of better temporal resolution of the time of the injury than that which is obtained with imaging.

Typical EEG signs of white matter injury are unilateral or bilateral positive sharp waves in the central region (so-called positive Rolandic sharp waves). In 1972 Cukier *et al.* reported positive Rolandic sharp waves in the EEGs of preterm infants with periventricular hemorrhage [42]. The findings were confirmed several years later in a further study which used CT diagnosis of intraventricular hemorrhage (IVH) [43]. These waveforms are characteristic electropositive sharp waves over the Rolandic (central) regions (C_3–C_4) of the brain that can occur as isolated sharp waves or in trains (Fig. 9.2). The designation of a type-B positive Rolandic sharp wave requires a single but clear and definite paroxysmal discharge, positive in polarity with a steep initial slope and sharp peak, suddenly arising out of the background rhythm with a duration of between 60 and 200 ms but usually 60–100 m [44,45]. Type-A Rolandic waves are smaller, occur in runs, and can be seen in the EEG of normal babies. It has been suggested that type-B positive Rolandic sharp waves (PRSW) only occur when there is evidence of white matter damage [46,47,48]. One French group found that PRSW detection improved the sensitivity of ultrasound scanning for the diagnosis of cystic PVL from 78.3% to 88% [46]. The incidence of PRSW in cohort studies of preterm infants has varied from 7% to 38%. Positive Rolandic sharp waves appear earlier than the cysts of PVL imaged with ultrasound, but the exact temporal (or any) relationship between PRSW and the ultrasound appearance of a flare is unknown. Watanabe *et al.* suggest than PRSW appear about 6 days after the insult, emerging as the background depression of the EEG, which occurs in response to the acute insult, resolves [49].

Hughes *et al.* found that there was an increased detection rate of sharp waves if the temporal areas of the brain were also monitored [44]. The incidence of temporal sharp waves plus PRSW was 67%. Some authors have disputed the significance of temporal sharp waves in preterm babies [50], particularly when they are few in number, short in duration, and disappear within a few days of birth [49]. Positive temporal sharp waves occur in up to 22% of babies of 29–30 weeks' gestation and about 12% of those born at 31–32 weeks; some studies found them to be even more common, and present in 55% of babies born at 21–32 weeks [51].

Sharp waves have also been detected in the frontal and occipital regions, and were considered predictive of mild PVL, unless occurring in more than one region when the prognosis was worse [52]. A discontinuous pattern in the EEG has been reported during early neonatal life in babies who later developed PVL [53]. These Japanese authors describe an evolving pattern of background abnormality, which allowed them to implicate antenatal events in 20% of their cases, and perinatal events in 50% [54,55]. Calculation of the EEG spectral edge frequency, usually defined as the frequency below which 90% of the EEG power exists, can be done easily with modern cotside continuous EEG monitors. So far only one study has suggested that this might be of any prognostic value, with a lower frequency being found in babies who later developed white matter injury [56].

Diagnostic categories resulting from screening

Normal

For more information on recognizing the normal appearances of cranial imaging with ultrasound and MRI in premature babies, see Chapter 6. It is always worthwhile recording at least some of the normal images permanently.

Prognosis after normal imaging in the neonatal period

For prognostic purposes most would classify as normal babies whose ultrasound scans showed no abnormality or only mild echodensities present for less than a week. A meta-analysis of 11 follow-up studies reporting the outcome for over 1200 preterm babies showed that a normal cranial ultrasound was associated with a 3%–4% risk of major disability, usually CP [57]. The prognosis for learning difficulty is less optimistic, and relates to the gestational age. As discussed elsewhere in this chapter, the importance of subtle white matter injury that can be detected with MRI but not ultrasound is under active investigation.

Germinal matrix-intraventricular hemorrhage

The germinal matrix is formed from neuroepithelial cells in the wall of the lateral ventricle, and occupies a surprisingly large volume of the preterm brain in this region [58] (Fig. 9.3a–c). This region is an important source of

undifferentiated glial cell precursors (glioblasts) which proceed to migrate into the developing neocortex [59]. These cells are abundant until about 34 weeks and then regress, although small pockets remain. Pathologists have long recognized the frequent existence of bleeding into this periventricular matrix layer in preterm infants, sometimes involving the choroid plexus. The most common site for germinal matrix bleeding to occur is in the caudothalamic region, adjacent to the foramina of Munro (Fig. 4.8). Bleeding into the lateral ventricle at term usually arises mainly from the choroid plexus or the thalamus (pp. 119–122). Larroche and others considered that bleeding into the germinal matrix was a consequence of stasis and engorgement of the deep cerebral veins [61,62]. The terminal vein has a configuration involving a U turn, and the angle at which the thalamo-striate and choroid veins join into the internal veins at the foramina of Munro is sharp, which may account for the propensity for bleeding at this point (Fig. 9.4a). The aterial supply of the germinal matrix is via the branches of the lateral striate arteries and Heubner's artery (Fig. 9.4b). After a prolonged and heated debate between those who considered that germinal matrix bleeding was arterial in origin and those who thought that it was venous, the venous theory is once more in the ascent [64]. This fits neatly with the explanation for the association of GMH-IVH with parenchymal venous infarction (see below).

Terminology and classification

In the past "periventricular hemorrhage" was often used as a generic term, embracing germinal matrix hemorrhage, intraventricular hemorrhage and hemorrhage into the periventricular white matter. This term is not sufficiently precise and in our view has led to misunderstanding between professionals, and between professionals and parents. We prefer to use the term "germinal matrix-intraventricular hemorrhage" (GMH-IVH) to describe bleeding which is isolated to the germinal matrix, and to include uncomplicated intraventricular hemorrhage – that is, where there is blood in the ventricular cavity but no ventriculomegaly. Using this terminology clearly separates GMH-IVH from parenchymal lesions. Parenchymal lesions are no longer thought to result from extrusion of intraventricular blood under pressure into the substance of the brain, and further study has revealed different types of parenchymal abnormality, so that we prefer a nomenclature that does not lump these conditions together. Although the Papile classification had the merit of simplicity it was designed to grade a single CT scan, and had the disadvantage of assuming that all abnormalities of the preterm brain were part of a single spectrum. This view is now known to be incorrect; further, the system took no account of the evolution over time which can be seen with serial imaging. Finally, the classification was hierarchal, assuming (incorrectly) that ventriculomegaly was always a stage in the process from grade I to grade IV hemorrhage, and that a parenchymal lesion was always the end-stage. For these reasons, we recommend that this system be abandoned. This was the recommendation made in the first edition of this book, which has since been supported by Paneth and many others [65].

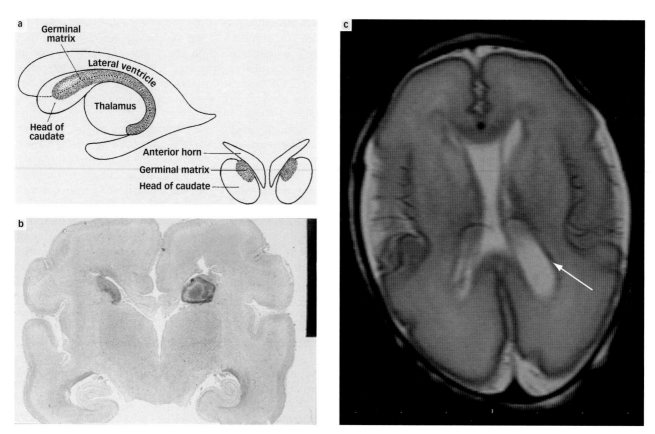

Fig. 9.3a–c. **(a)** Diagram showing the volume of brain occupied by the germinal matrix, and its position. Adapted from Grant, 1986 with permission [60]. **(b)** Pathological specimen showing the normal germinal matrix capillary bed on the left, with a germinal matrix bleed on the right. **(c)** Axial T$_2$-weighted MR image showing the extent of the germinal matrix (smooth rim of T$_2$ hypotensity, arrow) in a preterm baby.

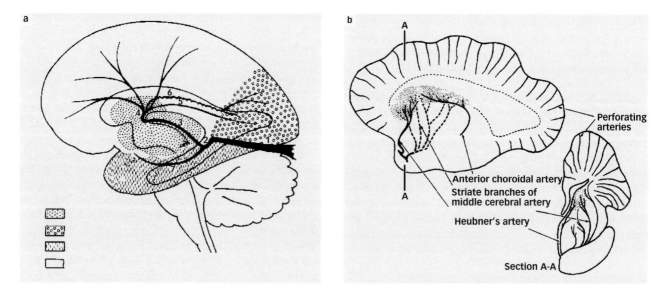

Fig. 9.4a,b. **Schematic representation of brain territories drained by the vein of Galen and their tributaries; hatched and stippled areas have a double venous drainage: toward the deep system of Galen and toward the basilar system. (1) Sinus rectus, (2) ampulla Galen, (3) paired small veins of Galen or internal cerebral veins, (4) terminal vein in the subependymal germinative zone at the level of the foramen of Monro, (5) thalamostriate vein, (6) choroidal vein, (7) basilar vein. From Larroche [61] and Hambleton and Wigglesworth [63], with permission.**

Table 9.3. Factors associated with an increased risk of germinal matrix-intraventricular hemorrhage (GMH-IVH) in preterm infants. IUGR, intrauterine growth retardation; CTG, cardiotocography; PET, pre-eclamptic toxemia; PROM, prolonged rupture of membranes; RDS, respiratory distress syndrome; SVC, superior vena cava.

Factor	Reference
Prenatal factors	
Lack of exposure to antenatal steroids	[27,29,66,67,68,69,70,71]
Maternal aspirin therapy	[72]
Maternal smoking	[73,74]
Reason for prematurity other than PET	[75]
Male sex	[27,76]
Vaginal delivery (contentious, may be related to lower gestational age)	[67,77,78,79]
Very preterm delivery	Virtually all studies show inverse correlation with gestational
Thrombophilia, e.g., Factor V Leiden heterozygosity	age [80]
Placental abnormalities; IUGR, abnormal Doppler studies, abnormal CTG	[81,82,83]
PROM, chorioamnionitis, high interleukin 6 levels – note that some say moderately elevated cytokine levels are beneficial	[84,85]
Factors at delivery	
Birth depression; asphyxia; acidosis	[27,86,87,88]
Birth trauma; bruising	[89]
Postnatal factors	
RDS, particularly if complicated by:	Virtually all studies show a relationship between GMH-IVH and RDS requiring mechanical ventilation
pneumothorax	[77,86,90,91,92,93]
hypercarbia	[77,86,90,94,95,96]
acidosis, bicarbonate therapy	[74,77,91]
hypoxia	[74,97]
Hypotension, low right ventricular output, low SVC flow	[79,98,99,100,101,102]
Fluctuating cerebral blood flow, fluctuating blood pressure, low cerebral blood flow	[103,104,263,264,265]
Coagulation disturbance (prematurity/bruising/sepsis); association with pulmonary hemorrhage	[77,106,107]
Tolazoline therapy	[77]
Patent ductus arteriosus (low BP, cerebral steal)	[108,109]

Etiology

Bleeding into the germinal matrix is thought to arise from venous stasis with underlying changes in cerebral blood flow. Premature babies often have an increase in intracranial venous pressure associated with their respiratory disease and accompanying need for artificial ventilation, and on top of that their cerebral blood flow (and venous pressure) fluctuates as they "fight the ventilator," and/or develop hypotension, pneumothorax, acidosis, and patent ductus arteriosus. Preterm babies often have thrombocytopenia and a coagulopathy with poor autoregulation of cerebral blood flow (CBF). All these clinical factors, and more, have been implicated in the genesis of GMH-IVH (Table 9.3). Studies from the early 1980s onwards have shown associations of respiratory distress syndrome (RDS), pneumothorax, hypercarbia, and coagulopathy with GMH-IVH [77,90,110]. Some of the implicated causative agents may be co-travelers, but careful timing studies confirm that many of the factors included in Table 9.3 are genuine antecedents. The occurrence of GMH-IVH is tightly linked to gestational age, and is more common the more preterm the baby; unilateral parenchymal infarction is now very rare after 28 weeks of gestation. The contribution of vaginal delivery remains debatable; one recent study observed that the effect of vaginal delivery disappeared when adjustment was made for chorioamnionitis, raising the interesting hypothesis that preterm vaginal delivery is a marker for intrauterine infection [78]. Given that most very preterm babies whose mothers have pre-eclampsia are delivered by caesarean section this plausible hypothesis would also explain the paradoxical protection which pre-eclamptic toxemia (PET) apparently offers.

Incidence and timing

The incidence of GMH-IVH continues to reduce over time (Fig. 9.1), although a plateau may have been reached. The current incidence of GMH-IVH plus parenchymal lesions is around 25% for babies born weighing <1500 g, a figure reached

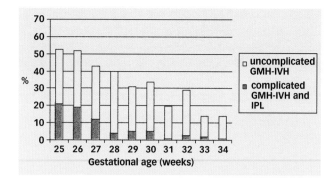

Fig. 9.5. **Incidence of GMH-IVH by gestation. Data from [112]. IPL, intraparenchymal lesion.**

by the early 1990s and reported in the large New Jersey study [111]. In a study of 1600 very low birthweight babies the incidence was 41% in those born at < 26 weeks; 20% at 26–28 weeks; and 8% at >28 weeks [112] (Fig. 9.5). The large French "Epipage" study enrolled 2667 babies born at 22–32 weeks of gestation, and reported very similar findings with uncomplicated GMH-IVH in about 20% of the survivors, with 40% of those below 26 weeks' gestation being affected [113]. In summary, over the last decade, rates of IVH have declined from 49% to 20%, however rates have remained at 25%–30% for very low birthweight (<1500 g) infants and they are highest in extremely low birth weight (<1000 g) infants [114,115].

The vast majority of GMH-IVH occurs very early in postnatal life, with at least 75% of cases diagnosed by 72 hours of age or earlier [111,116]. In 10%–20% of babies further progression takes place over the next 24–48 hours [117].

In a study of over 1000 preterm babies born in New Jersey in 1984–87 repeated cranial ultrasound scanning was performed as near as possible to 4 hours, 24 hours, and 7 days. Although this study was limited to babies weighing <2 kg at birth, it has major strengths because it was large, population based, and prospective. Of the 1079 babies studied 265 developed IVH; 95 had bleeding present on the first scan, and a further 49 on the second [111]. In a study which is now largely historical, Szymonowicz and Yu [118] scanned all babies of birth weight less than 1250 g who were admitted to a neonatal unit in Melbourne over an 8-month period in 1982. Babies were scanned daily for 4 days and then weekly. The overall incidence of IVH was high in this study at 60%; 96% of germinal matrix hemorrhage and 79% of intraventricular hemorrhage had occurred by 48 hours [118]. In another Australian study 77% of all GMH-IVH was present on the first scan, at 8 hours [119]. Some have suggested that the epidemiology of very early GMH-IVH differs from that relating to later-appearing bleeds, with obstetric and perinatal factors being more important in the early developing lesions [89], and ischemia-reperfusion a factor in later appearing lesions [79].

Natural history of GMH-IVH
Hemorrhage into the germinal matrix eventually resorbs leaving a small, subependymal cyst (Fig. 9.6a,b). A subependymal cyst is of no consequence, but must be distinguished from a connatal pseudocyst, which can sometimes be seen lying along the floor of the frontal horn of the lateral ventricle (p. 229 *et seq.*). As intraventricular bleeding resolves an echodense line, rather like a pencil-line, can often be identified with ultrasound outlining the walls of the lateral ventricles. This probably represents hemosiderin deposit, and supports an earlier diagnosis of GMH-IVH.

Ultrasound and MRI appearances of GMH-IVH
The characteristic ultrasound appearances of GMH-IVH are shown in Figs. 9.6 and 9.7, and the MRI appearances in Fig. 9.6b and Fig. 9.7c. Germinal matrix hemorrhage is usually indicated by an echoreflective area in the caudo thalamic groove. It is important to distinguish this from the normal appearances of a small echoreflective area seen in this region, which arises from normal choroid plexus "tucking" into the caudo thalamic groove. Echodensity in this region appearing after 30 days has also been described in babies with chronic lung disease receiving steroids, in whom it probably does not represent bleeding into the germinal matrix [121]. Intraventricular hemorrhage is marked by an echoreflective opacity within the ventricular cavity, usually adherent to the germinal matrix at the head of the caudate nucleus (Fig. 9.7a,b) but occasionally mobile when the head is moved (Fig. 9.7d). There is often abnormal echoreflectivity in the third and fourth ventricle visible on coronal images, presumably indicating the presence of clotted blood.

Accuracy of ultrasound and MR diagnosis of GMH-IVH
There is a lack of concordance between observers in any test involving pattern recognition, and a recent audit showed that only 59% (range 45%–71%) of observers (mainly specialist pediatric registrars with little or no specific training) correctly interpreted a set of six common ultrasound abnormalities [122]. The Australia and New Zealand neonatal network have reported similar problems with image interpretation [123]. Unsurprisingly the inter-observer agreement for the diagnosis of germinal matrix hemorrhage is worse than that for the identification of either intraventricular or parenchymal lesions [124]. However, there was agreement about the broad diagnostic category in 92% of cases in the Pinto study. There was similar level of agreement between 8 Texan observers reporting on 180 scans [125], although agreement for GMH-IVH was poor with a kappa of only 0.26, and only 4 of 20 sonograms were interpreted with perfect agreement by all observers. False-positive diagnosis of germinal matrix hemorrhage was also a problem in the study by Hope *et al.* [126]. The subjective nature of ultrasound interpretation remains problematic, both for clinical and research purposes. Repeat imaging, with review and consensus, and constant training and updating remain the key to minimizing disagreement. In our opinion the results of ultrasound imaging should not be conveyed to parents without review and a repeat, particularly if the results suggest the possibility of an adverse prognosis.

Ultrasound cannot reliably detect lesions below 0.5 cm, but was found to be 100% sensitive and 91% specific for germinal matrix hemorrhage larger than this detected at autopsy [127].

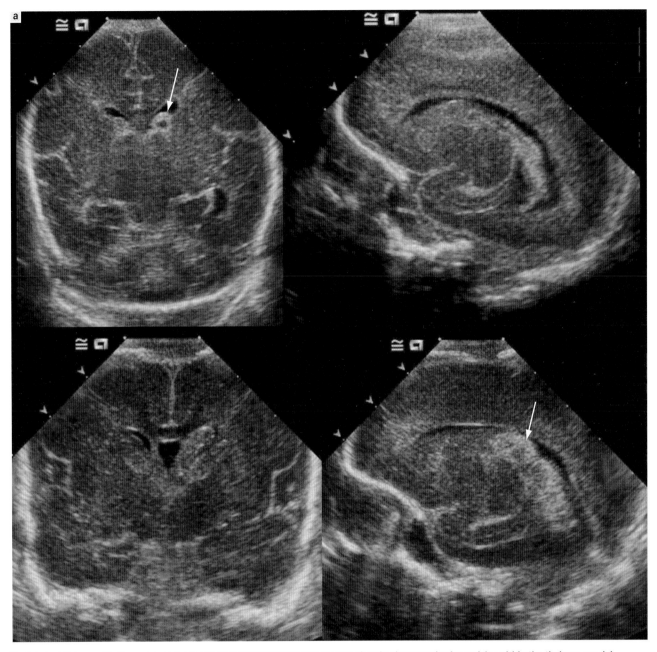

Fig. 9.6a,b. **(a) Top and bottom row coronal and parasagittal ultrasound images showing increased echogenicity within the thalamo-caudal notch in keeping with germinal matrix hemorrhage (arrow).**

A more recent US study reported less impressive results when ultrasound diagnosis was compared to autopsy detection of GMH-IVH; only 9 of 15 cases were detected and there were 5 false-positive sonograms [128].

Magnetic resonance imaging has better inter-observer agreement than ultrasound for the diagnosis of GMH-IVH [129]. Fairly good correlation between MRI and ultrasound for the diagnosis of GMH-IVH and parenchymal lesions, including cystic PVL, has been shown in comparative studies [130,131,132]. So far, the results of correlating MRI in life with

autopsy findings are good, but as yet relatively few babies or fetuses who were imaged with MRI in life have undergone autopsy [133,134].

Prognosis after imaging showing uncomplicated GMH-IVH in the neonatal period

Most follow-up studies have found that the risk of a major disability, usually spastic diplegic cerebral palsy, is the same (about 4%–5%) in groups of preterm survivors who were found to have uncomplicated GMH-IVH as in preterm babies with

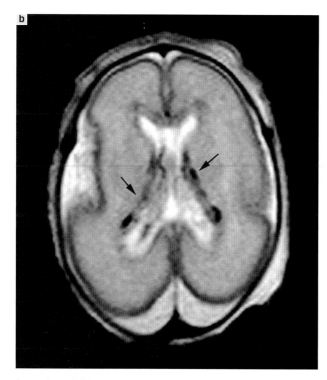

Fig. 9.6. **(cont.) (b) Axial T$_2$-weighted image showing MRI showing germinal matrix hemorrhage (arrows). With permission of Counsell** *et al.* **[120].**

persistently normal ultrasound imaging [135,136,137,138,139 140]. In a geographical cohort of 699 babies of birthweight 500–1249 g born in Alberta, Canada, between 1987 and 1990 none of the 16 with a neonatal diagnosis of isolated GMH-IVH were disabled at 2 years [141]. The results of the New Jersey study are somewhat different, and in this study 37/149 (25%) with uncomplicated GMH-IVH had disabling cerebral palsy at 2 years of age [9]. This was a much higher risk than in the group with persistently normal cranial ultrasound scans, and high when compared with other studies, even the more recent study from Cleveland [142].

Further, the 6-year follow-up of one cohort showed that there was also a risk of a low IQ, with an odds ratio of 4 (1.2–18.6) [143]. There was no link with psychiatric disorders [144]. The attributable risk of GMH-IVH for learning disability (US mental retardation) was 5% (for comparison the attributable risk ascribed to a parenchymal lesion was 50%). Recent data from the post surfactant era, with smaller more immature infants surviving, suggest that extremely low birthweight (ELBW) infants with uncomplicated GMH-IVH on cranial ultrasound have significantly lower mean Mental Development Index (MDI) scores (45% had MDI <70), higher rates of major neurologic abnormalities (13%), and neurodevelopmental impairments at 20 months compared with infants with normal cranial ultrasound findings [142]. These rates of impairment were significantly higher in this ELBW group with GMH-IVH than in the unaffected babies, and were higher than the rates seen in ELBW babies with normal ultrasound scans in other studies, which report rates of around 9% for cerebral palsy and 25% for MDI <70 [145]. Other groups around the world have not found the outcome for infants with uncomplicated GMH-IVH to be significantly different from those without, even when follow-up was extended to 8 years of age [140]. The mechanism of brain injury in uncomplicated GMH-IVH which has been proposed is that of impaired cortical development. At 10–20 weeks' gestation, the germinal matrix is a source of neuronal precursor cells; following this point and during the time when very low birthweight (VLBW) infants are born, the germinal matrix is a source of undifferentiated glial precursor cells (glioblasts) which will migrate [146]. Some of these cells give rise to oligodendroglia, the absence of which may affect myelination. Others will mature into astrocyte precursor cells, necessary for cortical development. Subplate neurons are a transient cell population that undergo programmed cell death, and in humans the subplate zone peaks at 24 weeks of gestation, undergoes dissolution in the third trimester, and is largely absent after 6 months of postnatal age [147]. Subplate neurons become incorporated into mature synaptic networks, and these cells are also vulnerable to injury during preterm life, particularly from hypoxic ischemia [148].

Increasing evidence suggests that GMH-IVH may result in extensive brain injury especially if sustained early on in gestation. Using MRI, Vasileiadis demonstrated a 16% reduction in cortical gray matter volume at term-corrected age in a cohort of infants with uncomplicated GMH-IVH, but no neurodevelopmental follow-up information is yet available from this cohort [149].

Our current advice to parents whose baby has been discovered to have uncomplicated GMH-IVH is that their baby is at slightly higher risk of an adverse neurodevelopmental outcome than if no abnormality had been found, but that this risk is not greatly increased above the baseline risk related to gestational age. We say this only with the proviso that the ultrasound scan at discharge does not show significant brain atrophy (increased interhemispheric distance, widened subarachnoid space, and enlarged ventricles), in which case we are more cautious. Magnetic resonance imaging at term may soon be more readily available to all, and in our center it does allow us to refine the prognosis in individual cases (see "Periventricular white matter injury").

Hemorrhagic parenchymal infarction and porencephalic cyst

The white matter of the preterm brain can be damaged as a result of focal destruction, usually the end-stage of a much larger area of coagulation necrosis in an area of hemorrhagic infarction. This parenchymal destruction roughly equates to the Papile "grade IV" intraventricular hemorrhage, and is part of the spectrum that we would classify as an intraparenchymal lesion (IPL). These globular areas of parenchymal damage are thought to arise because of obstruction to the venous drainage in the periventricular white matter caused by the presence of blood clot in the germinal matrix. Postmortem findings confirm venous infarction (Fig. 9.8), and MRI confirms the fan-shaped distribution of these lesions even more clearly than ultrasound [62,150].

When a focal area of damage in the parenchyma of the brain is imaged with ultrasound it usually appears as an area of increased echoreflectivity in the first instance. It is often difficult to know whether the abnormal appearance has resulted from hemorrhage, or infarction, or a combination of the two. As a result, we prefer to use the general term "intraparenchymal lesion" (IPL) to describe these abnormalities. We believe that imaging appearances should be described in terms of their degree of echoreflectivity, size, laterality, location, and evolution rather that in pseudo-pathological language which makes assumptions about the etiology – "ischemic lesion," for example.

Etiology

The neuropathology of a hemorrhagic periventricular infarction (HPI), a common form of IPL, consists of a large region of hemorrhagic necrosis in the periventricular white matter dorsal and lateral to the external angle of the lateral ventricle. Over half the lesions are asymmetric and around 8% are associated with a large IVH. Careful neuropathologic studies have shown that in most cases this lesion is a hemorrhagic infarction [151]. The original germinal matrix hemorrhage is thought to lead to obstruction of the terminal veins (Fig. 9.4a), leading to periventricular ischemia and then hemorrhagic infarction. The prevention of these lesions depends entirely on the prevention of GMH-IVH.

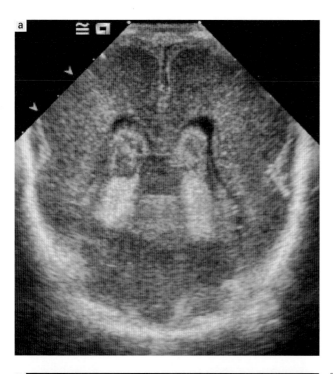
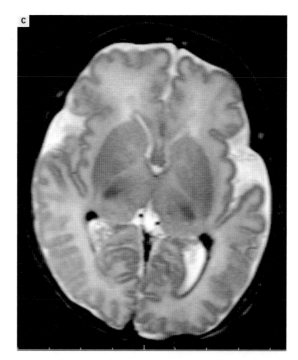
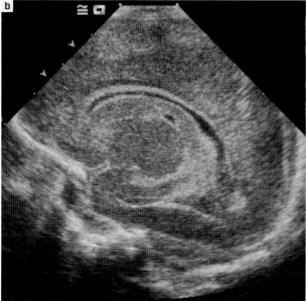

Fig. 9.7a–d. **Ultrasound appearance of bleeding into the lateral ventricle arising from the germinal matrix (a) coronal (b) parasagittal images. (c) Axial T$_2$-weighted MR image shows signal hypointensities in keeping with hemorrhage lining the ventricular ependyma and ventricle. (d) Parasagittal ultrasound images showing GMH-IVH and mobile clot within the ventricle. Hemosiderin lining the walls of the lateral ventricle after earlier GMH-IVH.**

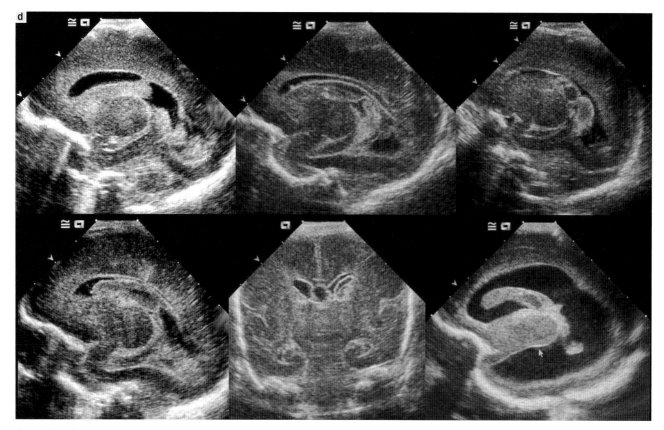

Fig. 9.7. **(cont.)**

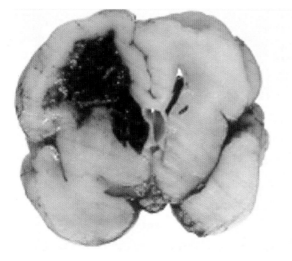

Fig. 9.8. **Pathological specimen showing a hemorrhagic parenchymal lesion consistent with a venous infarction, in a preterm brain.**

Incidence and timing

Like GMH-IVH, IPLs mostly occur during early neonatal life, although an IPL was present at birth in 16% in one study. The lesions were still echoreflectant at birth and probably recent in most, although 3% had a resolving IPL or porencephalic cyst at delivery [152]. The vast majority of the parenchymal lesions (80%–90%) developed within 96 hours after birth. Despite the

decline in incidence of GMH-IVH since the early 1980s (see section on GMH-IVH, p. 180), IPL remains a significant problem especially in infants of less than 750 g birthweight.

Natural history and prognosis

More than half of the babies who have a porencephalic cyst will develop a hemiplegia on the opposite side in childhood, but their function is often surprisingly good and their intelligence can be normal [153]. Anterior lesions carry a better prognosis than parieto-occipital porencephalic cysts [152]. The chance of a good intellectual outcome is reduced if there is co-existing bilateral ventriculomegaly. Magnetic resonance imaging may assist in refining the prognosis, because infants with a unilateral lesion who also have abnormal signal from myelination in the posterior limb of the internal capsule (PLIC) at term have a higher chance of developing hemiplegia than those with normal signal from myelin in the PLIC [152,154]. The abnormal myelin probably represents Wallerian degeneration.

Ultrasound and MRI appearances

A globular echoreflective lesion in the white matter in the region of the corona radiata, which is unilateral and associated with a GMH-IVH on the same side, is likely to represent an HPI, a specific form of IPL (Fig. 9.9). As discussed, these lesions usually arise as a result of obstruction of the venous drainage and consequent infarction of the white matter, but this cannot be assumed from the ultrasound appearances. The periventricular IPL appears initially as a fan-shaped structure (Figs. 9.9, 9.10a) which usually evolves into a porencephalic cyst (Figs. 9.9, 9.10a and b). The lesions can be quite small and anterior to the trigone, in which case the prognosis is usually better (Fig. 9.10c). The distinction from the small bilateral cysts of periventricular leukomalacia is important because the prognosis is very different. Children with porencephalic cysts, even large ones, can do well whereas the less impressive cysts of periventricular leukomalacia indicate more severe white matter destruction with a worse prognosis.

Periventricular white matter injury

Cystic periventricular leukomalacia and diffuse periventricular white matter injury

Periventricular white matter injury (PWMI) is now the most common type of brain injury in preterm infants and is the major cause of chronic neurodevelopmental and cognitive impairment in survivors of preterm birth [155,156]. The spectrum of PWMI ranges from focal cystic necrotic periventricular

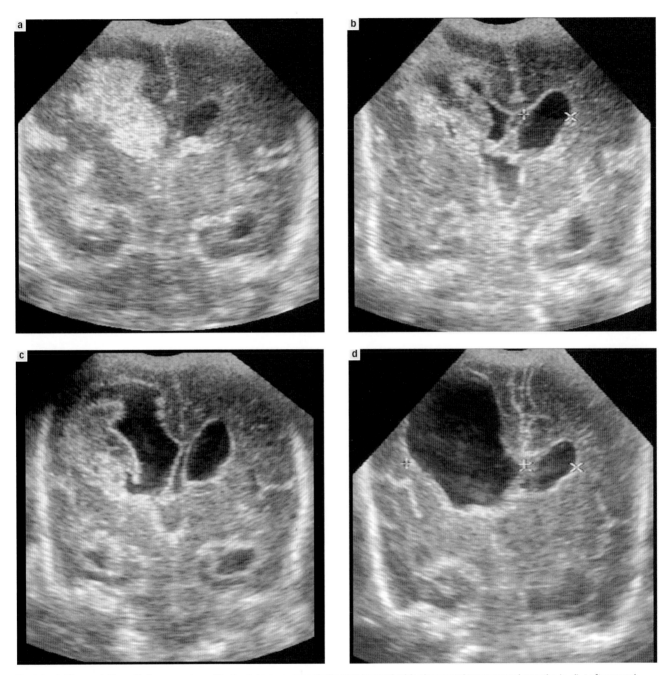

Fig. 9.9a–d. **The evolution of intraparenchymal lesion into a porencephalic cyst imaged with ultrasound over several months (a–d). Left coronal ultrasound on top row (a) shows a wedge-shaped area of increased echogenicity adjacent to the right lateral ventricle and GMH-IVH within that ventricle. Subsequent images on top row (b) and bottom row (c, d) show the evolution of the intraparenchymal lesion into a porencephalic cyst and the resolution of the GMH-IVH.**

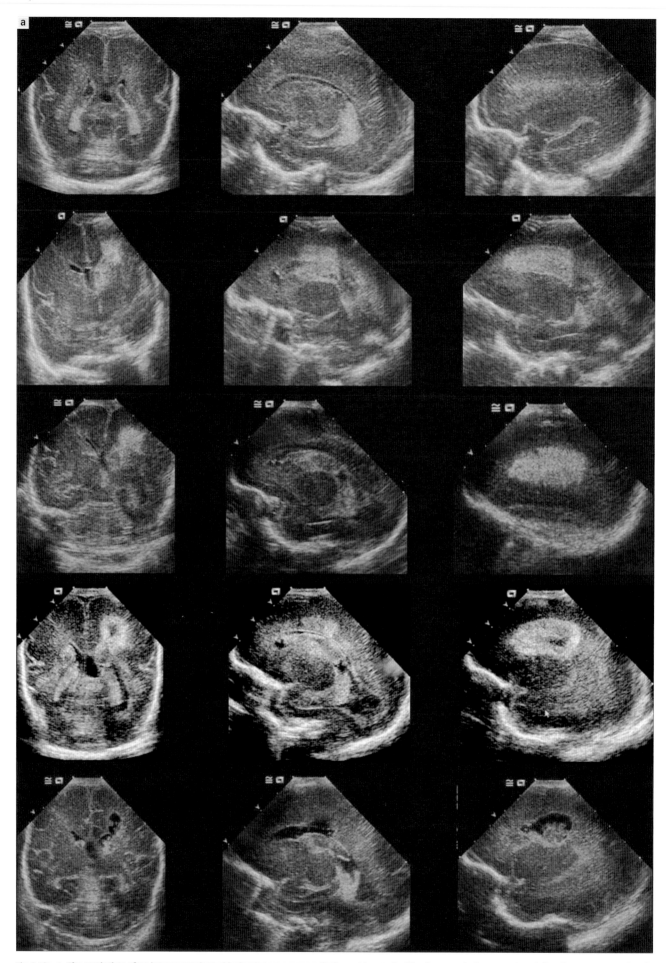

Fig. 9.10a–c. **The evolution of an intraparenchymal lesion into a porencephalic cyst imaged with ultrasound of a premature infant born at 26 weeks of gestational age. (a) Top row shows ultrasound images taken on day 1, followed by ultrasound images of day 3, day 5, day 10 and bottom row day 53 (term-equivalent age). Note the evolution of the area of increased echogenicity adjacent to the lateral left ventricle into a porencephalic cyst over 53 days.**

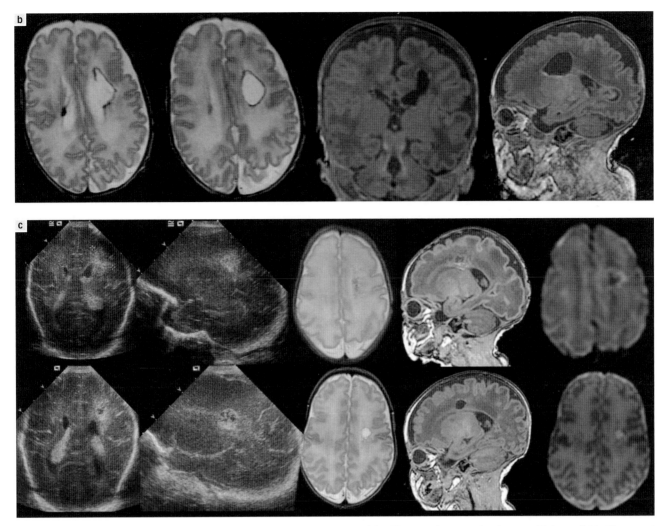

Fig. 9.10. (cont.) (b) The MR images of the same baby at term: the two axial T$_2$-weighted images, the coronal and parasagittal T$_1$-weighted images at term-equivalent age show a periventricular infarction involving the left frontal lobe in continuity with the ventricle, with a rim of T$_2$ hypotensity and patchy T$_1$-weighted hypertensities in keeping with mature blood products. There is also intraventricular hemorrhage. These are the appearances of a left porencephalic cyst. (c) Top row images of a premature infant of 28 weeks of gestational age at 34 corrected gestational age; bottom row at term-equivalent age. Top row shows coronal and left parasagittal ultrasound image. There is a wedge-shaped area of increased echogenicity adjacent to the left lateral ventricle. Axial T$_2$-weighted MR image shows multiple serpiginous hypointense structures in keeping with thrombosed veins. Sagittal T$_1$-weighted image shows early cavitation and hemorrhagic change. Apparent diffusion coefficient map shows a region of restricted diffusion. Bottom row images show progression to cavitation on ultrasound and MRI. Apparent diffusion coefficient map shows signal in keeping with free diffusion within the cavity.

lesions (periventricular leukomalacia, PVL) to diffuse PWMI [156] which on MRI studies may be associated with DEHSI of the white matter on conventional T$_2$-weighted scans [32,33]. The spectrum also includes ventriculomegaly and reduction in white matter volume, enlarged subarachnoid space and immature gyral development [36,37]. Cystic PVL may be accompanied by diffuse PWMI or occur as an isolated lesion. The period of most risk for PWMI is between 23 and 32 weeks' postconceptional age; the highest risk is in infants of lower gestational ages and birthweights (500–1000 g). Premature infants with PWMI are also at increased risk of other forms of brain injury, notably GMH-IVH and intraparenchymal injury. As previously described, the refinement of medical care of the extremely preterm infant has resulted in a

significant reduction in the incidence of all forms of GMH-IVH, whereas the incidence of PWMI is not decreasing and is now the major problem facing VLBW infants [157]. Furthermore, the spectrum of PWMI has changed in the last two decades: the incidence of cystic PVL has declined significantly and diffuse PWMI is the predominant lesion [34,158,159]. In these recent series cystic PVL lesions accounted for fewer than 5% of cases. This shift in the pattern of disease reflects the survival of smaller and smaller infants who are born during a stage of developmental vulnerability in the periventricular white matter [160].

Periventricular leukomalacia was first described by Banker and Larroche in 1962; they observed that "leukomalacia," long

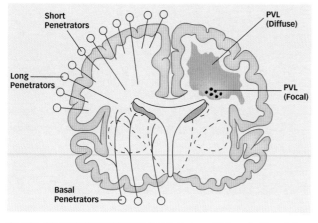

Fig. 9.11. **Diagram illustrating the border zone which probably exists in the preterm brain between the ventriculofugal and ventriculopedal arterial supplies. Adapted from Volpe [156].**

recognized by adult neuropathologists and seen by Virchow (1867) and Parrot (1868–77) in the autopsied brains of babies, was particularly common in the periventricular zone of premature babies who died [161]. As neonatal intensive care was not yet developed, their sample was represented by preterm infants who died after periods of apnea or cardiac arrest, and the studies were mostly restricted to infants of 34 weeks' gestation and above. They went on to study well over 200 cases [162]. The diagnosis of PVL is a pathological one, and the histological findings are those of a patchy focal coagulation necrosis. Early on there is a cellular reaction with microglial cells surrounding the damaged area, which fills with nuclear debris and can cavitate. Areas of calcification and gliosis are found within a few weeks. Macroscopically the lesions appear as small pearly white spots, usually in the periventricular zone, standing out against the cream-colored background of the brain. The site of the lesions led Larroche to conclude that they were ischemic, because they were situated in regions where there are only limited and small anastomoses between the major arteries of the brain. This "vascular theory" continues to be popular, and initial support was provided by further study of the arterial supply of the neonatal brain, apparently demonstrating a border zone between the ventriculofugal and ventriculopedal vessels [163] (Fig. 9.11; from Volpe [156]). Recent experimental evidence suggests that although perturbations in cerebral blood flow are necessary, they are not sufficient to damage the periventricular white matter and cellular maturational factors related to susceptible oligodendrocyte progenitor cells play a greater role in the genesis of PWMI [157].

In the early stages of injury, diffuse PWMI is distinguished by the presence of numerous reactive microglia in the periventricular white matter. The primary population of degenerating cells within diffuse lesions are pre-myelinating oligodendroglia (i.e., oligodendrocyte (OL) progenitor cells). In contrast to cystic PVL, diffuse PWMI is characterized by a marked depletion of OL progenitor cells, ranging from 50% to 90%. Microglia, astrocytes, and axons appear to be more resistant to injury than pre-oligodendrocytes. At later stages diffuse PWMI lesions contain numerous reactive astrocytes (gliosis). Diffuse

Table 9.4. Factors associated with an increased risk of white matter damage in preterm infants.

Factor	Reference
Prenatal factors	
Lack of exposure to antenatal steroids	[71,164,165,166,167]
Prolonged rupture of membranes	[168,169,170,171]
Exposure to tocolysis	[172]
Chorioamnionitis, especially funisitis (see below)	[168,169,173,174,175,176] [83,170]
Funisitis	[177,178,179]
Multiple pregnancy	[168,169,170,180,181]
Intrauterine growth restriction	[82]
Perinatal factors	
Antepartum hemorrhage, placental abruption	[97,182,183,184,185]
Abnormal CTG	[170,186]
Emergency caesarean section	[187]
Low Apgar score, cord blood acidosis	[188]
Postnatal factors	
Septicemia	[166]
Hypocarbia	[172,189,190,191,192,193,194 195,196,197,198]
Hyperbilirubinemia (found in very few studies, little biological plausibility)	[169,189]
Patent ductus arteriosus	[187,199]
Necrotizing enterocolitis	[187]

PWMI thus appears to be a form of PVL that is initiated through targeted injury to the OL lineage with relative sparing of other glial or axonal elements [157].

Etiology

Larroche described finding PVL in 197 of 802 preterm brains examined at autopsy between 1967 and 1974, and she recognized a link with RDS, septicemia, kernicterus, congenital heart disease, and maternal diabetes. The term babies with PVL who she studied at autopsy were more likely to be growth retarded. Time has attested to the quality of these careful early observations; many of the factors implicated in recent clinical studies are the same as those first observed by Larroche over 30 years ago (Table 9.4). There is increasing realization that in many cases the problem originates antenatally, with chorioamnionitis (especially funisitis), placental insufficiency, antepartum hemorrhage, and intrauterine hypoxia all being implicated. Autopsy evidence suggested that white matter damage was antenatal in 31% of a cohort of 83 babies in Oxford [200]. Placental insufficiency, with abnormal umbilical artery flow demonstrated with Doppler, ominous CTG, and reduced fetal movements, was a frequent antecedent of white matter lesions in a series from Utrecht, with about 22% of all cases considered to have arisen antenatally [81]. One group in Japan claim to have diagnosed periventricular echo-density with fetal ultrasound [201]. Placental insufficiency with intrauterine growth retardation (IUGR) is a risk factor for pre-term white matter damage, although there is still a great deal of uncertainty regarding the right time to deliver affected fetuses. Most fetal medicine experts would regard absent or reversed flow in the ductus venosus as a preterminal change, but the evidence from the GRIT trial [202] does not support early delivery when there is uncertainty.

Animal models of PVL have been developed, designed to imitate situations reflecting the current theories for the etiology of the condition. Withdrawal of a sufficient volume of blood to cause hypotension in 113-day fetal sheep was followed by histological evidence of PVL [203]. The effect was thought to mimic that of placental separation. Similar changes have been produced by bilateral carotid ischemia lasting 30 minutes [204,205], or repeated umbilical cord occlusion in the near-term fetal sheep [206]. In-utero-sustained hypoxia ischemia has been modeled in the pregnant rabbit and leads to hypotonia and postural defects in the products of the pregnancy, and these observed effects are accompanied by a reduction in white matter volume and a reduction in fractional anisotropy measured by magnetic resonance diffusion tensor imaging [207]. *Escherichia coli* toxin has been used to study the protective effect of pretreatment with interleukin and tumor necrosis factor (TNF) alpha in pups, and injection of *E. coli* into the uterine horns of pregnant rabbits also produces white matter damage in the fetuses [208]. Small fetal and neonatal animal models have generally been uninformative due to the paucity of cerebral white matter and a propensity for mixed gray and white matter injury. In addition a broad spectrum of injury is seen following uniform ischemic insults within species as well as differences in histopathology between species in response to similar experimental conditions. Recent work done by Back in the immature sheep fetus (0.65 gestation) has provided novel information about regional cerebral blood flow and insult topography [157].

Vascular theory

The main vascular supply to the preterm cerebral white matter is thought to be via long and short penetrating arteries (Fig. 9.11) [156]. A reduction in cerebral blood flow could produce ischemia in the vascular end zones, the periventricular region. The neonate is known to have a very low baseline cerebral blood flow, and sick newborns have a "pressure-passive" circulation, placing them at high risk of ischemia [209,210]. It has been proposed that deep-seated focal cystic necrotic lesions of PVL arise from severe and persistent ischemia in vascular end zones of long penetrating arteries. The occurrence of less severe or briefer episodes of ischemia in the more superficial territory of the short penetrating arteries may account for diffuse PWMI. The main blows to this otherwise attractive hypothesis are the failure to identify the necessary arterial end zones, and the lack of convincing evidence

showing that hypotension is a risk factor for PVL [211]. Some would say that blood pressure bears a poor relationship to cerebral blood flow, and they have a point [212]. However, an extensive search has failed to identify ventriculofugal vessels [213,214]. There is now very strong evidence that hypocarbia is associated with PVL (Table 9.4), and this does lend some support to the vascular hypothesis because hypocarbia is such a potent cerebral vasoconstrictor.

Experimental models using the fetal sheep support the notion that human periventricular white matter may be particularly vulnerable to global cerebral hypoperfusion because the duration of cerebral ischemia was a critical factor required to generate a graded spectrum of PWMI [215]. However, when addressing the vascular end zone hypothesis, it was observed that gradients of ischemia between the cerebral cortex and periventricular white matter may not be sufficiently large to account for selective injury to the latter [215]. The current opinion among experts in the field is that cellular maturational factors related to susceptible OL progenitors are likely to play a greater role than vascular factors in defining the topography of the injury [157].

Oligodendroglial theory

There is now a large body of evidence suggesting that the late OL progenitor cell is the major potential target in PWMI, leading to disrupted maturation of the OL lineage. The developmental window of highest risk for PWMI (23–32 weeks' postconceptional age) coincides with a period of human cerebral white matter development during which there is a major population of late oligodendroglial progenitors [160]. Experimental studies have shown that the developmental predilection for PWMI to occur during prematurity is related to both the timing of the appearance and regional distribution of susceptible pre-oligodendrocytes – this may explain why parts of the preterm white matter appear more vulnerable [215]. The decline in risk for PWMI coincides with the onset of a wave of differentiation of pre-oligodendrocytes to immature OLs that initiate myelination in the periventricular white matter [216]. A cartoon devised by Back which summarizes current thinking regarding stages of development in the OL lineage is shown in Fig. 9.12 [157].

Oligodendrocyte progenitor cells are extremely vulnerable to oxidative stress and hypoxia ischemia. The fetal cerebral white matter is rich in membrane lipids that are readily oxidized. In addition the developing white matter may be more vulnerable to oxidative damage due to a delay in the expression of antioxidant enzymes superoxide dismutase, catalase, and glutathione peroxidase [217]. In support of this, recent studies have shown that significant oxidative damage can be detected in human periventricular white matter that displays histopathological features of PWMI [218]. Interestingly, oxidative damage selectively targeted the white matter and spared the cerebral cortex, consistent with the notion that PWMI arises in part from hypoxia ischemia related to vascular end zones [219]. Oligodendrocytes play a central role in central nervous system iron metabolism and so may be at risk for iron-mediated oxygen radical toxicity. This is of relevance to preterm infants as the risk of PWMI is increased in infants with

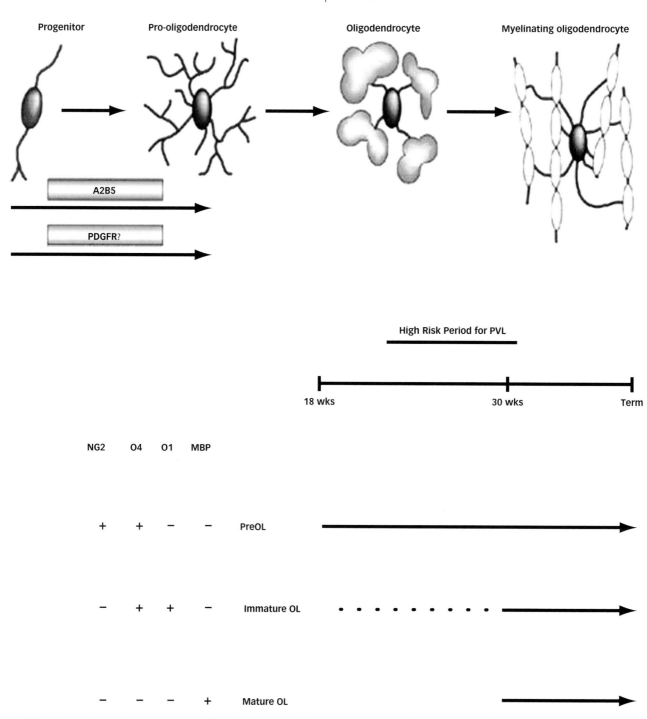

Fig. 9.12. Cartoon showing the development of the oligodendrocyte lineage related to gestational age, devised from the work of Back [157].

GMH-IVH [156]. GMH-IVH increases the availability of free iron in the spinal fluid and is one further mechanism for the potential generation of toxic free radicals [220].

The OL progenitors are particularly susceptible to glutamate-mediated receptor toxicity (mediated by both receptor-dependent and receptor-independent mechanisms). In addition to this susceptibility, the timing of glutamate receptor expression coincides with the window of cerebral white matter vulnerability. Increased expression of the GluR4 subunit occurs between 23 and 32 weeks' gestation in human parietal white matter and is expressed on both pre-oligodendrocytes and immature OLs [221]. Although further research is needed, it is proposed that glutamate release from cells of the OL lineage and axons in response to perinatal hypoxia ischemia could trigger white matter injury via activation of receptors on adjacent pro-oligodendrocytes. At present it is not known whether axonal damage occurs as a consequence of damage to the pre-oligodendrocytes, or vice-versa, or whether the insult which causes the damage in the first place insults pre-oligodendrocytes and causes axonal damage at the same time [222].

Neuroinflammatory mechanisms

Multiple lines of investigation support the notion that alterations in neuroinflammatory mediators exacerbate PWMI. Activated microglia release a number of cytokines, tumor necrosis factor, and interferon-γ that are directly toxic to pre-oligodendrocytes and in combination their toxicity is synergistic [223]. Although a correlation between maternal–fetal infection, PWMI, and the subsequent development of CP has been proposed [224] several recent studies have failed to support this relationship in premature infants because of a lack of evidence for either intrauterine exposure to infection or inflammatory cytokines in neonatal blood [225,226]. However, many clinical studies show an increased risk of PVL after prolonged membrane rupture with or without chorioamnionitis, and/or later neonatal sepsis [11,168,173] and some authors suggest that sepsis is the most important factor, more important than hypoxic ischemia [227]. The association between a fetal inflammatory response, usually demonstrated by the presence of funisitis, is stronger than the link with chorioamnionitis alone [174,177,178,179]. The link between necrotizing enterocolitis (particularly requiring surgery) and PVL also implicates cytokines [228]. Epidemiological studies suggest that the pro-inflammatory cytokines interleukin-1 beta (IL-1β), IL-6 and tumor necrosis factor alpha are all increased in neonatal blood and/or amniotic fluid in babies who develop PVL and CP [229,230,231]. High levels of IL-18 in cord blood have also been described in association with later preterm white matter damage [232].

Endotoxin and cytokines are further implicated in a pathway leading to hypotension and reduced cerebral blood flow in the preterm infant, thus increasing the risk of ischemic damage. In various neonatal models, endotoxin led to arterial hypotension and PWMI [233]. Other studies however have not demonstrated any change in cerebral blood flow with endotoxin [234]; rather endotoxin was found to sensitize the brain to hypoxic-ischemic injury. Interestingly, the timing of exposure to endotoxin can also reduce rather than exacerbate injury in both adult and perinatal animals due to ischemic tolerance.

Several pro-inflammatory cytokines damage the periventricular white matter through peroxynitrite-mediated toxicity to the OL lineage. Further studies are needed to define how neuroinflammatory mediators and cerebral ischemia may interact to promote PWMI.

Incidence and timing

Cystic PVL

Whereas cystic PVL was more common a decade or more ago, with advances in neonatal intensive care such as surfactant therapy, new ventilator strategies and use of pharmacological agents such as antenatal steroids and indomethacin, overt cystic lesions are now rare [235]. Cystic PVL is consistently described in about 5% of babies less than 30–32 weeks imaged with ultrasound [113]. Resch *et al.* reported their experience over 10 years in one center in Austria, where cystic PVL was found in 98/3187

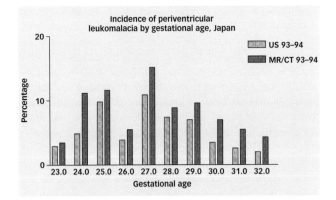

Fig. 9.13. **The incidence of periventricular leukomalacia diagnosed with ultrasound and MRI in a national study in Japan. Data from [28].**

(3%) of all babies, 4% of those less than 32 weeks' gestation [236]. In Osaka, Japan, the incidence was only 2% at less than 34 weeks [183]. The routine use of MRI is more common in Japan, and a national survey reported an incidence of cystic PVL diagnosed with ultrasound of 4.8%–4.9%, increasing to 7.7%–7.9% when MRI and/or CT were used [28]. The incidence peaked at around 27 weeks, but the relationship with gestational age was not as marked as that seen for GMH-IVH (Fig. 9.13).

Diffuse PWMI

Diffuse PWMI, including white matter signal abnormalites on T_2-weighted MR images, ventriculomegaly and delayed myelination, has been described in up to 70% of very preterm infants [32,34,36,159,237]. In the most recent and largest series studied (167 preterm infants <30 weeks' gestational age at birth), 72% of infants had diffuse PWMI – 51% mild, 17% moderate, and 4% severe [159]. In addition 49% had gray matter abnormalities. Diffuse PWMI has been associated with proven sepsis and inotrope use [36]. One study using serial MRI in infants <30 weeks' gestational age from the first week of life demonstrated that diffuse PWMI was usually not detected until term or near term-corrected age [32]. The authors concluded that although brain injury may occur antenatally, it often becomes clinically detectable only later in or beyond the neonatal period. This may also explain the higher positive predictive value of MRI compared to cranial ultrasound for CP [15]. The clinical correlate of diffuse PWMI has not yet been fully characterized and this is an area of active research; however, it is noteworthy that the high incidence of diffuse PWMI is similar to the high frequency (~50%) of later cognitive and behavioral deficits in VLBW infants. It is possible that the high frequency of cognitive behavioral problems on follow-up of preterm infants who do not show major abnormalities on cranial ultrasound are related to diffuse PWMI.

Natural history of periventricular white matter injury

Cystic PVL

In the neonatal period the evolution of parenchymal lesions helps to determine the probable pathology, which is important for prognosis. Periventricular cysts can persist for several months, but they usually disappear eventually, although there is a permanent glial scar. This can be seen at autopsy [238,239] or imaged with MR. Late MR shows delayed myelination in babies with PVL, with a reduction in white matter bulk and glial reaction. The ventricles are often scalloped by sulci abutting directly onto the ventricular wall because of the reduction in buffering white matter, or squared off because periventricular cystic lesions have become incorporated into the lateral ventricles. Glial scarring shows on MR as high T_2 signal, and is well seen with FLAIR (fluid attenuated inversion recovery) sequences. The increased signal intensity usually extends right down to the ventricular wall, which may help to distinguish preterm from term periventricular white matter damage (p. 000). Only MR can detect signal change from myelin in the region of the internal capsule, which may fail to appear by term-equivalent age; this failure is associated with the development of CP [240,241]. Abnormalities of the deep gray matter were not found by Inder and colleagues, but others have seen thalamic changes accompanying PVL [242,243].

Diffuse PWMI

A comprehensive survey of cerebral abnormalities in preterm infants studied with serial MRI scans starting with an initial scan as soon as possible after birth has provided unique information on the natural history of white matter abnormalities [32,33]. The most common abnormalities seen on the initial MRI were: GMH, GMH-IVH, ventricular dilatation, punctuate white matter lesions, and cerebellar hemorrhagic lesions. No baby demonstrated DEHSI on the initial scan, however 80% had DEHSI present in the white matter on the MRI at term-equivalent age. This suggests that the multiple immunological, nutritional, pharmacological and other stresses of premature

exposure to an extrauterine environment may affect the normal brain development trajectory. In the study by Dyet and colleagues there was no relationship between DEHSI and ventricular dilatation or the standard deviation score for head circumference, suggesting that the pathologic process does not necessarily involve white matter atrophy [33].

Ultrasound and MRI appearances

Diagnosis of white matter lesions with ultrasound was first described almost 20 years ago [244,245,246,247]. The first MR descriptions soon followed [248], but much remains to be learnt about this important problem and there is still no agreement about classification systems suitable for use in imaging studies.

Flare

This abnormality appears on ultrasound and is diagnosed when the affected area of parenchyma appears as echoreflective ("bright") as the choroid. The appearances need to be considered and contrasted with the normal periventricular "blush" which occurs in the peritrigonal region of the brain, because the area around the trigone is the most likely to be involved. The main challenge of ultrasound diagnosis of "flare" lies in trying to distinguish what is abnormal from the normal periventricular blush or halo. A normal appearance (Chapter 4) is of an area of increased echoreflectivity fanning out from around the posterior horn of the ventricles, with an indistinct border and with persisting fine, brush stroke "gracile" lines within it (Fig. 4.10). A coarse, blotchy echoreflective area (usually peritrigonal) with a better defined outer border and without gracile lines within it and which is as echoreflective as the choroid or bone is abnormal (Fig. 9.14c). The

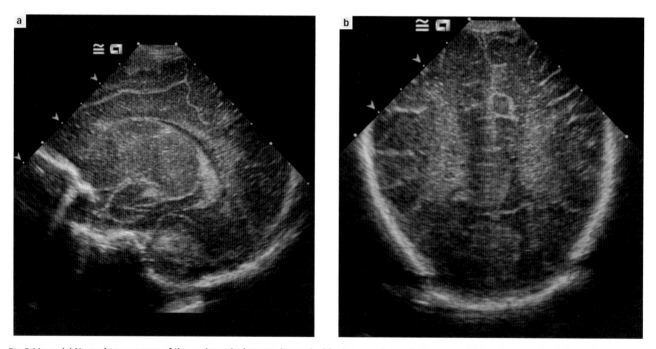

Fig. 9.14a–c. (a) Normal appearance of the periventricular zone imaged with ultrasound seen in the coronal (a) and parasagittal planes (b). (c) A periventricular "flare" with echodensity in the peritrigonal area which is as dense as the choroid plexus and lacks the normal pattern of gracile lines within it, with a blotchy outer border in a coronal and parasagittal ultrasound scan.

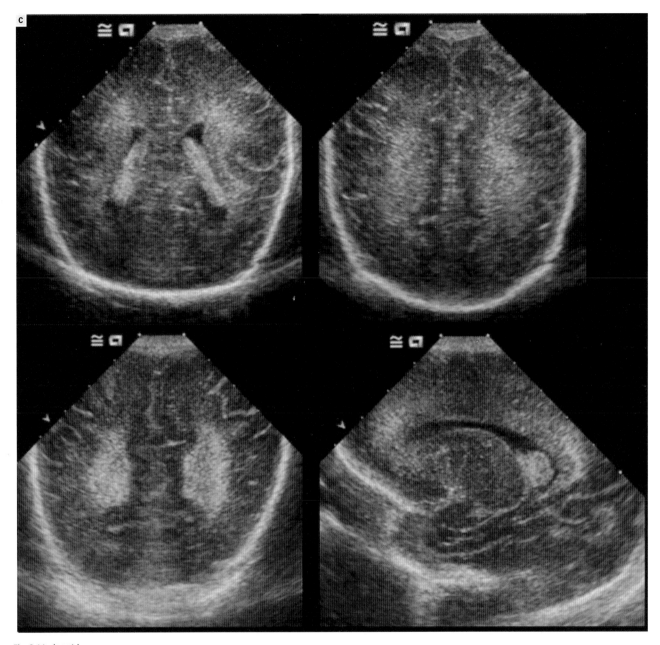

Fig. 9.14. **(cont.)**

appearances should be confirmed in two planes before being accepted as genuine. In general it is considered that a "flare" appears 24–48 hours after an insult, but there is very little precision in this and high-quality systematic studies are lacking. Once seen, the appearances can persist from 2 days to more than 14 days. After that time, the flare may disappear leaving very little abnormality in its wake, or ventriculomegaly and/or cystic change in the parenchyma may emerge. The prognosis depends crucially on the duration and the evolution of the flare, and may also depend on the homogeneity.

Sie *et al.* attempted MR confirmation of sonographic white matter abnormality in 53 babies (not all preterm) with areas of increased echodensity [249]. Magnetic resonance imaging showed hemorrhagic white matter lesions, usually distributed along the ventricle, in 32 babies. The MRI abnormalities were particularly common in babies with inhomogenous flare on ultrasound which lasted for more than a week; MRI provided additional information in 68%. Dual imaging of a further cohort of 76 babies showed that MRI provided additional information in 22% [130].

It is not possible from a single study to determine whether a flare will resolve, or whether the area of brain will develop the multiple cysts of PVL, or a single large IPL. A globular unilateral triangular echoreflective area with the apex of triangle at lateral border of lateral ventricle, with a GMH-IVH on the same side, is more likely to be an area of hemorrhagic

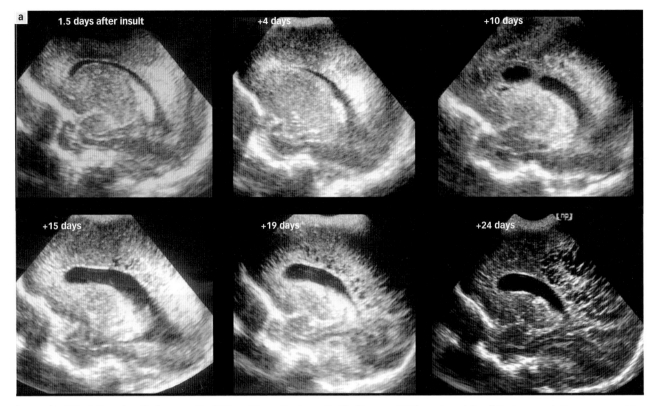

Fig. 9.15a,b. **(a) Evolution of cystic degeneration in the white matter imaged with ultrasound. This preterm baby girl, who was a twin, was several days old when a hypoxic-ischemic insult occurred. The first ultrasound image was done 1.5 days afterwards and showed an area of increased echoreflectivity in the periventricular area which evolved into cystic white matter over time.**

infarction and to evolve into a porencephalic cyst that communicates with the lateral ventricle. Areas of bilateral homogenous abnormal echoreflectivity in the periventricular zone, with loss of gracile lines and no GMH-IVH, are more likely to evolve into multicystic white matter damage. Studies have suggested that cranial ultrasound has a poor sensitivity in the detection of diffuse PWMI, the commonest form of brain injury in the preterm infant. As discussed, this may explain why neonatal brain MRI before discharge was better than cranial ultrasound in predicting CP in VLBW infants [15].

Cystic PVL

Hill *et al.* were probably the first to diagnose cystic PVL with ultrasound [250]. Cystic change can follow flare, in general at around 2–4 weeks (10 days at the earliest), or appear without any preceding abnormality, sometimes very late in the infant's hospital stay [251]. One Japanese study which used EEG to time the initiating insult described a median time to cyst formation of 18 days, with a range of 10–39 days [252], and it is the case that the first cysts are often seen well after 35 days of age [253]. This Dutch group found that the time from flare to cyst was shorter (mean 21 days) when bilateral cystic PVL developed than when it was unilateral or asymmetrical (35 days).

The location of white matter abnormalities which are most likely to correspond with a pathological finding of PVL are along the ventricular body and in the region of the trigone,

mainly posterior. Cysts can vary in size and location, from one or two tiny microcysts only 0.2–0.5 cm in size in the frontal lobe, through several cysts less than 0.5 cm diameter in the parieto-occipital lobe, into bilateral occipital cysts larger than 0.5 cm in diameter (Fig. 9.15a,b). The latter carries the worst prognosis. Linda de Vries has suggested a grading system for PVL that has been widely adopted (Table 9.5), but with the advent of MRI and the realization that ultrasound is very insensitive for the detection of neonatal white matter injury this probably needs revision. The appearances of cystic white matter change on a histological specimen are shown in Fig. 9.16.

Diffuse PWMI

Cranial ultrasound has been shown to have poor sensitivity in the detection of diffuse PWMI, which can only be detected by MR imaging [158] (Fig. 9.17). The appearance of periventricular "caps" can also be seen with MRI and is thought to represent a layer of migrating glial cells [255] (Fig. 9.18). More recent cranial ultrasound studies have related signs of brain atrophy or suboptimal brain growth (enlarged subarachnoid space, widened interhemispheric fissure, reduced complexity of gyral folding) on sequential cranial ultrasound with neurodevelopmental outcome at 3 years of age [26]: infants without major lesions but with signs of atrophy at discharge had significantly worse neurocognitive outcomes. It is likely that

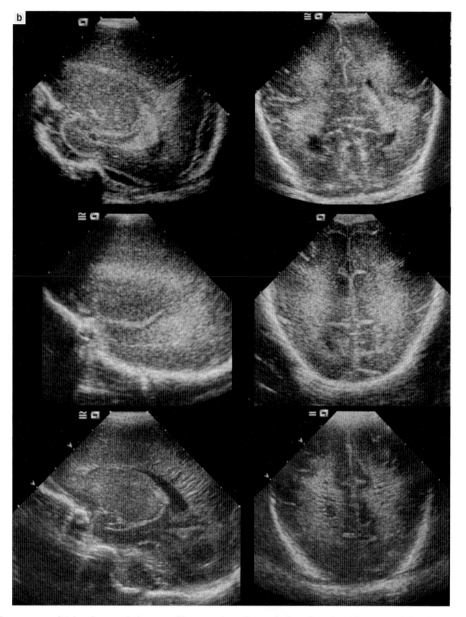

Fig. 9.15. (cont.) (b) These parasagittal and coronal ultrasound images show the evolution of cystic white matter injury in a preterm infant born at 30 weeks of gestation, the recipient twin of twin-to-twin transfusion syndrome. The images are taken over a period of two weeks.

further quantitative studies that assess brain growth on cranial ultrasound will improve the detection of diffuse PWMI, but at present MRI is by far the most sensitive imaging method.

Diffuse PWMI has been assessed both qualitatively and quantitatively using MRI. One of the first qualitative studies used the term "diffuse and excessive high signal intensity" (DEHSI) to describe the visual assessment of the white matter on conventional T_2-weighted MR images. DEHSI was present in 22/29 ex-preterm babies imaged at term [32], generally appeared after 27 weeks' post-conceptional age, and was associated with ventricular dilatation and squaring of ventricles and an enlarged interhemispheric space. The subjective nature of this finding must be emphasized; however, the Hammersmith group subsequently described the association between DEHSI

and increased apparent diffusion coefficients (ADC) within the white matter on diffusion-weighted imaging, with ADC values of DEHSI being similar to those in the white matter of infants with cystic PVL [34]. The nature of DEHSI is not known for certain; the signal change may represent vasogenic edema, oligodendrocyte damage, or reduced axonal diameter. The Leeds group did not find DEHSI as often as in the Hammersmith series, but their cohort were imaged at 36 weeks and the appearance does appear to be more common at around term-equivalent age [256].

Other quantitative techniques such as diffusion tensor imaging have been used to quantify white matter injury in preterm infants with normal conventional MR images [257,258]. These studies show that the impact of preterm brain injury probably extends beyond tissue loss, also permanently affecting the development of fiber tracts. Terrie Inder's group have devised a very helpful scoring system for the objective classification of both white and gray matter abnormality and gyral development [159]. The extremely immature infant of <26 weeks' gestation had a pattern of injury characterized by ventriculomegaly and a marked reduction in white matter volume, enlarged subarachnoid space and immature gyral development (Fig. 9.19). In the whole group, abnormalities in gray matter development were associated with the presence of white matter abnormalities. The cause of the alteration of gray matter development in association with white matter injury is unknown but is thought to relate to a disturbance in cortical development. This disturbance may arise from input deprivation and output isolation of overlying gray matter secondary to white matter injury, as suggested by the studies by Marin-Padilla, who demonstrated distinct alterations in the morphology and organization of neurons in the cortex overlying PVL [259]. Fiber development in cerebral white matter is probably crucial to gyral development, hence the disruption that MRI tractography studies suggest is associated with PWMI is likely to have important global effects on cerebral function. Studies

quantifying cortical folding in preterm infants at term have demonstrated that the cortical volume or folding complexity is reduced in preterm versus term infants and add weight to this hypothesis [260,261].

Quantitative studies from Inder's large cohort (using post-acquisition MR-processing techniques, tissue segmentation methods and three-dimensional renderings) have shown that preterm birth was associated with reduced total cerebral tissue volumes when MRIs at term were compared to term controls [37,158]. The impairments in cerebral development included significant reductions in cerebral cortical and deep nuclear gray matter volumes in ex-preterm infants when compared to term-born children. The reductions in cerebral gray matter were accompanied by almost a doubling of the intracerebral volume of CSF and were related to the presence of cerebral white matter injury [37]. Factors associated with reductions in total cerebral volume included the degree of immaturity at birth, white matter injury, intrauterine growth restriction, and exposure to postnatal dexamethasone. Using a combination of conventional imaging, diffusion-weighted imaging, and deformation-based morphometry (DBM), which uses image registration and statistical analysis to quantify structural differences between groups, the Hammersmith group identified volume reduction of the thalamus and lentiform nuclei in association with preterm birth only in infants with diffuse PWMI defined by abnormal ADC values [262]. The same group used neuroinformatic tools to determine the relationship between cortical surface area and cerebral volume and demonstrated that the cortical surface area was related to cerebral volume; increasing prematurity and male gender were associated with a lower scaling exponent [261]. Workers at Yale have also demonstrated that ex-preterm children have reduced regional cortical volumes at 8 years of age compared to control children [263,264]. The reductions were particularly marked in the premotor, sensorimotor, mid-temporal, and parieto-occipital regions of the brain, the corpus callosum, the basal ganglia and the hippocampi, and reductions in these

Table 9.5. Classification of periventricular and subcortical leukomalacias based on ultrasound findings [254].

Grade I	Periventricular echodense area present for 7 days or more
Grade II	Periventricular echodense areas evolving into lateralized frontoparietal cysts
Grade III	Periventricular echodense areas evolving into multiple cysts in the parieto-occipital white matter
Grade IV	Echodense areas in the deep white matter with evolution into multiple subcortical cysts

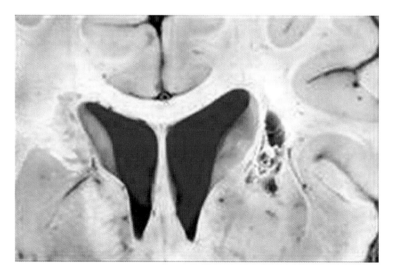

Fig. 9.16. **Pathological specimen showing cystic change in the periventricular white matter.**

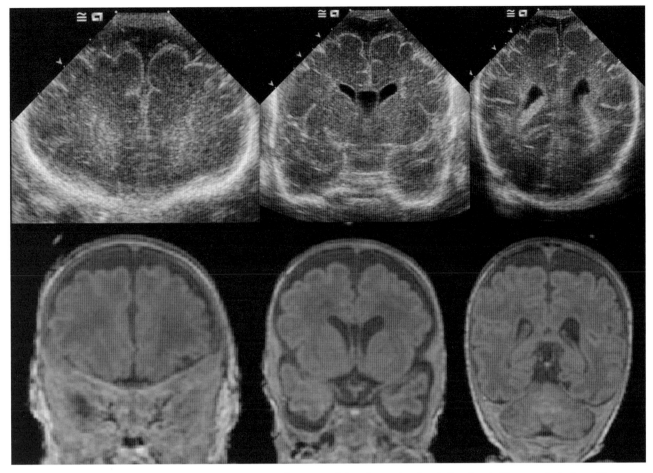

Fig. 9.17. **A set of coronal ultrasound and T$_1$-weighted images of a preterm infant (24 weeks of gestational age) at term-equivalent age. The images show prominent subarachnoid spaces and a cavum septum pellucidum. If head growth is poor and other white matter abnormalities are found on MRI, the increased extracerebral space might be indicative of cerebral atrophy.**

areas correlated with a lower IQ. A reduction in hippocampal volume may be responsible for memory problems later on [265].

Punctate white matter lesions

The finding of punctate white matter lesions is so far limited to MR images, usually at term, although the Leeds group have described them earlier when they may be benign [35,266]. The nature of these lesions remains to be defined, and they may represent micro-hemorrhagic change, or possibly the presence of lipids from myelin breakdown. The lesions tend to occur in clusters or in a linear pattern in the deep white matter of the centrum semiovale [256]. Further follow-up studies are awaited, and we have not included a specific section on prognosis of these lesions because most of the existing follow-up studies have reported on the outcome in infants whose punctate lesions accompanied other abnormalities in the white matter demonstrated with MRI.

Post-hemorrhagic hydrocephalus and ventriculomegaly

See Chapter 11 for further discussion and images showing ventriculomegaly, both progressive and non-progressive, and information about the prognosis of shunted hydrocephalus and antenatally diagnosed ventriculomegaly.

Accuracy and level of agreement in the diagnosis of parenchymal lesions

Early claims that ultrasound could detect 28%–80% of histologically proven PVL appear to be unfounded [126,127]. Diagnosis of GMH-IVH and parenchymal lesions with ultrasound remains much more reliable than the recognition of subtle white matter damage. Early ultrasound studies report good correlation with autopsy changes, but most of the lesions had a hemorrhagic component which is now less common. De Vries used ultrasonography correctly to identify 13 of 18 cases later confirmed to have PVL at autopsy [238], but others report more disappointing results. Expert re-interpretation of large numbers of ultrasound images collected by the Australia and New Zealand Neonatal Network suggested that there was significant under-reporting of white matter abnormalities in all units [123].

Most comparative MR studies report good correlation with ultrasound for the diagnosis of cystic PVL, although even MR

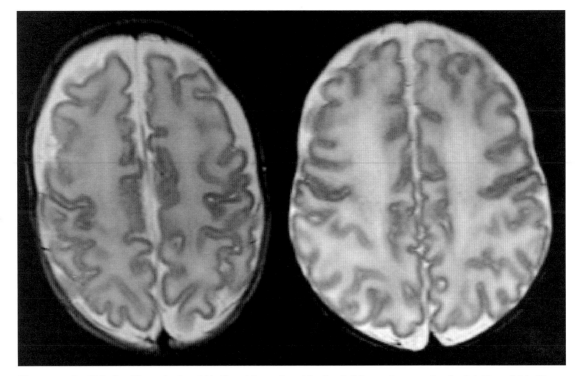

Fig. 9.18. **Diffuse excessive high signal intensity (DEHSI) in the white matter at the level of the centrum semiovale. Axial T$_2$-weighted image on the left shows normal signal intensity in the white matter, whereas DEHSI is present in the right image.**

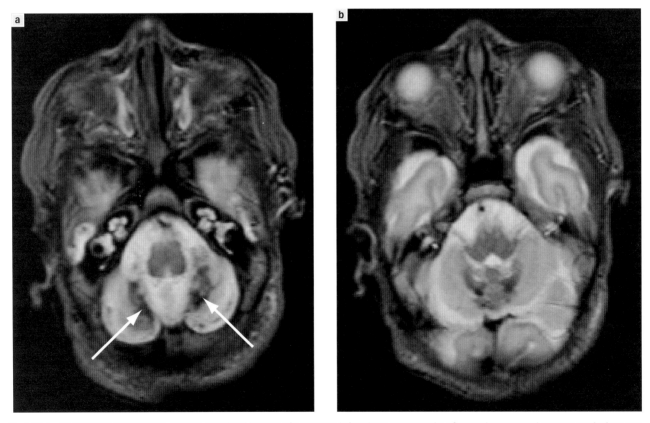

Fig. 9.19a,b. **Cerebellar hemorrhages.** Axial T$_2$-weighted images of a preterm infant born at 23 weeks of gestation scanned at term-equivalent age show bilateral hemispheric hemorrhages (arrow) and cerebellar volume loss.

probably underestimates the extent of the gliosis [267]. Far more white matter lesions are diagnosed with MRI later on than are found in early neonatal life with ultrasound [131,268,269], and it is now obvious that ultrasound has significant limitations in the detection of diffuse PWMI [158,270]. The recent Japanese national study also described a consistently higher rate of white matter abnormality when babies were imaged with MRI than with ultrasound, and ultrasound probably only detects the "tip of the iceberg" (Fig. 9.13). The problem may not be restricted to the white matter: Terrie Inder found that many preterm babies without any suggestion of overt white matter injury imaged with ultrasound had reduced cortical gray matter demonstrable with MRI at term, with immature gyral development and enlarged subarachnoid spaces, and the discrepancy was even more marked in those who also had abnormal ultrasound appearances [36,37].

Prognosis after imaging showing flare, cystic PVL and diffuse PWMI

Flare

The prognosis of "flare" relates to whether the abnormality resolves rapidly or persists for longer than 14 days before disappearing, and to some extent on whether the appearances are homogenous. Transient echoreflective lesions were associated with an increased risk of later neurodevelopmental problems in even the earliest series [272,273]. Unfortunately the definition of a "prolonged" echodensity varies from more than 7 days to more than 14 days, and the classification of De Vries allows for the development of small cysts in the lowest grade (Table 9.5) [254]. Echoreflectivity persisting for more than 14 days occurred in 7.5% of the babies imaged by the Dutch group, 23% of whom developed diplegia [274]. Similar results were reported in the French EPIPAGE study, with 17% of those who had persisting echodensities (defined as present for more than 14 days with no cyst formation) developing CP [139]. The most adverse prognosis of "flare" was reported in the Alberta series, with a 50% risk of CP after even transient periventricular echodensity [141]. In spite of these varying results, there does appear to be general agreement that the prognosis of a flare which persists for less than a week is good.

Our advice would be to repeat the imaging frequently when a flare is diagnosed, and to be circumspect in giving a prognosis until the situation after 2–3 weeks is clear. The prognosis of a flare which resolves completely in less than a week is probably good, equivalent to a normal scan (see above). There is a risk of CP – perhaps around 20% – when the flare persists for more than 2 weeks and particularly if ventriculomegaly emerges (see above). The risk of subsequent problems is of course higher if cysts appear.

Cystic PVL

Widespread cortical echolucency remains the most reliable early imaging predictor of CP which can be detected with ultrasound, a finding that has strengthened considerably since the first edition of this book [9,139,141,275]. The addition of several large cohorts to the earlier follow-up studies has served only to consolidate the initially depressing results [9,141,253]. The vast majority of babies who have bilateral echolucent lesions in the white matter of the occipital lobes develop CP, usually spastic diplegia or quadriplegia often with associated intellectual and visual problems. Involvement of the anterior-parietal-occipital regions, or the occipito-parietal region bilaterally is particularly associated with a high risk of CP and learning difficulties [236,276,277]. Most babies who have bilateral occipito-parietal cysts visualized with ultrasound later develop CP, whereas only about 5%–6% of those with isolated anterior cysts do so. The risk of an IQ <70 is about 50% with fronto-parietal-occipital damage but is less (25%) with cysts in a single area [143], and is reduced to about 12% when that area is confined to the frontal lobe. Unilateral cystic PVL was followed by CP in 35% of children in the French cohort study of almost 2000 preterm babies, whereas bilateral cystic PVL was associated with cerebral palsy in 75% [139]; rather lower than the CP rates of 75% (unilateral PVL) and 99% (bilateral occipital PVL) reported in many series.

White matter damage diagnosed during preterm life also increases the risk of later psychiatric problems such as attention deficit hyperactivity disorder (ADHD). Whilst these conditions are commonly reported in ex-preterm cohorts whatever the ultrasound diagnosis, a neonatal diagnosis of a parenchymal lesion and/or ventricular enlargement increases the risk [144]. Cerebral visual impairment and later epilepsy are also quite common, and there can be secondary optic disc changes due to optic nerve hypoplasia which adds to the visual loss from cortical and optic radiation damage [278]. Magnetic resonance imaging follow-up studies so far confirm the ultrasound results, although large geographical cohort studies are awaited [279].

Our current advice regarding the prognosis of cystic PVL would be to base counseling on repeated imaging, if possible with information from MRI at term, including an analysis of the signal from myelin in the posterior limb of the internal capsule. For babies with small cysts confined to the anterior periventricular white matter the prognosis is generally good, with a definite possibility of an entirely normal outcome. The majority (but not all) of those with "medium" sized and more widespread lesions will usually develop some form of disability, including spastic diplegic CP (many retaining the ability to walk), learning difficulties, or ADHD. Again, MRI at term can help in refining this prognosis. Babies with extensive bilateral occipito-parietal cystic PVL continue to fare badly, with virtually all of them developing severe CP, usually spastic quadriplegic CP, with learning difficulties; many acquire epilepsy and/or have significant visual impairment.

Diffuse PWMI

In follow-up of a large series of infants studied [159] where 72% of infants demonstrated diffuse PWMI, an increasing severity of PWMI at term equivalent age was associated with poorer performance on the cognitive and psychomotor scales of the Bayley scales of infant development II as well as with increased risks of severe cognitive delay, severe motor delay, CP, and neurosensory impairment. Children with more severe white matter abnormalities had a higher number of neurodevelopmental impairments than children with less severe or no abnormalities. Gray matter abnormalities were also associated with an increased risk of severe cognitive delay, psychomotor delay and CP, but to a lesser extent than white matter abnormalities. These findings were independent of abnormalities on cranial ultrasound and of other perinatal factors and confirm the relevance of early structural brain abnormalities for subsequent neurodevelopemental risk spanning across neurologic, cognitive, and motor domains.

In a preterm cohort studied with serial scans, 30% of infants demonstrated ventriculomegaly on their first scan just after birth and 39% had ventricular dilatation on their final scan. Indeed lateral ventricle size is included as one of the scoring items in the Inder white matter score and ventriculomegaly, along with a widened extracerebral space, is typically associated with PWMI. Dyet and co-workers, however, saw no difference in DQs between infants with and without ventricular dilatation on their first and term MRIs [33]. There was no difference between post-hemorrhagic and non-hemorrhagic causes. However when only infants with IVH were considered, those who developed ventricular dilatation subsequently had significantly lower DQS compared to infants who did not develop ventricular dilatation. Indeed, Vollmer and colleagues from UCLH report on long-term disabilities in babies with non-progressive post-hemorrhagic ventriculomegaly [280]. They (and others) have hypothesized that excess non-protein-bound "free" iron released into the CSF after GMH-IVH may be toxic to the developing white matter via the production of reactive oxygen species [220]. Others suggest that the reason for ventriculomegaly does not matter, because the finding represents a sign of cortical and white matter injury in any event, and so far no correlation has been demonstrated between the levels of non-protein-bound iron and degree of white matter damage, or outcome [220,281].

Many studies support the increasingly accepted notion that moderate to severe non-progressive ventriculomegaly with irregular ventricular margins is often an indicator of diffuse PWMI, and is associated with an adverse outcome including at school age [38,143,280]. A large GMH-IVH is virtually always accompanied by a degree of ventriculomegaly at some point in time, and later MRI reveals permanent ventricular dilatation with periventricular white matter loss in a proportion. Over half of ex-preterm children who had enlarged ventricles by term-equivalent age had IQ scores of less than 70 in the outcome study of the indomethacin prevention trial; there were 11 such children who were compared to 246 without enlarged ventricles [281]. Most of the ex-preterm survivors from UCLH with ventriculomegaly also had GMH-IVH, and 66 such children were followed to school age, when their IQ was significantly lower (mean performance IQ 91) than the group with entirely normal cranial ultrasound scans early on [280]. Motor function was also assessed, and disabling motor impairment was also much more common in the ventriculomegaly GMH-IVH group than in those with normal scans, being present in 16%. The survivors of the indomethacin prevention trial were carefully imaged and followed-up, and those with ventriculomegaly (defined as a lateral midbody ventricular diameter of more than 1 cm on a sagittal scan) had a 30% incidence of CP [282].

Given the current state of knowledge, we would counsel parents whose preterm baby was found on cranial ultrasound at term-equivalent age to have persisting moderate to severe ventriculomegaly and signs of brain atrophy or poor growth of the white matter that there was a definite risk (~50% overall) of learning difficulty and poor school performance, with a mean reduction of around 10 IQ points and a possibility of a more significant reduction. A recent study has shown that signs of brain atrophy can be detected by cranial ultrasound at discharge and such infants perform poorly. We would also say that if there was no focal lesion seen on imaging the risk of motor deficit was higher than for a preterm baby with no cranial ultrasound abnormality, but it was still most likely that the baby would not develop CP. We would modify that risk if the baby was also born at less than 26 weeks' gestation because of the high background risk for this group. We would be much more optimistic when counseling the parents of a baby born at more than 28 weeks' gestation who had developed only mild non-progressive ventriculomegaly than in the case of a 24-week-gestation baby with moderate ventriculomegaly. We would offer to perform MRI at term-equivalent age if the parents wanted more information; the absence of DEHSI at term is a good prognostic sign, albeit present in only 20% of the group of ex-preterms at term.

Large studies comparing MRI with 1- and 2-year neurodevelopmental outcomes have now been published [33,38,283], and 6-year outcome studies are in progress. The results show that MRI at term-equivalent age has an important role in improving the identification of infants at high risk for subsequent neurodevelopmental impairment. Many large neonatal units are now routinely imaging preterm babies at term-equivalent age with MRI – at UCLH it is our current practice to offer this to all parents of infants born at less than 32 weeks' gestation. We have found it useful to adopt a qualitative scoring system of the white and gray matter development and abnormalities based on that used by Inder [36,283].

Cerebellar lesions

Terminology and classification

Recent studies suggest an important role for the cerebellum in the development of cognitive and social functions – it is realized that the high density of neurons contained within the cerebellum makes an important contribution to overall intellectual function. With use of MRI, in particular volumetric techniques, some interesting data are emerging. Cerebellar volumes at term-equivalent age were reduced in those infants who demonstrated PWMI on MRI [284]. This effect on cerebellar growth was independent of prematurity in this study. Other groups have confirmed the effect of PWMI on cerebellar growth even in the absence of direct cerebellar injury [285]. These data suggest that the long-term neurodevelopmental disabilities seen in survivors of premature birth may be attributable in part to impaired cerebellar development.

Etiology

The etiology of the cerebellar lesions which are now being increasingly recognized with MRI is not yet certain. The suggestion has been made that some are due to hemorrhage into germinal matrix tissue which is present in the cerebellum.

Incidence and timing

In a preterm cohort studied with serial MRI scans, cerebellar hemorrhagic lesions were present in 7% of infants [256]. Cerebellar lesions were related to low gestational age and birthweight and vaginal delivery, and were more common in those who died before follow-up. Most lesions were unilateral and half were associated with IVH. Cerebellar atrophy developed in two-thirds [33].

Cerebellar hemorrhage is quite common in preterm babies, occurring in 10%–25% in one old autopsy study [286]. More recent screening ultrasound studies suggest that cerebellar hemorrhage can be seen in at least 3% of very low birthweight babies [287,288,289]. Magnetic resonance imaging has revealed non-hemorrhagic lesions of the cerebellum in preterm babies; some are cases of secondary atrophy probably resulting from infarction of the inferior cerebellar arteries [290,291,292].

Ultrasound and MRI appearances

An ultrasound and MRI study in Austria described three patterns of cerebellar abnormality in preterm babies: volume reduction of the cerebellar hemispheres with a small but preserved vermis; volume reduction of the hemispheres with a ballooned fourth ventricle, and a small deformed vermis; and a normal-shaped cerebellum which was very reduced in volume [293]. These authors found hemosiderin in the posterior fossa in some cases, but more often the symmetry and morphology of the lesions suggested to them that the cause was a combination of a destructive disorder and developmental arrest. There were apparent similarities to Dandy-Walker variant or pontocerebellar hypoplasia on some of the images. The Leeds group described rather smaller lesions, mainly small unilateral foci or punctate lesions towards the periphery of the cerebellar hemispheres. More attention will undoubtedly need to be paid to cerebellar lesions in future. An example of the MRI appearances of lobar cerebellar hemorrhage in a preterm baby is given in Fig. 9.19a,b.

Prognosis of cerebellar lesions

There is increasing evidence that the cerebellum plays an important part in cognition in addition to its role in coordinating movement and adjustment of posture. Survivors of preterm birth with cerebellar hemorrhage tended to have lower DQ especially if there was subsequent cerebellar atrophy [33]. Other studies have shown that children with CP who are born preterm often show cerebellar lesions [294], although it is unclear whether the lesions are the primary cause of adverse outcome. Cerebellar abnormalities (reduced volumes) were associated with adverse outcome only when supratentorial lesions were seen [295]. Small cerebellar hemorrhages without associated lesions or volume reduction may not be of major prognostic significance, but much more work is required in this area before a reliable prognosis can be given to parents [296].

Treatment and prevention of conditions detected with screening in preterm babies

At the present time there is no treatment that can reduce the risk of neurodevelopmental sequelae in babies found to have cerebral lesions on ultrasound or MR screening. Given the plasticity of the neonatal brain, it would be comforting to think that this will not always be the case. Considerable progress has been made in understanding the pathogenesis of PWMI and identifying maturation-dependent cellular and molecular mechanisms of PWMI. The worryingly high incidence of diffuse PWMI appears to be related to both the timing and the appearance and regional distribution of susceptible OL progenitor cells. Identification of these cells as the main target in diffuse PWMI will provide the guidance and rationale for the development of neuroprotective therapies for the premature infant. The prevention of cerebral ischemia in critically ill infants is an important avenue of clinical research. The extreme vulnerability of OL progenitor cells to oxidative stress has led some research groups to consider the use of antioxidant therapy in preterm infants. This is an exciting and active research area; robust reliable neuroimaging tools are required for prognosis and also for monitoring the effects of interventions.

The best preventive treatment is to avoid preterm birth, or at least to delay delivery sufficiently long enough to allow a full course of antenatal steroids to be given. There is no evidence so far that early delivery should be attempted when the membranes are ruptured in order to try to avoid cytokine damage. Currently, we do not recommend any postnatal intervention apart from high-quality neonatal intensive care, with all the dedication and obsession that this entails. Indomethacin prophylaxis looked promising for a while, but the follow-up studies have been disappointing [297]. Early "prophylactic" physiotherapy has not been shown to be of any benefit either.

References

1. Papile L-A, Burstein J, Burstein R, Koffler H. Incidence and evolution of subependymal and intraventricular haemorrhage: a study of infants with birthweights less than 1500 g. *J Pediatr* 1978; **92**: 529–34.

2. Lacey DJ, Topper WH, Buckwald S, Zorn WA, Berger PE. Preterm very-low-birth-weight neonates: relationship of EEG to intracranial hemorrhage, perinatal complications, and developmental outcome. *Neurology* 1986; **36**: 1084–7.

3. Batton DG, DeWitte DB, Boal DK, Nardis EE, Maisels MJ. Incidence and severity of intraventricular hemorrhage: 1981–84. *Am J Perinatol* 1986; **3**: 353–6.

4. Strand C, Laptook AR, Dowling S *et al* Neonatal intracranial hemorrhage: 1. Changing pattern in inborn low birth weight infants. *Early Human Dev* 1990; **23**: 117–28.

5. Hanigan WC, Morgan AM, Anderson RJ *et al.* Incidence and neurodevelopmental outcome of periventricular hemorrhage and hydrocephalus in a regional population of very low birth weight infants. *Neurosurgery* 1991; **29**: 701–6.

6. Batton DG, Holtrop P, DeWitte D, Pryce C, Roberts C. Current gestational age-related incidence of major intraventricular hemorrhage. *J Pediatr* 1994; **125**: 623-5.

7. Synnes AR, Chien L-Y, Peliowski A, Baboolal R, Lee SK. Variations in intraventricular hemorrhage incidence rates among Canadian neonatal intensive care units. *J Pediatr* 2001; **138**: 525-31.

8. Ment LR, Bada HS, Barnes P *et al.* Practice parameter: neuroimaging of the neonate. Report of the quality standards subcommittee of the American Academy of Neurology and the Practice Committee of the Child Neurology Society. *Neurology* 2002; **58**: 1726-38.

9. Pinto-Martin JA, Riolo S, Cnaan A, Holzman C, Susser MW, Paneth N. Cranial ultrasound prediction of disabling and nondisabling cerebral palsy at age two in a low birth weight population. *Pediatrics* 1995; **95**: 249-54.

10. O'Shea TM, Klinepeter KL, Dillard RG. Prenatal events and the risk of cerebral palsy in very low birth weight infants. *Am J Epidemiol* 1998; **147**: 362-9.

11. Wheater M, Rennie JM. Perinatal infection is an important risk factor for cerebral palsy in very low birth weight infants. *Dev Med Child Neurol* 2000; **42**: 364-7.

12. Maas YGH, Mirmiran M, Hart AAM, Koppe JG, Aroiagno RL, Spekreijse H. Predictive value of neonatal neurological tests for developmental outcome of preterm infants. *J Pediatr* 2000; **137**: 100-6.

13. de Vries LS, van Haastert IL, Rademaker KJ, Koopman C, Groenendaal F. Ultrasound abnormalities preceding cerebral palsy in high risk preterm infants. *J Pediatr* 2004; **144**: 815-820.

14. Leijser LM, de Vries LS, Cowan FM. Using cerebral ultrasound effectively in the newborn infant. *Early Hum Dev* 2006; **82(12)**: 827-35.

15. Mirmiran M, Barnes PD, Keller K *et al.* Neonatal brain magnetic resonance imaging before discharge is better than serial cranial ultrasound in predicting cerebral palsy in very low birth weight preterm infants. *Pediatrics* 2004; **114(4)**: 992-8.

16. Dubowitz LMS, Dubowitz V, Palmer PG, Miller G, Fawer C-L, Levene MI. Correlation of neurological assessment in the preterm newborn infant with outcome at age 1 year. *J Pediatr* 1984; **105**: 452-6.

17. Harding D, Kuschel C, Evans N. Should preterm infants born after 29 weeks' gestation be screened for intraventricular haemorrhage? *J Paediatr Child Health* 1998; **34**: 57-9.

18. Chess PR, Chess MA, Manuli MA, Guillet R. Screening head ultrasound to detect intraventricular hemorrhage in premature infants. *Pediatr Radiol* 1997; **27**: 305-8.

19. Townsend SF, Tumack CM, Thilo EH, Merenstein GB, Rosenberg AA. Late neurosonographic screening is important to the diagnosis of periventricular leukomalacia and ventricular enlargement in preterm infants. *Pediatr Radiol* 1999; **29**: 347-52.

20. Hecht S, Filly RA, Callen PW, Wilson-Davis SL. Intracranial hemorrhage: late onset in the preterm neonate. *Radiology* 1983; **149(697)**: 699.

21. Perlman JM, Rollins N. Surveillance protocol for the detection of intracranial abnormalities in premature neonates. *Arch Pediatr Adolesc Med* 2000; **154**: 822-6.

22. Nwafor-Anene VN, DeCristofaro JD, Baumgart S. Serial head ultrasound studies in preterm infants: how many normal studies does one infant need to exclude significant abnormalities. *J Perinatol* 2003; **23**: 104-10.

23. Allikn M, Matsumoto H, Santhouse AM *et al.* Cognitive and motor function and the size of the cerebellum in adolescents born very pre-term. *Brain* 2001; **124**: 60-6.

24. Counsell S, Boardman JP. Differential brain growth in the infant born preterm: current knowledge and future developments from brain imaging. *Semin Fetal Neonatal Med* 2005; **10**: 403-10.

25. Anderson NG, Laurent I, Woodward LJ, Inder TE. Detection of impaired growth of the corpus callosum in premature infants. *Pediatrics* 2006; **118(3)**: 951-60.

26. Horsch S, Muentjes C, Franz A, Roll A. Ultrasound diagnosis of brain atrophy is related to neurodevelopmental outcome in preterm infants. *Acta Paediatr* 2005; **94**: 1815-21.

27. Heuchan AM, Evans N, Henderson-Smart DJ, Simpson JM. Perinatal risk factors for major intraventricular haemorrhage in the Australian and New Zealand neonatal network, 1995-1997. *Arch Dis Child* 2002; **86(2)**: F86-F90.

28. Fujimoto S, Togari H, Takashima S *et al.* National survey of periventricular leukomalacia in Japan. *Acta Paediatr Jpn* 1998; **40**: 239-43.

29. Harding JE, Miles FKI, Becroft DMO, Allen BC, Knight DB. Chest physiotherapy may be associated with brain damage in extremely premature infants. *Paediatrics* 1998; **132**: 440-4.

30. Williams AN, Sunderland R. Neonatal shaken baby syndrome: an aetiological view from Down Under. *Arch Dis Child* 2002; **86**: F29-F30.

31. The HiFi Study Group. High-frequency oscillatory ventilation compared with conventional mechanical ventilation in the treatment of respiratory failure in preterm infants. *N Engl J Med* 1989; **320**: 88-93.

32. Maalouf EF, Duggan PJ, Rutherford MA *et al.* Magnetic resonance imaging of the brain in a cohort of extremely preterm infants. *J Pediatr* 1999; **135**: 351-7.

33. Dyet LE, Kennea N, Counsell SJ *et al.* Natural history of brain lesions in extremely preterm infants studied with serial magnetic resonance imaging from birth and neurodevelopmental assessment. *Pediatrics* 2006; **118(2)**: 536-48.

34. Counsell SJ, Allsop JM, Harrison MC *et al.* Diffusion-weighted imaging of the brain in preterm infants with focal and diffuse white matter abnormality. *Pediatrics* 2003; **112(1)**: 1-7.

35. Childs A-M, Cornette L, Ramenghi LA *et al.* Magnetic resonance and cranial ultrasound characteristics of periventricular white matter abnormalities in newborn infants. *Clin Radiol* 2001; **56**: 647-55.

36. Inder TE, Wells SJ, Mogridge NB, Spencer C, Volpe JJ. Defining the nature of the cerebral abnormalities in the premature infant: a qualitative magnetic resonance imaging study. *J Paediatr* 2003; **143**: 171-9.

37. Inder TE, Warfield SK, Wang H, Huppi PS, Volpe JJ. Abnormal cerebral structure is present at term in premature infants. *Pediatrics* 2005; **115**: 286-94.

38. Miller SP, Ferriero DM, Leonard C *et al.* Early brain injury in premature newborns detected with magnetic resonance imaging is associated with adverse early neurodevelopmental outcome. *J Paediatr* 2005; **147**: 609-16.

39. Tharp BR, Scher MS, Clancy RR. Serial EEGs in normal and abnormal infants with birth weights less than 1200 grams – a prospective study with long term follow-up. *Neuropediatrics* 1989; **20**: 64-72.

40. Bejar R, Coen RW, Merritt TA *et al.* Focal necrosis of the white matter (periventricular leukomalacia): sonographic, pathologic, and electroencephalographic features. *Am J Neuroradiol* 1986; **7**: 1073-80.

41. Connell J, de Vries LS, Oozeer R, Dubowitz LMS, Dubowitz V. Predictive value of early continuous electroencephalogram monitoring in ventilated infants with intraventricular hemorrhage. *Pediatrics* 1988; **82**: 337-43.

42. Cuckier F, Andre M, Monod N, Dreyfus-Brisac C. Apport de l'EEG au diagnostic des hemorrhagies intra-ventriculaires du premature. *Rev EEG Neurophysiol* 1972; **2**: 318-22.

43. Clancy R, Tharp BR, Enzmann D. EEG in premature infants with intraventricular hemorrhage. *Neurology* 1984; **34(583)**: 590.

44. Hughes JR, Guerra R. The use of the EEG to predict outcome in premature infants with positive sharp waves. *Clin Electroencephalogr* 1994; **25**: 127-35.

45. Hughes JR. Electro-clinical correlations of positive and negative sharp waves on the temporal and central areas in premature infants. *Clin Electroencephalogr* 1991; **22**: 30-9.

46. Marret S, Parain D, Samson-Dollfus D. Positive Rolandic waves and periventricular leukomalacia in the newborn. *Neuropediatrics* 1986; **17**: 199-202.

47. Novotny EJ, Tharp BR, Coen RW, Bejar R, Enzmann D, Vaucher YE. Positive Rolandic sharp waves in the EEG of the premature infant. *Neurology* 1997; **37**: 1481–6.

48. Baud O, d'Allest A-M, Lacaze-Masmonteio T *et al.* The early diagnosis of periventricular leukomalacia in premature infants with positive Rolandic sharp waves on serial electroencephalography. *J Pediatr* 1998; **132**: 813–17.

49. Watanabe K, Hayakawa F, Okumura A. Neonatal EEG: a powerful tool in the assessment of brain damage in preterm infants. *Brain Dev* 1999; **21**: 361–72.

50. Scher MS, Bova JM, Dokianakis SG, Steppe DA. Positive temporal sharp waves on EEG recordings of healthy neonates: a benign pattern of dysmaturity in pre-term infants at post-conceptional term ages. *Electroencephalogr Clin Neurophysiol* 1994; **90**: 173–8.

51. Vecchierini-Blineau MF, Nogues B, Louvet S, Desfontaines O. Positive temporal sharp waves in electroencephalograms of the premature newborn. *Neurophysiol Clin* 1996; **26**: 350–62.

52. Okumura A, Hayakawa F, Kato T *et al.* Abnormal sharp transients on electroencephalograms in preterm infants with periventricular leukomalacia. *J Paediatr* 2003; **143**: 26–30.

53. Hayakawa F, Okumura A, Kato T, Kuno K, Watanabe K. Disorganized patterns: chronic-stage EEG abnormality of the late neonatal period following severely depressed EEG activities in early preterm infants. *Neuropediatrics* 1997; **28**: 272–5.

55. Hayakawa F, Okumura A, Kato T, Kuno K, Watanabe K. Determination of timing of brain injury in preterm infants with periventricular leukomalacia with serial neonatal electroencephalography. *Pediatrics* 1999; **104**: 1077–88.

56. Inder TE, Buckland L, Williams CE *et al.* Lowered electroencephalographic spectral edge frequency predicts the presence of cerebral white matter injury in premature infants. *Pediatrics* 2003; **111**: 27–33.

57. Ng PC, Dear PRF. The predictive value of a normal ultrasound scan in the preterm baby – a meta-analysis. *Acta Paediatr Scand* 1990; **79**: 286–91.

58. Battin MR, Maalouf EF, Counsell SJ *et al.* Magnetic resonance imaging of the brain in very preterm infants: visualization of the germinal matrix, early myelination, and cortical folding. *Pediatrics* 1998; **101**: 957–62.

59. Marin-Padilla M. Developmental neuropathology and impact of perinatal brain damage. I: Hemorrhagic lesions of neocortex. *J Neuropathol Exp Neurol* 1996; **55**: 758–73.

60. Grant EG. Sonography of the premature brain. *Neuroradiology* 1986; **28**: 476–90.

61. Larroche J-C. *Developmental Pathology of the Neonate*, 1st edn. Amsterdam, Excerpta Medica, 1977.

62. Gould SJ, Howard S, Hope PL, Reynolds EOR. Periventricular intraparenchymal cerebral haemorrhage in preterm infants: the role of venous infarction. *J Pathol* 1987; **151**: 197–202.

63. Hambleton G, Wigglesworth JS. Origin of intraventricular haemorrhage in the preterm infant. *Arch Dis Child* 1976; **51**: 651–9.

64. Ghazi-Birry HS, Brown WR, Moody DM, Challa VR, Block SM, Reboussin DM. Human germinal matrix: venous origin of hemorrhage and vascular characteristics. *Am J Neuroradiol* 1997; **18**: 219–29.

65. Paneth N. Classifying brain damage in preterm infants. *J Pediatr* 1999; **134(5)**: 527–9.

66. Kari MA, Hallman M, Eronen M, Teramo K, Virtanen M, Koivisto M. Prenatal dexamethasone treatment in conjunction with rescue therapy of human surfactant: a randomized placebo-controlled multicentre study. *Pediatrics* 1994; **93**: 730–6.

67. Ment LR, Oh W, Ehrenkranz RA, Philip AGS, Duncan CC, Makuch RW. Antenatal steroids, delivery mode, and intraventricular hemorrhage in preterm infants. *Am J Obstet Gynecol* 1995; **172**: 795–800.

68. Crowley P. Corticosteroids prior to preterm delivery. In: Neilson JP, Crowther CA, Hodnett ED, Hofmeyr GJ, Kierse MJNC, eds. *Pregnancy and Childbirth Module of the Cochrane Collaboration* 3rd edn. Oxford, Update Software, 1997.

69. Cooke RWI. Trends in incidence of cranial ultrasound lesions and cerebral palsy in very low birthweight infants 1982–1993. *Arch Dis Child* 1999; **80**: F115–F117.

70. Shankaran S, Bauer CR, Bain R, Wright LL, Zachary J. Relationship between antenatal steroid administration and grade III and IV intracranial hemorrhage in low birth weight infants. *Am J Obstet Gynecol* 1995; **173**: 305–11.

71. Canterino JC, Verma U, Visintainer PF, Elimian A, Klein SA, Tejani H. Antenatal steroids and neonatal periventricular leukomalacia. *Obstet Gynecol* 2001; **97**: 135–9.

72. Rumak CM, Guggenheim MA, Peterson RG, Johnson ML, Braithwaite WR. Neonatal IVH and maternal use of aspirin. *Obstet Gynecol* 1981; **58**: 52S–5S.

73. Spinillo A, Ometto A, Bottino R, Piazzi G, Iasci A, Rondini G. Antenatal risk factors for germinal matrix hemorrhage and intraventricular hemorrhage in preterm infants. *Eur J Obstet Gynecol Reprod Biol* 1995; **60**: 13–19.

74. Bada HS, Korones SB, Perry EH *et al.* Frequent handling in the neonatal intensive care unit and intraventricular hemorrhage. *J Pediatr* 1990; **117**: 126–31.

75. Kuban KCK, Leviton A, Pagano M, Fenton T, Strassfield R, Wolff M. Maternal toxemia is associated with reduced incidence of germinal matrix hemorrhage in premature babies. *J Child Neurol* 1992; **7**: 70–6.

76. Szymonowicz W, Yu VYH, Wilson FE. Antecedents of periventricular haemorrhage in infants weighing 1250 g or less at birth. *Arch Dis Child* 1984; **59**: 13–17.

77. Thorburn RJ, Lipscomb AP, Stewart A *et al.* Timing and antecedents of periventricular haemorrhage and of cerebral atrophy in very preterm infants. *Early Hum Dev* 1982; **7**: 221–38.

78. Hansen A, Leviton A. Labor and delivery characteristics and risks of cranial ultrasonographic abnormalities among very-low-birth-weight infants. *Am J Obstet Gynecol* 1999; **181**: 997–1006.

79. Osborn DA, Evans N, Kluckow M. Hemodynamic and antecedent risk factors of early and late periventricular/intraventricular hemorrhage in premature infants. *Pediatrics* 2003; **112**: 33–9.

80. Petaja J, Hiltunen L, Fellman V. Increased risk of intraventricular hemorrhage in preterm infants with thrombophilia. *Pediatr Res* 2001; **49**: 643–6.

81. de Vries LS, Eken P, Groenendaal F, Rademaker KJ, Hoogervorst B, Bruinse HW. Antenatal onset of haemorrhagic and/or ischaemic lesions in preterm infants: prevalence and associated obstetric variables. *Arch Dis Child Fetal Neonatol Ed* 1998; **78**: f51–f56.

82. Viscardi RM, Sun C-CJ. Placental lesion multiplicity: risk factor for IUGR and neonatal cranial ultrasound abnormalities. *Early Hum Dev* 2001; **62**: 1–10.

83. Verma U, Tejani N, Klein S *et al.* Obstetric antecedents of intraventricular hemorrhage and periventricular leukomalacia in the low birth weight neonate. *Am J Obstet Gynecol* 1997; **176**: 275–81.

84. Vergani P, Patane L, Doria P *et al.* Risk factors for neonatal intraventricular haemorrhage in spontaneous prematurity at 32 weeks gestation or less. *Placenta* 2000; **21**: 402–7.

85. Heep A, Behrendt D, Nitsch P, Fimmers R, Bartmann P, Dembinski J. Increased serum levels of interleukin 6 are associated with severe intraventricular haemorrhage in extremely premature infants. *Arch Dis Child* 2003; **88(6)**: 501–4.

86. Wallin LA, Rosenfeld CR, Laptook AR *et al.* Neonatal intracranial haemorrhage II: risk factor analysis in an inborn population. *Early Hum Dev* 1990; **23**: 129–37.

87. Ment LR, Oh W, Philip AGS *et al.* Risk factors for early intraventricular hemorrhage in low birthweight infants. *J Pediatr* 1992; **121**: 776–83.

88. Victory R, Penava D, da Silva O, Natale R, Richardson B. Umbilical cord pH and base excess values in relation to neonatal morbidity for infants delivered preterm. *Am J Obstet Gynaecol* 2003; **189**: 803–7.

89. Leviton A, Pagano M, Kuban KCK, Krishnamoorthy KS, Sullivan KF, Alfred EN. The epidemiology of germinal matrix haemorrhage during the first half day of life. *Dev Med Child Neurol* 1991; **33**: 138–45.

90. Linder N, Haskin O, Levit O *et al*. Risk factors for intraventricular hemorrhage in very low birth weight premature infants: a retrospective case-control study. *Pediatrics* 2003; **111(5)**: e590–e595.

91. Tzogalis D, Fawer CL, Wong Y, Calame A. Risk factors associated with the development of peri-intraventricular haemorrhage and periventricular leukomalacia. *Helvet Paediatr Acta* 1988; **43**: 363–76.

92. Hill, A, Perlman JM, Volpe JJ. Relationship of pneumothorax to occurence of IVH in the premature newborn. *Pediatrics* 1982; **69**: 144–5.

93. Lipscomb AP, Thorburn RJ, Reynolds EOR *et al*. Pneumothorax and cerebral haemorrhage in preterm infants. *Lancet* 1981; **i**: 414–16.

94. Cooke RWI. Factors associated with periventricular haemorrhage in very low birthweight infants. *Arch Dis Childhood* 1981; **56**: 425–31.

95. Fabres J, Carlo WA, Phillips V, Howard G, Ambalavanan N. Both extremes of arterial carbon dioxide pressure and the magnitude of fluctuations in arterial carbon dioxide pressure are associated with severe intraventricular hemorrhage in preterm infants. *Pediatrics* 2007; **119(2)**: 299–305.

96. Kaiser JR, Gauss CH, Pont MM, Williams DK. Hypercapnia during the first 3 days of life is associated with severe intraventricular hemorrhage in very low birth weight infants. *J Perinatol* 2006; **26**: 279–85.

97. Weindling AM, Wilkinson AR, Cook J, Calvert SA, Fok T-F, Rochefort MJ. Perinatal events which precede periventricular haemorrhage and leucomalacia in newborn. *Br J Obstet Gynaecol* 1985; **92**: 1218–23.

98. Miall-Allen VM, de Vries LS, Whitelaw AG. Mean arterial blood pressure and neonatal cerebral lesions. *Arch Dis Child* 1987; **62**: 1068–9.

99. Bada HS, Krones SB, Perry EH *et al*. Mean arterial blood pressure changes in premature infants and those at risk for periventricular hemorrhage. *J Pediatr* 1990; **117**: 607–14.

100. Watkins AMC, West CR, Cooke RWI. Blood pressure and cerebral haemorrhage and ischaemia in very low birthweight infants. *Early Hum Dev* 1989; **19**: 103–10.

101. D'Souza SW, Janakova H, Minors D *et al*. Blood pressure, heart rate, and skin temperature in preterm infants: association with periventricular haemorrhage. *Arch Dis Child* 1995; **72**: F162–F167.

102. Kluckow M, Evans N. Low superior vena cava flow and intraventricular haemorrhage in preterm infants. *Arch Dis Child* 2000; **82(3)**: f188–f194.

103. Perlman JM, McMenamin JB, Volpe JJ. Fluctuating cerebral blood flow velocity in respiratory distress syndrome: relation to the development of intraventricular hemorrhage. *N Engl J Med* 1983; **309**: 204–9.

104. Miall-Allen VM, de Vries LS, Dubowitz LMS, Whitelaw AGL. Blood pressure fluctuation and intraventricular hemorrhage in the preterm infants of less than 31 weeks gestation. *Pediatrics* 1989; **83**: 657–61.

105. Meek JH, Tyszczuk L, Elwell CE, Wyatt JS. Low cerebral blood flow is a risk factor for severe intraventricular haemorrhage. *Arch Dis Child* 1999; **80**: F15–F18.

106. McDonald MM, Johnson ML, Rumack CM, *et al*. Role of coagulopathy in newborn ICH. *J Pediatr* 1984; **74**: 26–31.

107. Bassan H, Benson CB, Limperopoulos C *et al*. Ultrasonographic features and severity scoring of periventricular hemorrhagic infarction in relation to risk factors and outcome. *Pediatrics* 2006; **117(6)**: 2111–17.

108. Shortland DB, Trounce JQ, Levene MI, Archer LNJ, Evans DH, Shaw DE. Patent ductus arteriosus and cerebral circulation in preterm circulation in preterm infants. *Dev Med Child Neurol* 1990; **32**: 386–93.

109. Evans N, Kluckow M. Early ductal shunting and intraventricular haemorrhage in ventilated preterm infants. *Arch Dis Child* 1996; **75**: f183–f186.

110. Cooke RWI. Factors associated with periventricular haemorrhage in very low birthweight infants. *Arch Dis Child* 1981; **56**: 425–31.

111. Paneth N, Pinto-Martin J, Gardiner J *et al*. Incidence and timing of germinal matrix/intraventricular hemorrhage in low birth weight infants. *Am J Epidemiol* 1993; **137**: 1167.

112. Kuban K, Sanocka U, Leviton A *et al*. White matter disorders of prematurity: association with intraventricular haemorrhage and ventriculomegaly. *J Pediatr* 1999; **134**: 539–46.

113. Larroque B, Marret S, Ancel PY *et al*. White matter damage and intraventricular hemorrhage in very preterm infants: the EPIPAGE study. *J Paediatr* 2003; **143**: 477–83.

114. Lemons JA, Bauer CR, Oh W *et al*. Very low birth weight outcomes of the National Institute of Child Health and Human Development Neonatal Research Network, January 1995 through December 1996. *Pediatrics* 2001; **107(1)**: e1–e8.

115. Horbar JD, Badger GJ, Carpenter JH *et al*. Trends in mortality and morbidity for very low birth weight infants, 1991–1999. *Pediatrics* 2002; **110**: 143–51.

116. Dolfin T, Skidmore MB, Fong KW, Hoskins EM, Shennan AT. Incidence, severity, and timing of subependymal and intraventricular hemorrhages in preterm infants born in a perinatal unit as detected by serial real-time ultrasound. *Pediatrics* 1983; **71**: 541–6.

117. Levene MI, de Vries LS. Extension of neonatal intraventricular haemorrhage. *Arch Dis Child* 1984; **59**: 631–6.

118. Szymonowicz W, Yu VYH. Timing and evolution of periventricular haemorrhage in infants weighing 1250 g or less at birth. *Arch Dis Child* 1984; **59**: 7–12.

119. de Crespigny LC, Mackay R, Murton LJ, Roy RND, Robinson PH. Timing of neonatal cerebroventricular haemorrhage with ultrasound. *Arch Dis Child* 1982; **57**: 231–3.

120. Counsell SJ, Rutherford MA, Cowan FM, Edwards AD. Magnetic resonance imaging of preterm brain injury. *Arch Dis Child Fetal Neonatal Ed* 2003; **88**: F269–F274.

121. Smets K, De Kezel C, Govaert P. Subependymal caudothalamic groove hyperechogenicity and neonatal chronic lung disease. *Acta Paediatr* 1997; **86**: 1370–3.

122. Reynolds PR, Dale RC, Cowan FM. Neonatal cranial ultrasound interpretations: a clinical audit. *Arch Dis Child* 2001; **84**: f92–f95.

123. Harris DL, Bloomfield FH, Teele RL, Harding JE. Variable interpretation of ultrasonograms may contribute to variation in the reported incidence of white matter damage between newborn intensive care units in New Zealand. *Arch Dis Childhood Fetal Neonatal Ed* 2006; **91(1)**: 11–16.

124. Pinto J, Paneth N, Kazam E *et al*. Interobserver variability in neonatal cranial ultrasonography. *Pediatr Perinatal Epidemiol* 1988; **2**: 43–58.

125. Corbett SS, Rosenfeld CR, Laptook AR *et al*. Intraobserver variability in the assessment of neonatal cranial ultrasound. *Early Hum Dev* 1991; **27**: 9–17.

126. Hope PL, Gould SJ, Howard S, Hamilton PA, Costello AM, Reynolds EOR. Precision of ultrasound diagnosis of pathologically verified lesions in the brains of very preterm infants. *Dev Med Child Neurol* 1988; **30**: 457–71.

127. Carson SC, Hertzberg BS, Bowie JD, Burger PC. Value of sonography in the diagnosis of intracranial hemorrhage and periventricular leukomalacia: a postmortem study of 35 cases. *Am J Radiol* 1990; **155**: 595–601.

128. Adcock LM, Moore PJ, Schlesinger AE, Armstrong DL. Correlation of ultrasound with postmortem neuropathologic studies in neonates. *Pediatr Neurol* 1998; **19**: 263–71.

129. Blankenberg FG, Loh N-N, Bracci P *et al*. Sonography, CT, and MR imaging: a prospective comparison of neonates with suspected intracranial ischemia and hemorrhage. *Am J Neuroradiol* 2000; **21**: 213–18.

130. Blankenberg FG, Norbash AM, Lane B, Stevenson DK, Bracci PM, Enzmann DR. Neonatal intracranial ischemia and hemorrhage: diagnosis with US, CT, and MR imaging. *Radiology* 1996; **199**: 253–9.

131. Maalouf EF, Duggan PJ, Counsell SJ *et al*. Comparison of findings on cranial ultrasound and magnetic resonance imaging in preterm infants. *Pediatrics* 2001; **107**: 719-27.

132. Debillon T, N'Guyen S, Quere MP, Moussaly F, Roze JC. Limitations of ultrasonography for diagnosing white matter damage in preterm infants. *Arch Dis Child* 2003; **88(4)**: 275-9.

133. Felderhoof-Mueser U, Rutherford MA, Squier WV *et al*. Relationship between MR imaging and histopathological findings of the brain in extremely sick preterm infants. *Am J Neuroradiol* 1999; **20**: 1349-57.

134. Whitby EH, Paley MN, Cohen M, Griffiths PD. Postmortem MR imaging of the fetus: an adjunct or a replacment for conventional autopsy? *Semin Fetal Neonatal Med* 2005; **10(5)**: 475-84.

135. Rennie JM. *Neonatal Cerebral Ultrasound*, 1st edn. Cambridge, Cambridge University Press, 1997.

136. Stewart A, Reynolds EOR, Hope PL *et al*. Reliability of neurodevelopmental disorders estimated from ultrasound appearances of brains of very preterm infants. *Dev Med Child Neurol* 1987; **29**: 3-11.

137. Goldstein RB, Filly RA, Hecht S, Davis S. Noncystic "increased" periventricular echogenicity and other mild cranial sonographic abnormalities: predictors of outcome in low birthweight infants. *J Clin Ultrasound* 1989; **17**: 553-62.

138. Weisglas-Kuperus N, Baerts W, Fetter WPF, Sauer PJJ. Neonatal cerebral ultrasound, neonatal neurology and perinatal conditions as predictors of neurodevelopmental outcome in very low birthweight infants. *Early Hum Dev* 1992; **31**: 131-48.

139. Ancel P-Y, Livinec L, Larroque B *et al*. Cerebral palsy among very preterm children in relation to gestational age and neonatal ultrasound abnormalities: the EPIPAGE cohort study. *Pediatrics* 2006; **117(3)**: 828-35.

140. Sherlock RL, Anderson PJ, Doyle LW. Neurodevelopmental sequelae of intraventricular haemorrhage at 8 years of age in a regional cohort of ELBW/very preterm infants. *Early Hum Dev* 2005; **81**: 909-16.

141. Aziz K, Vickar DB, Suave RS, Etches P, Pain KS, Robertson CMT. Province based study of neurologic disability of childen weighing 500-1249g at birth in relation to neonatal cerebral ultrasound findings. *Pediatrics* 1995; **95**: 837-44.

142. Patra K, Wilson-Costello D, Taylor HG, Mercuri-Minich N, Hack M. Grades I-II intraventricular hemorrhage in extremely low birth weight infants: effects on neurodevelopment. *J Paediatr* 2006; **149**: 169-73.

143. Whitaker AH, Feldman JF, van Rossem R *et al*. Neonatal cranial ultrasound abnormalities in low birth weight infants: relation to cognitive outcomes at 6 years of age. *Pediatrics* 1996; **98**: 719-29.

144. Whitaker AH, VanRossem R, Feldman JF *et al*. Psychiatric outcomes in low birth weight children at age 6 years: relation to neonatal cranial ultrasound abnormalities. *Arch Gen Psychiatry* 1997; **54**: 847-56.

145. Laptook AR, O'Shea TM, Shankaran S, Bhaskar B. Adverse neurodevelopmental outcomes among extremely low birth weight infants with a normal head ultrasound: prevalence and antecedents. *Pediatrics* 2005; **115(3)**: 673-80.

146. Kostovic I, Jovanov-Milosevic N. The development of cerebral connections during the first 20 to 45 weeks' gestation. *Semin Fetal Neonatal Med* 2006; **11(6)**: 415-22.

147. McQuillen PS, Ferriero DM. Selective vulnerability in the developing central nervous system. *Pediatr Neurol* 2004; **30**: 227-35.

148. Volpe JJ. Subplate neurons - missing link in brain injury of the premature infant? *Pediatrics* 1996; **97**: 112-13.

149. Vasileiadis GT, Gelman N, Han VK *et al*. Uncomplicated intraventricular hemorrhage is followed by reduced cortical volume at near-term age. *Pediatrics* 2004; **114**: e367-e372.

150. Counsell S, Maalouf EF, Rutherford MA, Edwards AD. Periventricular haemorrhagic infarct in a preterm neonate. *Eur J Pediatr Neurol* 1999; **3**: 25-8.

151. Takashima S, Takashi M, Ando Y, Pathogenesis of periventricular white matter haemorrhage in preterm infants. *Brain Dev* 1986; **8**: 25-30.

152. de Vries LS, Roelants-van Rijn AM, Rademaker KJ, van Haastert IC, Beek FJA, Groenendaal F. Unilateral parenchymal haemorrhagic infarction in the preterm infant. *Eur J Pediatr Neurol* 2001; **5**: 139-49.

153. Blackman JA, McGuinness GA, Bale JF, Smith WL. Large postnatally acquired porencephalic cysts: unexpected developmental outcomes. *J Child Neurol* 1991; **6**: 58-64.

154. de Vries LS, Groenendaal F, van Haastert IC, Eken P, Rademaker KJ, Meiners LC. Asymmetrical myelination of the posterior limb of the internal capsule in infants with periventricular haemorrhagic infarction: an early predictor of hemiplegia. *Neuropediatrics* 1999; **30**: 314-19.

155. Ferriero D. Neonatal brain injury. *New Engl J Med* 2004; **351**: 1985-95.

156. Volpe JJ. Neurobiology of periventricular leukomalacia in the premature infant. *Pediatr Res* 2001; **50**: 553-62.

157. Back SA. Perinatal white matter injury: the changing spectrum of pathology and emerging insights into pathogenetic mechanisms. *Mental Retard Dev Disabil Res Rev* 2006; **12**: 129-40.

158. Inder TE, Anderson NJ, Spencer C, Wells S, Volpe JJ. White matter injury in the premature infant: a comparison between serial cranial sonographic and MR findings at term. *Am J Neuroradiol* 2003; **24**: 805-9.

159. Woodward LJ, Anderson PJ, Austin NC, Howard K, Inder TE. Neonatal MRI to predict neurodevelopmental outcomes in preterm infants. *New Engl J Med* 2006; **355**: 685-94.

160. Back SA, Luo NL, Borenstein NS, Levine JM, Volpe JJ, Kinney HC. Late oligodendrocyte progenitors coincide with the developmental window of vulnerability for human perinatal white matter injury. *J Neurosci* 2001; **21(4)**: 1302-12.

161. Banker BQ, Larroche JC. Periventricular leukomalacia of infancy. A form of neonatal anoxic encephalopathy. *Arch Neurol* 1962; **7**: 386-410.

162. Larroche J-C. Lesions of haemorrhagic type, mainly venous. *Dev Pathol Neonate Amsterdam, Excerpta Medica*, 1977; 354-98.

163. Van Den Bergh R, Van Der Eecken H. *Anatomy and Embryology of Cerebral Circulation. Progress in Brain Research*, 30th edn. Amsterdam, Elsevier, 1968; 1-25.

164. Baud O, Foix-L'Helias L, Kaminski M *et al*. Antenatal glucocorticoid treatment and cystic periventricular leukomalacia in very premature infants. *N Engl J Med* 1999; **341**: 1190-6.

165. Leviton A, Dammann O, Allred EN *et al*. Antenatal corticosteroids and cranial ultrasonographic abnormalities. *Am J Obstet Gynecol* 1999; **181(4)**: 1007-17.

166. Vermeulen GM, Bruinse HW, Gerards LJ, de Vries LS. Perinatal risk factors for cranial ultrasound abnormalities in neonates born after spontaneous labour before 34 weeks. *Obstet Gynaecol* 2001; **94**: 290-5.

167. Agarwal R, Chiswick ML, Rimmer S *et al*. Antenatal steroids are associated with a reduction in the incidence of cerebral white matter lesions in very low birthweight infants. *Arch Dis Child Fetal Neonatol Ed* 2002; **86**: F96-F101.

168. Zupan V, Gonzalez P, Lacaze Masmonteil T *et al*. Periventricular leukomalacia: risk factors revisited. *Dev Med Child Neurol* 1996; **38**: 1061-7.

169. Resch B, Vollaard E, Maurer U, Haas J, Rosegger H, Muller W. Risk factors and determinants of neurodevelopmental outcome in cystic periventricular leucomalacia. *Eur J Pediatr* 2000; **159**: 663-70.

170. de Vries LS, Eken P, Groenendaal F, Ardemaker KJ, Hoogervorst B, Bruinse HW. Antenatal onset of haemorrhagic and/or ischaemic lesions in preterm infants: prevalence and associated obstetric variables. *Arch Dis Child* 1998; **78**: f51-f56.

171. Burguet A, Monnet E, Pauchard JY et al. Some risk factors for cerebral palsy in very premature infants: importance of premature rupture of membranes and monochorionic twin placentation. *Biol Neonate* 1999; **75**: 177–86.

172. Kubota H, Ohsone Y, Oka F, Sueyoshi T, Takanashi J, Kohno Y. Significance of clinical risk factors of cystic periventricular leukomalacia in infants with different birthweights. *Acta Paediatr* 2001; **90**: 302–8.

173. Wu YW, Colford JM. Chorioamnionitis as a risk factor for cerebral palsy. *J Am Med Assoc* 2000; **284(11)**: 1417–24.

174. Leviton A, Paneth N, Reuss ML et al. Maternal infection, fetal inflammatory response, and brain damage in very low birth weight infants. *Pediatr Res* 1999; **46**: 566–75.

175. Dammann O, Leviton A. Maternal intrauterine infection, cytokines, and brain damage in the preterm newborn. *Pediatr Res* 1997; **42**: 1–8.

176. De Felice C, Toti P, Laurini RN et al. Early neonatal brain injury in histological chorioamnionitis. *J Pediatr* 2001; **138**: 101–4.

177. Redline RW, O'Riordan A. Placental lesions associated with cerebral palsy and neurologic impairment following term birth. *Arch Pathol Lab Med* 2000; **124**: 1785–91.

178. Wharton KN, Pinar H, Stonestreet BS et al. Severe umbilical cord inflammation – a predictor of periventricular leukomalacia in very low birth weight infants. *Early Hum Dev* 2004; **77**: 77–87.

179. Yoon BH, Romero R, Park JS et al. The relationship among inflammatory lesions of the umbilical cord (funisitis), umbilical cord plasma interleukin 6 concentration, amniotic fluid infection, and neonatal sepsis. *Am J Obstet Gynecol* 2000; **183**: 1124–9.

180. Bejar R, Vigliocco G, Gramajo H, Solana C, Benirschke K, Berry C. Antenatal origins of neurologic damage in newborns II. Multiple gestations. *Am J Obstet Gynecol* 1990; **162**: 1230–6.

181. Larroche J-C. Brain damage in monozygous twins. *Biol Neonate* 1990; **57**: 261–78.

182. Itakura A, Kurauchi O, Hayakawa F, Matsuzawa K, Mizutani S, Tomoda Y. Timing of periventricular leukomalacia using neonatal electroencephalography. *Int J Gynecol Obstet* 1996; **55**: 111–15.

183. Kumazaki K, Nakayama M, Sumida Y et al. Placental features in preterm infants with periventricular leukomalacia. *Pediatrics* 2002; **109**: 650–5.

184. Calvert SA, Hoskins EM, Fong KW, Forsyth SC. Etiological factors associated with periventricular leukomalacia. *Acta Paediatr Scand* 1987; **75**: 254–9.

185. Gibbs JM, Weindling AM. Neonatal intracranial lesions following placental abruption. *Eur J Pediatr* 1994; **153**: 195–7.

186. Ito T, Kadowaki K, Takahashi H, Nagata N, Makio A, Terakawa N. Clinical features of cardiotocographic findings for premature infants with antenatal periventricular leukomalacia. *Early Hum Dev* 1997; **47**: 195–201.

187. de Vries LS, Regev R, Dubowitz LMS, Whitelaw A, Aber VR. Perinatal risk factors for the development of extensive cystic leukomalacia. *Am J Dis Child* 1988; **142**: 732–5.

188. Low A, Panagiotopoulos C, Derrick EJ. Newborn complications after intrapartum asphyxia with metabolic acidosis in the preterm fetus. *Am J Obstet Gynecol* 1995; **172(3)**: 805–10.

189. Ikonen RS, Janas MO, Koivikko MJ, Laippala P, Kuusinen EJ. Hyperbilirubinaemia, hypocarbia and periventricular leukomalacia in preterm infants. *Acta Paediatr Scand* 1991; **81**: 802–7.

190. Fujimoto S, Togari H, Yamaguchi N, Mizutami F, Suzuki S, Sobajima H. Hypocarbia and cystic periventricular leukomalacia in preterm infants. *Arch Dis Child* 1994; **71**: F107–F110.

191. Graziani LJ, Spitzer AR, Mitchell DG et al. Mechanical ventilation in preterm infants: neurosonographic and developmental studies. *Pediatrics* 1992; **90**: 515–22.

192. Wiswell TE, Graziani LJ, Kornhauser MS et al. Effects of hypocarbia on the development of cystic periventricular leukomalacia in premature infants treated with high-frequency jet ventilation. *Pediatrics* 1996; **98**: 918–24.

193. Dammann O, Allred EN, Kuban KCK et al. Hypocarbia during the first 24 postnatal hours and white matter echolucencies in newborns less than/equal to 28 weeks gestation. *Pediatr Res* 2001; **49(3)**: 388–93.

194. Liao S-L, Lai S-H, Chou Y-H, Kuo C-Y. Effect of hypocapnia in the first three days of life on the subsequent development of periventricular leukomalacia in premature infants. *Acta Paediatr* 2001; **42(2)**: 90–3.

195. Okumura A, Hayakawa F, Itomi K et al. Hypocarbia in preterm infants with periventricular leukomalacia: the relation between hypocarbia and mechanical ventilation. *Pediatrics* 2001; **107(3)**: 469–75.

196. Giannakopoulou C, Korakaki E, Manoura A et al. Significance of hypocarbia in the development of periventricular leukomalacia in preterm infants. *Pediatr Int* 2004; **46**: 268–73.

197. Shankaran S, Langer JC, Kazzi SN, Laptook AR, Walsh M. Cumulative index of exposure to hypocarbia and hyperoxia as risk factors for periventricular leukomalacia in low birth weight infants. *Pediatrics* 2006; **118(4)**: 1654–9.

198. Murase M, Ishida A. Early hypocarbia of preterm infants: its relationship to periventricular leukomalacia and cerebral palsy, and its perinatal risk factors. *Acta Paediatr* 2005; **94**: 85–91.

199. Pladys P, Beuchee A, Wodey E, Treguier C, Lassel L, Betremieux P. Patent ductus arteriosus and cystic periventricular leucomalacia in preterm infants. *Acta Paediatr* 2002; **90**: 309–15.

200. Murphy DJ, Squier MV, Hope PL, Sellers S, Johnson A. Clinical associations and time of onset of cerebral white matter damage in very preterm babies. *Arch Dis Child* 1996; **75**: F27–F32.

201. Yamamoto N, Utsu M, Serizawa M et al. Neonatal periventricular leukomalacia preceded by fetal periventricular echodensity. *Fetal Diagn Ther* 2000; **15**: 198–208.

202. The GRIT study group. Infant wellbeing at 2 years of age in the growth restriction intervention trial (GRIT): multicentred randomised controlled trial. *Lancet* 2004; **364**: 513–20.

203. Matsuda T, Okuyama K, Cho K et al. Induction of antenatal periventricular leukomalacia by hemorrhagic hypotension in the chronically instrumented fetal sheep. *Am J Obstet Gynecol* 1999; **181**: 725–30.

204. Reddy K, Mallard C, Guan J et al. Maturational change in the cortical response to hypoperfusion injury in the fetal sheep. *Pediatr Res* 1998; **43**: 674–82.

205. Petersson KH, Pinar H, Stopa EG et al. White matter injury after cerebral ischemia in ovine fetuses. *Pediatr Res* 2002; **51**: 768–76.

206. Ohyu J, Marumo G, Ozawa H et al. Early axonal and glial pathology in fetal sheep brains with leukomalacia induced by repeated umbilical cord occlusion. *Brain Dev* 1999; **21**: 248–52.

207. Drobyshevsky A, Derrick M, Wyrwicz AM et al. White matter injury correlates with hypertonia in an animal model of cerebral palsy. *J Cereb Blood Flow Metab* 2007; **27(2)**: 270–81.

208. Debillon T, Gras-Leguen C, Verielle V et al. Intrauterine infection induces programmed cell death in rabbit periventricular white matter. *Pediatr Res* 2000; **47**: 736–42.

209. Boylan G, Young K, Panerai RB, Rennie JM, Evans DH. Dynamic cerebral autoregulation in sick newborn infants. *Pediatr Res* 2000; **48**: 12–17.

210. Tsuji M, Saul P, du Plessis A et al. Cerebral intravascular oxygenation correlates with mean arterial pressure in critically ill premature infants. *Pediatrics* 2000; **108(4)**: 625–32.

211. Dammann O, Allred EN, Kuban KCK et al. Systemic hypotension and white-matter damage in preterm infants. *Dev Med Child Neurol* 2002; **44**: 82–90.

212. Tyszczuk L, Meek JH, Elwell CE, Wyatt JS. Cerebral blood flow is independent of mean arterial blood pressure in preterm infants undergoing intensive care. *Pediatrics* 1998; **102**: 337–41.

213. Kuban KCK, Gilles F. Human telencephalic angiogenesis. *Ann Neurol* 1985; **17**: 539–48.

214. Nelson MD, Gonzalez-Gomez I, Gilles FH. The search for human telencephalic ventriculofugal arteries. *Am J Neuroradiol* 1991; **12**: 223–8.

215. Riddle A, Luo NL, Manese M *et al*. Spatial heterogeneity in oligodendrocyte lineage maturation and not cerebral blood flow predicts fetal ovine periventricular white matter injury. *J Neurosci* 2006; **26(11)**: 3045–55.

216. Back SA, Luo NL, Borenstein NS, Volpe JJ, Kinney HC. Arrested oligodendrocyte lineage progression during human cerebral white matter development: dissociation between the timing of progenitor differentiation and myelinogenesis. *J Neuropathol Exp Neurol* 2002; **61(2)**: 197–211.

217. Baud O, Greene AE, Li J, Wang H, Volpe JJ, Rosenberg PA. Glutathione peroxidase-catalase cooperativity is required for resistance to hydrogen peroxide by mature rat oligodendrocytes. *J Neurosci* 2004; **24(7)**: 1531–40.

218. Haynes RL, Folkerth RD, Keeff RJ *et al*. Nitrosative and oxidative injury to premyelinating oligodendrocytes in periventricular leukomalacia. *J Neuropathol Exp Neurol* 2003; **62(5)**: 441–50.

219. Back SA, Luo NL, Mallison RA *et al*. Selective vulnerability of preterm white matter to oxidative damage defined by F2-isoprostanes. *Ann Neurol* 2005; **58(1)**: 108–20.

220. Savman K, Nilsson UA, Blennow M, Kjellmer I, Whitelaw A. Non-protein-bound iron is elevated in cerebrospinal fluid from preterm infants with posthemorrhagic ventricular dilatation. *Pediatr Res* 2001; **49(2)**: 208–12.

221. Follett PL, Deng W, Dai W *et al*. Glutamate receptor-mediated oligodendrocyte toxicity in periventricular leukomalacia: a protective role for topiramate. *J Neurosci* 2004; **24(18)**: 4412–20.

222. Dammann O, Hagberg H, Leviton A. Is periventricular leukomalacia an axonopathy as well as an oligopathy? *Pediatr Res* 2001; **49(4)**: 453–7.

223. Agresti C, D'Urso D, Levi G. Reversible inhibitory effects of interferon-gamma and tumour necrosis factor-alpha on oligodendroglial lineage cell proliferation and differentiation in vitro. *Eur J Neurosci* 1996; **8(6)**: 1106–16.

224. Hagberg H, Mallard C. Effect of inflammation on central nervous system development and vulnerability. *Curr Opin Neurol* 2005; **18**: 117–23.

225. Nelson KB, Grether JK, Damabrosia JM *et al*. Neonatal cytokines and cerebral palsy in very preterm infants. *Pediatr Res* 2003; **53**: 600–7.

226. Grether JK, Nelson KB, Walsh E, Willoughby RE, Redline RW. Intrauterine exposure to infection and the risk of cerebral palsy in very premature infants. *Arch Pediatr Adolesc Med* 2003; **157(1)**: 26–32.

227. Graham EM, Holcroft CJ, Rai KK, Donohue PK, Allen MC. Neonatal cerebral white matter injury in preterm infants is associated with culture positive infections and only rarely with metabolic acidosis. *Am J Obstet Gynecol* 2004; **191**: 1305–10.

228. Hintz SR, Kendrick DE, Stoll BJ *et al*. Neurodevelopment and growth outcomes of extremely low birth weight infants after necrotizing enterocolitis. *Pediatrics* 2005; **115(3)**: 696–703.

229. Yoon BH, Romero R, Yang SH *et al*. Interleukin-6 concentration in umbilical cord plasma are elevated in neonates with white matter lesions associated with periventricular leukomalacia. *Am J Obstet Gynecol* 1996; **174**: 1433–40.

230. Yoon BY, Jun JK, Romero R *et al*. Amniotic fluid inflammatory cytokines (interleukin-6, interleukin-1beta, and tumor necrosis factor alpha), neonatal brain white matter lesions, and cerebral palsy. *Am J Obstet Gynecol* 1997; **177**: 19–26.

231. Baud O, Emilie D, Pelletier E *et al*. Amniotic fluid concentrations of interleukin-1beta, interleukin-6 and TNF-alpha in chorioamnionitis before 32 weeks of gestation: histological associations and neonatal outcome. *Br J Obstet Gynaecol* 1999; **106**: 72–7.

232. Minagawa K, Tsuji Y, Ueda H, Koyama K, Okumura H, Hashimoto-Tamaoki T. Possible correlation between high levels of IL-18 in the cord blood of preterm infants and neonatal development of periventricular leukomalacia and cerebral palsy. *Cytokine* 2002; **17**: 164–70.

233. Hagberg H, Peebles D, Mallard C. Models of white matter unjury: comparison of infections, hypoxic-ischemic, and excitotoxic insults. *Mental Retardation Dev Disabil Res Rev* 2002; **8**: 30–8.

234. Eklind S, Mallard C, Leverin A-L *et al*. Bacterial endotoxin sensitizes the immature brain to hypoxic-ischemic injury. *Eur J Neurosci* 2001; **13**: 1101–106.

235. Hamrick SEG, Miller SP, Leonard C *et al*. Trends in severe brain injury and neurodevelopmental outcome in premature newborn infants: the role of cystic periventricular leukomalacia. *J Pediatr* 2004; **145**: 593–9.

236. Resch B, Vollaard E, Maurer U, Haas J, Rosegger H, Muller W. Risk factors and determinants of neurodevelopmental outcome in cystic periventricular leucomalacia. *Eur J Pediatr* 2000; **159**: 663–70.

237. Leviton A, Gilles F. Ventriculomegaly, delayed myelination, white matter hypoplasia, and periventricular leukomalaia: how are they related? *Pediatr Neurol* 1996; **15**: 127–36.

238. de Vries LS, Wigglesworth JS, Regev R, Dubowitz LMS. Evolution of periventricular leukomalacia during the neonatal period and infancy: correlation of imaging and postmortem findings. *Early Hum Dev* 1988; **17**: 205–19.

239. Rodriguez J, Claus D, Verellen G, Lyon G. PVL: ultrasonic and neuropathologic correlation. *Dev Med Child Neurol* 1990; **32**: 347–55.

240. Roelants-van Rijn AM, Croenendaal F, Beek FJA, Eken P, van Haastert IC, de Vries LS. Parenchymal brain injury in the preterm infant: comparison of cranial ultrasound, MRI and neurodevelopmental outcome. *Neuropediatrics* 2002; **32**: 80–9.

241. Cowan FM, de Vries LS. The internal capsule in neonatal imaging. *Semin Fetal Neonatal Med* 2005; **10(5)**: 461–74.

242. Yokochi K. Thalamic lesions revealed by MR associated with periventricular leukomalacia and clinical profiles of subjects. *Acta Paediatr* 1997; **86**: 493–6.

243. Lin Y, Okumura A, Hayakawa F, Kato T, Kuno K, Watanabe K. Quantitative evaluation of thalami and basal ganglia in infants with periventricular leukomalacia. *Dev Med Child Neurol* 2001; **43**: 481–5.

244. Levene MI, Wigglesworth JS, Dubowitz V. Haemorrhagic periventricular leukomalacia in the neonate: a real time ultrasound study. *Pediatrics* 1983; **71**: 794–7.

245. Guzzetta F, Shackleford GD, Volpe S, Perlman JM, Volpe JJ. Periventricular echodensities in the newborn period: critical determinant of neurologic outcome. *Pediatrics* 1986; **78**: 955–1006.

246. Bozynski MEA, Nelson MN, Matalon TAS *et al*. Cavitary periventricular leukomalacia: incidence and short term outcome in infants weighing < 1200 grams at birth. *Dev Med Child Neurol* 1985; **27**: 572–7.

247. Bowerman RA, Donn SM, DiPietro MA, D'Amato CJ, Hicks SP. Periventricular leukomalacia in the preterm newborn infant: sonographic and clinical features. *Radiology* 1984; **151**: 383–8.

248. Flodmark O, Lupton B, Li D *et al*. MR imaging of periventricular leukomalacia in childhood. *Am J Neuroradiol* 1989; **10**: 111–18.

249. Sie LT, van der Knaap MS, van Wezel-Meijler G, Taets van Amerongen AHM, Lafeber HN, Valk J. Early MR features of hypoxic-ischemic brain injury in neonates with periventricular densities on sonograms. *Am J Neuroradiol* 2000; **21**: 852–61.

250. Hill A, Melson GL, Clark HB, Volpe JJ. Haemorrhagic periventricular leukomalacia: diagnosis by real time ultrasound and correlation with autopsy findings. *Pediatrics* 1982; **69**: 282–4.

251. Andre P, Thebaud B, Delavaucoupet J *et al.* Late-onset cystic periventricular leukomalacia in premature infants: a threat until term. *Am J Perinat* 2001; **18(2)**: 79-86.

252. Kubota T, Okumura A, Hayakaa F *et al.* Relation between the date of cyst formation observable on ultrasonography and the timing of injury determined by serial electroencephalography in preterm infants with periventricular leukomalacia. *Brain Dev* 2001; **23**: 390-4.

253. Pierrat V, Duquennoy C, van Haastertt IC, Ernst M, Guilley N, de Vries LS. Ultrasound diagnosis and neurodevelopmental outcome of localised and extensive cystic periventricular leucomalacia. *Arch Dis Child* 2001; **84(3)**: f151-f156.

254. de Vries LS, Eken P, Dubowitz LMS. The spectrum of leucomalacia using cranial ultrasound. *Behav Brain Res* 1992; **49**: 1-6.

255. Childs A-M, Ramenghi LA, Evans DJ *et al.* MR features of developing periventricular white matter in preterm infants: evidence of glial cell migration. *Am J Neuroradiol* 1998; **19**: 971-6.

256. Arthur R. Magnetic resonance imaging in preterm infants. *Paediatr Radiol* 2006; **36**: 593-607.

257. Huppi PS, Murphy B, Maier SE *et al.* Microstructural brain development after perinatal cerebral white matter injury assessed by diffusion tensor magnetic resonance imaging. *Pediatrics* 2001; **107(3)**: 455-60.

258. Arzomanian Y, Mirmiran M, Barnes PD *et al.* Diffusion tensor brain imaging findings at term-equivalent age may predict neurologic abnormalities in low birth weight preterm infants. *Am J Neuroradiol* 2003; **24**: 1646-53.

259. Marin-Padilla M. Developmental neuropathololgy and impact of perinatal brain damage. II. White matter lesions of the neocortex. *J Neuropathol Exp Neurol* 1997; **56(3)**: 219-35.

260. Ajayi-Obe M, Saeed N, Cowan FM, Rutherford MA, Edwards AD. Reduced development of cerebral cortex in extremely preterm infants. *Lancet* 2000; **356**: 1162-4.

261. Kappellou O, Counsell SJ, Kennea N *et al.* Abnormal cortical development after premature birth shown by altered allometric scaling of brain growth. *PLoS Med* 2006; **3(8)**: e265.

262. Boardman JP, Counsell SJ, Rueckert D *et al.* Abnormal deep grey matter development following preterm birth detected using deformation based morphometry. *NeuroImage* 2006; **32(1)**: 70-8.

263. Peterson BS, Vohr B, Staib LH *et al.* Regional brain volume abnormalities and long-term cognitive outcome in preterm infants. *J Am Med Assoc* 2000; **285(15)**: 1939-47.

264. Peterson BS, Anderson AW, Ehrenkrantz R *et al.* Regional brain volumes and their later neurodevelopmental correlates in term and preterm infants. *Pediatrics* 2003; **111(5)**: 939-48.

265. Isaacs EB, Lucas A, Chong WK *et al.* Hippocampal volume and everyday memory in children of very low birth weight. *Pediatr Res* 2000; **47**: 713-20.

266. Cornette LG, Tanner SF, Ramenghi LA *et al.* Magnetic resonance imaging of the infant brain: anatomical characteristics and clinical significance of punctate lesions. *Arch Dis Child* 2002; **86(3)**: 171-7.

267. Schouman-Claeys E, Henry-Feugeas M-C, Roset F *et al.* Periventricular leukomalacia: correlation between MR imaging and autopsy findings during the first 2 months of life. *Radiology* 1993; **189**: 59-64.

268. Stewart AL, Rifkin L, Amess PN *et al.* Brain structure and neurocognitive and behavioural function in adolescents who were born very preterm. *Lancet* 1999; **353**: 1653-7.

269. Cooke RWI, Abernethy LJ. Cranial magnetic resonance imaging and school performance in very low birthweight infants in adolescence. *Arch Dis Child* 1999; **81**: F116-F121.

270. Miller SP, Cozzio CC, Goldstein RB *et al.* Comparing the diagnosis of white matter injury in premature newborns with serial MR imaging and transfontanel ultrasonography findings. *Am J Neuroradiol* 2003; **24**: 1661-9.

272. Graham M, Levene MI, Trounce JQ, Rutter N. Prediction of cerebral palsy in very low birthweight infants: prospective ultrasound study. *Lancet* 1987; **ii**: 593-4.

273. Appleton RE, Lee REJ, Hey EN. Neurodevelopmental outcome of transient neonatal echodensities. *Arch Dis Child* 1990; **65**: 27-9.

274. Jongmans M, Henderson S, de Vries LS, Dubowitz L. Duration of periventricular densities in preterm infants and neurologic outcome at 6 years of age. *Arch Dis Child* 1993; **69**: 9-13.

275. Holling EE, Leviton A. Characteristics of cranial ultrasound white-matter echolucencies that predict disability: a review. *Dev Med Child Neurol* 1999; **41**: 136-9.

276. Fazzi E, Orcesi S, Caffi L, Ometto A, Rondini G, Telesca C. Neurodevelopmental outcome at 5-7 years in preterm infants with periventricular leukomalacia. *Neuropediatrics* 1994; **25**: 134-9.

277. Rogers B, Msall M, Owens T *et al.* Cystic periventricular leukomalacia and type of cerebral palsy in preterm infants. *J Pediatr* 1994; **125**: S1-S8.

278. Lanzi G, Fazzi E, Uggetti C *et al.* Cerebral visual impairment in periventricular leukomalacia. *Neuropediatrics* 1998; **29**: 145-50.

279. Aida N, Nishimura G, Hachiya Y, Matsui K, Takeuchi M, Itani Y. MR imaging of perinatal brain damage: comparison of clinical outcome with initial and follow-up MR findings. *Am J Neuroradiol* 1998; **19**: 1909-21.

280. Vollmer B, Roth S, Riley K *et al.* Neurodevelopmental outcome of preterm infants with ventricular dilatation with and without associated haemorrhage. *Dev Med Child Neurol* 2006; **48**: 348-52.

281. Ment LR, Vohr B, Allan W *et al.* The etiology and outcome of cerebral ventriculomegaly at term in very low birth weight preterm infants. *Pediatrics* 1999; **104**: 243-8.

282. Allan WC, Vohr B, Makuch RW, Kasz KH, Ment LR. Antecedents of cerebral palsy in a multicenter trial of indomethacin for intraventricular hemorrhage. *Arch Pediatr Adolesc Med* 1997; **151**: 580-5.

283. Woodward LJ, Anderson PJ, Austin NC, Howard K, Inder TE. Neonatal MRI to predict neurodevelopmental outcomes in preterm infants. *N Engl J Med* 2006; **355**: 685-94.

284. Shah DK, Anderson PJ, Carlin JB *et al.* Reduction in cerebellar volumes in preterm infants: relationship to white matter injury and neurodevelopmental outcome at two years of age. *Pediatr Res* 2006; **60(1)**: 97-102.

285. Limperopoulos C, Soul JS, Haidar H *et al.* Impaired trophic interactions between the cerebellum and the cerebrum among preterm infants. *Pediatrics* 2005; **116(4)**: 844-50.

286. Grunnet ML, Shields WD. Cerebellar haemorrhage in preterm infants. *J Pediatr* 1975; **88**: 605-8.

287. Mercuri E, He J, Curati WL, Dubowitz LMS, Cowan FM, Bydder GM. Cerebellar infarction and atrophy in infants and children with a history of premature birth. *Pediatr Radiol* 1997; **27**: 139-43.

288. Merrill JD, Piecuch RE, Fell SC, Barkovich AJ, Goldstein RB. A new pattern of cerebellar hemorrhages in preterm infants. *Pediatrics* 1998; **102**: 1-5.

289. Limperopoulos C, Benson CB, Bassan H *et al.* Cerebellar hemorrhage in the preterm infant: ultrasonographic findings and risk factors. *Pediatrics* 2005; **116**: 717-24.

290. Bodensteiner JB, Johnsen MD. Cerebellar injury in the extremely premature infant: newly recognised but relatively common outcome. *J Child Neurol* 2004; **19**: 139-42.

291. Johnsen SD, Tarby TJ, Lewis KS, Bird R, Prenger E. Cerebellar infarction: an unrecognised complication of low birthweight. *J Child Neurol* 2002; **17**: 320-4.

292. Johnsen SD, Bodensteiner JB, Lotze TE. Frequency and nature of cerebellar injury in the extremely premature survivor with cerebral palsy. *J Child Neurol* 2005; **20**: 60-4.

293. Messerschmidt A, Brugger PC, Boltshauser E *et al.* Disruption of cerebellar development: potential complication of extreme prematurity. *Am J Neuroradiol* 2005; **26**: 1659–67.

294. Johnson S D, Tarby T J, Lewis K S, Bird R, Prenger E. Cerebellar infarction: an unrecognised complication of low birthweight. *J Child Neurol* 2002; **17**: 320–4.

295. Srinivasan L, Allsop J, Counsell SJ, Boardman JP, Edwards AD, Rutherford M. Smaller cerebellar volumes in very preterm infants at term-equivalent gestational age are associated with the presence of supratentorial lesions. *Am J Neuroradiol* 2006; **27**: 573–9.

296. Miall LS, Cornette LG, Tanner SF, Arthur RJ, Levene MI. Posterior fossa abnormalities seen on magnetic resonance brain imaging in a cohort of newborn infants. *J Perinatol* 2003; **23**: 396–403.

297. Schmidt B, Davis P, Moddemann D *et al.* Long-term effects of indomethacin prophylaxis in extremely low birth weight infants. *N Engl J Med* 2001; **344(26)**: 1966–72.

Chapter 10 | Common maternal and neonatal conditions that may lead to neonatal brain imaging abnormalities

NICOLA J. ROBERTSON,
CORNELIA F. HAGMANN, *and*
JANET M. RENNIE

Introduction

The superb anatomical detail, gray–white matter differentiation, subtle volume differences, and metabolic information available from magnetic resonance studies of the newborn brain have revolutionized our understanding of the trajectory of normal development and the effect of prenatal and postnatal factors. It is increasingly recognized that an adverse prenatal or postnatal environment can have profound effects on the normal course of brain development, leading to long-term consequences in brain structure, behavior, cognition, and neurology.

This chapter is divided into three sections. The first section describes two common maternal conditions that may lead to neonatal cerebral injury. Being a twin, for example, may influence the trajectory of brain development merely by the sharing of a placenta and the effect of common placental anastomoses on the brain. Substance or alcohol abuse, an increasing problem in western countries, influences brain development in subtle ways; there has been much interest recently in the way that environmental influences acting during early development shape risk in later life. This is termed *epigenetics* and refers to the system of inheritance that does not involve changes in the primary DNA sequence but which can nevertheless be transmitted through cell lineages and can result in altered gene expression (for review see [1]). In the current era where brain magnetic resonance imaging (MRI) is possible in infants at risk, we are able to study the phenotypes of certain environmental influences. Due to lack of space, we have not been able to discuss other maternal problems that can lead to fetal brain injury, such as road traffic accidents, anaphylaxis, or serious maternal illness particularly liver disease. Nor have we been able to discuss the effects of drugs such as sodium valproate. The effect of in utero viral infection is discussed in Chapter 13.

The second section deals with neonatal conditions that may lead to brain injury. This section is by no means comprehensive and only the commoner conditions have been discussed, in particular those problems such as hyperbilirubinemia and hypoglycemia, which occur following birth when specific problems may be manifest during the transition from fetal to extrauterine life. The brain imaging abnormalities that may be observed in infants with congenital heart disease are also included here, although it is increasingly recognized that such infants may have abnormal in utero brain development as evidenced by altered brain metabolism and microstructure shortly after birth and before heart surgery [2].

The final section discusses specific brain abnormalities that may be detected in apparently well neonates on a postnatal ward or as part of a pathological process – lenticulostriate vasculopathy and subependymal pseudocysts. Non-specific cranial ultrasound abnormalities are in fact surprisingly common: a cranial ultrasound study of newborn infants admitted to a postnatal ward directly after birth and regarded as normal by obstetric and pediatric staff demonstrated ultrasound abnormalities in as many as 20% [3]. Ischemic lesions such as periventricular and thalamic densities were the most common finding (8%) followed by hemorrhagic lesions (6%). These ultrasound abnormalities were associated with deviant patterns on the neurological examination. Another larger cranial ultrasound study reported a 0.26% prevalence of *major* brain lesions in apparently normal term infants: two cases of germinal matrix-intraventricular hemorrhage (GMH-IVH), one temporal lobe hemorrhage, two cases of agenesis of the corpus callosum, and one middle cerebral artery infarct [4]. Cohorts of apparently normal term infants are now being studied with brain MRI; a recent study at 3 T demonstrated intracranial hemorrhage (mainly posterior fossa subdural or parenchymal hemorrhage in the occipital lobe) in 26% of vaginal births [5]. Magnetic resonance imaging is more sensitive than ultrasound imaging at detecting abnormalities, especially in the posterior fossa. "Screening" of the brains of all term-born newborn babies with ultrasound or MRI is not currently clinically indicated. "Screening" preterm babies is widely practiced and is discussed in Chapter 9.

Neonatal Cerebral Investigation, eds. Janet M. Rennie, Cornelia F. Hagmann and Nicola J. Robertson. Published by Cambridge University Press. © Cambridge University Press 2008.

Maternal conditions that may lead to neonatal cerebral injury

Multiple pregnancy

Incidence and terminology

The incidence of twin pregnancies in the UK is 14.4 per 1000 births [6]. Twin pregnancies have a ninefold increased risk of cerebral palsy, and triplet pregnancies a 47-fold increased risk [7]. The higher relative risk for cerebral damage is due to the higher incidence of premature birth and low birth weight in twin and triplet sets. In addition, the configuration of placental vascular anastomoses is an important factor in the derivation of brain damage in monochorionic (MC) twins [8].

Approximately one-third of twin pregnancies are monozygotic; most share a single MC placenta. It is well known that perinatal morbidity and mortality in MC twins is 3–5 times more common than in dichorionic (DC) twins [9,10]. Much of the increased risk of adversity is related to two main factors: the presence of vascular anastomoses leading to twin-to-twin transfusion syndrome (TTTS) and the effect of one twin dying in utero on the surviving twin [11]. Studies have shown evidence of cerebral white matter lesions (see Chapter 9) in one-third of MC infants at birth, particularly those complicated by TTTS and co-twin demise [9,12]. In a study comparing the prevalence of cranial ultrasound abnormalities from 85 MC and 94 DC twins in relation to chorionicity and discordant birth weight, MC twins had a sevenfold higher risk of white matter lesions compared to dichorionic twins [13]. In babies with discordant birth weights, TTTS and co-twin death had independent effects on the incidence of white matter lesions. Interestingly, discordant birth weight babies had a threefold higher risk of developing cerebral white matter lesions compared with those with concordant birth weight; this supports the evidence that a >30% birth weight discordance identifies babies who are at risk for adverse outcome [14]. Some studies have suggested that intrauterine growth retardation (IUGR) in MC twins is associated with a higher incidence of neurological damage [15,16].

A recent population-based study comparing long-term outcomes of MC TTTS pregnancies with a contemporaneous regional comparison cohort has added important information to the field. Children born very preterm in the TTTS group had significantly lower intelligent quotient (IQ) scores than non-TTTS twins or singletons who were also born very preterm. In this study there was no increased prevalence of cerebral palsy in TTTS children [17]. There was no difference between donor and recipients in terms of outcome.

Prognosis and counseling

Parents need to be counseled during pregnancy about the three- to fourfold higher risk of neurological impairment in MC twins compared to gestation-age matched DC twins. Prenatal factors such as TTTS, discordant birth weight and co-twin death influence the risk of an adverse neurodevelopmental outcome in MC twins. However, many children have a good outcome. Normal postnatal cranial imaging can provide some reassurance although not of course a guarantee, and we would offer postnatal ultrasound and MRI to twins who had required treatment for TTTS, who were sole survivors or who were born significantly preterm. We do not currently offer to image all sets of twins born above 35 weeks' gestation who remain well. We would counsel parents based on the result of the imaging; the spectrum of lesions is covered in Chapter 8 and 9.

Substance and alcohol abuse

Incidence

The 2002–2003 US National Survey on Drug Use on Health found that of pregnant women aged 15–44, 4.3% used illicit drugs, 18% tobacco, and 9.8% alcohol. The cost to society is vast and includes long-lasting effects on the developing brain. The pattern of anomalies following exposure to large amounts of alcohol were first reported by Lemoine and colleagues in France in 1968 [18]. In 1980, Rosett established criteria which are still widely used for fetal alcohol syndrome: (1) pre- and postnatal growth restriction; (2) dysfunction of the central nervous system (CNS); (3) a particular pattern of craniofacial characteristics [19]. Fetal alcohol syndrome represents only one end of a spectrum of disturbed fetal development following prenatal exposure to heavy alcohol; some children are only partially affected and are described as exhibiting fetal alcohol effects.

Neonatal brain imaging following fetal alcohol exposure

In infants who were exposed to heavy maternal alcohol consumption, brain MRI has revealed a range of abnormalities which include hypoplasia of the vermis of the cerebellum, a thin hypoplastic corpus callosum, small hippocampi, and wide cortical sulci [20,21]. Small brain size has been consistently reported [22], as well as regional brain volume differences. Prenatal alcohol exposure disproportionately affects midline craniofacial and brain structures; abnormalities of the corpus callosum include complete and partial agenesis, smaller callosal volumes or alterations in callosal shape [23,24]. Microstructural abnormalities in the corpus callosum have been observed with diffusion tensor imaging in fetal alcohol syndrome [25]. Fetal alcohol syndrome is also associated with a range of neurocognitive deficits which include areas such as attention, memory, learning, language, and motor skills.

Neonatal brain imaging following fetal cocaine exposure

A study investigating cranial ultrasound findings in 39 term and near-term infants with fetal exposure to cocaine demonstrated no increase in the incidence of cranial ultrasound abnormalities compared with 39 matched control infants [26], although changes in the flow velocity of the anterior cerebral artery consistent with the vasoconstrictive effects of the drug were documented. Other studies have confirmed that fetal cocaine exposure does not lead to increased incidence of congenital brain malformations [27], although heavy cocaine exposure was associated with a higher risk of subependymal hemorrhage on cranial ultrasound [28,29]. The long-term implications of these subtle abnormalities in the neonatal period remain to be determined.

Neonatal conditions that may lead to brain injury

Hypoglycemia

Incidence and terminology

Hypoglycemia is the most common metabolic disorder to affect the newborn infant. The precise definition of neonatal hypoglycemia remains unclear; however, there is clearly evidence that hypoglycemia can cause encephalopathy and result in permanent brain injury [30]. Because of the controversy surrounding the definition of hypoglycemia, it is difficult to ascertain the prevalence of hypoglycemia in at-risk groups [31]. Using one level for blood glucose concentrations (2.6 mmol/l), Lucas *et al.* [32] reported a prevalence of 67%, whereas a more recent study of normal term and preterm infants reported prevalences of 10% and 4% respectively [33].

Pathophysiology

Blood glucose levels fall immediately after birth but rise a few hours later either spontaneously or in response to feeding; this pattern is considered to be normal. No study has ever been able to address the precise degree and duration of hypoglycemia which might prove harmful to the human neonate, and of course no such study will ever be done. As with hypoxic ischemia, there is considerable variability between babies with regard to exacerbating and protective factors. Several factors make the newborn brain *less* vulnerable to hypoglycemic damage compared to the mature adult brain. These factors include the following:

1. Glycogen stored in astrocytes may supply glucose to the neuron in times of short supply from the bloodstream [34]. This may be of greatest importance during labor when placental transport ceases.
2. Newborn babies can use alternative fuels to glucose during hypoglycemia. For example, during the establishment of feeds, ketone bodies, β-hydroxybutyrate, and acetoacetate can supplement glucose to maintain normal cerebral metabolism [35,36,37]; in addition amino acids, free fatty acids, lactate, and pyruvate enter the immature brain through specific transport mechanisms on the blood–brain barrier [38,39]. "Switching off" ketone body production probably occurs when a supplementary formula feed is given, hence the advice to avoid formula wherever possible when mothers are trying to establish breast feeding [40].
3. The cerebral glucose utilization rate in the neonate is low (~18 μmol. min^{-1}. 100 g^{-1}) increasing almost fourfold in the first 6 years. The cerebral metabolic rate for glucose is highest in the thalamus and subcortical areas in the newborn, which contrasts with the mature uniform pattern of glucose utilization [41].
4. An increase in cerebral blood flow associated with hypoglycemia has been observed in newborn puppies; this may be a protective response that maintains net substrate delivery to the brain; this response has also been observed in human newborn infants (Fig. 10.1) [42,43].

It is generally believed that brief self-limiting episodes of hypoglycemia are of no neurological significance if they are

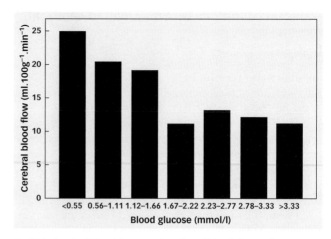

Fig. 10.1. **Cerebral blood flow as a function of blood glucose in 25 newborn infants measured 2 hours after birth. Cerebral blood flow was measured by xenon clearance. Modified from Pryds *et al.* (1988) [43].**

not accompanied by clinical signs or other complications. However, there is no doubt that prolonged symptomatic hypoglycemia can damage the neonatal brain. By the time a baby presents with abnormal signs there has often been a long period of preceding asymptomatic hypoglycemia, and the whole history often goes back 12–24 hours. The biochemical effects of prolonged hypoglycemia include the following: a reduction in the cerebral metabolic rate (CMR) of glucose and oxygen, a reduction in phosphocreatine (PCr), adenosine triphosphate (ATP) and phospholipds, an increase in CMR lactate, and an increase in intracellular Ca^{2+} and extracellular K^+, ammonia, glutamate, and aspartate. Hypoglycemia is an excitotoxic condition, with the increased levels of aspartate and glutamate binding to N-methyl-D-aspartate (NMDA) receptors and opening Ca^{2+}-permeable channels [44]. This leads to a cellular Ca^{2+} influx which leads to neuronal death beginning in neuronal dendrites. As no anerobic metabolism occurs there is no acidosis or infarction.

Clinical presentation

Clinical manifestations of hypoglycemia relate to the secretion of epinephrine and include tremor, seizures, apnea, irritability, hypotonia, high-pitched cry, and poor feeding. At-risk babies include those who are small-for-gestational-age, infants of diabetic mothers, and babies who are stressed by hypoxic ischemia or sepsis.

Neuropathology

Pathological studies from the 1960s clearly describe the neuropathological features of hypoglycemic brain injury in series of affected newborns [45,46]. Anderson and her colleagues described acute degeneration of neurons and glial cells throughout the cerebral cortex with the occipital lobes being most affected. In contrast to the findings in hypoxic ischemia, involvement of the cortex at the base of the cerebral sulci (ulegyria) was not a feature [46]. Banker studied the brains of three

Table 10.1. Summary of MRI reports linking neonatal hypoglycemia to occipital brain injury. Adapted from Filan *et al.* (2006) [53].

Author	Spar [54]	Aslan [55]	Barkovich [56]	Traill [57]	Murakami [58]	Kinnala [41]	Cakmakci [59]	Filan [53]
No. of cases (those with occipital injury)	1 (1)	1 (1)	5 (5)	2 (2)	8 (7)	18 (3)	1 (1)	4 (4)
Gestation (weeks)	Term	Term		Term	37–41	35–42	36	36–40
Age at first MR scan	19 days	10 days	13–27 days	10 months	9 months to 9 years	2–39 days	–	4–7 days
Seizures at presentation	1	1	5	2	6	0	1	3
Outcome data	None	Disability and decreased VEP	None	2 disability 1 visual deficit	8 disability 4 visual deficit	1 disability	normal	1 disability and visual deficit

infants who died some time after neonatal hypoglycemia: microcephaly was associated with wide sulci and atrophic gyri.

Determinants of neuronal injury in neonatal hypoglycemia

As yet there is no explanation for the observed vulnerability of the occipital region although it is possible that it relates to a regional developmental deficit in the expression or function of the glucose membrane transporter proteins.

It is known that the presence of alternative brain fuels – ketones, lactate, fatty acids, and amino acids – may explain the apparent tolerance in the infant brain to relative glucose restriction in the neonatal period. In infants with hyperinsulinism, the absence of ketones may increase the vulnerability of the newborn brain to injury during periods of metabolic stress. Indeed, there is evidence of a potential role of hyperinsulinism in brain injury because a high incidence of neurodisability (33%) and epilepsy (25%) is seen in the survivors [47,48].

Experimental and human data suggest an enhanced vulnerability to ischemic injury with hypoglycemia [49,50]. These data (and others) suggest that degrees of ischemia and hypoglycemia that alone would not cause brain injury might do so when acting together.

EEG in neonatal hypoglycemia

As yet there are no specific EEG changes described which consistently accompany hypoglycemia. Other neurophysiological studies have shown changes; in one such study [51] the mean increase in latency of brainstem-evoked response was 8% baseline, however each of the five infants studied had a different blood glucose level below which the latency increased (1.9–2.6 mmol/l). The authors concluded that while each subject had a different hypoglycemic threshold for neurophysiological change, no baby had abnormal responses at a blood level of 2.6 mmol/l or above and the authors concluded that this should be considered the safe level [51].

Cranial ultrasound in neonatal hypoglycemia

Magnetic resonance imaging is vastly superior to cranial ultrasound for the detection of parieto-occipital injuries consequent to neonatal hypoglycemia [52,53]. Currently, imaging with ultrasound cannot reliably detect damage associated with hypoglycemia, although scanning via the posterior fontanelle using modern ultrasound machines may prove more sensitive.

MRI studies in neonatal hypoglycemia

Within the last 15 years several MRI case series of severe newborn hypoglycemia have been published – these are summarized in Table 10.1. A consistent pattern of injury affecting predominantly the occipital lobes and posterior parietotemporal regions is described [52,53,54,55,56,57,58,59]. A recent case series using diffusion-weighted imaging revealed extensive areas of restricted diffusion within the occipital cortex and white matter, corpus callosum and optic radiations on apparent diffusion coefficient (ADC) maps within the first week [53], which corresponded to abnormal occipital white matter signal on early T_2-weighted images (Fig. 10.2 [53]). On follow-up scans generalized occipital lobe atrophy with thin atrophic gyri and increased white matter signal intensity is observed (Fig. 10.3).

Counseling and prognosis

One retrospective study of preterm babies suggested that hypoglycemia (defined as blood glucose below 2.6 mmol/l) for at least 5 days was associated with neurodevelopmental impairment [32]. These data cannot be extrapolated to term-born babies, or applied to infants in the current era with improved nutrition.

There can be no doubt that prolonged symptomatic hypoglycemia can cause permanent brain injury. Adverse outcomes include learning difficulties, visual impairment, and epilepsy including West's syndrome [60,61]. We would offer MRI to babies who had hypoglycemic seizures and counsel parents according to the results. We do not offer MRI to babies

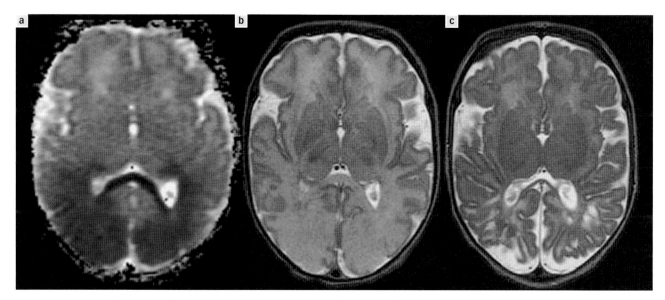

Fig. 10.2a–c. **Apparent diffusion coefficient (ADC) trace map (a) and T$_2$-weighted image (b) from a 36-week-gestation infant who developed symptomatic hypoglycemia on day 4 and was scanned on day 6. The follow-up scan on day 44 is shown in (c). Reproduced with permission from Filan et al. (2006) [53].**

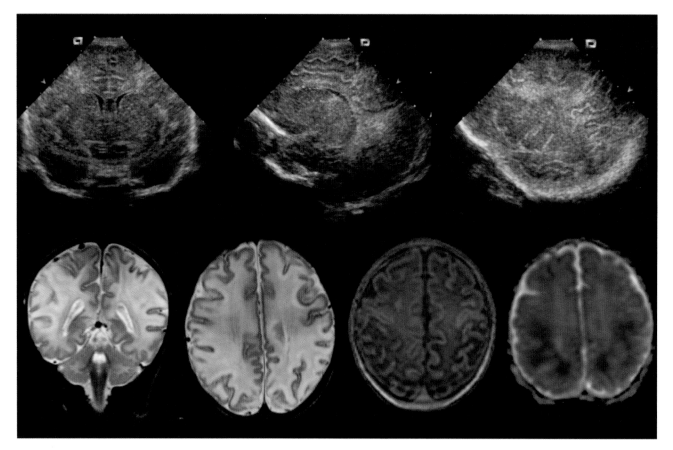

Fig. 10.2d. **Upper row: Coronal and parasagittal ultrasound images of a term infant at 4 days of age show patchy areas of increased echogenicity in the white matter, particularly in the parieto-occipital area. This infant had prolonged hypoglycaemia on day 3 after birth, blood glucose on re-admission was 0.1 mmol/l. Bottom row: Coronal and axial T$_2$ w, axial T$_1$w MR images and ADC trace map from the same infant on day 10. Diffusely abnormal signal intensity is seen in the white matter in addition to extensive parieto-occipital cortical infarction. Several areas of laminar cortical necrosis can be seen. On the ADC trace map (MR image on the bottom right), areas of restricted diffusion are seen in the parieto-occipital white matter.**

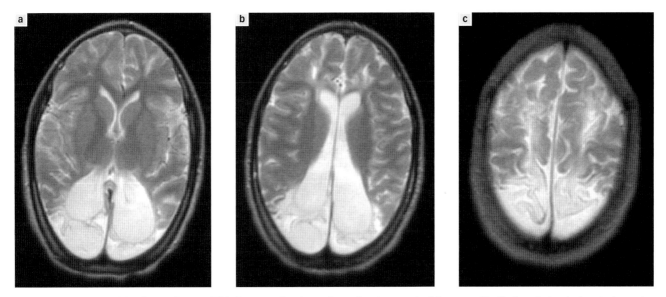

Fig. 10.3a–c. **Axial T$_2$-weighted scans from a child of 8 years showing regions of mature cerebral damage with gliosis and atrophy in anterior and deep watershed regions (in keeping with partial prolonged hypoxic ischemic encephalopathy). The baby had a serum glucose of zero recorded when he collapsed at the age of 9 hours, having taken virtually no feed since birth (emergency caesarean for fetal distress). Posteriorly the damage extends beyond arterial watershed territories in keeping with cerebral infarction due to hypoglycemia. The child was disabled by spastic quadriplegic cerebral palsy, developmental delay and epilepsy.**

who had short periods of asymptomatic hypoglycemia whose neonatal neurological examination is normal, and would counsel that they were not at risk of sequelae due to the low blood glucose.

Jaundice

Incidence and terminology

Clinical jaundice, which becomes visible in a white-skinned baby when total serum bilirubin (TSB) levels reach 85–120 μmol/l, is the most common clinical sign in neonatal medicine. More than 60% of otherwise healthy newborns and almost all preterm infants develop clinical jaundice during the first week of life. The usual peak TSB occurs between 72 and 120 hours – in the current era of early postnatal discharge, most infants have been discharged from hospital by this time. Hyperbilirubinemia typically resolves by 7–10 days of age and the outcome is usually benign. However, severe hyperbilirubinemia, defined as TSB above the 95th percentile for age in hours (high-risk zone), occurs in 8%–9% of infants in the first week, with ~4% affected after 72 hours [62] (Fig. 10.4). Without intervention, a progressive increase in TSB levels to >99th percentile for age in hours puts otherwise healthy babies at risk of bilirubin-induced brain damage. The estimated incidence of brain injury due to bilirubin toxicity is 1 in 30 000 infants [63].

Jaundice is thought to have been first described in Chinese pediatric texts as early as 1100 AD [64]. The term kernicterus, "jaundice of the nuclei," was introduced in the 1900s as a description of the yellow staining of basal ganglia in infants who died with severe jaundice – many of these with severe rhesus disease [65]. Treatment of severe neonatal jaundice

became possible with the introduction of exchange transfusion in the 1940s. The serendipitous discovery of the therapeutic effect of light on neonatal jaundice in 1958 resulted in the widespread use of phototherapy [66]. Indeed there was a virtual disappearance of kernicterus in industrialized countries following the introduction of phototherapy in the 1960s. Hyperbilirubinemia and subsequent bilirubin-induced brain injury re-emerged as an important clinical problem in the 1990s due to increased breast-feeding rates, early hospital discharges, and a more relaxed approach to jaundice and phototherapy levels. New terminology has recently been introduced and the classical clinical expression of kernicterus can be divided into *acute bilirubin encephalopathy* and *chronic bilirubin-induced neurologic dysfunction (BIND)* [67]. BIND refers to a wide spectrum of disorders caused by severe hyperbilirubinemia; the insult is an elevated TSB level that exceeds the infant's neuroprotective defences and results in neuronal injury, primarily of the basal ganglia, hippocampus and cerebellum, and brainstem nuclei for oculomotor function and hearing.

Pathophysiology

All human neonates experience temporary physiological jaundice due to the immaturity of hepatic conjugation and transport processes for unconjugated bilirubin (UCB). The antioxidant properties of these modest elevations of plasma UCB are probably neuroprotective [68]. In some newborns, hyperbilirubinemia develops when the rate of bilirubin production via the breakdown of heme by the reticuloendothelial system exceeds the rate of elimination, mostly by conjugation. Genetic, racial,

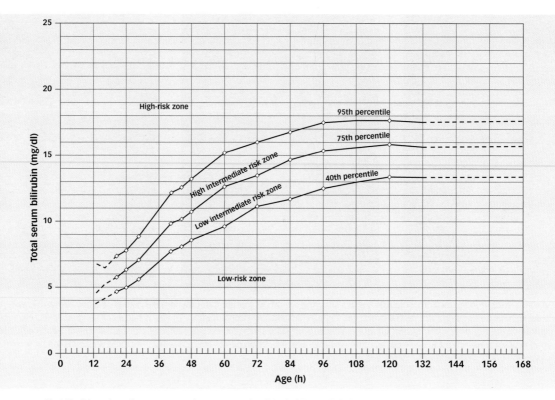

Fig. 10.4. **Hour-specific bilirubin values from a group of over 13 000 healthy babies and their risk designation based on their hour-specific serum bilirubin values. The high-risk zone is designated by the 95th percentile track; the intermediate-risk zone is subdivided into upper and lower risk zones by the 75th percentile track; the low-risk zone is defined by the 40th percentile track. The conversion of mg/dl to μmol/l requires multiplication by 17.1. Reproduced with permission from Bhutani** *et al.* **(1999) [62].**

and environmental factors affect the equilibria between these processes. Generally, early-onset severe hyperbilirubinemia is associated with increased bilirubin production, while late-onset hyperbilirubinemia is often associated with delayed bilirubin elimination with or without increased bilirubin production (Table 10.2).

Unconjugated bilirubin is fat soluble, crosses cell membranes, and is potentially neurotoxic. Phototherapy employs blue wavelengths of light and detoxifies bilirubin, facilitating its excretion by routes other than conjugation in the liver (water-soluble photo-isomers are excreted in the bile and urine without conjugation). There is no evidence that neurotoxicity occurs at a specific bilirubin concentration. The critical level in an otherwise healthy baby is influenced by the postnatal age, maturity, duration of hyperbilirubinemia, and rate of TSB rise. Factors that predispose infants to acute bilirubin encephalopathy at lower TSB values include: "near term" gestation (35 to <38 weeks), hypoalbuminemia, disruption of the blood–brain barrier (asphyxia or trauma), hemolysis, infection, hypoglycemia, and other factors such as drugs that interfere with albumin binding to bilirubin (for example, sulphisoxazole was the cause of many cases of kernicterus in the 1960s) [63,69]. Several studies have demonstrated that boys are more susceptible than girls to the adverse effects of neonatal hyperbilirubinemia [70]. A number of investigators have presented evidence that unbound or "free" bilirubin is a more appropriate predictor of neurotoxicity, although at present there are no commercially available assays for unbound bilirubin. Some Japanese and American studies have suggested that levels of >0.8 μg/dl of unbound bilirubin are associated with an increasing risk of BIND [71].

Clinical presentation
A significantly elevated TSB is a neonatal emergency because of the potential neurotoxic effects: if there are clinical signs of an encephalopathy immediate action is essential if permanent damage is to be avoided.

Acute bilirubin encephalopathy
The presenting signs of acute bilirubin encephalopathy (ABE) can be subtle and non-specific. The early presenting signs of ABE consist of decreased feeding, lethargy, variable abnormal tone (hypo- and hypertonia), and high-pitched cry. If untreated these may progress to increasing hypotonia with retrocollis and opisthotonus (Fig. 10.5). Advanced signs include bicycling movements, irritability, crying, seizures, setting sun sign, fever, and death. Volpe has described a scoring system for grading the severity of ABE to document the progression of signs (Table 10.3). Increasing scores are indicative of worsening BIND, which becomes progressively irreversible [67]. Prompt and effective intervention during the early phases of ABE can prevent sequelae, i.e., rapid reduction of the bilirubin

Table 10.2. Differential diagnosis of hyperbilirubinemia based on pathophysiology of presentation. Adapted from Smitherman *et al.* (2006) [63].

Early-onset hyperbilirubinemia (age <72 hours)		Late-onset hyperbilirubinemia (age >72 hours and <2 weeks)
First 24 hours of life	First week	> 1 week of life
Direct Coombs positive isoimmune erythroblastosis:	Benign idiopathic jaundice (physiologic; <40th percentile)	Prolonged idiopathic jaundice (breast milk jaundice; TSB <13 mg/dl)
• Rhesus disease		
• minor blood group incompatibilities	Sepsis (viral or bacterial)	Sepsis (viral or bacterial)
• ABO (often the direct Coombs negative)	Increased enteropathic circulation	Functional gastrointestinal tract abnormalities
Direct Coombs negative	Disorders of bilirubin metabolism	
• G6PD deficiency	• UG1TA1 gene polymorphism (delayed conjugation)	
• Intrinsic red blood cell defect	• Co-inheritance of UG1TA1 polymorphism with G6PD deficiency, ABO incompatibility, spherocytosis	
• spherocytosis		
• elliptocytosis	• Crigler-Naajar syndromes: I and II	
• hemoglobinopathies	• others	
	Metabolic disorders	
	• Galactosemia	
	• alpha-1-antitrypsin deficiency	
	• storage disorders	
	• others	
	Enclosed hemorrhages	Cystic fibrosis
	• cephalohematoma, subaponeurotic hemorrhage	Hypothyroidism
	• bruising	

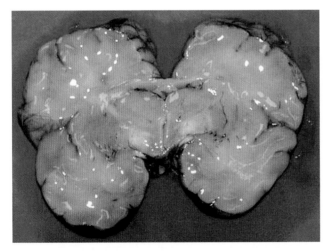

Fig. 10.5. **Pathological specimen from a term infant who died as a result of bilirubin-induced neuronal damage. The yellow-stained regions include the basal ganglia (particularly the globus pallidus and subthalamic nucleus) and hippocampus.**

load by a combination of intensive phototherapy and exchange transfusion. The rate of progression of clinical signs will depend on several factors including the rate of rise in bilirubin, duration of hyperbilirubinemia, serum albumin, level of unbound bilirubin, and presence of co-existing morbidities. Death may result from respiratory failure and progressive coma or seizures.

Chronic bilirubin-induced neurologic dysfunction

Typically, chronic bilirubin-induced neurologic dysfunction (BIND) presents as extrapyramidal movement disorders (dystonia and athetosis), gaze abnormalities, auditory disturbances (especially sensorineural hearing loss), and enamel dysplasia of the decidual teeth. Cognitive deficits are unusual but may be severe – they may reflect inaccurate assessment of intelligence in children with hearing, co-ordination and communication problems. The mortality approaches 10%. In the acute period, detection of abnormalities of the brainstem auditory-evoked response is a very sensitive indicator of BIND; it has been suggested that the auditory system may be the most sensitive neural system to BIND. In most cases the auditory disturbance is a bilateral high-frequency loss.

Determinants of neuronal injury

The imprecise relationship between total serum bilirubin levels and adverse neurological outcome has stimulated research to identify more accurate markers of bilirubin toxicity.

Prematurity

Premature infants are considered to be more prone to BIND than full-term infants. Elevated bilirubin levels appear in some studies to be a risk factor for hearing loss in premature babies. The high incidence of bilateral sensorineural deafness in a population of sick very low birth weight infants

Table 10.3. Clinical progression of acute bilirubin encephalopathy, from Volpe [72]. An incremental score is assigned for each clinical sign to obtain a maximum bilirubin-induced neurologic dysfunction (BIND) score of 9. Infants with scores of 4–6 usually have reversible acute bilirubin encephalopathy (ABE). A progression to a higher score is indicative of worsening BIND [67].

Clinical evaluation	Non-specific, subtle	Progressive toxicity	Advanced toxicity
Score for a clinical sign in each column	1	2	3
Ranges of scores	1–3	4–6	7–9
Mental status	Sleepy + poor feeding	Lethargy + irritability feeding	Semi-coma or seizures
Muscle tone	Slight decrease	Hyper- or hypotonia depending on arousal state or mild nuchal/truncal arching	Markedly increased (opisthotonus), or bicycling movements
Cry	High pitched	Shrill	Inconsolable

Table 10.4. Major differences in topography of neuropathology between BIND and hypoxic ischemic injury in the term infant. Adapted from Volpe [72].

Brain region	BIND	Hypoxic-ischemic encephalopathy
Cerebral cortex and/ or periventricular white matter	–	+
Basal ganglia		
• Caudate-putamen	–	+
• Globus pallidus	+	–
Hippocampus	Sectors CA 1, 2	Sector CA 1
Thalamus	Subthalamic nucleus	Anterior and lateral nuclei
Substantia nigra	Reticulata	Compacta
Cochlear nuclei	+	–
Dentate nuclei	+	–

with serum bilirubin levels > 240 µmol/l was reduced when lower thresholds for intervention were used [73]. Other studies have suggested that the "coexistence of risk factors for hearing loss may be more important than the individual risk factors themselves" as sensorineural hearing loss was more likely if acidosis occurred when peak serum bilirubin levels were >200 µmol/l or if peak bilirubin levels coincided with aminoglycoside use. Recently, the specific vulnerability to BIND of "late preterm infants" has been highlighted [74]. Unsuccessful and suboptimal lactation was the most frequent experience in late preterm infants who developed kernicterus. The potential incidence of BIND is higher in the late preterm infant due to an increased vulnerability and the fact that many are mistakenly cared for as healthy term infants.

Acidosis
Acidosis can influence bilirubin entry into the brain by promoting precipitation into partially polar lipid membranes [75] and increasing cerebral blood flow and therefore contact time between brain endothelium and bilirubin [76].

Neuropathology
The hallmarks of acute bilirubin encephalopathy are bilirubin staining of neurons and neuronal necrosis leading to permanent gliosis. Bilirubin staining occurs in a characteristic topography (Fig. 10.5 and Table 10.4). The regions most commonly affected are the basal ganglia (particularly the globus pallidus and subthalamic nucleus), hippocampus, substantia nigra, cranial nerve nuclei (particularly the oculomotor, vestibular, cochlear, and facial nerve nuclei), brainstem nuclei (particularly the reticular formation of the pons and olivary nucleus), the dentate nuclei of the cerebellum, and anterior horn cells of the spinal cord. Much has been learned about the neuropathology of hyperbilirubinemia from the Gunn rat animal model of hyperbilirubinemia. This model, described by Gunn in 1938, is a mutant jaundiced rat of Wistar strain lacking activity of the uridine diphosphate glucuronyltransferase (UDPGT) enzyme that is responsible for conjugating unconjugated bilirubin. The clinical course and neuropathology associated with bilirubin encephalopathy are similar to those seen in humans. The neurotoxicity of bilirubin is confirmed by the remarkable similarities in the topography of bilirubin staining and neuronal necrosis in full-term or preterm infants with marked hyperbilirubinemia, in some preterm infants without hyperbilirubinemia (but with a combination of other associated risk factors) and the homozygous Gunn rat. Brain pigmentation lasts 7–10 days; during this time neuronal injury evolves.

The distribution of neuronal injury generally corresponds closely to the distribution of bilirubin staining; this distribution of injury with BIND is different to that seen in hypoxic-ischemic injury [72] (Table 10.4). For example, the cerebral cortex and periventricular white matter are generally not affected in BIND. The early neuronal changes in BIND consist of swollen granular cytoplasm, microvacuolation, and disruption of neuronal and nuclear membranes followed by neuronal loss and astrocytosis [77]. Affected regions become permanently gliotic. The early basophilic, swollen neurons of bilirubin injury differ from the shrunken eosinophilic neuron of hypoxic-ischemic encephalopathy.

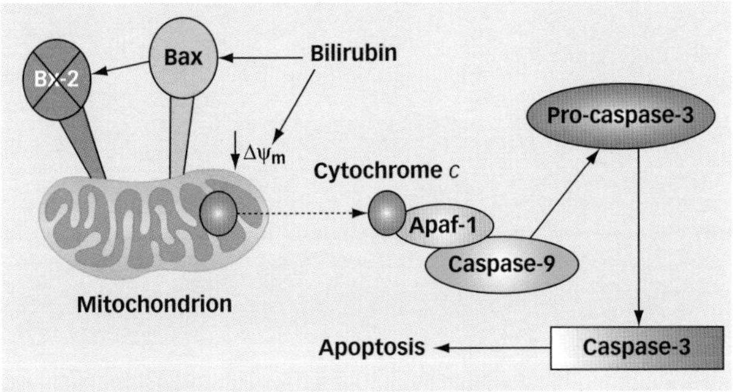

Fig. 10.6. **Schematic representation of bilirubin-induced apoptosis via the mitochondrial pathway. Exposure of rat neurons to unconjugated bilirubin resulted in a decrease in mitochondrial transmembrane potential, leading to the release of cytochrome c. Cytosolic cytochrome c then binds to the apoptosis protease activating factor-1 (Apaf-1) triggering the activation of caspase-9. Caspase-9 cleaves and activates pro-caspase-3 to the active form which results in the execution of the apoptosis cascade. Unconjugated bilirubin will also disrupt membrane function, lower action potentials and disturb neurotransmitter synthesis and transmission. Cell death occurs via other pathways in addition to the apoptosis pathway. Reproduced with permission from Ostrow** *et al.* **(2004) [79].**

Molecular basis of bilirubin-induced neurotoxicity

The molecular mechanisms of bilirubin toxicity are only beginning to be understood [78,79]. Exposure to high levels of unconjugated bilirubin is toxic to astrocytes and neurons, and leads to complex alterations in several vital cell functions, resulting in cell death with a mixed picture of apoptosis and necrosis. Unconjugated bilirubin damages mitochondrial membranes, leads to swelling and release of cytochrome c into the cytosol. Several cell death pathways are involved: bilirubin-induced apoptosis in neurons via the mitochondrial pathway is shown in Fig. 10.6. Unconjugated bilirubin will also disrupt membrane function, lower action potentials, and disturb neurotransmitter synthesis and transmission. Neuronal vulnerability depends on both gestation and postnatal age, possibly reflecting the functional status of specific brain areas at the time of the metabolic insult.

The EEG and other neurophysiological tests

Reversible depressive effects of bilirubin on neuronal function have been shown using auditory-nerve- and brainstem-evoked potentials, visual-evoked potentials and somatosensory-evoked potentials [80,81]. Experimental unilateral bilirubin encephalopathy was associated with decreased amplitude and flattening of the EEG [82]. A more recent study concluded that exposure to hyperbilirubinemia transiently delayed the EEG maturation in term newborn infants [83].

Brain imaging studies in BIND

Cranial ultrasound

Bilateral hyperechogenic signals from globus pallidi have been observed in some infants where serial cranial ultrasound scanning has been performed, particularly in preterm infants who develop BIND [84] (Fig. 10.7). In this case (a 25-week gestation preterm infant) the pallidal hyperintensity was confirmed on T_1-weighted MRI at a corrected age of term. In general, ultrasound is not reliable for the detection of kernicteric brain injury, which requires MRI for confirmation.

MRI and MRS

The diagnosis of BIND is facilitated by the use of MRI – both the localization of the abnormal signal intensity and the evolution over time. The symmetrical involvement of the globus pallidus seen as a hyperintense signal on T_1-weighted MRI is a common and characteristic finding of acute bilirubin encephalopathy [85]. Serial MRI studies have documented a shift from acute mainly T_1 hypersignal (Fig. 10.8) to permanent T_2 hypersignal in the globus pallidus during the late neonatal period [84] (Fig. 10.9). Reports vary, but it is thought that the loss of the hyperintense T_1 signal occurs between the first and third weeks [84]. Similar observations of permanent changes on T_2-weighted imaging of the globus pallidus were also reported in preterm infants [86,87]. Indeed, many of the MRI reports of globus pallidal involvement in BIND include preterm infants, suggesting that pallidal injury in BIND is not dependent on the specific gestation of the infant. Other conditions causing abnormal signal of the globus pallidus on MRI need to be considered, e.g., carbon monoxide, manganese intoxication or a mitochondriopathy. A summary of the MR descriptions of BIND in the literature is in Table 10.5.

Proton (^{1}H) magnetic resonance spectroscopy has been used to study infants with hyperbilirubinemia. A decreased Naa/Cho ratio, indicating neuronal injury, and an abnormally high Lac/Naa ratio were found in an infant with MRI changes in the globus pallidus and who developed cerebral palsy [95]. Despite the abnormal globus pallidus signal intensity on the T_1-weighted MRI, the diffusion-weighted imaging was normal. Another recent study suggests that BIND has a characteristic metabolic signature detectable on ^{1}H MRS; ratios of taurine, glutamate, glutamine, and *myo*-inositol relative to creatine were elevated, whereas the ratio of choline to creatine was decreased compared to normal values at a similar maturational stage [96].

Counseling and prognosis

Babies who develop abnormal neurological signs (Table 10.3) associated with high unconjugated bilirubin levels are at risk of permanent sequelae and should be imaged with MRI. MRI evidence of damage in the globi pallidi is associated with dystonic tetraplegic cerebral palsy, and these children are often severely disabled by their involuntary movements (www.pickonline.org). They are usually hearing impaired and often have upgaze palsy, but their intellect is usually preserved. These children require very specialized schooling and support to maximize their potential. Some children who were later considered to be damaged by kernicterus have normal MRIs [97], hence the need for caution when counseling parents whose baby was symptomatic but has normal imaging. Occasionally, kernicterus can develop in preterm babies who have levels of bilirubin below those which would

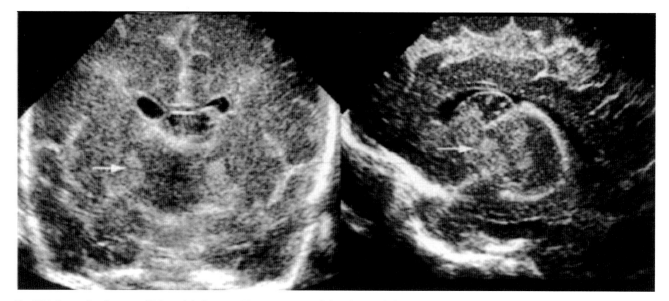

Fig. 10.7. Coronal and parasagittal cranial ultrasound in an ex-preterm infant (25 weeks' gestation) at a corrected age of 32 weeks. A bilateral echogenicity was observed in both globi pallidi (arrows). This was confirmed on MRI at term-corrected age. Reproduced with permission from Govaert *et al.* (2005) [84].

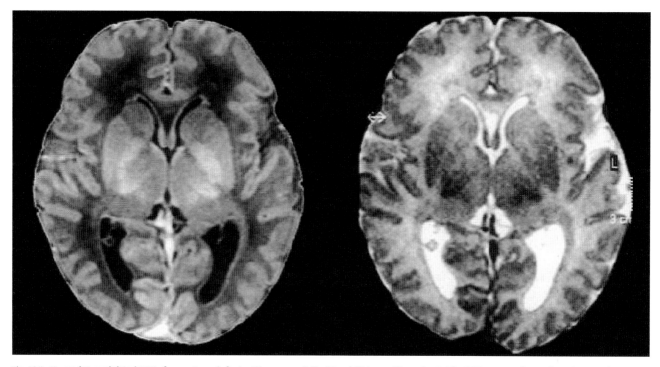

Fig. 10.8. T_1- and T_2-weighted MRIs from a term infant with a serum bilirubin of 776 mmol/l on day 2. The MRI was performed on day 6 and demonstrates a high signal in globus pallidus on T_1, but only a mildly hyperintense signal on T_2. This is in contrast to the permanent increase in signal intensity seen on T_2-weighted images after the early neonatal period associated with gliosis in the following MRIs in Fig 10.9. Reproduced with permission from Govaert *et al.* (2005) [84].

be expected to cause damage and whose clinical signs are so subtle that the diagnosis is not suspected at the time ("low-bilirubin kernicterus"). Increased use of MRI in preterm cohorts will shed more light on this topic and hopefully begin to elucidate risk factors.

Congenital heart disease

Incidence and terminology

Congenital heart disease (CHD) is a common cause of childhood morbidity and occurs in 6–8 per 1000 live births; up to

Table 10.5. Published MRI series detailing the age at MRI and the MRI findings in neonatal cases of severe hyperbilirubinemia. Adapted from Govaert *et al.* (2003) [84]. MRI studies in the early neonatal period generally demonstrate a hyperintense signal in the globus pallidus; the loss of this signal occurs between weeks 1 and 3 after birth leading to a long-term increased signal in the globus pallidus (+ subthalamic nucleus) on T_2 imaging. $\Delta+$, increase of signal intensity; $\Delta-$, no change in signal intensity; $\Delta?$, information unclear; Pallidal, globus pallidus; subthal, subthalamus also affected in a similar way to the globus pallidus.

Author	Term or preterm	Age at MRI	MR findings T_1	MR findings T_2
Penn *et al.* [88]	Term	16 days	$\Delta++$	Pallidal $\Delta+$
Yokochi [89]	Term × 3	3, 7, 12 years		Pallidal $\Delta+$
Martich-Kriss *et al.* [90]	Term	18 days/6 months		Pallidal $\Delta+$
Worley *et al.* [91]	Term	7 months		Pallidal $\Delta+$
Steinborn *et al.* [92]	Term	2.5 years		Pallidal and subthal $\Delta+$
Harris *et al.* [93]	Term × 2	5, 9 days	Pallidal $\Delta+$	
Sugama *et al.* [87]	Preterm × 2	1 year, 10 months, 5 months		Pallidal $\Delta+$
	Term × 1	4 years		Pallidal and subthal $\Delta+$
Okumura *et al.* [86]	Preterm × 2	5, 9 months		Pallidal $\Delta+$
Yilmaz and Ekinci [94]	Term × 8	3–53 months	Normal	Pallidal $\Delta+$
Govaert *et al.* [84]	Preterm × 1	38 weeks	Pallidal and subthal $\Delta+$ Normal	$\Delta-$
	Preterm × 4	12–22 months	Pallidal and subthal $\Delta+$ Normal	Pallidal and subthal $\Delta+$
	Term × 1 (G6PD deficient)	6 days	Pallidal and subthal $\Delta+$	Pallidal and subthal $\Delta+$
	Term × 2	3 months		Pallidal and subthal $\Delta+$
		6–12 days		Pallidal $\Delta+$
Groenendaal *et al.* [95]	Term × 5	1–7 days	Normal × 4	$\Delta?$
			Pallidal $\Delta+$ × 1	$\Delta?$

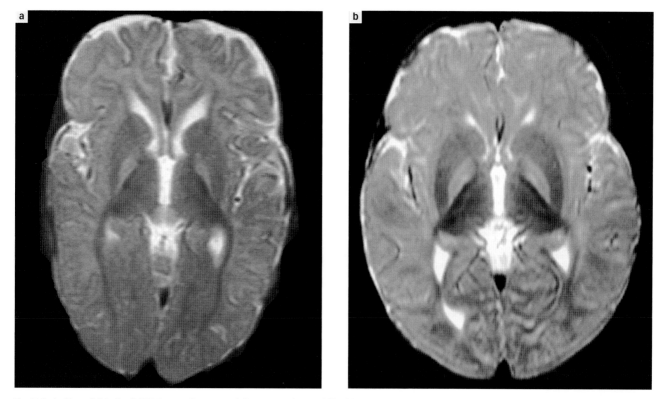

Fig. 10.9a,b. T_2-weighted axial MRI scans in mature injury secondary to bilirubin toxicity. (a) The scan is from a child of 9 months of age showing bilateral symmetrical increased signal within the globus pallidi with volume loss. This child had been born preterm, and developed "low bilirubin" kernicterus during the neonatal course. The child was disabled, with athetoid cerebral palsy and sensorineural deafness requiring aiding. (b) The scan is from a child of a year, who had undergone an exchange transfusion in the neonatal period for a peak serum bilirubin of 720 µmol/l due to hemolysis secondary to ABO incompatibility. There are similar appearances but without the volume loss, and, like the child whose scan is shown in (a), this child had athetoid cerebral palsy and sensorineural deafness requiring aiding.

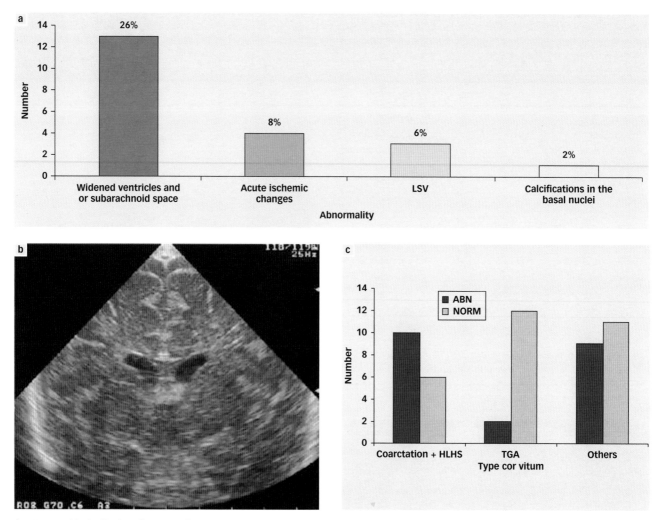

Fig. 10.10a–c. **(a)** Distribution of preoperative cerebral abnormalities on cranial ultrasound in infants with major congenital heart disease (CHD). **(b)** Preoperative cranial ultrasound scan in a patient with coarctation of the aorta. The coronal view through the third ventricle shows enlarged ventricles and widened subarachnoid space. This was the commonest cerebral abnormality on cranial ultrasound, occurring in 26% of cases. **(c)** Distribution of cerebral abnormalities according to type of CHD in 50 full-term infants with major CHD. Reproduced with permission from te Pas *et al.* (2005) [103].

50% of these children require open heart surgery to correct their defect. Several studies have shown that up to 50% of childhood survivors of CHD have impairments in several domains: fine motor skills, visuo-spatial skills, and cognition [98,99,100]. Although the incidence of neurodevelopmental impairment in newborns with CHD is as important as more commonly recognized conditions such as perinatal asphyxia and even prematurity, we are only beginning to understand the basis for these global deficits.

Studies of brain injury in newborns with CHD have mainly reported on aspects of treatment regarding surgery and cardiopulmonary bypass, however long-term neurodevelopmental deficits are seen even with attempts to normalize the cerebral blood flow during surgery [101]. Recently it has been recognized that more than half of newborns with CHD have neurological abnormalities prior to surgery and these abnormalities are a significant risk for later neurodevelopmental impairment [102].

Cranial ultrasound

A high incidence of cranial ultrasound abnormalities has been found preoperatively in newborn infants with CHD [103,104]. In the study by Te Pas from the Netherlands, 42% of full-term infants with major CHD admitted to Neonatal Intensive Care Units (NICU) had abnormal cranial ultrasound prior to surgery [103]. Widening of the ventricular and subarachnoid spaces was the most common abnormality and was seen in one-quarter of cases (Fig. 10.10a,b). Lenticulostriate vasculopathy (LSV) was seen in 6%; parenchymal echodensities and intraventricular hemorrhage (IVH) were also common. Compared to a similarly studied cohort of low-risk patients, there was a much higher incidence in patients with CHD. Van Houten also demonstrated abnormalities on cranial ultrasound in 59% of CHD infants compared to 14% of controls [104]; most of the abnormalities were diagnosed before surgery. Certainly, compared to the published cohorts of apparently well infants undergoing cranial ultrasound in whom ∼25% exhibit

Table 10.6. Timing and classification of cerebral injury on pre- and postoperative MRI in a series of 62 infants with congenital heart disease (CHD). Reproduced with permission from McQuillen *et al.* (2007) [106]. WMI, white matter injury; HI, hypoxic ischemia.

Timing of injury	Non-cystic WMI	Stroke	Intraventricular hemorrhage	Global HI
Preoperative (*n* = 62)	11 (18%)	13 (21%)	5 (8%)	0 (0%)
Postoperative (*n* = 53)	14 (26%)	5 (9%)	0 (0%)	0 (0%)

an abnormality [3], the incidence of cranial ultrasound abnormalities in infants with CHD prior to surgery appears to be almost double.

It is possible that brain abnormalities are more frequent in certain types of CHD; in one study cerebral abnormalities were more frequently seen in infants with hypoplastic left heart syndrome (HLHS) and coarctation of the aorta than in infants with transposition of the great arteries (TGA) [103] (Fig. 10.10c). Larger studies are needed to confirm this, but different patterns of altered antenatal blood flow may explain this difference in cerebral abnormality rates in different types of CHD.

There is mounting evidence that newborns with CHD have had impaired in utero brain growth possibly related to impaired cerebral oxygen delivery prenatally [105]. Cerebral atrophy takes several weeks to develop, and LSV probably also takes several weeks before it is visible on cranial ultrasound.

MRI and MRS in CHD
In the largest series of infants with CHD studied with MRI before and after neonatal surgery, more than one-third of newborns with CHD had brain injury before cardiac surgery [106]; this was most commonly stroke and was associated with balloon atrial septostomy [102]. An additional third of newborns acquired brain injury during or shortly after cardiac surgery; this was most commonly white matter injury and was particularly common in infants with single ventricle physiology and aortic arch obstruction [106]. The timing and types of cerebral injury in 62 infants with CHD studied prospectively with MRI are shown in Table 10.6 and MRI examples (pre- and postoperatively in different cardiac conditions) are shown in Fig. 10.11. The basal ganglia/thalamus or watershed pattern of injury was not observed in any newborn with CHD.

An abnormal brain microstructure and metabolism has been observed after birth in many newborns with CHD using diffusion-weighted imaging and ^{1}H MRS. The metabolic abnormalities in CHD include an elevated brain lactate and lower Naa/Cho [2,107]. In a recent study comparing 41 infants with congenital heart disease (29 with TGA and 12 with single ventricle physiology) with 16 control newborns of similar gestational age, those with congenital heart disease had a decrease of 10% in the ratio of *N*-acetylaspartate to choline ($p = 0.03$), an increase of 28% in the ratio of lactate to choline ($p = 0.08$), an increase of 4% in average diffusivity ($p < 0.001$), and a decrease of 12% in white-matter fractional anisotropy ($p < 0.001$) [108]. White matter injury is typically the pattern of injury observed in the premature newborn, yet full-term infants with CHD have a very high incidence of white matter injury with similar characteristics to the preterm infant. It has been suggested that this delayed development may be due to impaired in utero cerebral oxygen delivery.

Prognosis and counseling
The high incidence of cerebral abnormalities warrants routine cranial ultrasound in all newborn infants with CHD prior to surgery. Some units are able to offer pre-surgery MRI, but this depends on the stability of the infant. Parents need to be counseled regarding the increased risk for cognitive, fine motor and visuo-spatial abnormalities in infants with CHD and told that the cause for the neurological sequelae are complex and depend on fetal, preoperative, intraoperative, and postoperative factors. As more is learned about the specific characteristics of brain injury in CHD and emerging therapies for the prevention of brain injury are translated into clinical practice, the outcome for these infants in the future may improve.

Vascular birth marks: Sturge Weber syndrome
Sturge Weber syndrome (SWS) is a congenital neurocutaneous disorder with a facial capillary malformation (port wine stain), abnormal blood vessels of the brain (leptomeningeal angioma), or abnormal blood vessels in the eye predisposing to glaucoma [109]. The etiology of SWS remains unclear and no patterns of inheritance have been identified, although the sporadic and focal nature of SWS suggests the presence of a somatic mutation.

EEG in SWS
The typical EEG is asymmetric with the affected hemisphere showing a reduction in voltage and slowing of the background activity [110]. The asymmetry becomes more obvious as the atrophy of the hemisphere progresses.

Brain imaging in SWS
Computed tomography (CT) scanning is still used to demonstrate intracranial calcifications. Magnetic resonance imaging with gadolinium enhancement is used to demonstrate the leptomeningeal angioma. Magnetic resonance angiography shows diminution of the caliber of the arteries, thickening of the internal veins, an increase in the size of the choroid plexus, and an absence of the superficial hemispheric veins on the affected side [111]. High-resolution BOLD (blood-oxygen-level-dependent) MR venography has been shown to help with early diagnosis of this condition, which is an important goal [112]. Diffusion MRI has been reported to show restricted diffusion and high ADC in the affected area [113]. Magnetic resonance perfusion imaging has been shown to be useful in the assessment of SWS [114]. Despite the recent advances in neuroimaging and increased knowledge of the molecular pathology of SWS, a full understanding of the neurological progression in SWS and ways to prevent this are still unknown.

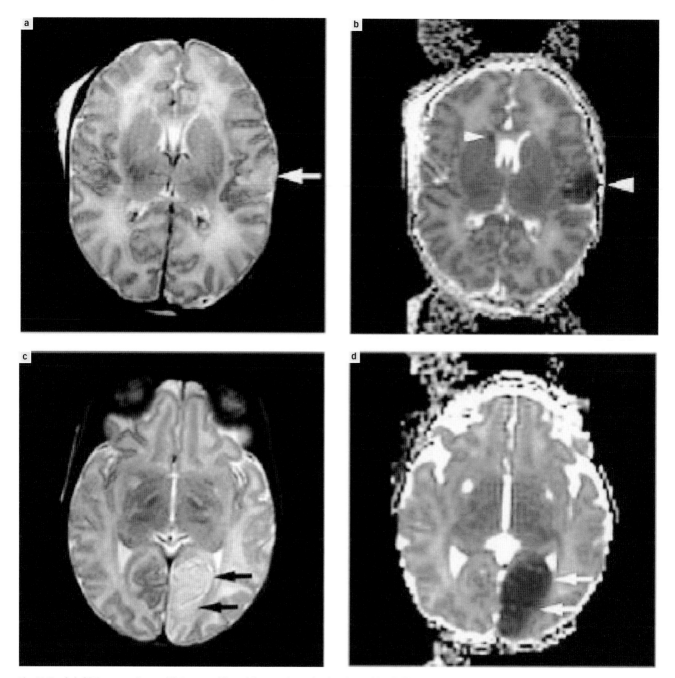

Fig. 10.11a–f. (a,b) Term newborn with transposition of the great arteries (TGA) requiring balloon atrial septostomy on day 1, imaged 48 hours later. On the T$_2$-weighted image (a) a subtle region of signal abnormality with sulcal effacement and loss of the cortical ribbon (arrow) in the distribution of a branch of the left middle cerebral artery is seen. (b) A corresponding hypointense region consistent with restricted diffusion (large arrow) is seen on the diffusivity map (arrowhead). (c,d) Term newborn with unbalanced complete atrioventricular septal defect (AVSD) imaged postoperatively on day 18, 7 days after a Norwood procedure. (c) T$_2$-weighted MRI scan shows a region of signal hyperintensity and swelling involving the left mesial occipital lobe in the territory of the posterior cerebral artery (black arrows) with reduced diffusivity (d). The appearances are those of an acute infarct.

Specific brain abnormalities that may be detected in apparently well neonates on a postnatal ward

Lenticulostriate vasculopathy

Incidence and clinical implications

Lenticulostriate vasculopathy (LSV) was first described by Grant in 1985 [115]. LSV is the description given to hyperechoic lenticulostriate arteries in the basal ganglia and thalamus and was first described on CT and cranial ultrasound images [115]. LSV can be unilateral or bilateral and has either a punctate pattern or a branching linear pattern – described as "branched candlestick stripes" (Fig. 10.12) [116,117,118,119]. The incidence of LSV is 0.4% of all liveborn neonates and 1.9%–5.8% of ill neonates [116,120,121,122]. In a prospective study of 1184 infants admitted to NICU during a 3-year period, the incidence

224

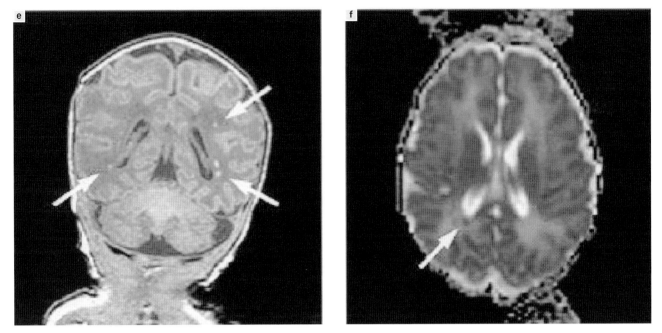

Fig. 10.11. (cont.) (e,f) Term newborn with TGA imaged postoperatively on day 16, 8 days after arterial switch procedure. Multiple foci of T_1 hyperintensity are seen on the coronal image (arrows). Some foci have reduced diffusivity ((f), arrow). Reproduced with permission from McQuillen *et al.* (2007) [106].

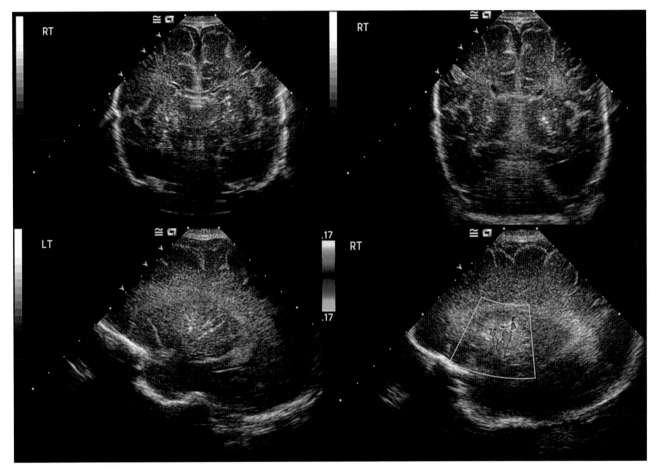

Fig. 10.12. **Top row:** coronal ultrasound scans from an expreterm infant (24 weeks of gestation) at term-equivalent age with hyperechoic lenticulostriate arteries in the basal ganglia and thalamus (lenticulostriate vasculopathy). Both a punctate pattern (left coronal view) and linear branching pattern (right coronal view) can be visualized. Bottom row: sagittal ultrasound scans demonstrating bright linear branched candlestick stripes from the vessels supplying the basal ganglia and thalamus (left sagittal view). The vessel patency and vascular nature of these basal ganglia and thalamic echogenicities is confirmed on color Doppler (right sagittal view).

Table 10.7. Fetal and neonatal conditions associated with lenticulostriate vasculopathy (LSV). TTTS, Twin-to-twin transfusion syndrome.

Neonatal and fetal conditions associated with LSV	Representative publications supporting this association
Fetal and neonatal infections	
CMV	De Vries et al. (2004) [123]
	Estroff et al. (1992) [124]
Rubella	Chang et al. (1996) [125]
HIV	Bode and Rudin (1995) [126]
Toxoplasma	Virkola et al. (1997) [127]
Syphilis	Wang et al. (1995) [116]
Hypoxia ischemia	Coley et al. (2000) [128]
Bacterial meningitis	Wang et al. (1995) [116]
Multiple births (TTTS)	De Vries et al. (1995) [129]
Congenital heart disease	Coley et al. (2000) [128]
	Hughes et al. (1991) [119]
Neonatal lupus	Cabañas et al. (1996) [130]
Infantile sialidosis	Ries et al. (1992) [131]
Fetal alcohol or drug exposure	Wang et al. (1995) [116]
Encephalitis	Wang et al. (1995) [116]
Chromosomal abnormalities	
Trisomy 21	Wang et al. (1995) [116]
Trisomy 13	Chabra et al. (1997) [132]
	Kriss and Kriss (1996) [133]
Congenital malformations	Coley et al. (2000) [128]
	Cabañas et al. (1994) [118]
	Kriss and Kriss (1996) [133]

of LSV was 2.45%. The cases were compared with 42 matched controls; except for more multiple births, neonates with LSV did not show more adverse findings than their matched controls [122].

Lenticulostriate vasculopathy is not thought to cause problems itself but is a marker for certain conditions (Table 10.7). There are many retrospective studies reporting an association of LSV with fetal and neonatal infections (mainly cytomegalovirus) [125,134], chromosomal abnormalities [133,135], hypoxic ischemia [128], CHD [128], fetal alcohol or drug exposure [119], congenital malformations, neonatal lupus erythematosus [130], twin-to-twin transfusion [129], hydrops fetalis, and infants of diabetic mothers.

Fetal intracranial hemodynamics may play a role in the pathogenesis of LSV. For example, a fetus at 31 weeks' gestation was found to have echogenic vessels in the thalami and basal ganglia [124]. The blood flow in the lenticulostriate arteries supplying the thalamus and basal ganglia is high in utero as there is active proliferation in the germinal matrix regions near the caudothalamic grooves [136]. It has been proposed that trivial insults may produce vascular changes in

these regions with high blood flow, but damage to the brain itself is limited because of the abundant blood flow [116]. LSV is merely an indicator of non-specific early insults to the developing brain.

Histopathology

Most of the lenticulostriate arteries that are involved in LSV are medium-sized, and have thickened and hypercellular walls with no associated fibrosis. Typically there is an intramural and perivascular deposition of a basophilic material, iron and calcium, and frequently there are also signs of vessel wall damage.

Brain imaging studies

Cranial ultrasound

In normal infants the small arteries supplying the basal ganglia are indistinct from the brain parenchyma. Bright, linear, branched candlestick stripes, termed LSV, have been reported in these regions in more than 200 infants in the English literature. Cranial ultrasound is the best tool for detecting LSV; vessel patency can be confirmed on color Doppler. The vascular nature of these basal ganglia and thalamic echogenicities is shown on Doppler ultrasound in Fig. 10.12, bottom right. In contrast with cranial ultrasound, CT is less sensitive at detecting the increased attenuation of vessels in the thalamus or basal ganglia in LSV series [116]. LSV may progress, stay the same or resolve [116,121].

Magnetic resonance imaging

Magnetic resonance imaging is less sensitive than cranial ultrasound in detecting LSV [116]. In one series, however, MRI showed areas of linear increased signal in regions corresponding to the thalamus and basal ganglia in 4 of 23 cases with LSV diagnosed on ultrasound [128].

Prognosis and counseling

Follow-up studies have reported a neurodevelopmental delay in 19%–55% of infants with LSV diagnosed in the newborn period; this wide range probably reflects the diverse associations of LSV [117,138]. In one series, idiopathic LSV on cranial ultrasound in infancy predicted the development of neuropsychiatric disorders later in childhood [139]; this needs to be confirmed in larger studies. It is generally thought that in the absence of underlying conditions such as fetal TORCH (Toxoplasmosis, Other agents, Rubella, CMV, Herpes simplex) infections, chromosomal abnormalities, malformations or hypoxia ischemia survival without adverse clinical outcome is the rule in newborns in whom LSV is detected.

Subependymal pseudocysts

Incidence and clinical implications

Subependymal pseudocysts are found in 0.5%–5.2% of newborn infants on cranial ultrasound or autopsy [140]. The condition was first described by Larroche in 22 autopsy cases [141]. The terms *germinolytic pseudocyst*, *germinal matrix pseudocyst* or *germinal layer pseudocyst* all mean the same thing; in this chapter we

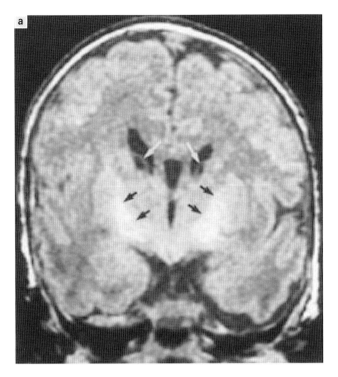

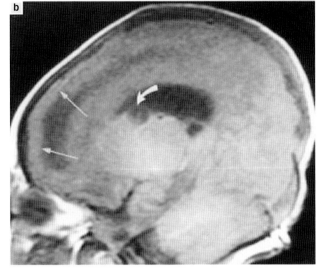

Fig. 10.13a–c. **T$_1$-weighted coronal (a) and sagittal (b) MRI scans from an infant with Zellweger syndrome. Subependymal pseudocysts can be seen in both views. The bilateral subependymal pseudocysts can be easily seen in the autopsy specimen of Zellweger syndrome in (c). Reproduced with permission from Barkovich and Peck (1997) [137].**

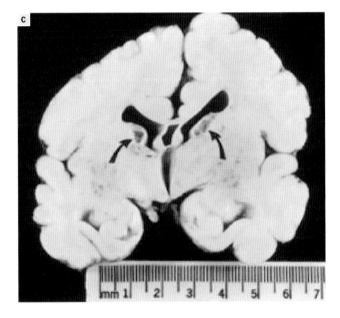

The term *pseudocyst* is used because of the absence of epithelial lining of the cyst wall. They are thought to be the result of antenatal germinal matrix regression or germinolysis. Cysts probably occur following hemorrhage or microinfarction of the germinal matrix. In preterm infants SEPCs are often located at the caudothalamic notch and, less frequently, around the frontal horns of the lateral ventricles [143]. It is thought that those SEPCs situated in the anterior horns of the lateral ventricles are formed earlier than those forming in the caudothalamic notch, as the germinal matrix is present in the frontal horns up to around 28 weeks' gestation and in the caudothalamic notch until 34–35 weeks' gestation. The advent of high-resolution antenatal ultrasound has permitted the detection of SEPCs prenatally, showing that they arise in prenatal life [144].

Associated congenital abnormalities such as cardiac defects have been identified [145,146] and congenital viral infections, especially rubella and cytomegalovirus infection, are associated with SEPCs [147,148,149,150]. Subependymal pseudocysts are described in some metabolic disorders, especially Zellweger syndrome (Fig. 10.13a–c) [151] and organic acidemias such as glutaric aciduria type 1 [152]. See Table 10.8 for the fetal and neonatal conditions associated with SEPCs.

Imaging

Cranial ultrasound

Subependymal pseudocysts are easily detected by ultrasound in the neonatal period. Typically they appear as tear-shaped echolucent areas adjacent to the caudothalamic groove on

will use the term subependymal pseudocyst (SEPC). The term SEPC is used for cysts seen within or adjacent to the lateral walls of the anterior horns of the ventricles or in the head of the caudate nuclei. They may be difficult to differentiate from strands that appear to run across the anterior horns of the lateral ventricles. The term "periventricular" should not be used as this may be mistaken for periventricular leukomalacia [142].

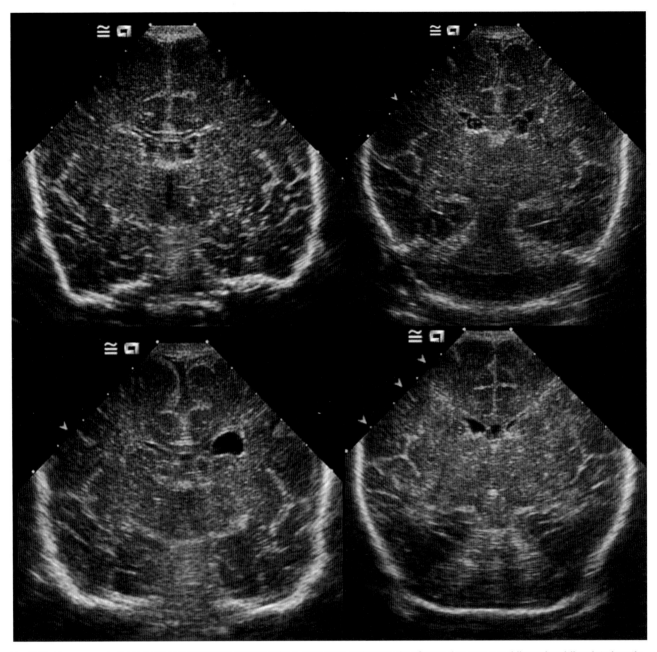

Fig. 10.14. **Four coronal ultrasound images in three preterm infants born at 34 and 35 weeks of gestation. Top row: bilateral multiloculated cystic formation within the caudo-thalamo groove. These cysts were observed on the admission cranial ultrasound scan. TORCH screen was negative. Bottom row: unilateral round cysts adjacent to the anterior horn of the lateral ventricle. As seen in these images subependymal pseudocysts (SEPCs) can mimic a widened frontal horn, but they are integrated in the ventricle.**

the floor of the lateral ventricle (Figs. 10.14, 10.15). Serial cranial ultrasound studies have shown that SEPCs resolve or diminish in size (on average 23 weeks after the initial cranial ultrasound) [153].

Magnetic resonance imaging
Subenpendymal pseudocysts can be visualized on MRI (Fig. 10.16).

Counseling and prognosis
When pseudocysts are isolated then they regress spontaneously and their prognosis is good [143,145,153,157,158]. If there are associated cerebral abnormalities present then the risk for neurodevelopmental impairment is dependent on the nature of these abnormalities. It is important to make the distinction between pseudocysts and cystic periventricular leukomalacia.

Table 10.8. Fetal and neonatal conditions associated with subependymal pseudocysts (SEPCs).

Fetal and neonatal conditions associated with SEPCs	Representative publications supporting this association
Following GMH-IVH: these appear within 1–2 weeks and are relatively short-lived	Ramenghi *et al.* (1997) [143]
Idiopathic in preterm infants: occasionally caudothalamic SEPCs appear in preterm infants ~4 weeks after birth apparently not related to GMH-IVH or infection	Larcos *et al.* (1994) [153]
Viral infection:	
CMV testing for CMV is mandatory for any cyst not related to GMH-IVH	De Vries *et al.* (2004) [123]
Rubella	
Toxoplasma	
HIV	
Multiple births (TTTS)	
Metabolic disorders	Twomey *et al.* (2003) [152]
Organic acidemias (glutaric aciduria type 1, methylmalonic acidemia)	van Straaten *et al.* (2005) [154]
Mitochondrial spectrum disorders: complex I, IV, pyruvate dehydrogenase deficiency	Russel *et al.* (1995) [151]
Zellweger syndrome	Barkovich *et al.* (1997) [137]
Neonatal lupus syndrome	Zuppa *et al.* (2004) [155]
Maternal substance abuse (cocaine)	Cohen *et al.* (1994) [156]

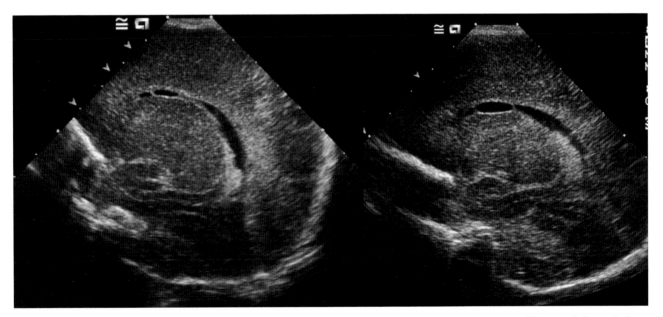

Fig. 10.15. **Lateral parasagittal cranial ultrasound scans in two preterm infants of 34 weeks of gestation (right image of the same infant as in the left lower image of Fig. 10.14; left image of the same infant as in right lower image in Fig. 10.14). As shown here on parasagittal images the cysts appear elongated and are often formed in one or two parts separated by thin septa.**

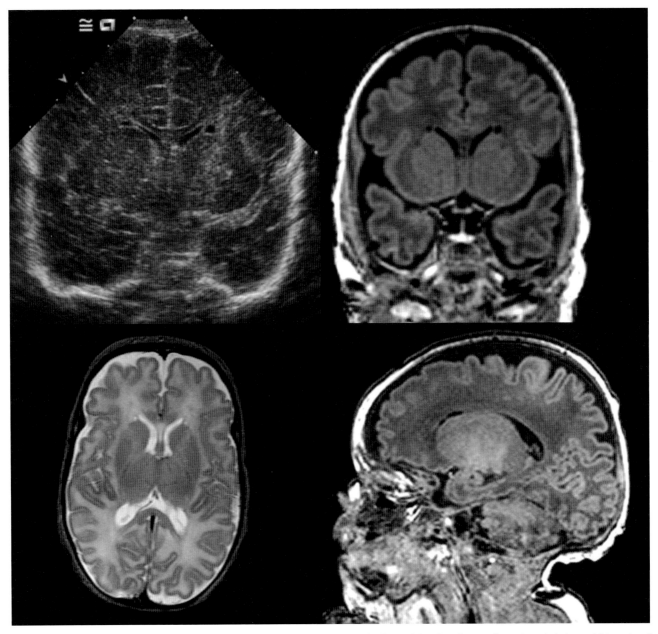

Fig. 10.16. **Coronal ultrasound, coronal T$_1$-weighted, axial T$_2$-weighted and, parasagittal T$_1$-weighted MR image of a preterm twin born at 26 weeks of gestation scanned at term-equivalent age. The cysts appeared at around 1 month of age; they were bilateral and adjacent to the frontal horn of the lateral ventricle.**

References

1. Cutfield W, Hofman P, Mitchell M, Morison I. Could epigenetics play a role in the developmental origins of health and disease? *Pediatr Res* 2007; **61(5 pt 2)**: 68R–75R.

2. Miller S, McQuillen P, Vigneron D *et al.* Preoperative brain injury in newborns with transposition of the great arteries. *Ann Thorac Surg.* 2004 **77(5)**: 1698–706.

3. Mercuri E, Dubowitz L, Brown S, Cowan F. Incidence of cranial ultrasound abnormalities in apparently well neonates on a postnatal ward: correlation with antenatal and perinatal factors and neurological status. *Arch Dis Child Fetal Neonatal Ed* 1998; **79(3)**: F185–9.

4. Wang L, Huang C, Yeh T. Major brain lesions detected on sonographic screening of apparently normal term neonates. *Neuroradiology* 2004; **46**: 368–73.

5. Looney C, Smith J, Merck L *et al.* Intracranial hemorrhage in asymptomatic neonates: prevalence on MR images and relationship to obstetric and neonatal risk factors. *Radiology* 2007; **242(2)**: 535–41.

6. OPCS 1997 Birth Statistics. *Review of the Register General on Births and Patterns of Family Building in England and Wales.* London, HMSO, 1997.

7. Petterson B, Nelson K, Watson L, Stanley F. Twins, triplets, and cerebral palsy in births in Western Australia in the 1980s. *Br Med J* 1993; **307(6914)**: 1239–43.

8. Bajoria R, Wee L, Anwar S, Ward S. Outcome of twin pregnancies complicated by single intrauterine death in relation to vascular anatomy of the monochorionic placenta. *Hum Reprod* 1999; **14**(8): 2124–30.

9. Bejar R, Vigliocco G, Gramajo H et al. Antenatal origin of neurologic damage in newborn infants. II. Multiple gestations. *Am J Obstet Gynecol* 1990; **162**(5): 1230–6.

10. Benirschke K, Kim C. Multiple pregnancy. 2. *N Engl J Med* 1973; **288**(25): 1329–36.

11. Pharoah P, Cooke T. Cerebral palsy and multiple births. *Arch Dis Child Fetal Neonatal Ed* 1996; **75**(3): F174–7.

12. Grafe M. Antenatal cerebral necrosis in monochorionic twins. *Pediatr Pathol* 1993; **13**(1): 15–19.

13. Adegbite A, Castille S, Ward S, Bajoria R. Prevalence of cranial scan abnormalities in preterm twins in relation to chorionicity and discordant birth weight. *Eur J Obstet Gynecol Reprod Biol* 2005; **119**(1): 47–55.

14. Cheung V, Bocking A, Dasilva O. Preterm discordant twins: what birth weight difference is significant? *Am J Obstet Gynecol* 1995; **172**(3): 955–9.

15. Yinon Y, Mazkereth R, Rosentzweig N, Jarus-Hakak A, Schiff E, Simchen M. Growth restriction as a determinant of outcome in preterm discordant twins. *Obstet Gynecol* 2005; **105**(1): 80–4.

16. Acosta-Rojas R, Becker J, Munoz-Abellana B et al. Twin chorionicity and the risk of adverse perinatal outcome. *Int J Gynaecol Obstet* 2007; **96**(2): 98–102.

17. Dickinson J, Duncombe G, Evans S, French N, Hagan R. The long term neurologic outcome of children from pregnancies complicated by twin-to-twin transfusion syndrome. *Br J Obstet Gynaecol* 2005; **112**(1): 63–8.

18. Lemoine P, Harrousseau H, Borteyru J, Menuet J. Les infants des parents alcoholoques. Anomalies observées. *A propos 127 cas. Ouest-Medical* 1968; **25**: 476–82.

19. Rosett H. A clinical perspective of the Fetal Alcohol Syndrome. *Alcohol Clin Exp Res* 1980; **4**(2): 119–22.

20. Autti-Rämö I, Autti T, Korkman M, Kettunen S, Salonen O, Valanne L. MRI findings in children with school problems who had been exposed prenatally to alcohol. *Dev Med Child Neurol* 2002; **44**(2): 98–106.

21. Riley E, McGee C, Sowell E. Teratogenic effects of alcohol: a decade of brain imaging. *Am J Med Genet C Semin Med Genet* 2004; **127**(1): 35–41.

22. Archibald S, Fennema-Notestine C, Gamst A, Riley E, Mattson S, Jernigan T. Brain dysmorphology in individuals with severe prenatal alcohol exposure. *Dev Med Child Neurol* 2001; **43**(3): 148–54.

23. Clark C, Li D, Conry J, Conry R, Loock C. Structural and functional brain integrity of fetal alcohol syndrome in nonretarded cases. *Pediatrics* 2000; **105**(5): 1096–9.

24. Bookstein F, Connor P, Huggins J, Barr H, Pimentel K, Streissguth A. Many infants prenatally exposed to high levels of alcohol show one particular anomaly of the corpus callosum. *Alcohol Clin Exp Res* 2007; **31**(5): 868–79.

25. Wozniak J, Mueller B, Chang P, Muetzel R, Caros L, Lim K. Diffusion tensor imaging in children with fetal alcohol spectrum disorders. *Alcohol Clin Exp Res* 2006; **30**(10): 1799–806.

26. King T, Perlman J, Laptook A, Rollins N, Jackson G, Little B. Neurologic manifestations of in utero cocaine exposure in near-term and term infants. *Pediatrics* 1995; **96**(2 Pt 1): 259–64.

27. Behnke M, Eyler F, Garvan C, Wobie K. The search for congenital malformations in newborns with fetal cocaine exposure. *Pediatrics* 2001; **107**(5): E74.

28. Frank D, McCarten K, Robson C et al. Level of in utero cocaine exposure and neonatal ultrasound findings. *Pediatrics* 1999; **104**(5 Pt 1): 1101–5.

29. Shankaran S, Lester BM, Das A et al. Impact of maternal substance use during pregnancy on childhood outcome. *Semin Fetal Neonatal Med* 2007; **12**(2): 143–50.

30. Vannucci R, Vannucci S. Hypoglycemic brain injury. *Semin Neonatol* 2001; **6**(2): 147–55.

31. Hawdon J. Metabolic disease: disorders of glucose homeostasis. In: Rennie JM, ed. *Roberton's Textbook of Neonatology*, 4th edn. London, Elsevier Churchill Livingstone, 2005; 853–865.

32. Lucas A, Morley R, Cole T. Adverse neurodevelopmental outcome of moderate neonatal hypoglycaemia. *Br Med J* 1988; **297**(6659): 1304–8.

33. Hawdon J, Ward Platt M, Aynsley-Green A. Patterns of metabolic adaptation for preterm and term infants in the first neonatal week. *Arch Dis Child Fetal Neonatal Ed* 1992; **67**: 357–65.

34. Eyre J, Stuart A, Forsyth R, Heaviside D, Bartlett K. Glucose export from the brain in man: evidence for a role for astrocytic glycogen as a reservoir of glucose for neural metabolism. *Brain Res Brain Res Rev* 1994; **635** (1–2): 349–52.

35. Owen O, Morgan A, Kemp H, Sullivan J, Herrera M, Cahill G. Brain metabolism during fasting. *J Clin Invest* 1967; **46**(10): 1589–95.

36. Hawkins R, Williamson D, Krebs H. Ketone-body utilization by adult and suckling rat brain in vivo. *Biochem J* 1971; **122**(1): 13–18.

37. Spitzer J, Weng J. Removal and utilization of ketone bodies by the brain of newborn puppies. *J Neurochem* 1972; **19**(9): 2169–73.

38. Cremer J, Cunningham V, Pardridge W, Braun L, Oldendorf W. Kinetics of blood–brain barrier transport of pyruvate, lactate and glucose in suckling, weanling and adult rats. *J Neurochem* 1979; **33**(2): 439–45.

39. Hellmann J, Vannucci R, Nardis E. Blood–brain barrier permeability to lactic acid in the newborn dog: lactate as a cerebral metabolic fuel. *Pediatr Res* 1982; **16**(1): 40–4.

40. de Rooy L, Hawdon J. Nutritional factors that affect the postnatal metabolic adaptation of full-term small- and large-for-gestational-age infants. *Pediatrics* 2002; **109**(3): E42.

41. Kinnala A, Suhonen-Polvi H, Äärimaa T et al. Cerebral metabolic rate for glucose during the first six months of life: an FDG positron emission tomography study. *Arch Dis Child Fetal Neonatal Ed* 1996; **74**(3): F153–7.

42. Anwar M, Vannucci R. Autoradiographic determination of regional cerebral blood flow during hypoglycemia in newborn dogs. *Pediatr Res* 1988; **24**(1): 41–5.

43. Pryds O, Greisen G, Friis-Hansen B. Compensatory increase of CBF in preterm infants during hypoglycaemia. *Acta Paediatr Scand* 1988; **77**(5): 632–7.

44. Volpe J. Hypoglycaemia and brain injury. In: Volpe J, ed. *Neurology of the Newborn*, 4th edn. Philadelphia, Saunders, 2001; 497–520.

45. Banker BQ. The neuropathological effects of anoxia and hypoglycemia in the newborn. *Dev Med Child Neurol* 1967; **9**(5): 544–50.

46. Anderson J, Milner R, Strich S. Effects of neonatal hypoglycaemia on the nervous system: a pathological study. *J Neurol Neurosurg Psychiatry* 1967; **30**(4): 295–310.

47. Meissner T, Wendel U, Burgard P, Schaetzle S, Mayatepek E. Long-term follow-up of 114 patients with congenital hyperinsulinism. *Eur J Endocrinol* 2003; **149**(1): 43–51.

48. Menni F, de Lonlay P, Sevin C et al. Neurologic outcomes of 90 neonates and infants with persistent hyperinsulinemic hypoglycemia. *Pediatrics* 2001; **107**(3): 476–9.

49. Glauser T, Rorke L, Weinberg P, Clancy R. Acquired neuropathologic lesions associated with the hypoplastic left heart syndrome. *Pediatrics* 1990; **85**(6): 991–1000.

50. Yager J, Brucklacher R, Vannucci R. Cerebral oxidative metabolism and redox state during hypoxia-ischemia and early recovery in immature rats. *Am J Physiol* 1991; **261**(4(2)): H1102–8.

51. Koh T, Eyre J, Aynsley-Green A. Neonatal hypoglycaemia – the controversy regarding definition. *Arch Dis Child* 1988; **63**(11): 1386–8.

52. Kinnala A, Rikalainen H, Lapinleimu H, Parkkola R, Kormano M, Kero P. Cerebral magnetic resonance imaging and ultrasonography findings after neonatal hypoglycemia. *Pediatrics* 1999; **103**(4(1)): 724–9.

53. Filan P, Inder T, Cameron F, Kean M, Hunt R. Neonatal hypoglycemia and occipital cerebral injury. *J Pediatr* 2006; **148**(4): 552–5.

54. Spar J, Lewine J, Orrison W. Neonatal hypoglycemia: CT and MR findings. *AJNR Am J Neuroradiol* 1994; **15**(8): 1477–8.

55. Aslan Y, Dinc H. MR findings of neonatal hypoglycemia. *AJNR Am J Neuroradiol* 1997; **18**(5): 994–6.

56. Barkovich A, Ali F, Rowley H, Bass N. Imaging patterns of neonatal hypoglycemia. *AJNR Am J Neuroradiol* 1998; **19**(3): 523–8.

57. Traill Z, Squier M, Anslow P. Brain imaging in neonatal hypoglycaemia. *Arch Dis Child Fetal Neonatal Ed* 1998; **79**(2): F145–7.

58. Murakami Y, Yamashita Y, Matsuishi T, Utsunomiya H, Okudera T, Hashimoto T. Cranial MRI of neurologically impaired children suffering from neonatal hypoglycaemia. *Pediatr Radiol* 1999; **29**(1): 23–7.

59. Cakmakci H, Usal C, Karabay N, Kovanlikaya A. Transient neonatal hypoglycemia: cranial US and MRI findings. *Eur Radiol* 2001; **11**(12): 2585–8.

60. Caraballo R, Sakr D, Mozzi M *et al.* Symptomatic occipital lobe epilepsy following neonatal hypoglycemia. *Pediatr Neurol* 2004; **31**(1): 24–9.

61. Hamano S, Tanaka M, Mochizuki M, Sugiyama N, Eto Y. Long-term follow-up study of West syndrome: differences of outcome among symptomatic etiologies. *J Pediatr* 2003; **143**(2): 231–5.

62. Bhutani VK JL, Sivieri EM. Predictive ability of a predischarge hour-specific serum bilirubin for subsequent significant hyperbilirubinemia in healthy term and near-term newborns. *Pediatrics* 1999; **103**(1): 6–14.

63. Smitherman H, Stark A, Bhutan V. Early recognition of neonatal hyperbilirubinemia and its emergent management. *Semin Fetal Neonatal Med* 2006; **11**(3): 214–24.

64. Fok T. Neonatal jaundice – traditional Chinese medicine approach. *J Perinatol* 2001; **21**(Suppl 1): S98–S100.

65. Arkwright J. A family series of fatal and dangerous cases of icterus neonatorum: fouteen cases in one family, with four survivors. *Edin Med J* 1902; **2**: 156–8.

66. Cremer R, Perryman P, Richards D. Influence of light on the hyperbilirubinaemia of infants. *Lancet* 1958; **1**(7030): 1094–7.

67. Johnson L, Brown A, VK B. BIND – a clinical score for bilirubin induced neurologic dysfunction in newborns. *Pediatric Suppl* 1999; **104**: 746–7.

68. Doré S, Snyder S. Neuroprotective action of bilirubin against oxidative stress in primary hippocampal cultures. *Ann N Y Acad Sci* 1999; **890**: 167–72.

69. MacDonald M. Hidden risks: early discharge and bilirubin toxicity due to glucose 6-phosphate dehydrogenase deficiency. *Pediatrics* 1995; **96**(4 **(Pt 1)**): 734–8.

70. Seidman D, Paz I, Stevenson D, Laor A, Danon Y, Gale R. Neonatal hyperbilirubinemia and physical and cognitive performance at 17 years of age. *Pediatrics* 1991; **88**(4): 828–33.

71. Nakamura H, Yonetani M, Uetani Y, Funato M, Lee Y. Determination of serum unbound bilirubin for prediction of kernicterus in low birth-weight infants. *Acta Paediatr Jpn* 1992; **34**(6): 642–7.

72. Volpe J. Bilirubin and brain injury. In: Volpe J, ed. *Neurology of the Newborn*. Philadelphia, Saunders, 2001; 521–46.

73. de Vries L, Lary S, Dubowitz L. Relationship of serum bilirubin levels to ototoxicity and deafness in high-risk low-birth-weight infants. *Pediatrics* 1985; **76**(3): 351–4.

74. Bhutani V, Johnson L. Kernicterus in late preterm infants cared for as term healthy infants. *Semin Perinatol* 2006; **30**(2): 89–97.

75. Brodersen R, Stern L. Deposition of bilirubin acid in the central nervous system – a hypothesis for the development of kernicterus. *Acta Paediatr Scand* 1990; **79**(1): 12–19.

76. Wennberg R. The blood–brain barrier and bilirubin encephalopathy. *Cell Mol Neurobiol* 2000; **20**(1): 97–109.

77. Ahab-Barmada M. *Hyperbilirubinaemia in the Newborn*. Ohio, Ross, 1983.

78. Hansen T. Bilirubin brain toxicity. *J Perinatol* 2001; **21**(Suppl 1): S48–51.

79. Ostrow J, Pascolo L, Brites D, Tiribelli C. Molecular basis of bilirubin-induced neurotoxicity. *Trends Mol Med* 2004; **10**(2): 65–70.

80. Nakamura H, Takada S, Shimabuku R, Matsuo M, Matsuo T, Negishi H. Auditory nerve and brainstem responses in newborn infants with hyperbilirubinemia. *Pediatrics* 1985; **75**(4): 703–8.

81. Chen Y, Kang W. Effects of bilirubin on visual evoked potentials in term infants. *Eur J Pediatr* 1995; **154**(8): 662–6.

82. Wennberg R, Hance A. Experimental bilirubin encephalopathy: importance of total bilirubin, protein binding, and blood-brain barrier. *Pediatr Res* 1986; **20**(8): 789–92.

83. Gürses D, Kiliç I, Sahiner T. Effects of hyperbilirubinemia on cerebrocortical electrical activity in newborns. *Pediatr Res* 2002; **52**(1): 125–30.

84. Govaert P, Lequin M, Swarte R *et al.* Changes in globus pallidus with (pre)term kernicterus. *Pediatrics* 2003; **112**(6 **Pt 1**): 1256–63.

85. Coskun A, Yikilmaz A, Kumandas S, Karahan O, Akcakus M, Manav A. Hyperintense globus pallidus on T1-weighted MR imaging in acute kernicterus: is it common or rare? *Eur Radiol* 2005; **15**(6): 1263–7.

86. Okumura A, Hayakawa F, Kato T, Itomi K, Mimura S, Watanabe K. Preterm infants with athetoid cerebral palsy: kernicterus? *Arch Dis Child Fetal Neonatal Ed* 2001; **84**(2): F136–7.

87. Sugama S, Soeda A, Eto Y. Magnetic resonance imaging in three children with kernicterus. *Pediatr Neurol* 2001; **25**(4): 328–31.

88. Penn AA, Enzmann DR, Hahn JS, Stevenson DK. Kernicterus in a full term infant. *Pediatrics* 1994; **93**: 1003–5.

89. Yokochi K. Magnetic resonance imaging in children with kernicterus. *Acta Paediatr* 1995; **84**: 937–9.

90. Martich-Kriss V, Kollias SS, Ball WS. MR findings in kernicterus. *Am J Neuroradiol* 1995; **16**: 819–21.

91. Worley G, Erwin CW, Goldstein RF, Provenzale JM, Ware RE. Delayed development of sensorineural hearing loss after neonatal hyperbilirubinemia: a case report with brain magnetic resonance imaging. *Dev Med Child Neurol* 1996; **38**: 271–8.

92. Steinborn M, Seelos KC, Heuck A, von Voss H, Reiser M. MR findings in a patient with kernicterus. *Eur Radiol* 1999; **9**(9): 1913–15.

93. Harris MC, Bernbaum JC, Polin JR, Zimmerman R, Polin RA. Developmental follow-up of breastfed term and near-term infants with marked hyperbilirubinaemia. *Pediatrics* 2001; **107**(5): 1075–80.

94. Yilmaz Y, Ekinci G. Thalamic involvement in a patient with kernicterus. *Eur Radiol* 2002; **12**(7): 1837–9.

95. Groenendaal F, van der Grond J, de Vries L. Cerebral metabolism in severe neonatal hyperbilirubinemia. *Pediatrics* 2004; **114**(1): 291–4.

96. Oakden W, Moore A, Blaser S, Noseworthy M. ¹H MR spectroscopic characteristics of kernicterus: a possible metabolic signature. *AJNR Am J Neuroradiol* 2005; **26**(6): 1571–4.

97. Yokochi K, Aiba K, Kodama M, Fujimoto S. Magnetic resonance imaging in athetotic cerebral palsied children. *Acta Paediatr Scand* 1991; **80**(8–9): 818–23.

98. Bellinger D, Wypij D, duDuplessis A *et al.* Neurodevelopmental status at eight years in children with dextro-transposition of the great arteries: the Boston Circulatory Arrest Trial. *J Thorac Cardiovasc Surg* 2003; **126**(5): 1385–96.

99. Hövels-Gürich H, Konrad K, Skorzenski D *et al.* Long-term neurodevelopmental outcome and exercise capacity after corrective surgery for tetralogy of Fallot or ventricular septal defect in infancy. *Ann Thorac Surg* 2006; **81**(3): 958–66.

100. Limperopoulos C, Majnemer A, Shevell M *et al.* Functional limitations in young children with congenital heart defects after cardiac surgery. *Pediatrics* 2001; **108**(6): 1325–31.

101. Karl T, Hall S, Ford G *et al.* Arterial switch with full-flow cardiopulmonary bypass and limited circulatory arrest: neurodevelopmental outcome. *J Thorac Cardiovasc Surg* 2004; **127**(1): 213–22.

102. McQuillen P, Hamrick S, Perez M *et al.* Balloon atrial septostomy is associated with preoperative stroke in neonates with transposition of the great arteries. *Circulation* 2006; **113**(2): 280–5.

103. Te Pas A, van Wezel-Meijler G, Bökenkamp-Gramann R, Walther F. Preoperative cranial ultrasound findings in infants with major congenital heart disease. *Acta Paediatr Jpn* 2005; **94**(11): 1597–603.

104. van Houten J, Rothman A, Bejar R. High incidence of cranial ultrasound abnormalities in full-term infants with congenital heart disease. *Am J Perinatol* 1996; **13**(1): 47–53.

105. Jouannic J, Benachi A, Bonnet D *et al.* Middle cerebral artery Doppler in fetuses with transposition of the great arteries. *Ultrasound Obstet Gynecol* 2002; **20**(2): 122–4.

106. McQuillen P, Barkovich A, Hamrick S *et al.* Temporal and anatomic risk profile of brain injury with neonatal repair of congenital heart defects. *Stroke* 2007; **38**(2 Suppl):736–41.

107. Mahle W, Tavani F, Zimmerman R *et al.* An MRI study of neurological injury before and after congenital heart surgery. *Circulation* 2002; **106**(12 Suppl 1): 1109–14.

108. Miller SP, McQuillen PS, Hamrick S *et al.* Abnormal brain development in newborns with congenital heart disease. *N Engl J Med* 2007; **357**(19): 1928–38.

109. Comi A. Advances in Sturge-Weber syndrome. *Curr Opin Neurol* 2006; **19**(2): 124–8.

110. Brenner R, Sharbrough F. Electroencephalographic evaluation in Sturge-Weber syndrome. *Neurology* 1976; **26**(7): 629–32.

111. Vogl T, Stemmler J, Bergman C, Pfluger T, Egger E, Lissner J. MR and MR angiography of Sturge-Weber syndrome. *AJNR Am J Neuroradiol* 1993; **14**(2): 417–25.

112. Mentzel H, Dieckmann A, Fitzek C, Brandl U, Reichenbach J, Kaiser W. Early diagnosis of cerebral involvement in Sturge-Weber syndrome using high-resolution BOLD MR venography. *Pediatr Radiol* 2005; **35**(1): 85–90.

113. Cakirer S, Yagmurlu B, Savas M. Sturge-Weber syndrome: diffusion magnetic resonance imaging and proton magnetic resonance spectroscopy findings. *Acta Radiol* 2005; **46**(4): 407–10.

114. Evans A, Widjaja E, Connolly D, Griffiths P. Cerebral perfusion abnormalities in children with Sturge-Weber syndrome shown by dynamic contrast bolus magnetic resonance perfusion imaging. *Pediatrics* 2006; **117**(6): 2119–25.

115. Grant E, Williams A, Schellinger D, Slovis T. Intracranial calcification in the infant and neonate: evaluation by sonography and CT. *Radiology* 1985; **157**(1): 63–8.

116. Wang H, Kuo M, Chang T. Sonographic lenticulostriate vasculopathy in infants: some associations and a hypothesis. *AJNR Am J Neuroradiol* 1995; **16**(1): 97–102.

117. Weber K, Riebel T, Nasir R. Hyperechoic lesions in the basal ganglia: an incidental sonographic finding in neonates and infants. *Pediatr Radiol* 1992; **22**(3): 182–6.

118. Cabañas F, Pellicer A, Morales C, García-Alix A, Stiris T, Quero J. New pattern of hyperechogenicity in thalamus and basal ganglia studied by color Doppler flow imaging. *Pediatr Neurol* 1994; **10**(2): 109–16.

119. Hughes P, Weinberger E, Shaw D. Linear areas of echogenicity in the thalami and basal ganglia of neonates: an expanded association. Work in progress. *Radiology* 1991; **179**(1): 103–5.

120. Shefer-Kaufman N, Mimouni F, Stavorovsky Z, Meyer J, Dollberg S. Incidence and clinical significance of echogenic vasculature in the basal ganglia of newborns. *Am J Perinatol* 1999; **16**(6): 315–19.

121. Chamnanvanakij S, Rogers C, Luppino C, Broyles S, Hickman J, Perlman J. Linear hyperechogenicity within the basal ganglia and thalamus of preterm infants. *Pediatr Neurol* 2000; **23**(2): 129–33.

122. Makhoul I, Eisenstein I, Sujov P *et al.* Neonatal lenticulostriate vasculopathy: further characterisation. *Arch Dis Child Fetal Neonatal Ed* 2003; **88**(5): F410–4.

123. de Vries LS, Gunardi H, Barth PG, Bok LA, Verboon-Maciolek MA, Groenendaal F. The spectrum of cranial ultrasound and magnetic resonance imaging abnormalities in congenital cytomegalovirus infection. *Neuropediatrics* 2004; Apr;**35**(2): 113–19.

124. Estroff J, Parad R, Teele R, Benacerraf B. Echogenic vessels in the fetal thalami and basal ganglia associated with cytomegalovirus infection. *J Ultrasound Med* 1992; **11**(12): 686–8.

125. Chang Y, Huang C, Liu C. Frequency of linear hyperechogenicity over the basal ganglia in young infants with congenital rubella syndrome. *Clin Infect Dis* 1996; **22**(3): 569–71.

126. Bode H, Rudin C. Calcifying arteriopathy in the basal ganglia in human immunodeficiency virus infection. *Pediatr Radiol* 1995; **25**(1): 72–3.

127. Virkola K, Lappalainen M, Valanne L, Koskiniemi M. Radiological signs in newborns exposed to primary *Toxoplasma* infection in utero. *Pediatr Radiol* 1997; **27**(2): 133–8.

128. Coley B, Rusin J, Boue D. Importance of hypoxic/ischemic conditions in the development of cerebral lenticulostriate vasculopathy. *Pediatr Radiol* 2000; **30**(12): 846–55.

129. de Vries L, Beek F, Stoutenbeek P. Lenticulostriate vasculopathy in twin-to-twin transfusion syndrome: sonographic and CT findings. *Pediatr Radiol* 1995; **25**(Suppl. 1): S41–2.

130. Cabañas F, Pellicer A, Valverde E, Morales C, Quero J. Central nervous system vasculopathy in neonatal lupus erythematosus. *Pediatr Neurol* 1996; **15**(2): 124–6.

131. Ries M, Deeg KH, Wölfel D, Ibel H, Maier B, Buheitel G. Colour Doppler imaging of intracranial vasculopathy in severe infantile sialidosis. *Pediatr Radiol* 1992; **22**(3): 179–81.

132. Chabra S, Kriss VM, Pauly TH, Hall BD. Neurosonographic diagnosis of thalamic/basal ganglia vasculopathy in trisomy 13 – an important diagnostic aid. *Am J Med Genet* 1997; **72**(3): 291–3.

133. Kriss V, Kriss T. Doppler sonographic confirmation of thalamic and basal ganglia vasculopathy in three infants with trisomy 13. *J Ultrasound Med* 1996; **15**(7): 523–6.

134. Tomà P, Magnano G, Mezzano P, Lazzini F, Bonacci W, Serra G. Cerebral ultrasound images in prenatal cytomegalovirus infection. *Neuroradiology* 1989; **31**(3): 278–9.

135. Herman T, Siegel M. Neurosonographic abnormalities in chromosomal disorders. *Pediatr Radiol* 1991; **21**(6): 398–401.

136. Pasternak J, Groothuis D. Regional variability of blood flow and glucose utilization within the subependymal germinal matrix. *Brain Res* 1984; **299**(2): 281–8.

137. Barkovich AJ, Peck WW. MR of Zellweger syndrome. *AJNR Am J Neuroradiol* 1997; **18**: 1163–70.

138. Ben-Ami T, Yousefzadeh D, Backus M, Reichman B, Kessler A, Hammerman-Rozenberg C. Lenticulostriate vasculopathy in infants with infections of the central nervous system sonographic and Doppler findings. *Pediatr Radiol* 1990; **20**(8): 575–9.

139. Wang H, Kuo M. Sonographic lenticulostriate vasculopathy in infancy with tic and other neuropsychiatric disorders developed after 7 to 9 years of follow-up. *Brain Dev* 2003; **25**(Suppl. 1): s43–7.

140. Makhoul I, Zmora O, Tamir A, Shahar E, Sujov P. Congenital subependymal pseudocysts: own data and meta-analysis of the literature. *Isr Med Assoc J* 2001; **3**(3): 178–83.

141. Larroche JC. Sub-ependymal pseudo-cysts in the newborn. *Biol Neonate* 1972; **21**(3): 170–83.

142. Brun N, Robitaille Y, Grignon A, Robinson B, Mitchell G, Lambert M. Pyruvate carboxylase deficiency: prenatal onset of ischemia-like brain lesions in two sibs with the acute neonatal form. *Am J Med Genet* 1999; **84**(2): 94–101.

143. Ramenghi LA, Domizio S, Quartulli L, Sabatino G. Prenatal pseudo-cysts of the germinal matrix in preterm infants. *J Clin Ultrasound* 1997; **25**(4): 169–73.

144. Malinger G, Lev D, Ben Sira L, Kidron D, Tamarkin M, Lerman-Sagie T. Congenital periventricular pseudocysts: prenatal sonographic appearance and clinical implications. *Ultrasound Obstet Gynecol* 2002; **20**(5): 447–51.

145. Rademaker KJ, De Vries LS, Barth PG. Subependymal pseudocysts: ultrasound diagnosis and findings at follow-up. *Acta Paediatr* 1993; **82**(4): 394–9.

146. Mito T, Ando Y, Takeshita K, Takada K, Takashima S. Ultrasonographical and morphological examination of subependymal cystic lesions in maturely born infants. *Neuropediatrics* 1989; **20**(4): 211–14.

147. Shaw CM, Alvord EC, Jr. Subependymal germinolysis. *Arch Neurol* 1974; **31**(6): 374–81.

148. Shackelford GD, Fulling KH, Glasier CM. Cysts of the subependymal germinal matrix: sonographic demonstration with pathologic correlation. *Radiology* 1983; **149**(1): 117–21.

149. de Vries LS, Verboon-Maciolek MA, Cowan FM, Groenendaal F. The role of cranial ultrasound and magnetic resonance imaging in the diagnosis of infections of the central nervous system. *Early Hum Dev* 2006; **82**(12): 819-25.

150. Herini E, Tsuneishi S, Takada S, Sunarini, Nakamura H. Clinical features of infants with subependymal germinolysis and choroid plexus cysts. *Pediatr Int* 2003; **45**(6): 692-6.

151. Russel IM, van Sonderen L, van Straaten HL, Barth PG. Subependymal germinolytic cysts in Zellweger syndrome. *Pediatr Radiol* 1995; **25**(4): 254-5.

152. Twomey E, Naughten E, Donoghue V, Ryan S. Neuroimaging findings in glutaric aciduria type 1. *Pediatr Radiol* 2003; **33**(12): 823-30.

153. Larcos G, Gruenewald S, Lui K. Neonatal subependymal cysts detected by sonography: prevalence, sonographic findings, and clinical significance. *AJR Am J Roentgenol* 1994; **162**(4): 953-6.

154. van Straaten HL, van Tintelen JP, Trijbels JM *et al.* Neonatal lactic acidosis, complex I/IV deficiency, and fetal cerebral disruption. *Neuropediatrics* 2005; **36**(3): 193-9.

155. Zuppa AA, Gallini F, De Luca D, Luciano R, Frezza S, de Turris PL, Tortorolo G. Cerebral ultrasound findings in neonatal lupus syndrome. *Biol Neonate* 2004; **86**(4): 230-4.

156. Cohen HL, Sloves JH, Laungani S, Glass L, DeMarinis P. Neurosonographic findings in full-term infants born to maternal cocaine abusers: visualization of subependymal and periventricular cysts. *J Clin Ultrasound* 1994; **22**(5): 327-33.

157. Zorzi C, Angonese I. Subependymal pseudocysts in the neonate. *Eur J Pediatr* 1989; **148**(5): 462-4.

158. Yamashita Y, Outani Y, Kawano Y, Horikawa M, Matsuishi T, Hashimoto T. Clinical analyses and short-term prognoses of neonates with subependymal cysts. *Pediatr Neurol* 1990; **6**(6): 375-8.

Chapter 11 | The baby with an enlarging head or ventriculomegaly

CORNELIA F. HAGMANN,
JANET M. RENNIE, *and*
NICOLA J. ROBERTSON

Introduction to the clinical problem

The widespread use of ultrasound imaging has completely changed the nature of neonatal practice in many areas, not least with regard to the diagnosis and management of hydrocephalus. It is very rare nowadays to be presented with a baby with a rapidly enlarging head circumference, dilated scalp veins and sunsetting eyes, because most cases are detected antenatally or detected in postnatal life before clinical signs develop. The widespread availability of ultrasound imaging means that it is no longer necessary to make the diagnosis by transillumination of the skull or air encephalography. The detection of ventriculomegaly in an asymptomatic fetus or neonate has created new challenges, because at the time of initial diagnosis it cannot be known whether progressive ventricular dilatation will develop.

The availability of imaging does not mean that postnatal measurement of the head circumference is redundant, and serial measurements are still vitally important in helping to determine whether the ventricles are enlarging progressively. Babies still present with large heads which are due to familial megalencephaly, and it is essential to measure the head circumference of both parents in a well baby with a big head before embarking on an expensive series of investigations which may not be necessary, and will only serve to worry the parents.

Ventriculomegaly may be congenital or acquired. In this chapter we discuss fetal ventriculomegaly, postnatally acquired ventricular dilatation, and the management and prognosis of non-progressive and progressive ventriculomegaly. Ventricular dilatation can be due to a heterogeneous group of pathologic processes including obstruction of cerebral fluid flow (obstructive hydrocephalus) or reduced reabsorption, primary neuronal loss, and abnormalities in brain development (Table 11.1). The distinction between ventricular dilatation due to cerebral atrophy and that secondary to raised intracranial pressure is the key to correct diagnosis and management of a baby found to have ventriculomegaly. In general the development of ventriculomegaly secondary to atrophy occurs slowly over weeks and is not associated with signs due to an increase in intracranial pressure or rapid head growth. Cerebral atrophy tends to be associated with irregularly shaped ventricles and there might be evidence of white matter loss or damage in the parenchyma. Antenatal diagnosed cerebral atrophy is likely to be associated with either microcephaly or normal head circumference with enlarged ventricles. Progressive ventricular dilatation tends to begin with trigonal enlargement and is associated with increasing occipito-frontal circumference, tense fontanelle, increased intracranial pressure (usually above 12 mmHg), and separation of the sutures. Signs of increased intracranial pressure include apnea, convulsions, irritability, poor feeding, and vomiting. Late signs include sunsetting of the eyes, bulging fontanelle and dilated scalp veins.

Fetal ventriculomegaly

Definition and incidence

Fetal ventriculomegaly is the most commonly detected abnormality of the fetal brain [1,2], and is detected in around 1–2 per 1000 fetuses [3]. Isolated ventriculomegaly occurs in about 0.39%–0.87% of births [4]. Ventriculomegaly is the single most sensitive marker for maldevelopment of the fetal central nervous system [1,2]. For these reasons, assessment of the ventricular size has become an important part of routine prenatal sonography [1,2]. There are a number of definitions of fetal ventriculomegaly, of which enlargement of the width of the lateral ventricular atrium is now the most widely accepted. The atrial diameter has been shown to be stable throughout gestation (Fig. 11.1) [2,5,6,7,8]. This measurement has also been shown to be less susceptible to measurement errors than others, and has proved highly reproducible. Any errors are usually small and tend to overestimate the atrial size [6].

The original study by Cardoza *et al.* recorded a mean atrial diameter of 7.6 mm with a standard deviation of 0.6 mm from 14 to 38 weeks of gestation [2]. Subsequent studies have shown similar values of the mean atrial diameters (5.4–6.6 mm with

Neonatal Cerebral Investigation, eds. Janet M. Rennie, Cornelia F. Hagmann and Nicola J. Robertson. Published by Cambridge University Press. © Cambridge University Press 2008.

Table 11.1. Causes of ventriculomegaly.

Congenital hydrocephalus
    Aqueduct stenosis
    Dandy Walker malformation
    Arnold Chiari malformation, usually associated with spina bifida
    Arachnoid cyst causing obstruction, e.g., in the quadrigeminal cisterns
    X-linked hydrocephalus
    Vein of Galen aneurysm
    Chromosomal disorders, e.g., trisomy 13, 18
Acquired hydrocephalus
    Intracranial hemorrhage
        Alloimmune thrombocytopenia
        Hemophilia
        Other inherited bleeding disorders, e.g., Christmas disease
        Late-onset vitamin K deficiency bleeding
        Alpha-1-antitrypsin deficiency
      Bleeding into a tumor or arteriovenous malformation
        Bleeding as a result of trauma during intrauterine life, at birth or later
    Intrauterine infection, e.g., with cytomegalovirus or toxoplasmosis
    Postmeningitic hydrocephalus
    Bony skull obstruction, e.g., Apert's, Pfeiffer's or Crouzon's syndrome
    Choroid plexus tumor causing cerebrospinal fluid overproduction
Cerebral atrophy causing ventriculomegaly
    Antenatal white matter destruction, e.g., twin-twin transfusion syndrome
    Postnatally acquired white matter damage

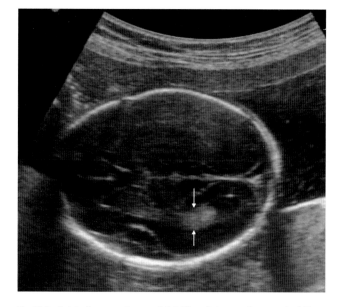

Fig. 11.1. **Axial ultrasound scan of fetal head shows placement of the calipers to measure ventricular atrial diameter.**

SD 1.2–1.4) [2,5,6,7,8,9,10]. The larger mean value of the original study by Cardoza is probably explained by the difference in method.

Male fetuses tend to have slightly larger ventricle size (atrial diameter 6.4 ± 1.3 mm) than female fetuses (5.8 ± 1.3 mm) [9,11,12]. Atrial diameters exceeding 10 mm (4 standard deviations above the mean), measured in a true transverse axial plane across the most posterior portion of choroid plexus from 14 weeks onwards, are defined as ventriculomegaly (Fig 11.1) [2,7,8,9,13]. Borderline ventriculomegaly is usually defined as an atrial width of 10–12 mm; mild ventriculomegaly, as atrial width of 12–15 mm; severe ventriculomegaly, as atrial width >15 mm. Borderline ventriculomegaly as a normal finding is more likely close to term for large fetuses and male fetuses, and some authors have even suggested that in male infants the upper limit of the ventricle size should be 12 mm [14].

Ventriculomegaly can be unilateral or bilateral. Asymmetry of the ventricles without dilatation can occur and be observed in normal fetuses, asymmetrical dilatation being defined as the size difference between the atria exceeding 2.4 mm [15].

Natural history of fetal ventriculomegaly

Fetal ventriculomegaly can resolve, persist or progress antenatally. Ventriculomegaly can be detected as early as 15 weeks of gestation or earlier and is usually detected at 20–24 weeks of gestation when the routine fetal anomaly scan is performed. In about one-third to two-thirds of cases ventriculomegaly resolves before birth [12,14,16,17,18,19,20,21,22,23]. Patel *et al.* performed serial ultrasounds on 26 fetuses with isolated mild ventriculomegaly, and fetal ventriculomegaly resolved in 38% ($n = 10$) and persisted in 62% ($n = 16$) [21]. Clinical data were available for 24 serially scanned fetuses (9 with resolution, 15 with stable diameters). Only 1 of these 9 had cognitive and motor delay. In comparison, 5/15 (33%) showed developmental delay [21]. Normal outcome was found significantly more often when ventriculomegaly improved than when it remained stable or worsened [20,24].

Causes and associations (concomitant brain anomalies)

Fetal ventriculomegaly can represent a normal variant or, as discussed, it can be due to any one of a number of disorders including hydrocephalus, neuronal loss, and abnormalities in brain development. Obstruction of normal cerebral fluid flow can be the result of a variety of processes such as Dandy Walker malformation, Arnold Chiari malformation, an arachnoid cyst causing obstruction, X-linked aqueductal stenosis, chromosomal anomalies (trisomy 13 and 18), and infection (toxoplasmosis, cytomegalovirus, varicella) (Table 11.1). Abnormalities of brain development include agenesis of the corpus callosum and holoprosencephaly. Other causes of ventriculomegaly are intracerebral hemorrhage or periventricular leukomalacia.

Data from several studies indicate that the associated anomalies account for most of the increased mortality and morbidity in fetuses with ventriculomegaly [3,5,13,14,16,18,21,25,26,27]. Vergani *et al.* found that an atrial width <12 mm was associated with other anomalies in only 6% of cases, compared with 56%

when the atrial width was >12 mm [14]. Other studies found that the incidence of associated anomalies is higher in fetuses having atria measuring 11–15 mm than in those with atria measuring 10 mm [20] [28,29]. Accompanying abnormalities are associated with a worse prognosis [5,27].

Chromosomal abnormalities associated with ventriculomegaly have been reported [3,14,18,28,30,31,32] and are more frequent in fetuses having atria measuring 11–15 mm [28,31]. The incidence of chromosomal abnormalities is strongly related to the presence of multisystem malformations [33]. Only 3% of fetuses with isolated ventriculomegaly as opposed to 36% of those with additional malformations had chromosomal defects [33]. Our current practice is to counsel the parents accordingly and offer karyotyping.

Management and investigation

Comprehensive and detailed fetal ultrasound imaging is the primary investigation in a fetus found to have ventriculomegaly, in order to detect associated fetal abnormalities. The importance of separating the cases of isolated mild ventriculomegaly from those with associated abnormalities in order to counsel accordingly about the prognosis is clear. However, certain exclusion of associated anomalies is not always easy, and counseling can be very challenging if there are equivocal findings. If mild fetal ventriculomegaly is found investigation should include targeted ultrasound imaging aimed at the detection of associated central nervous system (CNS) and other anomalies, karyotyping and screening for congenital infections and the presence of alloimmune thrombocytopenia.

The use of antenatal magnetic resonance imaging (MRI) for diagnosing associated CNS abnormalities in fetuses with ventriculomegaly has now been established in some centers for some years, but remains controversial. Offering MRI to all women whose fetuses were found to have mild ventriculomegaly would have major resource implications, and as yet expertise in the interpretation of fetal cerebral MRI is limited. Many authors agree that fetal MRI in the second and third trimesters can demonstrate CNS abnormalities which were not detected with ultrasound, which may influence the diagnosis and could thus be very useful in counseling patients [29,34,35,36,37,38,39,40,41]. In a recent French study MRI gave additional information in 5 of 106 of cases with mild fetal ventriculomegaly (10–12 mm, unilateral or bilateral); based on these findings parents could be informed that the risk of missing a CNS abnormality with ultrasound alone is around 5%–6% [42], but confirmation is needed. The Sheffield group reported obtaining additional information with fetal MR in 50% of the cases overall, 44% of those with mild ventriculomegaly, and 58% of those with severe ventriculomegaly. The authors acknowledge that this unusually high number was probably related to an inherent bias in the study sample (many fetuses had suboptimal ultrasound imaging and not all were scanned by experts) and the retrospective nature of the study [29]. In contrast, Malinger showed that specialist neurosonography had a higher sensitivity (96% vs. 85%) and higher specificity (87% vs. 80%) than MRI when compared to the referral ultrasound, with a positive predictive value

for neurosonography of 93% compared with 88% for MRI in the detection of associated CNS malformations [43,44]. The abnormality that is most often missed with ultrasound alone is agenesis of the corpus callosum (Fig. 11.2a,b), and it is important to remember that the development of the corpus callosum is not complete until after 20 weeks.

We currently recommend that if a brain abnormality is suspected with fetal ultrasound imaging the pregnant woman should be referred to a center with a multidisciplinary team. The team needs individuals with a high level of expertise in fetal medicine, neuroradiologists, neurosurgeons, and neonatologists who are able to discuss the findings, and arrange counseling and further management of the baby if necessary. We currently offer fetal MRI to selected cases, but not yet as a routine in cases with isolated borderline ventriculomegaly that is confirmed with specialist fetal neurosonography, normal karyotyping and no evidence of intrauterine infection or fetal thrombocytopenia. We do offer fetal MRI if there is any suspicion of another malformation (CNS or not) on ultrasound, or the ventriculomegaly is moderate to severe. If MRI is offered it is important to tell parents that ultrasound and fetal MRI might not detect some brain abnormalities early in pregnancy due to the lack of brain development at this time. For this reason, we and many other centers recommend repeated ultrasound imaging and we would consider repeating the fetal MRI. As a result parents need to be counseled that the diagnosis (and the prognosis) may change [24,45]. This uncertainty can prove understandably difficult for many parents to cope with.

Prognosis/Counseling

Before beginning counseling parents whose fetus is found to have fetal ventriculomegaly it is important to establish the following facts as far as possible:

- The severity of the ventriculomegaly (10–12 mm; 12–15 mm; >15mm)
- The gestation at which the diagnosis was first made and if there has been any progression
- The presence of any other abnormality (based on detailed ultrasound imaging of the fetus with MRI in appropriate cases)
- The karyotype and sex of the fetus
- Whether there is any evidence of alloimmune thrombocytopenia
- Whether there is any evidence of congenital infection.

The prognosis for fetuses with severe ventriculomegaly (>15 mm) is poor, particularly when the ventriculomegaly is associated with other abnormalities [20,25,46,47,48]. We, like others, continue to offer termination of pregnancy in this situation and if parents choose this option it is important to try to arrange a careful autopsy, considering postmortem MRI (Chapter 14). If parents choose to continue the pregnancy we arrange a neurosurgical consultation, and continue to monitor the fetus in order to determine the best choice regarding the place and mode of delivery.

Mild ventricular dilatation, whether bilateral or unilateral, continues to present a significant counseling challenge. Once further investigation has been undertaken (see above) there

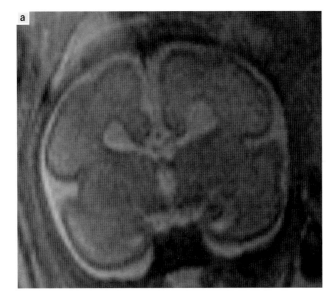

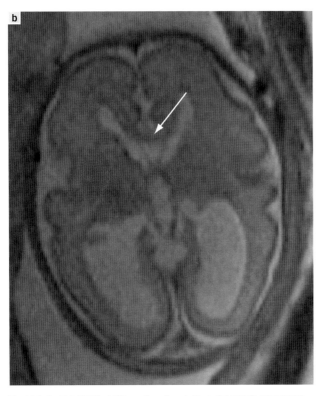

Fig. 11.2a,b. **Fetal MRI at 29 weeks of gestation.** Fetal MRI revealed in addition to mild ventriculomegaly, diagnosed by ultrasound, agenesis of the corpus callosum with the characteristic lateral convexity and separation of the frontal horns of the lateral ventricles seen on the coronal T_2-weighted MR image. The axial T_2-weighted image shows that the genu is present in keeping with partial agenesis (arrow). The trigones and occipital horns of the lateral ventricles are dilated, an appearance known as colpocephaly.

remains a sizeable number of cases in whom the diagnosis appears to be isolated mild ventriculomegaly although there is always uncertainty about cortical gyral abnormalities when scanning is performed in the second trimester. There is general agreement that the vast majority of children who had mild fetal ventriculomegaly function entirely normally, although as a population they are at an increased risk of developmental delay [16,19,26,49,50].

Furthermore, in most studies about the outcome of fetal ventriculomegaly the diagnosis of mild ventriculomegaly is based on measurements of only one ventricle [31]. It has been shown recently that isolated mild ventriculomegaly is often unilateral (usually left sided) and that mild unilateral ventriculomegaly has no effect on developmental outcome [11,32,51].

Some workers have differentiated 10–12 mm from 12–15 mm of enlargement, and to us this looks an increasingly worthwhile distinction: Vergani et al. reported a significantly lower rate of developmental delay when the atrial width was >10 mm and <12 mm (3%) than when it was 12–15 mm (25%) [14]. Other groups have reported similar results, with a significantly lower risk of adverse outcome when the atrial width is 10–12 mm [20,24,31,48]. Ouahba and colleagues found no difference in outcome between unilateral and bilateral mild ventriculomegaly, and in a study of 167 cases followed for 2 years 85% were normal overall, a figure which rose to 93% in the group with non-progressive dilatation that remained <12 mm [24]. Previous series have suggested that the neurological outcome of isolated unilateral ventriculomegaly is good [11,32]. Some authors suggest that different counseling should be offered for male and female fetuses, and in one study the risk of delayed development for a male fetus with isolated mild ventriculomegaly and normal karyotype was 5% whereas the risk for a female fetus increased to 23% [31].

In a systematic review of 30 papers reporting the outcome of fetuses with mild ventriculomegaly rates of developmental delay varied from mild impairment in 9% and moderate/severe impairment in 10% [50]. The duration of follow-up ranged from 1 month to 10 years, and there were no geographical cohort studies. It is crucial to continue follow-up beyond the second year of age because many of the skills deficits characteristic of mild impairment, such as learning disabilities, communication disorders, and attention deficits, are not apparent in infants and young children, and many of the studies report only very short follow-up. Further, reports of neurodevelopmental outcome are often based only on reviews of medical records and interviews with parents or health-care providers, not structured examinations. Using an objective tool administered in a blinded fashion the rate of developmental delay was found to be 36% at 21 months of age in children with mild fetal ventriculomegaly [49].

We currently counsel parents whose fetus is found to have isolated ventriculomegaly with atrial width of 10–15 mm that there is around a 10% risk of developmental delay, with a range in severity of outcome. Taking into account all the current information, we currently add that fetuses with isolated bilateral or unilateral ventriculomegaly with an atrial width of 10–12 mm dilatation have an extremely high chance of an entirely normal outcome, especially the male fetuses, whereas those with isolated bilateral ventriculomegaly of 12–15 mm or with asymmetrical dilatation of both ventricles still have a very good chance of being normal. However, the risk of developmental delay in this group is probably of the order of 15% overall, with 8% experiencing moderate to severe neurodevelopmental problems and the remaining 7% having only mild delay.

Postnatally acquired ventriculomegaly

Many of the conditions that can cause ventricular enlargement in prenatal life can also occur, or present, postnatally (Table 11.1). Intraventricular hemorrhage, for example, can occur in or ex utero due to alloimmune thrombocytopenia or trauma. The most frequent clinical problem is that of posthemorrhagic ventricular dilatation, which can progress rapidly or slowly to hydrocephalus requiring treatment. Much of this section is specific to this condition but methods of assessment and investigation are often relevant to ventriculomegaly caused by other conditions. As ever, it is important to distinguish ventriculomegaly due to atrophy from that due to cerebrospinal fluid (CSF) accumulation.

Etiology

Posthemorrhagic ventricular dilatation

The presence of blood within the ventricular system leads to the formation of multiple small clots, which impede the normal process of CSF circulation and reabsorption. These blood clots are demonstrable by ultrasound. There are some endogenous attempts to lyse blood clots in the CSF but such fibrinolysis is not very efficient [52] possibly due to low plasminogen concentration levels and high concentrations of plasminogen activator [53]. The subacute/chronic posthemorrhagic ventricular dilatation is related to obliterative arachnoiditis. Transforming growth factor β1 (TGF β1) is released into the CSF after intraventricular hemorrhage [54]. Over a period of 2–6 weeks TGF β1 stimulates the production of extracellular matrix proteins around the brainstem and the subarachnoid space [54]. Multiple blood clots may obstruct the ventricular system or the channels of reabsorption initially but lead to a chronic arachnoiditis of the basal cisterns involving the deposit of extracellular matrix in the foramina of the fourth ventricle, thus creating obstructive hydrocephalus. The same process can occur in the subarachnoid space, causing communicating hydrocephalus [55]. Periventricular white matter may then be injured from persistently raised pressure and edema [56], free radical damage from iron [57] or pro-inflammatory cytokines [58].

Other studies of infants with posthemorrhagic ventricular dilatation show damage due to ischemia, alterations in myelin and axons in white matter, together with physiological changes (impaired visual- and somatosensory-evoked potentials), consistent with cerebral white matter injury [59,60,61,62,63]. Furthermore, findings of cognitive defects support an effect of the ventricular dilatation on cerebral neurons [64,65].

Natural history of posthemorrhagic ventricular dilatation

Studies of the natural history of posthemorrhagic ventricular dilatation in the late 1980s suggested that about one-third of infants with intraventricular hemorrhage develop posthemorrhagic ventricular dilatation, usually within 10–20 days of the original bleed [61]. Of very low birth weight (VLBW) infants with posthemorrhagic ventricular dilatation, 85% subsequently had arrest of progression (spontaneous or induced by non-surgical intervention), and 15% required ventriculoperitoneal shunts for control of raised intracranial pressure [61]. In a study of preterm infants with a mean gestational age of 26.8 weeks born in 1994–1997, 49% of infants with intraventricular hemorrhage developed posthemorrhagic ventricular dilatation (25% progressive, 24% not progressive) [66]. Over time, 52% of the infants with progressive dilatation had arrest of progression either spontaneously (38%) or in response to non-surgical treatment (14%) whereas 34% required ventriculoperitoneal shunt insertion and 18% died [66]. The occurrence of the posthemorrhagic dilatation and the requirement for surgery were most strongly predicted by the severity of the intraventricular hemorrhage, occurring in 71% of infants with parenchymal lesions [66]. Only the grade of the intraventricular hemorrhage was significantly related to the likelihood of surgical intervention; hence, it is rare for an infant with intraventricular hemorrhage which is isolated to the germinal matrix to develop posthemorrhagic ventricular dilatation that requires surgical intervention [66,67]. Although the incidence of germinal matrix-intraventricular hemorrhage (GMH-IVH) has fallen significantly since the 1980s (Chapter 9) posthemorrhagic ventricular dilatation continues to present formidable management problems and carries a significant risk of adverse outcome [66].

Investigation of babies with ventricular dilatation

Clinical monitoring

Hopefully it goes without saying that regular measurements of head circumference plotted on the appropriate chart are essential, and regular neurological examinations should be performed.

Lumbar puncture

In our view a lumbar puncture is indicated in babies with ventricular dilatation. The risk of coning in the newborn period is minimal, although it can occur if there is a large collection in the posterior fossa and we would not perform a lumbar puncture in a baby with a large subdural hematoma with signs of raised intracranial pressure. Lumbar puncture is also contraindicated in babies whose platelet counts are below 100×10^9 /l because of the risk of a spinal subdural hematoma. In all other cases lumbar puncture should be performed because the information which can be obtained is very valuable for diagnosis and management. The CSF should be cultured to exclude meningitis, and it is important to consider fungal and viral meningitis. The CSF pressure can be measured directly at lumbar puncture, and is normally less than 5.5 mmHg or 7 cm water [56].

Hematological investigations

Babies with intracranial hemorrhage, in particular, need investigations aimed at excluding inherited or acquired bleeding disorders as the cause. A full coagulation screen should be performed, together with a blood count and film. If there is a suspicion of late-onset vitamin K deficiency bleeding (VKDB) then a request should be made for PIVKAs (proteins induced by vitamin K absence); a diagnosis of VKDB should also prompt a search for liver disease. Glutaric aciduria type I is a rare cause of subdural hematoma in infancy, but it is not standard practice to look for this as a cause of intracranial bleeding in the newborn period.

Ultrasound assessment of ventricular size

Ultrasound is the method of choice for monitoring the progress of ventriculomegaly and for assessing the rate of reduction of ventricular size after surgery. Ultrasound can also be used to check the position of a ventricular catheter. A large number of systems have been published, and the relative value of these is discussed in this section.

Linear measurements

The wide range of ventricular size that can be seen in the newborn is shown in Fig. 11.3. In order to define ventriculomegaly for incidence studies, to monitor progress, and to minimize inter-observer variability, a reproducible system of measurement is needed. Many different linear measurements of ventricular size have been published [68,69,70,71,72,73,74,75,76,77] (Fig. 11.4). London *et al.* made four linear measurements including the maximal span of the frontal horns, the width of the frontal horn at the level of the caudate nucleus, and the inter-caudate distance [71]. Allan *et al.* measured the diameter of the lateral ventricle at the mid body on a parasagittal scan [70]. The authors claimed that this measurement separated cases of progressive from non-progressive hydrocephalus, but did not study normal infants [70]. Poland carefully studied 67 normal infants but did not evaluate his measurement system in any babies with abnormal-sized ventricles [76]. Levene and Starte established a normal range of ventricular size from measurements of 273 preterm infants [74]. This index measures the distance from the falx to the lateral border of the lateral ventricle in a coronal view taken in the plane of the third ventricle (Fig. 11.5). This measurement is easy to understand and teach and is reproducible. As a consequence it has been widely adopted, and is usually termed the ventricular index. The original centile chart is reproduced as Fig. 11.6; unfortunately the normal range has never been extended beyond term-equivalent gestational age. Several studies of treatment of

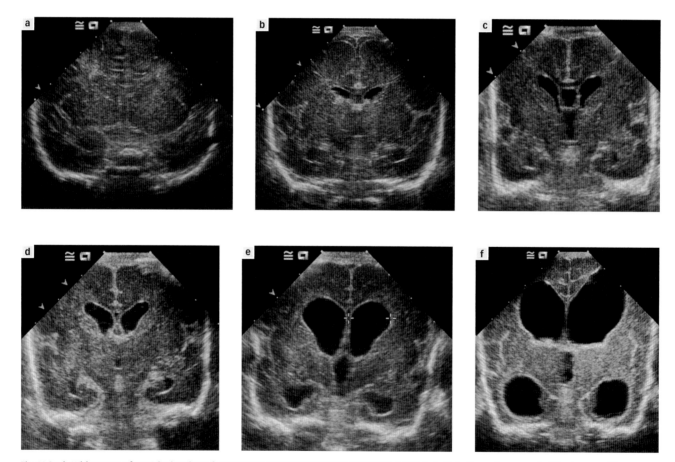

Fig. 11.3a–f. **Wide range of ventricular sizes, from normal to massively enlarged lateral ventricles. Note the enlargement of the temporal horns of the lateral ventricles in the last images; in normal ventricles these would not be apparent on this coronal view.**

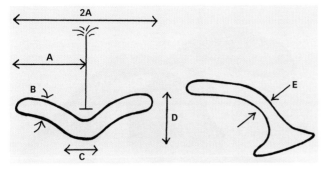

Fig. 11.4. **Different linear measurements which can be made from coronal and parasagittal scans** (reproduced with permission of Blackwell, from Levene *et al.* [78]. A: the ventricular index of Levene [69], Sauerbrei *et al.* [72], Lipscomb *et al.* [79]; 2A: Skolnick *et al.* [73], London *et al.* [71]; B: London *et al.* [71], Sauerbrei *et al.* [72]; C: London *et al.* [71]; D: Levene and Starte [74]; E: Allan *et al.* [80]; Quisling *et al.* [81].

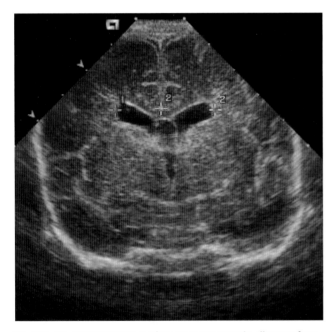

Fig. 11.5. **The ventricular index of Levene measures the distance from the falx to the border of the lateral ventricle in a coronal view taken in the plane of the third ventricle.**

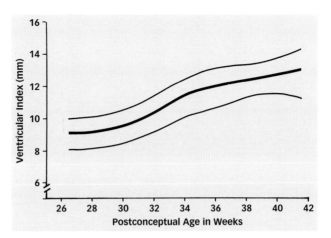

Fig. 11.6. **Centile chart of Levene ventriclular Index. Reproduced with permission from Levene, M. I. (1981). Measurement of the growth of the lateral ventricles in preterm infants with real-time ultrasound.** *Arch Dis Child* 56(12): 900–4 [69].

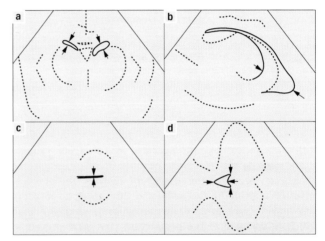

Fig. 11.7. **A line diagram showing linear measurements by ultrasound for the dimensions of the intracranial ventricles; the arrows indicate the correct position of the calipers and alignment. With permission from** *Arch Dis Child Fetal Neonatal Ed* 2000; 82:218–23; M. W. Davies, M. Swaminathan, S. L. Chuang, and F. R. Betheras [68].

posthemorrhagic ventricular dilatation after intraventricular hemorrhage used 4 mm above the 97th centile of Levene to define trial entry [82,83,84], and this has proved robust in many different centers.

Davies and his colleagues in Australia studied 120 preterm infants and provided reference ranges for linear measurements of the anterior horn width, thalamo-occipital distance of the lateral ventricle, the width of the third ventricle, and the width and length of the fourth ventricle in preterm infants between 23 to 33 weeks of gestational age (Fig. 11.7) [68]. Like Levene's ventricular index, these measurements are easily reproducible with minimal intra-observer and inter-observer variability [68]. Only the measurement of the fourth ventricle proved to have significant intra-observer variability. There was little change in the ventricular size between 23 and 32 weeks of gestation. These authors concluded that measurements of the anterior horn width >4 mm and thalamo-occipital distance >26 mm are abnormal in preterm infants less than 33 weeks of gestational age [68]. These additional measurements are now much used in the diagnosis and monitoring of the ventricular size, and we find them helpful. They have also been used to define trial entry in the trial of prevention of hydrocephalus after intraventricular hemorrhage in newborn infants by drainage, irrigation, and fibrinolytic therapy [82].

Area measurements

A two-dimensional measurement conveys more information than a one-dimensional measurement. Area calipers are now usually available on commercial ultrasound equipment,

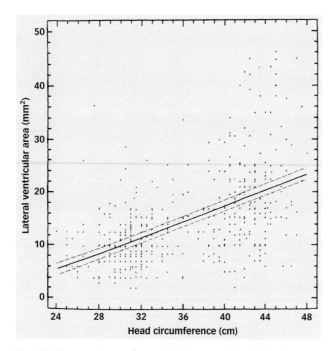

Fig. 11.8. **The normal range for ventricular area related to head circumference (on *x* axis). Reproduced with permission from E. Saliba, *et al.* (1990). Area of lateral ventricles measured on cranial ultrasonography in preterm infants: reference range. *Arch Dis Child* 65 (10 Spec No): 1029–32 [77].**

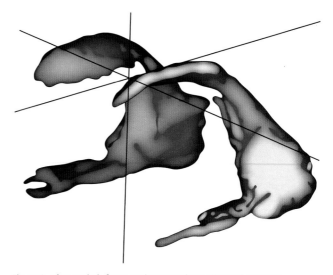

Fig. 11.9. **The study infants underwent three-dimensional (3D) ultrasound and MRI. The data were then reconstructed and segmented using an interactive segmentation program. This is a representative lateral ventricle segmentation of the 3D ultrasound from that study. Reproduced with permission from J. H. Gilmore *et al.* (2001). *Ultrasound Med. Biol.* 27 (No. 8): 1143–1146 [90].**

allowing the ventricle to be measured in two dimensions with ease. Tracing the ventricular area with electronic calipers at the cot-side may prolong the time of investigation but images can be stored for subsequent analysis. The practical difficulties including the additional time taken to measure area and the lack of an easily recognizable landmark with which to standardize the parasagittal view have prevented wide acceptance of area measurements. An additional problem is that when the ventricles are very large the boundaries are not always visible in the parasagittal or coronal plane. A normal range for area has been defined and used to study outcome (Fig. 11.8) [77]. During the first six weeks of life the mean postnatal head growth velocity was 0.53 cm/week with a mean postnatal ventricular area growth velocity of 0.39 mm² per week [77].

Volume measurements
Ultrasound has been shown to provide an accurate assessment of ventricular size. Brann *et al.* developed a cylindrical coordinate system to estimate ventricular volume based on two-dimensional ultrasound [85]. He showed, using volume measurements, that the rate of growth was greater in those who required intervention than in those with non-progressive ventriculomegaly. The differences were apparent from the third week of postnatal life [85], but this method has not been widely used. Studies of volumetric measurements of the ventricle have shown that three-dimensional ultrasound provides accurate and reliable measurements of ventricular volumes in term and preterm infants [86,87,88,89,90].

Nagdyman *et al.* demonstrated that head position influences left/right ventricle volume differences, but does not affect overall ventricle volume [87]. Gilmore *et al.* compared the ventricle volumes obtained by three-dimensional ultrasound with magnetic resonance imaging and found an excellent correlation between the volumes obtained using these two methods (Fig. 11.9) [90]. As yet volume estimation remains largely a research technique.

Doppler ultrasound studies of ventriculomegaly
The effect of raised intracranial pressure due to hydrocephalus on cerebral blood flow velocity (CBFV) is to elevate the systolic flow velocity and reduce the diastolic velocity. This increases the Pourcelot Index (PI = (peak systolic – end-disastolic velocity) / peak systolic velocity), and in the extreme situation the end-diastolic velocity is reduced to zero and the PI becomes 1. However, almost all the published studies report an increase in PI with posthemorrhagic and other forms of hydrocephalus [91,92,93,94,95], and most of the studies report observations from babies studied before and after ventriculoperitoneal shunting, rather than monitoring the change over time [96,97,98]. As a result serial measurements of PI have yet to find a clinical niche and do not add to the information obtained from serial occipito-frontal circumference measurements, and from serial ultrasound measurements of the ventricular index, the thalamo-occipital distance, the anterior horn width, and the width of the third ventricle.

Magnetic resonance imaging
In our view it is worthwhile performing MRI in babies with ventriculomegaly, in order to obtain additional information about white matter damage, which is not always visible with ultrasound. The MRI images give useful information prior to

surgery. In preterm babies with posthemorrhagic hydrocephalus the best prognostic information is obtained from MRI performed at term-corrected age (see Chapter 9).

Management

The aim of treatment in babies with ventricular dilatation is to protect the brain from damage secondary to raised intracranial pressure and minimize the need for a permanent shunt. Shunts are prone to complications such as infection and frequently require revision. Close monitoring is essential in order to distinguish the group with non-progressive ventriculomegaly from those whose ventricles will continue to enlarge and who are at risk of adverse effects of raised intracranial pressure. Once ventriculomegaly is recognized, surveillance of changes in ventricular size, rate of head growth, and clinical condition should be initiated. As discussed, we currently measure the ventricular index (in the mid-coronal view), the anterior width, the size of the third ventricle, and the thalamo-occipital distance since these measurements have the advantage of good inter-observer agreement and reproducibility. We do not currently measure area or use routine Doppler estimations of CBFV. We aim to perform ultrasound measurements thrice weekly, with daily head circumference measurements. Our practice is to perform lumbar puncture early on in the course of monitoring in order to exclude meningitis and to measure the CSF protein and pressure. It is important to continue to monitor babies with posthemorrhagic ventricular dilatation after discharge from hospital, because they can develop rapidly progressive hydrocephalus after many months.

The combination of rapidly enlarging ventricles and high intracranial pressure (>10 mmHg) with clinical signs of lethargy, apnea or convulsions is an indication for considering early surgical intervention. The best time for intervention in posthemorrhagic ventricular dilatation is still under debate. A retrospective study of early versus late treatment of posthemorrhagic ventricular dilatation from five neonatal units in the Netherlands showed that shunt insertion was significantly more frequent amongst infants in whom treatment was initiated once the ventricular width was 4 mm above the 97th centile (using the Levene ventricular index) (late treatment) [64] than in those treated earlier. It was also noted that those treated late were more likely to develop moderate to severe disabilities compared to those treated early [64]. The early treatment was varied, and included lumbar puncture, ventricular taps, placement of subcutaneous reservoir, and insertion of ventriculoperitoneal shunt. In view of these data a randomized controlled multicenter trial has been started comparing early and late intervention of posthemorrhagic ventricular dilatation. The "late" group will reach a ventricular size that is the same as that in the early ventriculomegaly trials, namely 4 mm above the 97th centile, whereas the "early" group will be treated at a ventricular size less than this, with a decision to treat based on progression of the ventriculomegaly and a "ballooning" shape of the ventricle. Once intervention has been started, only a few lumbar punctures are allowed in both groups, before insertion of a subcutaneous reservoir [64].

Prevention

At present there are no effective methods for preventing posthemorrhagic ventriculomegaly after GMH-IVH has developed, but it is important to reiterate the need for vitamin K prophylaxis in the newborn. At term, VKDB remains a relatively rare but important cause of intraventricular hemorrhage. In the future, early fibrinolysis may be aimed at prevention rather than cure in babies with intraventricular hemorrhage who are deemed to be at high risk of developing hydrocephalus.

Surgical intervention

Surgical treatment of posthemorrhagic dilatation includes external ventricular drain [99,100], subcutaneous ventricular reservoir placement [64,101,102,103], ventriculostomy, and ventriculoperitoneal shunt [104]. A formal ventriculoperitoneal shunt is the definitive and traditional treatment of most forms of hydrocephalus but it is not an option very early after intraventricular hemorrhage in extremely preterm infants because of the high risk of blockage, infection, and skin ulceration. Subcutaneous ventricular reservoir placement with repeated CSF drainage by needle puncture has been shown to be a safe procedure [67,101] and can be performed in neonatal intensive care units. An infection rate of 4%–8% is common when using ventricular reservoir devices [67,101]. Endoscopic third ventriculostomy is a technically demanding surgical option which has been applied to very few babies with posthemorrhagic hydrocephalus [105,106]. In infants with enlarging ventricles our decision to intervene is currently based on the development of signs suggesting raised intracranial pressure or a head circumference that is crossing centile lines.

Non-surgical intervention

Serial lumbar puncture

As the mechanism of posthemorrhagic dilatation is related to blockage of CSF channels by small blood clots, early removal of bloody CSF by lumbar puncture or even ventricular taps has been performed in small studies and a large multicenter study, but without beneficial effect [83,107,108,109].

Diuretic treatment

The use of acetazolamide and furosemide in an international randomized controlled trial of posthemorrhagic ventricular dilatation was associated with a higher rate of death or shunt insertions with a relative risk of 1.42 (95% confidence interval, CI, 1.06–1.90, $p = 0.026$), which is equivalent to one extra death or shunt insertion for every five infants allocated to the drug therapy. The treatment was associated with an increased neurological morbidity which was also shown at 1 year of age [84,110], and is now no longer considered appropriate management. Isosorbide is another historical treatment which worked on the diuresis principle and has been abandoned.

Fibrinolytic treatment

A review of 62 cases of intraventricular administration of fibrinolytic agents such as streptokinase or tissue plasminogen activator was unable to show any benefit [107]. One randomized controlled trial involving the intraventricular injection of streptokinase showed no reduction in the later need for shunt surgery [111]. As yet, this treatment is experimental.

Drainage, irrigation, and fibrinolysis

After a promising single-center pilot study of prevention of hydrocephalus by drainage, irrigation, and fibrinolytic therapy (DRIFT), a treatment which showed reduced shunt surgery and an improvement in mortality and disability rates [82], a multi-center randomized controlled study (the DRIFT trial) was commenced. The DRIFT treatment consists of the insertion of two ventricular catheters (one right frontal, one left occipital), intra-ventricular administration of tissue plasminogen activator and irrigation of the ventricles with artificial CSF for a median of 72 hours [55,82]. Drainage and irrigation may reduce ongoing brain injury by normalizing pressure, reducing free radical injury from non-protein-bound iron and reducing pro-inflammatory cytokines [112]. Standard treatment consisted of lumbar puncture and, when more than two lumbar punctures per day were necessary or when lumbar puncture failed to drain enough CSF, a ventricular reservoir was inserted. The trial was closed early after an interim analysis of the first 50% of infants conducted for the Data Monitoring and Safety Group [113]. This decision was based on the observation that 34% (12/34) of infants who received DRIFT had secondary intraventricular hemorrhage, compared with 8% (3/36) in the standard treatment group, a statistically significant difference. Additional evidence that this secondary hemorrhage was of clinical relevance is provided by the observation that 67% of infants in the DRIFT group had secondary intraventricular hemorrhage that required shunt surgery, whereas only 23% of the DRIFT group without secondary intraventricular hemorrhage required shunt surgery. No significant difference in primary outcome, shunt surgery or death was found between the two treatment groups [113].

Prognosis and counseling

Since the early days of shunt surgery, the mortality of hydro-cephalus has improved dramatically, and the rate of infection per operative procedure has also improved, with some centers reporting rates as low as 2%–4%. However, the neurodevelopmental outcome in infants with hydrocephalus continues to be generally poor, with about 75% of the children developing cerebral palsy and 50% learning disabilities, with a smaller percentage affected by epilepsy [114,115,116]. Hearing loss affects some 6% and visual impairment 9% of infants followed to 30 months of age [115]. Neuropsychiatric disorders including attention deficit hyperactivity disorder are also common and disabling.

In an early study in 1987 the main determinant of neuro-developmental outcome of posthemorrhagic ventricular dilatation seemed to be the presence or absence of parenchymal lesions [117]. These early results have been confirmed in more recent studies, with cerebral palsy developing in 2/10 infants with large intraventricular hemorrhage but no parenchymal lesion, compared to 11/13 infants with intraventricular hemorrhages and additional parenchymal lesions [118]. Similar results have been reported from Japan: 78 children with post-hemorrhagic hydrocephalus born between 1981 and 1999 were

followed for almost 10 years [119]. Only 16% had an entirely normal outcome, and the major determinant of outcome was the presence of a parenchymal lesion [119].

To summarize, the following general principles apply when counseling parents regarding the prognosis of their infant with posthemorrhagic ventricular dilatation:

- The prognosis for preterm babies with posthemorrhagic ventricular dilatation who require shunting is that the majority will have some form of disability:
  - cerebral palsy in at least 50%
  - learning difficulties in around 50%
  - epilepsy in around 30%
  - and visual impairment in 9%
- The presence of any lesion in the brain parenchyma worsens the outcome, with about 75% developing cerebral palsy
- The prognosis is worse for babies who require shunting than for those who do not
- Shunting in infancy carries a risk of infection, disconnection and blockage with about a half of babies requiring one or other repeat surgical procedure in the first year.

References

1. Filly RA, Cardoza JD, Goldstein RB, Barkovich AJ. Detection of fetal central nervous system anomalies: a practical level of effort for a routine sonogram. *Radiology* 1989; **172(2)**: 403–8.

2. Cardoza JD, Goldstein RB, Filly RA. Exclusion of fetal ventriculomegaly with a single measurement: the width of the lateral ventricular atrium. *Radiology* 1988; **169(3)**: 711–14.

3. Achiron R, Schimmel M, Achiron A, Mashiach S. Fetal mild idiopathic lateral ventriculomegaly: is there a correlation with fetal trisomy? *Ultrasound Obstet Gynecol* 1993; **3(2)**: 89–92.

4. Gupta JK, Bryce FC, Lilford RJ. Management of apparently isolated fetal ventriculomegaly. *Obstet Gynecol Surv* 1994; **49(10)**: 716–21.

5. Pilu G, Reece EA, Goldstein I, Hobbins JC, Bovicelli L. Sonographic evaluation of the normal developmental anatomy of the fetal cerebral ventricles: II. The atria. *Obstet Gynecol* 1989; **73(2)**: 250–6.

6. Heiserman J, Filly RA, Goldstein RB. Effect of measurement errors on sonographic evaluation of ventriculomegaly. *J Ultrasound Med* 1991; **10(3)**: 121–4.

7. Alagappan R, Browning PD, Laorr A, McGahan JP. Distal lateral ventricular atrium: reevaluation of normal range. *Radiology* 1994; **193(2)**: 405–8.

8. Farrell TA, Hertzberg BS, Kliewer MA, Harris L, Paine SS. Fetal lateral ventricles: reassessment of normal values for atrial diameter at US. *Radiology* 1994; **193(2)**: 409–11.

9. Patel MD, Goldstein RB, Tung S, Filly RA. Fetal cerebral ventricular atrium: difference in size according to sex. *Radiology* 1995; **194(3)**: 713–15.

10. Hilpert PL, Hall BE, Kurtz AB. The atria of the fetal lateral ventricles: a sonographic study of normal atrial size and choroid plexus volume. *AJR Am J Roentgenol* 1995; **164(3)**: 731–4.

11. Senat MV, Bernard JP, Schwarzler P, Britten J, Ville Y. Prenatal diagnosis and follow-up of 14 cases of unilateral ventriculomegaly. *Ultrasound Obstet Gynecol* 1999; **14(5)**: 327–32.

12. Mercier A, Eurin D, Mercier PY, Verspyck E, Marpeau L, Marret S. Isolated mild fetal cerebral ventriculomegaly: a retrospective analysis of 26 cases. *Prenat Diagn* 2001; **21(7)**: 589–95.

13. Filly RA, Goldstein RB, Callen PW. Fetal ventricle: importance in routine obstetric sonography. *Radiology* 1991; **181(1)**: 1–7.

14. Vergani P, Locatelli A, Strobelt N, Cavallone M, Ceruti P, Paterlini G, Ghidini A. Clinical outcome of mild fetal ventriculomegaly. *Am J Obstet Gynecol* 1998; **178(2)**: 218–22.

15. Achiron R, Yagel S, Rotstein Z, Inbar O, Mashiach S, Lipitz S. Cerebral lateral ventricular asymmetry: is this a normal ultrasonographic finding in the fetal brain? *Obstet Gynecol* 1997; **89(2)**: 233-7.

16. Bromley B, Frigoletto FD, Jr., Benacerraf BR. Mild fetal lateral cerebral ventriculomegaly: clinical course and outcome. *Am J Obstet Gynecol* 1991; **164(3)**: 863-7.

17. Breeze AC, Dey PK, Lees CC, Hackett GA, Smith GC, Murdoch EM. Obstetric and neonatal outcomes in apparently isolated mild fetal ventriculomegaly. *J Perinat Med* 2005; **33(3)**: 236-40.

18. Goldstein RB, La Pidus AS, Filly RA, Cardoza J. Mild lateral cerebral ventricular dilatation in utero: clinical significance and prognosis. *Radiology* 1990; **176(1)**: 237-42.

19. Goldstein I, Copel JA, Makhoul IR. Mild cerebral ventriculomegaly in fetuses: characteristics and outcome. *Fetal Diagn Ther* 2005; **20(4)**: 281-4.

20. Gaglioti P, Danelon D, Bontempo S, Mombro M, Cardaropoli S, Todros T. Fetal cerebral ventriculomegaly: outcome in 176 cases. *Ultrasound Obstet Gynecol* 2005; **25(4)**: 372-7.

21. Patel MD, Filly AL, Hersh DR, Goldstein RB. Isolated mild fetal cerebral ventriculomegaly: clinical course and outcome. *Radiology* 1994; **192(3)**: 759-64.

22. Toi A. Spontaneous resolution of fetal ventriculomegaly in a diabetic patient. *J Ultrasound Med* 1987; **6(1)**: 37-9.

23. Kelly EN, Allen VM, Seaward G, Windrim R, Ryan G. Mild ventriculomegaly in the fetus, natural history, associated findings and outcome of isolated mild ventriculomegaly: a literature review. *Prenat Diagn* 2001; **21(8)**: 697-700.

24. Ouahba J, Luton D, Vuillard E *et al.* Prenatal isolated mild ventriculomegaly: outcome in 167 cases. *Br J Obstet Gynaecol* 2006; **113(9)**: 1072-9.

25. Chervenak FA, Duncan C, Ment LR *et al.* Outcome of fetal ventriculomegaly. *Lancet* 1984; **2(8396)**: 179-81.

26. Mahony BS, Nyberg DA, Hirsch JH, Petty CN, Hendricks SK, Mack LA. Mild idiopathic lateral cerebral ventricular dilatation in utero: sonographic evaluation. *Radiology* 1988; **169(3)**: 715-21.

27. Nyberg DA, Mack LA, Hirsch J, Pagon RO, Shepard TH. Fetal hydrocephalus: sonographic detection and clinical significance of associated anomalies. *Radiology* 1987; **163(1)**: 187-191.

28. Tomlinson MW, Treadwell MC, Bottoms SF. Isolated mild ventriculomegaly: associated karyotypic abnormalities and in utero observations. *J Matern Fetal Med* 1997; **6(4)**: 241-4.

29. Morris JE, Rickard S, Paley MN, Griffiths PD, Rigby A, Whitby EH. The value of in-utero magnetic resonance imaging in ultrasound diagnosed foetal isolated cerebral ventriculomegaly. *Clin Radiol* 2007; **62(2)**: 140-4.

30. Greco P, Vimercati A, De Cosmo L, Laforgia N, Mautone A, Selvaggi L. Mild ventriculomegaly as a counselling challenge. *Fetal Diagn Ther* 2001; **16(6)**: 398-401.

31. Pilu G, Falco P, Gabrielli S, Perolo A, Sandri F, Bovicelli L. The clinical significance of fetal isolated cerebral borderline ventriculomegaly: report of 31 cases and review of the literature. *Ultrasound Obstet Gynecol* 1999; **14(5)**: 320-6.

32. Lipitz S, Yagel S, Malinger G, Meizner I, Zalel Y, Achiron R. Outcome of fetuses with isolated borderline unilateral ventriculomegaly diagnosed at mid-gestation. *Ultrasound Obstet Gynecol* 1998; **12(1)**: 23-6.

33. Nicolaides KH, Berry S, Snijders RJ, Thorpe-Beeston JG, Gosden C. Fetal lateral cerebral ventriculomegaly: associated malformations and chromosomal defects. *Fetal Diagn Ther* 1990; **5(1)**: 5-14.

34. Levine D, Barnes PD, Madsen JR, Abbott J, Mehta T, Edelman RR. Central nervous system abnormalities assessed with prenatal magnetic resonance imaging. *Obstet Gynecol* 1999; **94(6)**: 1011-19.

35. Levine D. Fetal magnetic resonance imaging. *Top Magn Reson Imaging* 2001; **12(1)**: 1-2.

36. Levine D. Magnetic resonance imaging in prenatal diagnosis. *Curr Opin Pediatr* 2001; **13(6)**: 572-8.

37. Levine D. Ultrasound versus magnetic resonance imaging in fetal evaluation. *Top Magn Reson Imaging* 2001; **12(1)**: 25-38.

38. Levine D, Barnes PD, Madsen JR, Li W, Edelman RR. Fetal central nervous system anomalies: MR imaging augments sonographic diagnosis. *Radiology* 1997; **204(3)**: 635-642.

39. Levine D, Barnes PD, Robertson RR, Wong G, Mehta TS. Fast MR imaging of fetal central nervous system abnormalities. *Radiology* 2003; **229(1)**: 51-61.

40. Whitby EH, Paley MN, Sprigg A *et al.* Comparison of ultrasound and magnetic resonance imaging in 100 singleton pregnancies with suspected brain abnormalities. *Br J Obstet Gynaecol* 2004; **111(8)**: 784-92.

41. Whitby E, Paley MN, Davies N, Sprigg A, Griffiths PD. Ultrafast magnetic resonance imaging of central nervous system abnormalities in utero in the second and third trimester of pregnancy: comparison with ultrasound. *Br J Obstet Gynaecol* 2001; **108(5)**: 519-26.

42. Salomon LJ, Ouahba J, Delezoide AL *et al.* Third-trimester fetal MRI in isolated 10- to 12-mm ventriculomegaly: is it worth it? *Br J Obstet Gynaecol* 2006; **113(8)**: 942-7.

43. Malinger G, Lev D, Lerman-Sagie T. Fetal central nervous system: MR imaging versus dedicated US - need for prospective, blind, comparative studies. *Radiology* 2004; **232(1)**: 306; author reply pp. 306-7.

44. Malinger G, Ben-Sira L, Lev D, Ben-Aroya Z, Kidron D, Lerman-Sagie T. Fetal brain imaging: a comparison between magnetic resonance imaging and dedicated neurosonography. *Ultrasound Obstet Gynecol* 2004; **23(4)**: 333-40.

45. Fogliarini C, Chaumoitre K, Chapon F *et al.* Assessment of cortical maturation with prenatal MRI. Part II: abnormalities of cortical maturation. *Eur Radiol* 2005; **15(9)**: 1781-9.

46. Breeze AC, Alexander PM, Murdoch EM, Missfelder-Lobos HH, Hackett GA, Lees CC. Obstetric and neonatal outcomes in severe fetal ventriculomegaly. *Prenat Diagn* 2007; **27(2)**: 124-9.

47. Twining P, Jaspan T, Zuccollo J. The outcome of fetal ventriculomegaly. *Br J Radiol* 1994; **67(793)**: 26-31.

48. Graham E, Duhl A, Ural S, Allen M, Blakemore K, Witter F. The degree of antenatal ventriculomegaly is related to pediatric neurological morbidity. *J Matern Fetal Med* 2001; **10(4)**: 258-63.

49. Bloom SL, Bloom DD, DellaNebbia C, Martin LB, Lucas MJ, Twickler DM. The developmental outcome of children with antenatal mild isolated ventriculomegaly. *Obstet Gynecol* 1997; **90(1)**: 93-7.

50. Laskin MD, Kingdom J, Toi A, Chitayat D, Ohlsson A. Perinatal and neurodevelopmental outcome with isolated fetal ventriculomegaly: a systematic review. *J Matern Fetal Neonatal Med* 2005; **18(5)**: 289-98.

51. Kinzler WL, Smulian JC, McLean DA, Guzman ER, Vintzileos AM. Outcome of prenatally diagnosed mild unilateral cerebral ventriculomegaly. *J Ultrasound Med* 2001; **20(3)**: 257-262.

52. Whitelaw A. Endogenous fibrinolysis in neonatal cerebrospinal fluid. *Eur J Pediatr* 1993; **152(11)**: 928-930.

53. Whitelaw A, Mowinckel MC, Abildgaard U. Low levels of plasminogen in cerebrospinal fluid after intraventricular haemorrhage: a limiting factor for clot lysis? *Acta Paediatr* 1995; **84(8)**: 933-6.

54. Whitelaw A, Christie S, Pople I. Transforming growth factor-beta 1: a possible signal molecule for posthemorrhagic hydrocephalus? *Pediatr Res* 1999; **46(5)**: 576-580.

55. Whitelaw A. Intraventricular haemorrhage and posthaemorrhagic hydrocephalus: pathogenesis, prevention and future interventions. *Semin Neonatol* 2001; **6(2)**: 135-46.

56. Kaiser AM, Whitelaw AG. Cerebrospinal fluid pressure during post haemorrhagic ventricular dilatation in newborn infants. *Arch Dis Child* 1985; **60(10)**: 920-4.

57. Savman K, Nilsson UA, Blennow M, Kjellmer I, Whitelaw A. Non-protein-bound iron is elevated in cerebrospinal fluid from preterm infants with posthaemorrhagic ventricular dilatation. *Pediatr Res* 2001; **49(2)**: 208-12.

58. Savman K, Blennow M, Hagberg H, Tarkowski E, Thoresen M, Whitelaw A. Cytokine response in cerebrospinal fluid from preterm

infants with posthaemorrhagic ventricular dilatation. *Acta Paediatr* 2002; **91(12)**: 1357–63.

59. De Vries LS, Pierrat V, Minami T, Smet M, Casaer P. The role of short latency somatosensory evoked responses in infants with rapidly progressive ventricular dilatation. *Neuropediatrics* 1990; **21(3)**: 136–9.

60. Wozniak M, McLone DG, Raimondi AJ. Micro- and macrovascular changes as the direct cause of parenchymal destruction in congenital murine hydrocephalus. *J Neurosurg* 1975; **43(5)**: 535–45.

61. Volpe J. *Neurology of the Newborn*, 4th edn. Philadelphia, Saunders, 2001.

62. Boillat CA, Jones HC, Kaiser GL, Harris NG. Ultrastructural changes in the deep cortical pyramidal cells of infant rats with inherited hydrocephalus and the effect of shunt treatment. *Exp Neurol* 1997; **147(2)**: 377–88.

63. Lary S, De Vries LS, Kaiser A, Dubowitz LM, Dubowitz V. Auditory brain stem responses in infants with posthaemorrhagic ventricular dilatation. *Arch Dis Child* 1989; **64 (1** Spec No): 17–23.

64. de Vries LS, Liem KD, van Dijk K *et al.* Early versus late treatment of posthaemorrhagic ventricular dilatation: results of a retrospective study from five neonatal intensive care units in The Netherlands. *Acta Paediatr* 2002; **91(2)**: 212–17.

65. Dykes FD, Dunbar B, Lazarra A, Ahmann PA. Posthemorrhagic hydrocephalus in high-risk preterm infants: natural history, management, and long-term outcome. *J Pediatr* 1989; **114(4 Pt 1)**: 611–18.

66. Murphy BP, Inder TE, Rooks V *et al.* Posthaemorrhagic ventricular dilatation in the premature infant: natural history and predictors of outcome. *Arch Dis Child Fetal Neonatal Ed* 2002; **87(1)**: F37–41.

67. Hudgins RJ, Boydston WR, Gilreath CL. Treatment of posthemorrhagic hydrocephalus in the preterm infant with a ventricular access device. *Pediatr Neurosurg* 1998; **29(6)**: 309–13.

68. Davies MW, Swaminathan M, Chuang SL, Betheras FR. Reference ranges for the linear dimensions of the intracranial ventricles in preterm neonates. *Arch Dis Child Fetal Neonatal Ed* 2000; **82(3)**: F218–23.

69. Levene MI. Measurement of the growth of the lateral ventricles in preterm infants with real-time ultrasound. *Arch Dis Child* 1981; **56(12)**: 900–4.

70. Allan WC, Holt PJ, Sawyer LR, Tito AM, Meade SK. Ventricular dilation after neonatal periventricular-intraventricular hemorrhage. Natural history and therapeutic implications. *Am J Dis Child* 1982; **136(7)**: 589–93.

71. London DA, Carroll BA, Enzmann DR. Sonography of ventricular size and germinal matrix hemorrhage in premature infants. *AJR Am J Roentgenol* 1980; **135(3)**: 559–64.

72. Sauerbrei EE, Digney M, Harrison PB, Cooperberg PL. Ultrasonic evaluation of neonatal intracranial hemorrhage and its complications. *Radiology* 1981; **139(3)**: 677–85.

73. Skolnick ML, Rosenbaum AE, Matzuk T, Guthkelch AN, Heinz ER. Detection of dilated cerebral ventricles in infants: a correlative study between ultrasound and computed tomography. *Radiology* 1979; **131(2)**: 447–51.

74. Levene MI, Starte DR. A longitudinal study of post-haemorrhagic ventricular dilatation in the newborn. *Arch Dis Child* 1981; **56(12)**: 905–10.

75. Helmke K, Winkler P. [Sonographically determined normal values of the intracranial ventricular system in the first year of life.] *Monatsschr Kinderheilkd* 1987; **135(3)**: 148–52.

76. Poland RL, Slovis TL, Shankaran S. Normal values for ventricular size as determined by real time sonographic techniques. *Pediatr Radiol* 1985; **15(1)**: 12–14.

77. Saliba E, Bertrand P, Gold F, Vaillant MC, Laugier J. Area of lateral ventricles measured on cranial ultrasonography in preterm infants: reference range. *Arch Dis Child* 1990; **65 (10** Spec No): 1029–32.

78. Levene MI, Williams JL, Fawer CL. Ultrasound of the infant's brain. *Clinics in Developmental Medicine, no. 92.* Spastics International Medical Publications. 1985 Oxford, Blackwell.

79. Lipscomb AP, Thorburn RJ, Stewart AL, Reynolds EO, Hope PL. Early treatment for rapidly progressive post-haemorrhagic hydrocephalus. *Lancet* 1983; **1(8339)**: 1438–9.

80. Allan WC, Holt PJ, Sawyer LR, Tito AM, Meade SK. Ventricular dilatation after neonatal periventricular-intraventricular hemorrhage. Natural history and therapeutic implications. *Am J Dis Child* 1982; **136(7)**: 589–93.

81. Quisling RG, Reeder JD, Setzer ES, Kande JV. Temporal comparative analysis of computed tomography with ultrasound for intracranial hemorrhage in premature infants. *Neuroradiology* 1983; **24(4)**: 205–11.

82. Whitelaw A, Pople I, Cherian S, Evans D, Thoresen M. Phase 1 trial of prevention of hydrocephalus after intraventricular hemorrhage in newborn infants by drainage, irrigation, and fibrinolytic therapy. *Pediatrics* 2003; **111(4 Pt 1)**: 759–765.

83. Ventriculomegaly Trial Group. Randomised trial of early tapping in neonatal posthaemorrhagic ventricular dilatation. *Arch Dis Child* 1990; **65 (1 Spec No)**: 3–10.

84. International PHVD Drug Trial Group. International randomised controlled trial of acetazolamide and furosemide in posthaemorrhagic ventricular dilatation in infancy. *Lancet* 1998; **352(9126)**: 433–40.

85. Brann B St, Wofsy C, Papile LA, Angelus P, Backstrom C. Quantification of neonatal cerebral ventricular volume by real-time ultrasonography. In vivo validation of the cylindrical coordinate method. *J Ultrasound Med* 1990; **9(1)**: 9–15.

86. Kampmann W, Walka MM, Vogel M, Obladen M. 3-D sonographic volume measurement of the cerebral ventricular system: in vitro validation. *Ultrasound Med Biol* 1998; **24(8)**: 1169–74.

87. Nagdyman N, Walka MM, Kampmann W, Stover B, Obladen M. 3-D ultrasound quantification of neonatal cerebral ventricles in different head positions. *Ultrasound Med Biol* 1999; **25(6)**: 895–900.

88. Csutak R, Unterassinger L, Rohrmeister C, Weninger M, Vergesslich KA. Three-dimensional volume measurement of the lateral ventricles in preterm and term infants: evaluation of a standardised computer-assisted method in vivo. *Pediatr Radiol* 2003; **33(2)**: 104–9.

89. Haiden N, Klebermass K, Rucklinger E *et al.* 3-D ultrasonographic imaging of the cerebral ventricular system in very low birth weight infants. *Ultrasound Med Biol* 2005; **31(1)**: 7–14.

90. Gilmore JH, Gerig G, Specter B *et al.* Infant cerebral ventricle volume: a comparison of 3-D ultrasound and magnetic resonance imaging. *Ultrasound Med Biol* 2001; **27(8)**: 1143–6.

91. Chadduck WM, Seibert JJ, Adametz J, Glasier CM, Crabtree M, Stansell CA. Cranial Doppler ultrasonography correlates with criteria for ventriculoperitoneal shunting. *Surg Neurol* 1989; **31(2)**: 122–8.

92. Chadduck WM, Crabtree HM, Blankenship JB, Adametz J. Transcranial Doppler ultrasonography for the evaluation of shunt malfunction in pediatric patients. *Childs Nerv Syst* 1991; **7(1)**: 27–30.

93. Taylor GA, Madsen JR. Neonatal hydrocephalus: hemodynamic response to fontanelle compression – correlation with intracranial pressure and need for shunt placement. *Radiology* 1996; **201(3)**: 685–9.

94. Quinn MW, Ando Y, Levene MI. Cerebral arterial and venous flow-velocity measurements in post-haemorrhagic ventricular dilatation and hydrocephalus. *Dev Med Child Neurol* 1992; **34(10)**: 863–9.

95. Pople IK, Quinn MW, Bayston R, Hayward RD. The Doppler pulsatility index as a screening test for blocked ventriculo-peritoneal shunts. *Eur J Pediatr Surg* 1991; **1** (Suppl **1**): 27–9.

96. Seibert JJ, McCowan TC, Chadduck WM *et al.* Duplex pulsed Doppler US versus intracranial pressure in the neonate: clinical and experimental studies. *Radiology* 1989; **171(1)**: 155–9.

97. Quinn MW, Levene MI. Changes in cerebral artery blood flow velocity after intermittent cerebrospinal fluid drainage. *Arch Dis Child Fetal Neonatal Ed* 1994; **70(2)**: F158–9.

98. Pople IK. Doppler flow velocities in children with controlled hydrocephalus: reference values for the diagnosis of blocked cerebrospinal fluid shunts. *Childs Nerv Syst* 1992; **8(3)**: 124–5.

99. Weninger M, Salzer HR, Pollak A *et al.* External ventricular drainage for treatment of rapidly progressive posthemorrhagic hydrocephalus. *Neurosurgery* 1992; **31(1)**: 52–7; discussion pp. 57–8.

100. Rhodes TT, Edwards WH, Saunders RL *et al*. External ventricular drainage for initial treatment of neonatal posthemorrhagic hydrocephalus: surgical and neurodevelopmental outcome. *Pediatr Neurosci* 1987; **13(5)**: 255-62.

101. Brouwer AJ, Groenendaal F, van den Hoogen A *et al*. The incidence of infections of ventricular reservoirs in the treatment of post haemorrhagic ventricular dilatation: a retrospective study (1992–2003). *Arch Dis Child Fetal Neonatal Ed* 2007; **92(1)**: F41-3.

102. Gaskill SJ, Marlin AE, Rivera S. The subcutaneous ventricular reservoir: an effective treatment for posthemorrhagic hydrocephalus. *Childs Nerv Syst* 1988; **4(5)**: 291-5.

103. McComb JG, Ramos AD, Platzker AC, Henderson DJ, Segall HD. Management of hydrocephalus secondary to intraventricular hemorrhage in the preterm infant with a subcutaneous ventricular catheter reservoir. *Neurosurgery* 1983; **13(3)**: 295-300.

104. Boynton BR, Boynton CA, Merritt TA, Vaucher YE, James HE, Bejar RF. Ventriculoperitoneal shunts in low birth weight infants with intracranial hemorrhage: neurodevelopmental outcome. *Neurosurgery* 1986; **18(2)**: 141-5.

105. Balthasar AJ, Kort H, Cornips EM, Beuls EA, Weber JW, Vles JS. Analysis of the success and failure of endoscopic third ventriculostomy in infants less than 1 year of age. *Childs Nerv Syst* 2007; **23(2)**: 151-5.

106. Koch-Wiewrodt D, Wagner W. Success and failure of endoscopic third ventriculostomy in young infants: are there different age distributions? *Childs Nerv Syst* 2006; **22(12)**: 1537-41.

107. Haines SJ, Lapointe M. Fibrinolytic agents in the management of posthemorrhagic hydrocephalus in preterm infants: the evidence. *Childs Nerv Syst* 1999; **15(5)**: 226-34.

108. Anwar M, Kadam S, Hiatt IM, Hegyi T. Serial lumbar punctures in prevention of post-hemorrhagic hydrocephalus in preterm infants. *J Pediatr* 1985; **107(3)**: 446-50.

109. Mantovani JF, Pasternak JF, Mathew OP *et al*. Failure of daily lumbar punctures to prevent the development of hydrocephalus following intraventricular hemorrhage. *J Pediatr* 1980; **97(2)**: 278-81.

110. Kennedy CR, Ayers S, Campbell MJ, Elbourne D, Hope P, Johnson A. Randomized, controlled trial of acetazolamide and furosemide in posthemorrhagic ventricular dilation in infancy: follow-up at 1 year. *Pediatrics* 2001; **108(3)**: 597-607.

111. Luciano R, Velardi F, Romagnoli C, Papacci P, De Stefano V, Tortorolo G. Failure of fibrinolytic endoventricular treatment to prevent neonatal post-haemorrhagic hydrocephalus. A case-control trial. *Childs Nerv Syst* 1997; **13(2)**: 73-6.

112. Whitelaw A, Cherian S, Thoresen M, Pople I. Posthaemorrhagic ventricular dilatation: new mechanisms and new treatment. *Acta Paediatr Suppl* 2004; **93(444)**: 11-14.

113. Whitelaw A, Evans D, Carter M *et al*. Randomized clinical trial of prevention of hydrocephalus after intraventricular hemorrhage in preterm infants: brain-washing versus tapping fluid. *Pediatrics* 2007; **119(5)**: e1071-8.

114. Fernell E, Hagberg G, Hagberg B. Infantile hydrocephalus epidemiology: an indicator of enhanced survival. *Arch Dis Child Fetal Neonatal Ed* 1994; **70(2)**: F123-8.

115. Ventricluomegaly Trial Group. Randomised trial of early tapping in neonatal posthaemorrhagic ventricular dilatation: results at 30 months. *Arch Dis Child Fetal Neonatal Ed* 1994; **70(2)**: F129-36.

116. Hoppe-Hirsch E, Laroussinie F, Brunet L *et al*. Late outcome of the surgical treatment of hydrocephalus. *Childs Nerv Syst* 1998; **14(3)**: 97-9.

117. Cooke RW. Determinants of major handicap in post-haemorrhagic hydrocephalus. *Arch Dis Child* 1987; **62(5)**: 504-6.

118. de Vries LS, Rademaker KJ, Groenendaal F *et al*. Correlation between neonatal cranial ultrasound, MRI in infancy and neurodevelopmental outcome in infants with a large intraventricular haemorrhage with or without unilateral parenchymal involvement. *Neuropediatrics* 1998; **29(4)**: 180-8.

119. Futagi Y, Suzuki Y, Toribe Y, Nakano H, Morimoto K. Neurodevelopmental outcome in children with posthemorrhagic hydrocephalus. *Pediatr Neurol* 2005; **33(1)**: 26-32.

Chapter 12 | The baby with an abnormal antenatal scan: congenital malformations

CORNELIA F. HAGMANN,
JANET M. RENNIE, *and*
NICOLA J. ROBERTSON

Introduction – clinical presentation

Increasingly, neonatologists are asked to advise women whose fetus is thought to have a congenital malformation of the brain or spinal cord because of abnormal antenatal ultrasound imaging. Counseling women and their partners in this situation is delicate and important work, but can be very difficult given the current state of knowledge about the natural history of antenatally diagnosed abnormalities and the imprecision of diagnosis. Antenatal magnetic resonance imaging (MRI) can assist, but this technique should not be used solely "for reassurance" – in our experience this can generate more problems than it solves. Our aim in this chapter is not only to provide examples of images including some rare conditions, but also to give guidance regarding further investigation and prognosis to help neonatologists who are faced with the management of a fetus and baby with a suspected cerebral malformation.

The commonest problems presenting to the neonatologist are agenesis of the corpus callosum, ventriculomegaly, and cystic lesions (arachnoid cysts, suspected Dandy Walker cysts or persisting choroid plexus cysts). Postnatally the findings of subependymal cysts and striate vasculopathy are also common. Midline lesions of the skin over the spinal cord are not rare. As a result we make no excuse for concentrating on these conditions, but we have chosen to present the material in a systematic way.

Disorders of prosencephalic development

The spectrum of pathology varies from profound derangement (aprosencephaly) to disturbances of the midline prosencephalic development (agenesis of the corpus callosum). A suggested classification is shown in Fig. 12.1 [1]. A spectrum of severity of facial dysmorphosis is observed in holoprosencephaly, which can vary from cyclopia, ethmocephaly, and cebocephaly to premaxillary agenesis, or simple cleft lip or hypotelorism [2]. It is now rare to see a newborn baby with the facial features of a single nostril, cyclops or a proboscis because the diagnosis is usually made antenatally and most parents choose termination of pregnancy. However, it is important to have an understanding of the disorder in order to assist fetal medicine colleagues in counseling, and because alobar holoprosencephaly can occur in the absence of any facial abnormality or with only a cleft lip and palate or hypotelorism [3].

Prosencephalic development can be considered in terms of three sequential events: porencephalic formation (aprosencephaly, atelencephaly), prosencephalic cleavage (holoprosencephaly, holotelencephaly), and midline prosencephalic development (agenesis of the corpus callosum, agenesis of the septum pellucidum, septo-optic dysplasia, septo-optic-hypothalamic dysplasia). Advances in genetics have revealed

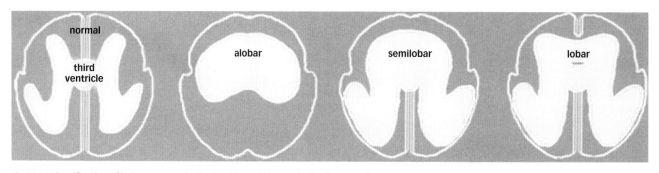

Fig. 12.1. **Classification of holoprosencephalic disorders. With permission from Leech, R. W. and Shuman, R. M. (1986). Holoprosencephaly and related midline cerebral anomalies: a review.** *J Child Neurol* **1(1): 3–18 [1].**

Neonatal Cerebral Investigation, eds. Janet M. Rennie, Cornelia F. Hagmann and Nicola J. Robertson. Published by Cambridge University Press. © Cambridge University Press 2008.

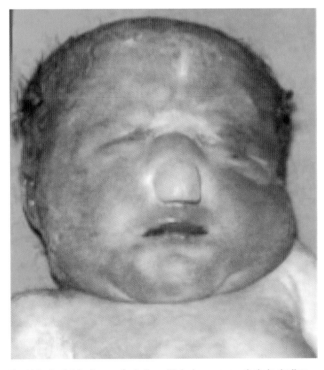

Fig. 12.2. **Pathology specimen of alobar holoprosencephaly demonstrating fused thalami and a monoventricle.**

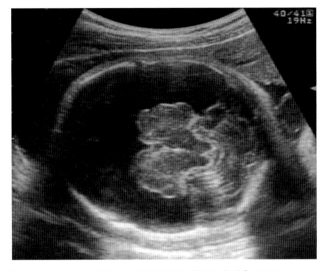

Fig. 12.4. **Antenatal ultrasound showing the typical features of holoprosencephaly with fused thalami and a large monoventricle.**

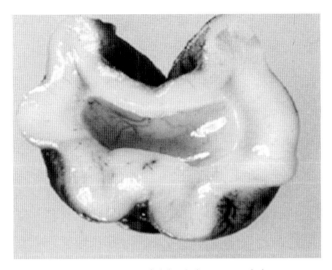

Fig. 12.3. **Facial features of a baby with holoprosencephaly including single nostril and hypotelorism.**

that homeobox genes, including sonic hedgehog (SHH) at the HPE3 locus causing an autosomal-dominant form of holoprosencephaly, are important in prosencephalic development [4].

Holoprosencephaly

The essential abnormality is a failure of the horizontal, transverse, and sagittal cleavage of the prosencephalon. Three variants may be distinguished (Fig. 12.2) [1]. The major pathological features of the most severe disturbance, alobar holoprosencephaly, include a single-sphered cerebral structure with a common ventricle (Fig. 12.2), a membranous roof over the third ventricle that is often distended into a large cyst posteriorly, the absence of olfactory bulbs and optic bulbs, accompanied by facial anomaly (Fig. 12.3). There may be a single median eye ("cyclops"), or severe hypotelorism, a single nostril nose (cebocephaly) with or without a proboscis and/or a cleft lip and palate (Fig. 12.3). The cases with the most severe facial deformity are generally associated with alobar holoprosencephaly. Onset of holoprosencephaly is no later than the fifth and sixth week of gestation. In a recent study in the north of England, the birth prevalence was 0.49 cases/10 000 births, with a higher prevalence of 1.2/10 000 registered births when fetal losses and terminations were included [5,6].

Imaging
Holoprosencephaly is usually diagnosed on antenatal ultrasound (Fig. 12.4). Postnatal cranial ultrasound reveals the single ventricle straddling fused thalami. The differentiation between the lobar and the semi lobar variants is easy with MRI, and is based on the detection of the posterior part of the falx and the interhemispheric fissure.

Clinical manifestation
Holoprosencephaly is particularly characteristic of trisomy 13 and 18. Clinical presentation depends upon the severity of the malformation. Careful examination of the parents is important as there is a rare autosomal-dominant form in which the carrier can have subtle midline defects such as ocular hypotelorism, single maxillary incisor tooth, anosmia, microcephaly or mental retardation.

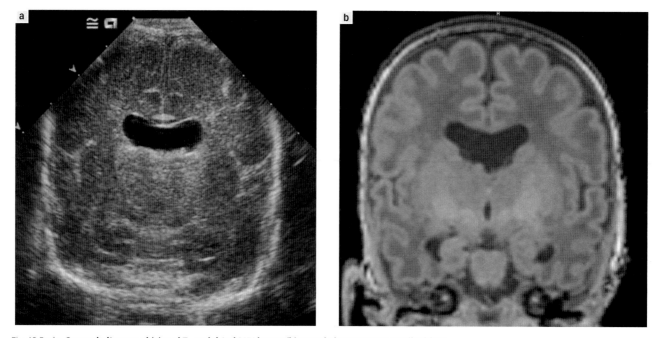

Fig. 12.5.a,b. **Coronal ultrasound (a) and T₁-weighted MRI image (b) reveal absent septum pellucidum.**

Counseling and prognosis

The prognosis of all but the most mildly affected cases is poor, and becomes obvious from the neonatal period with failure of neurological development, seizures, and death.

Agenesis of septum pellucidum

The septum pellucidum can be destroyed by hydrocephalus, or its absence can be associated with malformations of the brain such as septo-optic dysplasia. Thus the absence of the septum pellucidum can be an important clue to the presence of other abnormalities of prosencephalic development. Isolated absence of septum pellucidum (Fig. 12.5a,b) is rare compared to the absence of the septum pellucidum with associated brain abnormalities such as schizencephaly, holoprosencephaly and septo-optic dysplasia [7,8,9]. Barkovich *et al.* estimated the occurrence of isolated agenesis of the septum pellucidum as 2–3/10 000 individuals [7]. The full syndrome of septo-optic dysplasia includes absence of the septum pellucidum, optic nerve hypoplasia, absence or thinning of the corpus callosum, and hypothalamic–pituitary dysfunction. The falx is present in septo-optic dysplasia and usually absent in holoprosencephaly.

Imaging

The prenatal diagnosis of absence of septum pellucidum can be made with ultrasound, and the specific diagnosis of septo-pellucidum dysplasia is possible by fetal or postnatal MRI, although some caution is warranted in advising the parents since fetal or even early neonatal MRI is not sufficiently sensitive to detect mild degrees of hypoplasia of the optic nerve [10,11,12]. Because absence of the septum pellucidum can be associated with neuronal migration abnormalities or septo-optic dysplasia MRI should be obtained before counseling the parents.

Occasionally the two leaves of the septum pellucidum may fail to fuse and this is normal in preterm infants who have a large cavum septum pellucidum. However, if the structure is more than 10 mm wide in term infants further investigation with MRI is indicated; in one series of nine children eight had cognitive impairment and four had hypothalamic disturbances [13].

Clinical manifestation

The clinical features of absence of septum pellucidum depend on the associated abnormalities. Motor deficit, mental delay, blindness, and endocrine dysfunction are described in infants with absence of septum pellucidum and associated brain abnormalities, implying that in many reports where children were retarded the cause was due to the associated cerebral malformation rather than the absence of the septum pellucidum alone [9,14]. Nevertheless, some infants with isolated absence of septum pellucidum are reported to be neurologically abnormal [9,14]. In adult studies the absence of the septum pellucidum serves as a marker for cerebral dysfunction and has been described in various neuropsychiatric [15,16] and post-traumatic conditions [13,17].

Counseling and prognosis

The prognosis depends on whether the absent septum pellucidum is an isolated malformation, and we would not advise parents without additional information from postnatal or fetal MRI. Absence of septum pellucidum can be diagnosed by ultrasound from 20 weeks onwards, but some associated forebrain malformation and especially cortical dysplasia may not be detectable by ultrasound or fetal MRI before 30–32 weeks of gestation [11,18,19]. We have already noted the difficulty which may be encountered in reliably detecting optic nerve hypoplasia by fetal or early neonatal MRI. If the condition is truly isolated the prognosis is probably good. The finding of septo-optic dysplasia mandates referral for a full assessment of endocrine function, because hypothalamic and pituitary function are abnormal in 50%–90% of patients [20].

Agenesis of corpus callosum

The corpus callosum is the largest interhemispheric commissure (containing around 800 million fibers) that connects neocortical areas, integrating their functions. Development of the corpus callosum is a late event in ontogenesis, taking place between 12 and 18 weeks [21]. The growth of the corpus callosum can be monitored in utero, and occurs at the same time as much neuronal proliferation and migration. Agenesis of the corpus callosum may be either complete or partial and is rarely an isolated defect: it is usually seen in association with other nervous system abnormalities such as ventriculomegaly, interhemispheric cysts, Dandy Walker malformations, Chiari II malformation, encephalocele, holoprosencephaly, disorders of neuronal migration or extra-central nervous malformation [22,23,24,25,26]. Agenesis of the corpus callosum is more correctly termed dysgenesis because the fibers which normally cross the midline are not absent, but remain, forming the bundles of Probst on the internal aspect of the homolateral hemisphere (Fig. 12.6a). Agenesis of corpus callosum has been described in metabolic diseases such pyruvate dehydrogenase deficiency or non-ketotic hyperglycinemia. One important disorder characterized by agenesis of the corpus callosum in females is the Aicardi syndrome. Aicardi syndrome is defined as a triad of partial or complete agenesis of the corpus callosum, infantile spasms, and chorioretinal lacunae [27]. Other abnormalities such as neuronal migration, intracranial cysts or tumors and additional eye abnormalities have been described with Aicardi syndrome [27].

Imaging

The diagnosis is usually made by antenatal ultrasound and/or fetal MRI. There are controversial reports in the literature about the accuracy of diagnosing agenesis of the corpus callosum by antenatal ultrasound with reported detection rates as high as 66%–100% [28,29,30,31,32,33]. However, other groups postulate that agenesis of the corpus callosum is difficult to diagnose with ultrasound, especially in the second trimester [34,35], and false-positive [36,37] and false-negative diagnoses have been reported [37,38,39,40]. The conclusion of these reports is that fetal MRI is more sensitive than ultrasound in detecting agenesis of the corpus callosum and should be performed when it is suspected with ultrasound [35,38,39,41,42] (Fig. 12.6a,b). Fetal MRI is also important to rule out associated brain abnormalities of which the most common are interhemispheric cysts and gyral abnormalities.

The postnatal ultrasound appearances are characteristic (Fig. 12.6c,d). The normal corpus callosum is usually easily visualized in the midline with the pericallosal sulcus forming a clear "tram-like" band in the midline sagittal and coronal views [43]. In the absence of the corpus callosum the third ventricle often appears high and between the lateral ventricles

(this can vary), which are widely separated and of abnormal shape. The lateral ventricles appear like butterfly wings on the coronal views (Fig. 12.6a,c,e), with a lateral flat border [44]. There is a loss of the normal convexity of the medial borders of the anterior horns of the lateral ventricles, and in the posterior portion the atria and the occipital horns appear ballooned due to a persisting fetal configuration of the ventricles termed colpocephaly [45]. In the parasagittal view the cortical sulci radiate superiorly instead of horizontally, giving rise to a "sunburst" appearance (Fig 12.6d) [21]. Magnetic resonance imaging is indicated to evaluate associated neuronal migration disorder or other abnormalities, which may not have been seen on ultrasound, and to confirm the ultrasound findings (Fig. 12.6e,f).

Clinical manifestation

When agenesis of the corpus callosum is an isolated condition, infants may be asymptomatic [28,33,46,47,48]. Gupta and Lilford reported a 56% risk of developmental delay for children with agenesis of the corpus callosum when associated with other cerebral abnormalities and an 85% chance of a normal outcome in isolated agenesis of the corpus callosum [47]. Quite often it is associated with subtle to severe neurological deficits, generally appearing at school age with intellectual impairment, seizures, and behavioral disorders [22,46,49,50]. Follow-up studies have linked agenesis of the corpus callosum with neuropsychiatric disorders [50,51].

Infantile spasms are the most characteristic type of seizures for Aicardi syndrome and mental retardation a major feature. Neurological signs such as spastic hemiplegia are common in Aicardi syndrome [27].

Counseling and prognosis

As with agenesis of the septum pellucidum, it is vital to exclude other malformations before counseling regarding agenesis of the corpus callosum. If the abnormality is truly isolated then the prognosis is relatively good [47,48]. However, at school age, intellectual development tends to be at the lower end of the normal range, with subtle cognitive deficits [28,47,49]. If a second central nervous system (CNS) abnormality is found then the prognosis largely depends on the severity of that abnormality, but is often poor, although children with agenesis of the corpus callosum and giant interhemispheric arachnoid cyst can do well (Fig. 12.6g,h) [52]. Some have suggested that a more cautious prognosis should be given when a female fetus is found to have agenesis of the corpus callosum because of the risk of Aicardi syndrome, which does not occur in boys. The outcome of Aicardi syndrome is very severe in most cases but a spectrum of severity exists [27].

Abnormalities in the posterior fossa

Classically, posterior fossa cystic abnormalities have been divided into the Dandy Walker malformation, the Dandy Walker variant, and the mega cisterna magna. The Dandy Walker malformation consists of an enlarged posterior fossa with high position of the tentorium, hypogenesis or agenesis of the cerebellar vermis, and a cystic dilatation of the fourth ventricle. Many authors refer to Dandy Walker variant, but the term is used in so many different ways that it has caused confusion. Some authors use the term to refer to a hypoplastic inferior cerebellar vermis and a large cisterna magna without enlargement of the posterior fossa; others use it to refer to a Dandy-Walker-type malformation. In all these situations, the posterior fossa is not enlarged and the tentorium cerebelli is in its proper place. We agree with others, that the term "Dandy Walker variant" should no longer be used, and we would classify these abnormalities as cerebellar hypoplasia or dysplasia.

Dandy Walker malformation

The diagnosis of the "classic" Dandy Walker malformation consists of three major abnormalities: (1) enlarged posterior fossa with a high insertion of the tentorium cerebelli, (2) complete or partial agenesis of the cerebellar vermis, and (3) cystic dilatation of the fourth ventricle that fills nearly the posterior fossa. A tentorium in the correct anatomical position, not high, rules out a Dandy Walker malformation. Hydrocephalus may not become apparent for months or years after birth. Associated abnormalities are agenesis of the corpus callosum, aqueductal stenosis, cerebral neuronal heterotopias, abnormalities of inferior olivary or dentate nuclei.

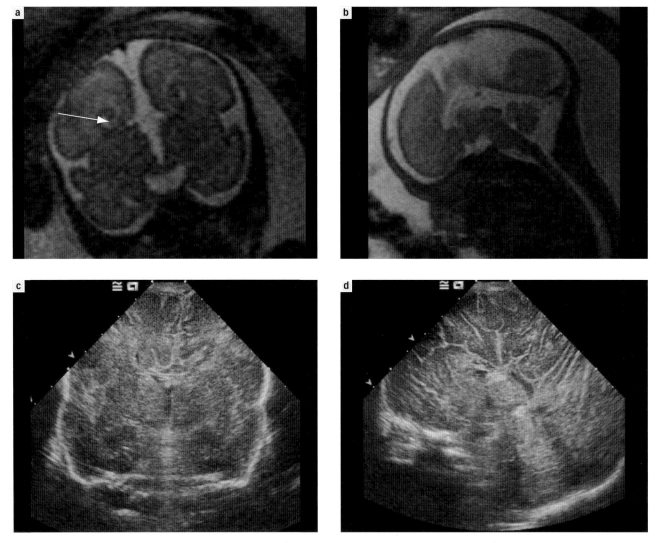

Fig. 12.6a–f. **The imaging characteristics of complete agenesis of the corpus callosum. (a,b) The appearances on fetal MRI (T$_2$-weighted images). (c,d) The appearances on neonatal cranial ultrasound images: (c) coronal and (d) sagittal midline image. (e,f) The postnatal T$_1$-weighted MRI appearances: (e) is a coronal view; (f) the midline sagittal. The coronal images (a,c,e) show the characteristic lateral convexity and separation of the frontal horns of the lateral ventricles and the upward extension of the third ventricle into the interhemispheric fissure between the lateral ventricles. On coronal MRI the bundle of Probst can be easily demonstrated (arrow in (a)). The postnatal sagittal MRI shows failure of formation of the cingulate gyrus with the cerebral sulci extending directly down to the roof of the lateral ventricle (white arrow); this is the correlate of the sunburst appearance seen ultrasound (f). (g,h) Coronal and axial T$_1$-weighted images show the absence of the corpus callosum with a large interhemispheric cyst, colpocephaly. The right lateral ventricles is effaced (arrow).**

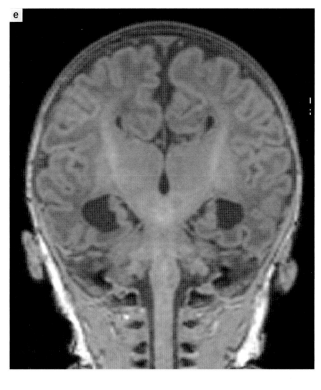

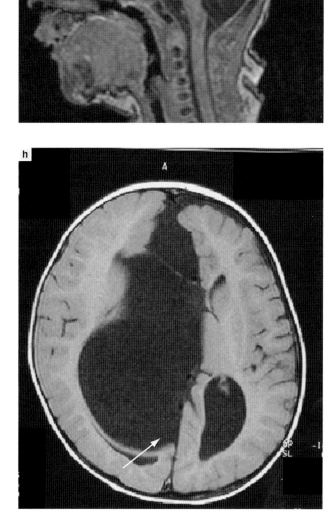

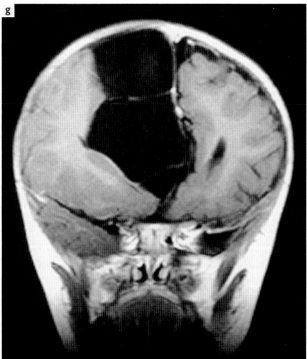

Fig. 12.6. **(cont.)**

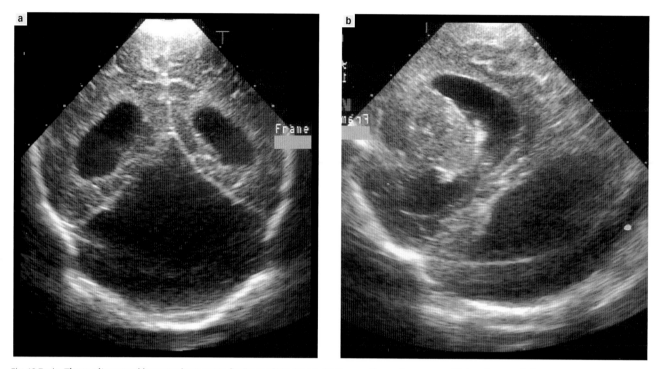

Fig. 12.7.a,b. **These ultrasound images show some findings of the Dandy Walker malformation: parsagittal and coronal ultrasound image with enlarged lateral ventricles and enlarged posterior fossa filled with a large CSF cyst.**

Imaging

Fetal or postnatal ultrasound can identify Dandy Walker malformation, the widening of the posterior fossa is best seen on a midline sagittal slice (Fig. 12.7a,b).

Clinical manifestation

Widespread use of antenatal and neonatal ultrasound has led to the identification of more cases in utero and in the neonatal period. After birth the baby should be referred to a neurosurgeon and regular head circumference measurements should be performed, because hydrocephalus develops within a few months in most cases. If undiagnosed antenatally, children under one year most often present with symptoms and signs of hydrocephalus and increased intracranial pressure, whereas children beyond one year usually present with delayed achievement of milestones, particularly walking and coordination [53]. Treatment options, when necessary, are cyst fenestration, ventriculo- and/or cystoperitoneal shunts and more recently endoscopic third ventriculostomy [54].

Counseling and prognosis

The neurodevelopmental outcome is related to both the severity of the malformation and the associated anomalies [55]. As with so many other conditions the prognosis is worse if there is a second CNS malformation [56,57,58]. Another prognostic factor seems to be gestational age at diagnosis, with poor prognosis if diagnosed before 21 weeks of gestation and a better prognosis if diagnosed later in gestation or postnatally [59,60].

Most large follow-up series of Dandy Walker syndrome report that the majority of the affected children have developmental delay although the severity varies, and about one-third of survivors are said to have an IQ of over 80 [56,58]. In other series, IQ was reported as normal in 54% children with isolated Dandy Walker malformation [61]. Normal lobulation of the vermis, in the absence of any supratentorial anomaly, appears to be a good prognostic factor in Dandy Walker malformation [62,63] whereas a dysgenetic vermis with only one or two recognizable lobes seems to be associated not only with poor neurodevelopmental outcome but also with other brain malformations (54).

Agenesis and hypoplasia of the cerebellum, including Joubert's syndrome

Cerebellar malformations are classified into abnormal formation (dysplasia) (Fig. 12.8a–f) and incomplete formation (hypoplasia) (Fig. 12.9) [64]. Incompletely formed or small, but otherwise normal appearing cerebella are considered as hypoplastic; cerebella with abnormally formed folia and fissures, as dysplastic. Normal values of the height of the cerebellum have been published with an average height of 15.4 mm at 28 weeks and an average height of 21 mm at term [65]. Generalized cerebellar hypoplasia occurs in the Dandy Walker complex, whereas generalized cerebellar dysplasia is often seen with congenital muscular dystrophies, congenital cytomegalovirus infection, and can be associated with lissencephaly or polymicrogyria.

Focal cerebellar dysplasia is described in Joubert's syndrome. In 1969, Joubert described four children with episodic hyperpnea, abnormal eye movement, ataxia, and mental retardation associated with agenesis of the cerebellar vermis, inherited in an autosomal-recessive manner [66]. Since then, many children with Joubert's syndrome have been described in the literature, confirming the original findings and establishing the "molar tooth sign" as the cardinal diagnostic imaging feature [67,68,69] (Fig. 12.10). Successful prenatal diagnosis of Joubert's syndrome is dependent on demonstrating vermis dysplasia, usually affecting the inferior vermis. The prenatal diagnosis of Joubert's syndrome and other posterior fossa malformation continues to be problematic, and fetal MRI at appropriate gestational can provide additional diagnostic information. For cerebellar, especially vermian abnormalities, fetal MRI should be performed only after 18 weeks of gestation, since potentially false-positive diagnoses may occur by scanning too early [70,71].

Mega cisterna magna, Blake's pouch cyst

Mega cisterna magna is difficult to diagnose since it is regarded as a normal variant corresponding to an expansion of the medullocerebellar cistern, which communicates freely with the subarachnoid space. The fetal cisterna magna is naturally wide [72] and widens throughout gestation before regressing postnatally. Mega cisterna magna can be differentiated from Dandy Walker malformation by the presence of a normal-sized and formed vermis, and a tentorium cerebelli in the correct position (see above). Cerebrospinal fluid collection in the posterior fossa should be termed mega cisterna magna only if there is no hydrocephalus or symptoms secondary to compression of the ventricular system [73]. Blake's cyst is a herniation

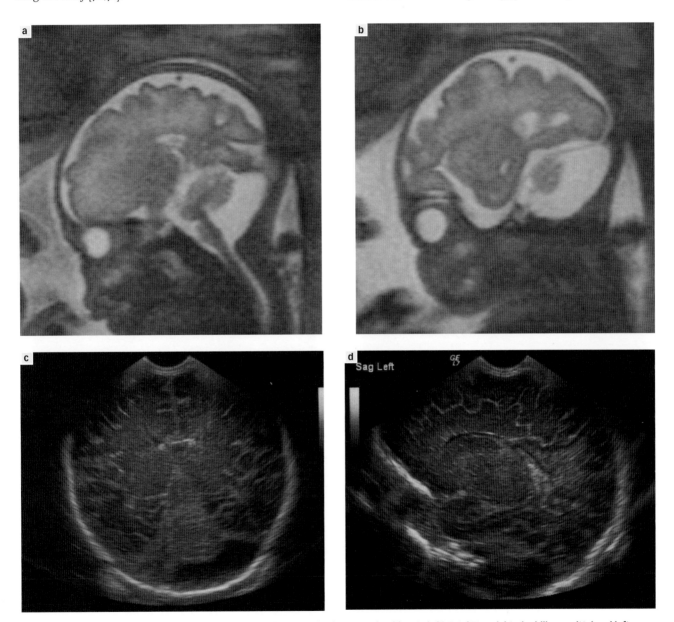

Fig. 12.8a–f. **Images showing left cerebellar hypoplasia with a posterior fossa arachnoid cyst. (a,b) Fetal T$_2$-weighted midline sagittal and left parasagittal MR image at 28 weeks of gestation. (c,d) Postnatal coronal and left parasagittal ultrasound at 38 weeks. (e,f) Postnatal T$_1$-weighted midline sagittal and axial MR image at 40 weeks of corrected gestational age. Postnatal ultrasound and MRI confirmed the antenatally diagnosed small left cerebellar hemisphere, a posterior fossa arachnoid cyst and a hypoplastic vermis.**

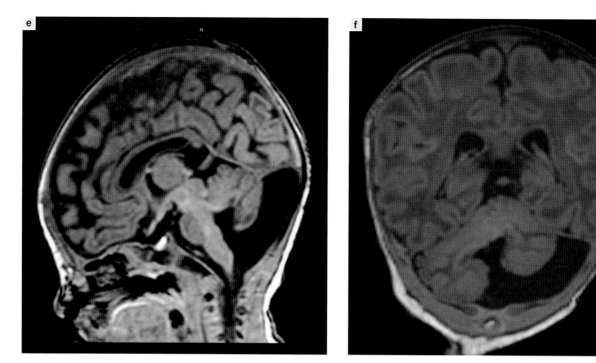

Fig. 12.8. **(cont.)**

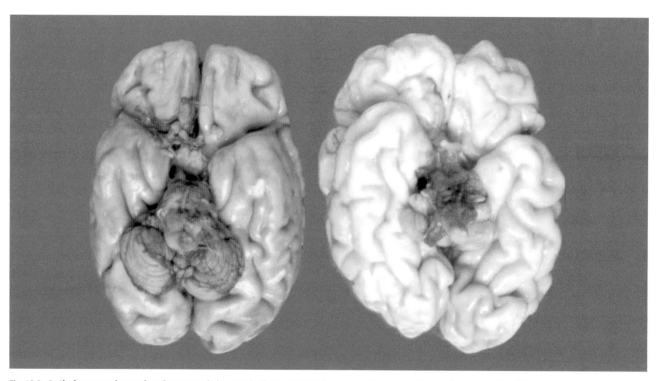

Fig. 12.9. **Pathology specimen showing normal size cerebellum on the left image and hypoplastic cerebellum on the right.**

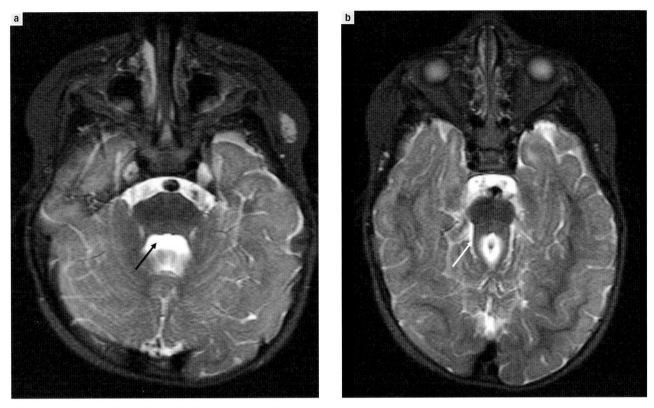

Fig. 12.10a,b. **Molar tooth sign. Child with clinical triad and radiological features of Joubert's syndrome. (a) Typical batwing appearance to the fourth ventricle (black arrow). (b) The prominent superior cerebellar peduncles with failure of the normal midline decussation (white arrow). This gives the typical "molar tooth" appearance. The midbrain is hypoplastic in this condition.**

of the inferior aspect of fourth ventricle through the foramen of Magendie into the vallecula and retrovermian cistern and can cause hydrocephalus [73] (Fig. 12.11a,b).

Disorders of neural tube development

Arnold Chiari malformation

Nearly every case of thoracolumbar, lumbar or lumbosacral myelomeningocele is accompanied by the Arnold Chiari malformation, which is central in the causation of hydrocephalus. This malformation includes inferior displacement of the medulla and fourth ventricle into cervical canal, elongation and thinning of the upper medulla and lower pons, inferior displacement of the lower cerebellum through the foramen magnum, and bony defects of the foramen magnum and upper cervical vertebrae. The Arnold Chiari malformation is associated with an aqueductal stenosis in up to 80% of cases [74] and with aqueductal atresia in an additional 10%.

Imaging

The Arnold Chiari malformation can be detected using ultrasound. Hydrocephalus is associated with Arnold Chiari malformation and there can be a loss of the septum pellucidum, which is often destroyed in the presence of long-standing prenatal hydrocephalus. Destruction of the septum pellucidum has to be distinguished from agenesis of the septum pellucidum (see above). In addition to brain MRI, all patients with

Arnold Chiari malformation should undergo spinal MR to detect hydromyelia [75].

Clinical presentation

The Arnold Chiari malformation is usually diagnosed because of the association with a neural tube defect. On occasion imaging performed for other signs – apnea or swallowing problems – reveals the abnormality. In a carefully studied series of infants with Arnold Chiari syndrome, one-third exhibited feeding disturbance (reflux, aspiration), laryngeal stridor, or apneic episode [76]. The median age of onset of midbrain symptoms is 3.2 months [77].

Counseling and prognosis

Generally, babies and children who have the Arnold Chiari malformation associated with spina bifida and hydrocephalus do not have specific neurological problems related to the Arnold Chiari malformation, and the prognosis relates to that of the neural tube defect and hydrocephalus. However, the constellation of stridor, apnea, cyanotic spells, and dysphagia is associated with a high mortality [78].

Cephalocele

Cephalocele is a midline defect of the skull that results in herniation of the cranial contents – either the meninges alone or both the meninges and brain. Meningoencephalocele refers to herniation of CSF, brain tissue, and meninges. Meningocele

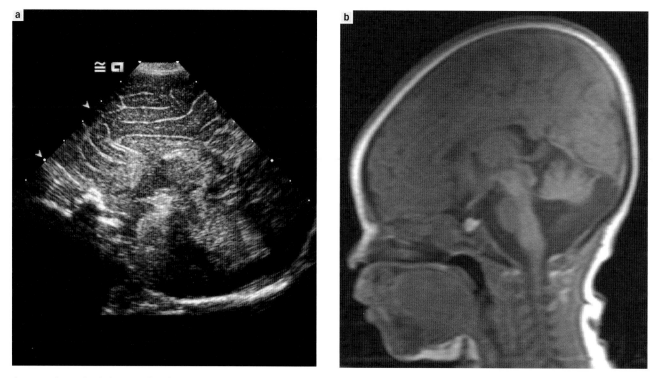

Fig. 12.11.a,b. **Sagittal ultrasound and T$_1$-weighted MR image showing a prominent Blake's pouch cyst; some authors may call this Dandy Walker variant.**

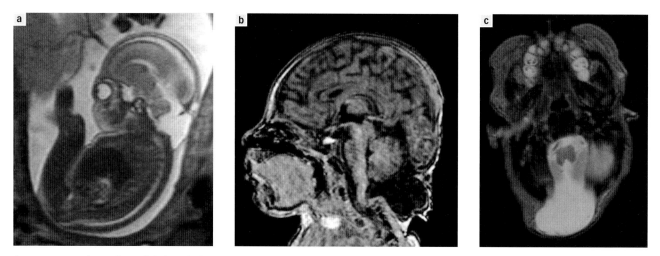

Fig. 12.12a–c. **Meningocele. Occipital cervical meningocele diagnosed antenatally. Note the short neck and subsequently Klippel-Feil was suspected. (a) Midline sagittal T$_2$-weighted image at 20 weeks of gestation. (b) Postnatal midline sagittal T$_1$-weighted image. (c) Postnatal axial T$_2$-weighted image showing the meningocele sac.**

refers to herniation of the meninges and CSF only (Fig. 12.12a–c). Skin-covered subscalp lesions that contain meninges or remnants of glial or neural tissue are termed atretic cephaloceles. Glioceles consist of CSF cysts lined by glial tissue. Most meningoencephaloceles are occipital, and the defect is thought to occur as a result of the failure of closure of the rostral end of the neural tube. Anterior encephaloceles are uncommon and more frequently reported in South-East Asia than in Europe or North America [79]. Occipital encephalocele can be part of a rare autosomal-recessive disorder, Meckel-Grubel syndrome, that is characterized by the classic triad of occipital encephalocele, polycystic kidneys, and axial polydactyly. Other associated malformations seen in this syndrome are microcephaly, microphthalmia, cleft lip and palate, and genital anomalies.

Imaging

The diagnosis is made prenatally by ultrasound and/or fetal MRI (Fig. 12.12a). Further CNS and abdominal imaging is indicated in order to examine the contents of the sac and to look for any associated malformation. Prenatal diagnosis of Meckel-Gruber syndrome is reliably made with ultrasound in the first trimester [80] and the state of the kidneys is important knowledge when confronted with counseling the parents. Postnatal MRI is indicated for planning surgery (Fig. 12.12b,c) and for diagnosing other abnormalities.

Clinical manifestation

The diagnosis is usually made in antenatal life, and after birth the condition is clinically obvious. Neurosurgical intervention is indicated in most cases.

Counseling and prognosis

Prognosis depends on the amount of protruding brain tissue and the associated malformations. Anterior encephaloceles tend to have better outcome than posterior ones [81]. If the lesion is an occipital or frontal meningocele then normal neurodevelopment is likely in over 50% of cases [82]. The prognosis depends on the volume of intracranial contents which are extruded, and is very poor if more than 50% of the brain volume is outside the skull. Meckel-Gruber syndrome is a lethal syndrome.

Occult spinal dysraphism

With the decline in the numbers of babies born with open neural tube defects, occult dysraphic states are of increasing importance in neonatal practice. We have confined the scope of this book to the brain, and more information on this topic can be found elsewhere.

Hydrocephalus

For information on diagnosis and counseling for hydrocephalus and ventriculomegaly see Chapter 11.

Malformation of cortical development

Malformation due to abnormal neuronal migration

Lissencephaly

Lissencephaly means "smooth brain" and refers to a paucity of gyral and sulcal development on the surface of the brain. Agyria is defined as an absence of gyri on the surface of the brain in association with a thick cortex and is synonymous with "complete lissencephaly." Pachygyria is defined as the presence of a few broad, flat gyri with thickened cortex and is synonymous with "incomplete lissencephaly." Lissencephaly is believed to result from a complete interruption of normal neuronal migration from the germinal matrix to the brain surface. Type I lissencephaly is also known as classical lissencephaly. Some patients with classical lissencephaly (agyria-pachygyria-complex) have a defect of the microtubule binding lissencephaly 1 (LIS1) gene at locus 17p13.3; a subset of the group with chromosome 17 mutations has characteristic facies and is classified as having Miller–Dieker syndrome. Other patients with classical lissencephaly have mutations of the doublecortin (DCX) gene at chromosome Xq22.3-q23; these

patients are typically boys whose mothers have heterotopia. About 75% of patients with lissencephaly have mutations of either 17p13.3 or Xq22.3–23 [83].

Type II, also known as cobble-stone lissencephaly, is characterized as HARD(E) syndrome (hydrocephaly, agyria, and retinal dysplasia) with or without encephalocele. It occurs in syndromes such as Fukuyama congenital muscular dystrophy, Finnish muscle eye brain disorder, and Walker–Warburg syndrome. Four genes have been associated with type II lissencephaly (POMT1 and POMT2 for Walker–Warburg, POMGnT1 for the Finish muscle eye brain disease, and fukutin for Fukuyama congenital muscular dystrophy). X-linked lissencephaly is associated with absent corpus callosum and ambiguous genitalia, which is caused by mutations of the ARX gene on chromosome Xp22.13 [84].

Imaging

Lissencephaly can be suspected by antenatal and postnatal ultrasound with findings such as absent parieto-occipital and calcarine fissures and abnormal Sylvian fissure indicative of underlying pathology [85,86] (Fig. 12.13a,b). There is usually a degree of ventriculomegaly, which raises suspicion. In the early second trimester, the normal brain is still smooth, and a diagnosis of delayed cortical development should not be considered before 20 weeks of gestation. In addition, the degree of cerebral involvement in lissencephaly varies; only the severe forms are likely to be detected by antenatal ultrasound. Magnetic resonance imaging can better depict pachygyria and subcortical band heterotopia, but even if fetal MRI is performed, mild forms of lissencephaly may not be detected if the examination is performed too early in pregnancy.

In patients with complete lissencephaly, MRI shows a smooth brain surface with diminished white matter and shallow, vertically orientated Sylvian fissures. These give the brain an appearance of figure-of-eight on axial images (Fig. 12.13c). In the incomplete lissencephaly areas of pachygyria are present together with agyria or normal cortex. Magnetic resonance imaging is able to detect associated brain malformation such as agenesis of the corpus callosum, heterotopia, and abnormalities in the posterior fossa.

Clinical manifestation

The clinical presentation of classical lissencephaly always features severe mental retardation, and diplegia, partial seizures and especially infantile spasms are the rule. Children with lissencephaly secondary to LIS1 and DCX mutations have similar neurological symptoms. Infantile seizures are common in severely affected children. The clinical features of type II lissencephaly include severe neurological dysfunction from birth, eye abnormalities and, in most, hydrocephalus.

Counseling and prognosis

The prognosis for babies diagnosed with lissencephaly is very poor and genetic counseling should be offered to the parents. Termination of pregnancy should be discussed if the diagnosis is made antenatally, and full neonatal intensive care is not indicated postnatally.

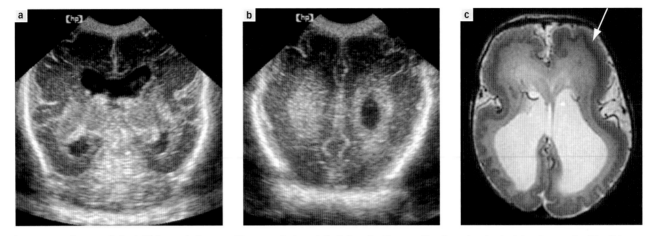

Fig. 12.13a–c. **Lissencephaly.** (a,b) Coronal ultrasound images of a term infant showing the paucity of gyral and sulcal development with mild ventriculomegaly. (c) Axial T$_2$-weighted MR image shows a shallow vertically oriented Sylvian fissure giving the brain a figure-of-eight appearance, with an unusual appearance of the cortical layers. Smooth underdeveloped cerebral gyri, the dark band (arrow) represents the layer of arrested neurons which have failed to reach outer cortex.

Malformation due to abnormal cortical organization and late migration

Schizencephaly

Schizencephaly is a severe cortical abnormality. In this condition there appears to be a complete agenesis of a portion of germinal matrix, leaving seams or clefts spanning from the cortical surface to the lateral ventricles edged by cortical gray matter. The lips of the clefts can become widely separated; they tend to occur in the regions of the Rolandic and Sylvian fissures, and involve predominantly frontal areas. The advent of MRI has contributed greatly to our understanding of anatomical and clinical aspects of schizencephaly. Some cases are caused by an environmental insult in the second trimester, in other cases the disorder is familial and may be associated with mutations of the EMX2 homeobox gene, located on chromosome 10q26 [87].

Imaging

It is not impossible to see the clefts on antenatal or postnatal ultrasound. The clue is often the presence of ventriculomegaly with colpocephaly, and the diagnosis can be confirmed either by fetal or postnatal MRI (Fig. 12.14a–d). For prognostic purposes, the patients are divided into unilateral and bilateral clefts, and open and fused lips.

If unilateral schizencephaly is suspected with antenatal ultrasound, fetal MRI should be performed to exclude the bilateral form of schizencephaly since this bilaterality does change the prognosis. Associated brain abnormalities such as absence of septum pellucidum or corpus callosal dysgenesis can be diagnosed by ultrasound and/or MRI, and migrational disorders such as heterotopia can be diagnosed by MRI.

Clinical manifestation

The most frequently presenting neonatal sign is asymmetrical muscle tone in the unilateral form, or childhood developmental delay when both hemispheres are involved [88]. Seizures can also be the first sign of the abnormality. Epilepsy is noted in 50%–80% of cases of schizencephaly, with onset before the age of 3 years in 81% of cases [89,90]. In most reports, seizures begin earlier and have worse outcome in patients with bilateral cleft, although seizures in unilateral ones are more frequent [90]. A neurological deficit is detected in almost half of the cases during the first year. The clinical (motor and cognitive outcome) features of schizencephaly are extremely variable and their severity is closely related to the size and bilaterality of the cleft. Children with unilateral schizencephaly often present with hemiparesis and mild mental delay. Children with bilateral cleft are usually tetraplegic with severe mental deficits [88,90]. Language impairment is seen in 60% of patients with unilateral clefts and 100% of children with bilateral clefts. The degree of malformation was not related to the severity of epilepsy in several studies [88,90].

Counseling and prognosis

The major prognostic factor is the bilaterality of the cleft and its location. From the discussion of the spectrum of clinical manifestations given above it can be seen that the prognosis of bilateral schizencephaly is poor. If there is a small unilateral closed-lip cleft without involvement of the motor cortex, the child is usually normal except for seizures [91]. In contrast, a motor defect was noted in 84%–100% of cases when the frontal lobe was involved, against only 29% if this was not the case [88,91,92]. A large unilateral cleft is likely to be associated with contralateral hemiplegic cerebral palsy, seizures, and severe learning disability. Genetic counseling should be offered to parents as the disorder is familial in some cases, and the parents should be offered MRI themselves.

Polymicrogyria

Polymicrogyria is characterized by a great number of small plications in the cortical surface. The multitude of small gyri

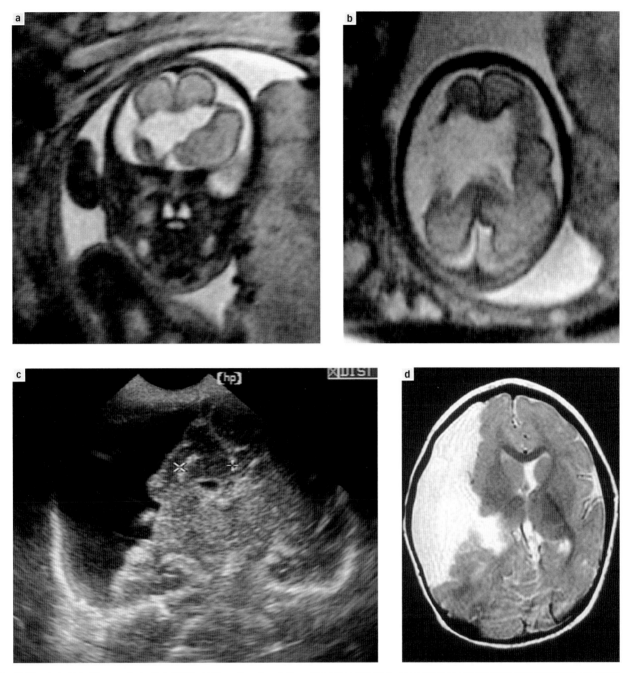

Fig. 12.14.a–d. **(a,b) Schizencephaly. Fetal MRI at 27 weeks of gestation. The antenatal ultrasound diagnosed unilateral cleft indicative of either unilateral schizencephaly or porencephalic cyst. Fetal MRI revealed bilateral schizencephaly with an open-lip cleft on the right side and a closed-lip cleft on the left side with gray matter lining the cleft. (c,d) Schizencephaly. Coronal ultrasound and axial T$_2$-weighted MR image showing unilateral open-lip schizencephaly in the neonatal period.**

is arranged in complicated festoon-like or glandular formations [21]. Polymicrogyria may affect the whole cortex, but more often they involve localized areas which often correspond to arterial territories. The layered and unlayered polymicrogyria are the two major histological variants. The non-layered type represents a disorder of neuronal migration, and thus appears no later than the fourth of fifth months of gestation. The layered type is a postmigrational disorder [21].

It is thought that polymicrogyria results from an insult to the brain that occurs toward the end of the neuronal migration period and during the early phase of cortical organization [93,94]. Several reported causes of polymicrogyria are thought to act through a final common pathway of perfusion failure, such as infectious fetopathies (e.g., cytomegalovirus) [95], maternal shock [96], or twin-to-twin transfusion syndrome [97,98].

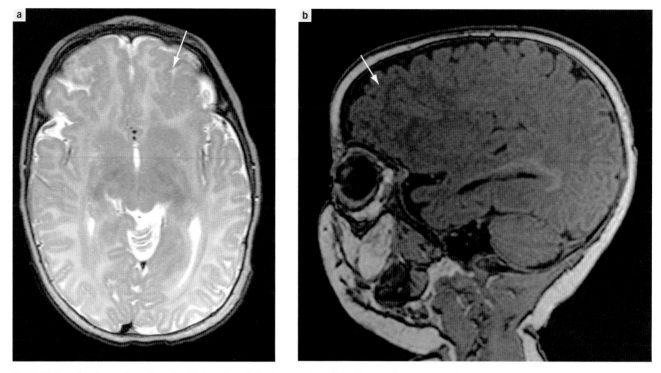

Fig. 12.15a,b. **Polymicrogyria. A 5-week-old, term-born infant presenting with seizures. These images show abnormal cortex with irregularity of the cortical–white matter junction. MRI diagnosed diffuse polymicrogyria affecting the left frontal (arrow), temporal and peri-Sylvian cortex as well as the right peri-Sylvian and frontal regions.**

Imaging

It is not surprising that polymicrogyria is very difficult to diagnose antenatally by fetal ultrasound, and so far very few cases have been reported [99,100,101,102,103,104,105,106]. In two case reports, polymicrogyria was suspected on antenatal ultrasound at 25 and 23 weeks' gestation because hyperechogenic lesions were seen; the diagnosis was confirmed with MRI and autopsy [102,104]. Given that the area of cortex which is involved can be very small, it is not likely that this diagnosis will ever be made easily in fetal life; even postnatal MRI can be difficult to interpret.

Polymicrogyria has a variable appearance on MRI studies depending on the technique used. On routine 5-mm, spin-echo sections, polymicrogyria has the appearance of thickened cortex with irregularity of the gray–white junction and therefore can mimic pachygyria [107]. Higher resolution of the cortex can be obtained by using thinner sections that reveal that the abnormality is composed of multiple, small gyri (Fig. 12.15a,b). As with schizencephaly, polymicrogyria may not be detected on antenatal ultrasound and/or fetal MRI if imaged too early in pregnancy or if the lesion is very small and localized. Postnatal imaging is warranted if antenatally polymicrogyria was suspected.

Clinical manifestation

The clinical features of polymicrogyria are non-specific and depend on the extent of the microgyric areas, their location, and presence of associated malformations. Small areas may not give rise to symptoms. The majority of children with polymicrogyria have severe learning difficulties, seizures, and abnormal neurological signs.

Congenital cystic lesions

Hydranencephaly

The whole of the anterior portion of both hemispheres is destroyed in this condition, thought to occur from an in utero occlusion of both carotid arteries or a massive hypotensive insult to the fetus (maternal collapse or death of monozygotic co-twin). There is a residual thin mantle of meninges and the skull is normally formed. The structures, which are supplied by the posterior cerebral circulation, are preserved, namely the brainstem, the occipital lobes, parts of the temporal lobes, and to some extent the basal ganglia.

Imaging

Prenatal diagnosis of hydranencephaly is suspected when there is a large fluid collection in the head with no recognizable cerebral cortex. It can be differentiated sonographically from holoprosencephaly by identifying the presence of dural attachments and distinctly separate thalami. In severe hydrocephalus, a rim of cerebral cortex around the cystic cavity and enlargement of the third ventricle may be visualized [108].

Counseling and prognosis

True hydranencephaly carries a dismal prognosis, and affected children usually die in infancy. Occasional long-term survivors are reported, but they are very disabled.

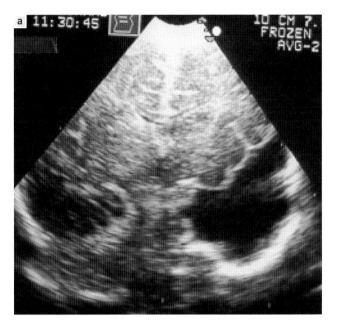

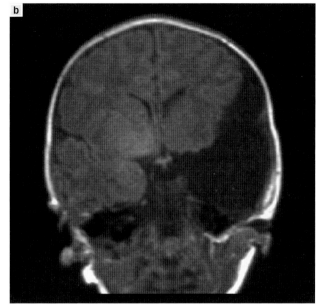

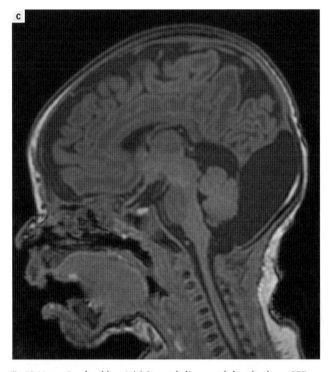

Fig. 12.16a–c. **Arachnoid cyst. (a) Coronal ultrasound showing large CSF-filled cyst in temporal lobe; (b) coronal T$_1$-weighted MR image showing arachnoid cyst in the middle cranial fossa; (c) arachnoid cyst in the posterior fossa and ambient cistern on this T$_1$-weighted midline sagittal view.**

Arachnoid cyst

Arachnoid cysts are benign congenital collections of fluid that develop within the arachnoid membrane. In many instances arachnoid cyst may be an incidental finding in children examined for head injury. But in recent years, the widespread use of antenatal ultrasound and the increasing use of fetal MRI have resulted in the frequent antenatal diagnosis of arachnoid cyst. The most common location is supratentorial (90%) within the middle cranial fossa (60%) with a predominance of the left hemisphere and along the Sylvian fissure [109,110]. Arachnoid cysts in the middle cranial fossa are usually of moderate size, and only 30% are reported to be large, occupying nearly the whole temporal fossa (Fig. 12.16a,b).

Posterior fossa cysts (Fig. 12.16c) are usually large and it is important to differentiate them from cysts of the Dandy Walker malformation. Arachnoid cysts do not lead to dilatation of the fourth ventricle. Postnatal evolving hydrocephalus is rare [111]. Suprasellar cysts may lead to obstructive hydrocephalus of the third ventricle at the level of the foramen of Munro, whereas hydrocephalus with posterior fossa cysts is caused by obstruction at the level of the fourth ventricle.

Interhemispheric cysts often reach a large size and are associated with dysgenesis or agenesis of the corpus callosum [52,55,112].

Arachnoid cysts have a higher incidence in patients with autosomal-dominant polycystic kidney disease; arachnoid cysts have been reported in as many as 8.1% of patients with this disorder [113].

Imaging

Ultrasound can diagnose arachnoid cysts in the usual position in the middle cranial fossa. Magnetic resonance imaging depicts arachnoid cysts as round to oval masses with signal intensity similar to that of CSF (Fig. 12.16a–c). Fetal MRI is probably worthwhile when an antenatal diagnosis of arachnoid cyst is made, in order to look for any other CNS malformation and to check that the diagnosis is correct before counseling the parents.

Clinical manifestation

Arachnoid cysts can cause symptoms if they expand and interfere with adjacent neuronal structures or CSF circulation. The current favored neurosurgical approach is to fenestrate the cyst, avoiding a permanent drain wherever possible. In childhood, headache and macrocrania are the most common clinical signs. In 31% of cases the children have epilepsy, and in these cases the cysts are virtually always located in the temporal region [114]; no epilepsy was noted in patients with arachnoid cysts in the posterior fossa [115]. The debate about cause and effect continues; some have argued that the temporal lobe is not properly formed whilst others maintain that all the effects are pressure-mediated.

Counseling and prognosis

Faced with the diagnosis of an isolated arachnoid cyst, particularly in the middle cranial fossa, we would give an optimistic prognosis to the parents [111,115]. We would counsel about the risk of epilepsy and the possible need for fenestration or shunt surgery [109,111,112,114,116]. Children who had arachnoid cysts diagnosed in fetal life should be followed-up, and repeat imaging should be considered and certainly performed if the head circumference enlarges, or seizures or abnormal neurological signs develop. This is because some arachnoid cysts can cause obstruction to CSF flow, in which case surgery is indicated. We would consider a routine repeat MRI at the age of a year or so in a baby with an arachnoid cyst closely related to the aqueduct (e.g., in the quadrigeminal cisterns) in order to detect any evidence of obstruction before signs developed. Many arachnoid cysts never cause any problems at all and remain clinically silent.

Congenital tumors

Although rare, congenital brain tumors represent 5%–12% of congenital neoplasia [117]. The most frequent histological diagnoses of congenital brain tumors are teratoma, benign astrocytoma, anaplastic astrocytoma, glioblastoma multiforme, medulloblastoma, and primitive neuroectodermal tumor. Discovery of a brain tumor in the neonatal period is very rare. They are more likely to come to light if they cause hydrocephalus; lipomas of the corpus callosum and choroid plexus papillomas have been described.

Congenital vascular lesions

The most frequent arterio-venous malformation in the newborn period is the aneurysm of the vein of Galen.

Aneurysm of the vein of Galen

Aneurysm of the vein of Galen is a vascular malformation within the brain, which is often associated with a high-flow arterio-venous fistula that can lead to high-output cardiac failure. The usual type occurs as a result of a dilatation of an embryological precursor of the vein of Galen. It is a rare but life-threatening condition; hence, this is an important diagnosis to make antenatally as immediate neonatal treatment can be life-saving.

Imaging

The sonographic appearances are well described. The aneurysm appears as a large cystic structure in the region of the third ventricle. The key to the recognition of this lesion is to demonstrate flow with Doppler in an echo-free cystic region, usually found in the midline above the third ventricle (Fig. 12.17a). Magnetic resonance imaging may help define the lesion (Fig. 12.17b,c) and can identify ischemic lesions that affect the outcome [118].

Clinical manifestation

The most important complication is heart failure, which can occur during fetal or neonatal life and adversely affects the prognosis. Cardiomegaly is present in 60% of the fetuses and is an important prognostic sign [119]. Babies who are asymptomatic should be referred to a center with special expertise for consideration of intravascular embolization of the lesion. In the UK there are two such designated centers (London and Glasgow), with further expertise available elsewhere in Europe, notably Paris.

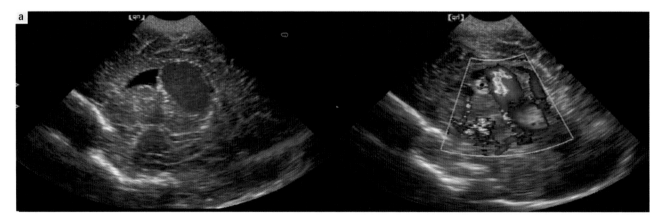

Fig. 12.17a–c. **Vein of Galen aneurysm. (a) Parasagittal ultrasound. Large hypoechogenic mass within the lateral ventricle as seen on this parasagittal ultrasound. Doppler studies show turbulent flow and arterio-venous connection. (b) Axial T$_2$-weighted MR image reveals marked enlargement of central venous structure. (c) MR angiogram demonstrates the vein of Galen malformation.**

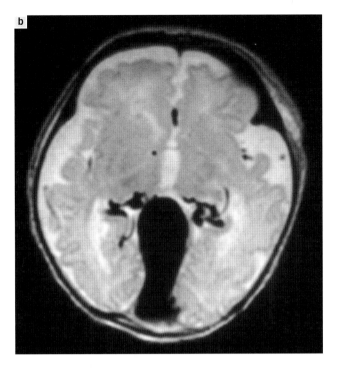

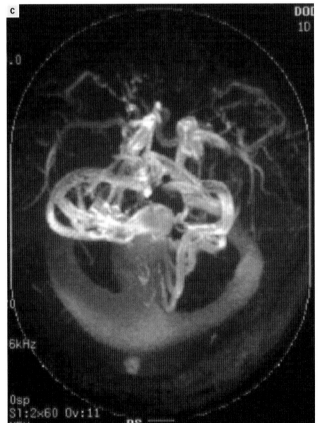

Fig. 12.17. **(cont.)**

Counseling and prognosis

The mortality of fetuses with hydrops and babies with severe heart failure is very high, and these babies do not usually survive long enough for transfer to a center for embolization. Without embolization the mortality of infants with this malformation and early cardiac failure is close to 100%. Since the introduction of embolization, 30%–45% survive, many with good neurodevelopmental outcome [120,121,122]. The presence of ischemic-hemorrhagic lesions will affect the prognosis, and evidence of such lesions on MRI is an important determinant of neonatal counseling regarding intervention.

References

1. Leech RW, Shuman RM. Holoprosencephaly and related midline cerebral anomalies: a review. *J Child Neurol* 1986; **1**(1): 3–18.
2. Demyer W, Zeman W, Palmer CG. The face predicts the brain: diagnostic significance of median facial anomalies for holoprosencephaly (arhinencephaly). *Pediatrics* 1964; **34**: 256–63.
3. Berry SA, Pierpont ME, Gorlin RJ. Single central incisor in familial holoprosencephaly. *J Pediatr* 1984; **104**(6): 877–80.
4. Roessler E, Belloni E, Gaudenz K *et al.* Mutations in the human Sonic Hedgehog gene cause holoprosencephaly. *Nat Genet* 1996; **14**(3): 357–60.
5. Pinar H, Tatevosyants N, Singer DB. Central nervous system malformations in a perinatal/neonatal autopsy series. *Pediatr Dev Pathol* 1998; **1**(1): 42–8.
6. Bullen PJ, Rankin JM, Robson SC. Investigation of the epidemiology and prenatal diagnosis of holoprosencephaly in the North of England. *Am J Obstet Gynecol* 2001; **184**(6): 1256–62.
7. Barkovich AJ, Norman D. Absence of the septum pellucidum: a useful sign in the diagnosis of congenital brain malformations. *AJR Am J Roentgenol* 1989; **152**(2): 353–60.
8. Kuhn MJ, Swenson LC, Youssef HT. Absence of the septum pellucidum and related disorders. *Comput Med Imaging Graph* 1993; **17**(2): 137–47.
9. Belhocine O, Andre C, Kalifa G, Adamsbaum C. Does asymptomatic septal agenesis exist? A review of 34 cases. *Pediatr Radiol* 2005; **35**(4): 410–18.
10. Malinger G, Lev D, Kidron D, Heredia F, Hershkovitz R, Lerman-Sagie T. Differential diagnosis in fetuses with absent septum pellucidum. *Ultrasound Obstet Gynecol* 2005; **25**(1): 42–9.
11. Lepinard C, Coutant R, Boussion F *et al.* Prenatal diagnosis of absence of the septum pellucidum associated with septo-optic dysplasia. *Ultrasound Obstet Gynecol* 2005; **25**(1): 73–5.
12. Pilu G, Sandri F, Cerisoli M, Alvisi C, Salvioli GP, Bovicelli L. Sonographic findings in septo-optic dysplasia in the fetus and newborn infant. *Am J Perinatol* 1990; **7**(4): 337–9.
13. Bodensteiner JB, Schaefer GB. Wide cavum septum pellucidum: a marker of disturbed brain development. *Pediatr Neurol* 1990; **6**(6): 391–4.
14. Williams J, Brodsky MC, Griebel M, Glasier CM, Caldwell D, Thomas P. Septo-optic dysplasia: the clinical insignificance of an absent septum pellucidum. *Dev Med Child Neurol* 1993; **35**(6): 490–501.
15. Filipovic B, Prostran M, Ilankovic N. Predictive potential of cavum septi pellucidi (CSP) in schizophrenics, alcoholics and persons with past head trauma. A post-mortem study. *Eur Arch Psychiatry Clin Neurosci* 2004; **254**(4): 228–30.
16. Kwon JS, Shenton ME, Hirayasu Y *et al.* MRI study of cavum septi pellucidi in schizophrenia, affective disorder, and schizotypal personality disorder. *Am J Psychiatry* 1998; **155**(4): 509–15.
17. Bodensteiner JB, Schaefer GB, Craft JM. Cavum septi pellucidi and cavum vergae in normal and developmentally delayed populations. *J Child Neurol* 1998; **13**(3): 120–1.
18. Pilu G, Tani G, Carletti A, Malaigia S, Ghi T, Rizzo N. Difficult early sonographic diagnosis of absence of the fetal septum pellucidum. *Ultrasound Obstet Gynecol* 2005; **25**(1): 70–2.

19. Supprian T, Sian J, Heils A, Hofmann E, Warmuth-Metz M, Solymosi L. Isolated absence of the septum pellucidum. *Neuroradiology* 1999; **41**(8): 563–6.

20. Hellstrom A, Aronsson M, Axelson C et al. Children with septo-optic dysplasia – how to improve and sharpen the diagnosis. *Horm Res* 2000; **53** (Suppl **1**): 19–25.

21. Volpe J. *Neurology of the Newborn*, 4th edn. Philadelphia, Saunders, 2001.

22. d'Ercole C, Girard N, Cravello L et al. Prenatal diagnosis of fetal corpus callosum agenesis by ultrasonography and magnetic resonance imaging. *Prenat Diagn* 1998; **18**(3): 247–53.

23. Parrish ML, Roessmann U, Levinsohn MW. Agenesis of the corpus callosum: a study of the frequency of associated malformations. *Ann Neurol* 1979; **6**(4): 349–54.

24. Barkovich AJ, Kjos BO. Gray matter heterotopias: MR characteristics and correlation with developmental and neurologic manifestations. *Radiology* 1992; **182**(2): 493–9.

25. Barkovich AJ, Norman D. Anomalies of the corpus callosum: correlation with further anomalies of the brain. *AJR Am J Roentgenol* 1988; **151**(1): 171–9.

26. Goldstein RB, La Pidus AS, Filly RA, Cardoza J. Mild lateral cerebral ventricular dilatation in utero: clinical significance and prognosis. *Radiology* 1990; **176**(1): 237–42.

27. Aicardi J. Aicardi syndrome. *Brain Dev* 2005; **27**(3): 164–71.

28. Pilu G, Sandri F, Perolo A et al. Sonography of fetal agenesis of the corpus callosum: a survey of 35 cases. *Ultrasound Obstet Gynecol* 1993; **3**(5): 318–29.

29. Malinger G, Zakut H. The corpus callosum: normal fetal development as shown by transvaginal sonography. *AJR Am J Roentgenol* 1993; **161**(5): 1041–3.

30. Malinger G, Lev D, Lerman-Sagie T. Is fetal magnetic resonance imaging superior to neurosonography for detection of brain anomalies? *Ultrasound Obstet Gynecol* 2002; **20**(4): 317–21.

31. Sonigo PC, Rypens FF, Carteret M, Delezoide AL, Brunelle FO. MR imaging of fetal cerebral anomalies. *Pediatr Radiol* 1998; **28**(4): 212–22.

32. Visentin A, Pilu G, Falco P, Bovicelli L. The transfrontal view: a new approach to the visualization of the fetal midline cerebral structures. *J Ultrasound Med* 2001; **20**(4): 329–33.

33. Vergani P, Ghidini A, Strobelt N, Locatelli A, Mariani S, Bertalero C, Cavallone M. Prognostic indicators in the prenatal diagnosis of agenesis of corpus callosum. *Am J Obstet Gynecol* 1994; **170**(3): 753–8.

34. Bennett GL, Bromley B, Benacerraf BR. Agenesis of the corpus callosum: prenatal detection usually is not possible before 22 weeks of gestation. *Radiology* 1996; **199**(2): 447–50.

35. Frates MC, Kumar AJ, Benson CB, Ward VL, Tempany CM. Fetal anomalies: comparison of MR imaging and US for diagnosis. *Radiology* 2004; **232**(2): 398–404.

36. Whitby E, Paley MN, Davies N, Sprigg A, Griffiths PD. Ultrafast magnetic resonance imaging of central nervous system abnormalities in utero in the second and third trimester of pregnancy: comparison with ultrasound. *Br J Obstet Gynaecol* 2001; **108**(5): 519–26.

37. Blaicher W, Prayer D, Mittermayer C et al. Magnetic resonance imaging in foetuses with bilateral moderate ventriculomegaly and suspected anomaly of the corpus callosum on ultrasound scan. *Ultraschall Med* 2003; **24**(4): 255–60.

38. Simon EM, Goldstein RB, Coakley FV et al. Fast MR imaging of fetal CNS anomalies in utero. *AJNR Am J Neuroradiol* 2000; **21**(9): 1688–98.

39. Levine D, Barnes PD, Madsen JR, Li W, Edelman RR. Fetal central nervous system anomalies: MR imaging augments sonographic diagnosis. *Radiology* 1997; **204**(3): 635–42.

40. Levine D, Barnes PD, Robertson RR, Wong G, Mehta TS. Fast MR imaging of fetal central nervous system abnormalities. *Radiology* 2003; **229**(1): 51–61.

41. Levine D, Trop I, Mehta TS, Barnes PD. MR imaging appearance of fetal cerebral ventricular morphology. *Radiology* 2002; **223**(3): 652–60.

42. Levine D, Barnes PD, Madsen JR, Abbott J, Mehta T, Edelman RR. Central nervous system abnormalities assessed with prenatal magnetic resonance imaging. *Obstet Gynecol* 1999; **94**(6): 1011–19.

43. Babcock DS. The normal, absent, and abnormal corpus callosum: sonographic findings. *Radiology* 1984; **151**(2): 449–53.

44. Skeffington FS. Agenesis of the corpus callosum: neonatal ultrasound appearances. *Arch Dis Child* 1982; **57**(9): 713–14.

45. Hernanz-Schulman M, Dohan FC, Jr., Jones T, Cayea P, Wallman J, Teele RL. Sonographic appearance of callosal agenesis: correlation with radiologic and pathologic findings. *AJNR Am J Neuroradiol* 1985; **6**(3): 361–8.

46. Goodyear PW, Bannister CM, Russell S, Rimmer S. Outcome in prenatally diagnosed fetal agenesis of the corpus callosum. *Fetal Diagn Ther* 2001; **16**(3): 139–45.

47. Gupta JK, Lilford RJ. Assessment and management of fetal agenesis of the corpus callosum. *Prenat Diagn* 1995; **15**(4): 301–12.

48. Francesco P, Maria-Edgarda B, Giovanni P, Dandolo G, Giulio B. Prenatal diagnosis of agenesis of corpus callosum: what is the neurodevelopmental outcome? *Pediatr Int* 2006; **48**(3): 298–304.

49. Moutard ML, Kieffer V, Feingold J et al. Agenesis of corpus callosum: prenatal diagnosis and prognosis. *Childs Nerv Syst* 2003; **19**(7–8): 471–6.

50. Taylor M, David AS. Agenesis of the corpus callosum: a United Kingdom series of 56 cases. *J Neurol Neurosurg Psychiatry* 1998; **64**(1): 131–4.

51. David AS, Wacharasindhu A, Lishman WA. Severe psychiatric disturbance and abnormalities of the corpus callosum: review and case series. *J Neurol Neurosurg Psychiatry* 1993; **56**(1): 85–93.

52. Griebel ML, Williams JP, Russell SS, Spence GT, Glasier CM. Clinical and developmental findings in children with giant interhemispheric cysts and dysgenesis of the corpus callosum. *Pediatr Neurol* 1995; **13**(2): 119–24.

53. Osenbach RK, Menezes AH. Diagnosis and management of the Dandy-Walker malformation: 30 years of experience. *Pediatr Neurosurg* 1992; **18**(4): 179–89.

54. Klein O, Pierre-Kahn A. [Focus on Dandy-Walker malformation.] *Neurochirurgie* 2006; **52**(4): 347–56.

55. Epelman M, Daneman A, Blaser SI et al. Differential diagnosis of intracranial cystic lesions at head US: correlation with CT and MR imaging. *Radiographics* 2006; **26**(1): 173–96.

56. Hirsch JF, Pierre-Kahn A, Renier D, Sainte-Rose C, Hoppe-Hirsch E. The Dandy-Walker malformation. A review of 40 cases. *J Neurosurg* 1984; **61**(3): 515–22.

57. Chang MC, Russell SA, Callen PW, Filly RA, Goldstein RB. Sonographic detection of inferior vermian agenesis in Dandy-Walker malformations: prognostic implications. *Radiology* 1994; **193**(3): 765–70.

58. Estroff JA, Scott MR, Benacerraf BR. Dandy-Walker variant: prenatal sonographic features and clinical outcome. *Radiology* 1992; **185**(3): 755–8.

59. Ulm B, Ulm MR, Deutinger J, Bernaschek G. Dandy-Walker malformation diagnosed before 21 weeks of gestation: associated malformations and chromosomal abnormalities. *Ultrasound Obstet Gynecol* 1997; **10**(3): 167–70.

60. Kolble N, Wisser J, Kurmanavicius J et al. Dandy-Walker malformation: prenatal diagnosis and outcome. *Prenat Diagn* 2000; **20**(4): 318–27.

61. Bernard JP, Moscoso G, Renier D, Ville Y. Cystic malformations of the posterior fossa. *Prenat Diagn* 2001; **21**(12): 1064–9.

62. Klein O, Pierre-Kahn A, Boddaert N, Parisot D, Brunelle F. Dandy-Walker malformation: prenatal diagnosis and prognosis. *Childs Nerv Syst* 2003; **19**(7–8): 484–9.

63. Boddaert N, Klein O, Ferguson N et al. Intellectual prognosis of the Dandy-Walker malformation in children: the importance of vermian lobulation. *Neuroradiology* 2003; **45**(5): 320–4.

64. Patel S, Barkovich AJ. Analysis and classification of cerebellar malformations. *AJNR Am J Neuroradiol* 2002; **23**(7): 1074–87.

65. Garel C. *MRI of the Fetal Brain*, 1st edn. Berlin, Springer-Verlag, 2004.

66. Joubert M, Eisenring JJ, Robb JP, Andermann F. Familial agenesis of the cerebellar vermis. A syndrome of episodic hyperpnea, abnormal eye movements, ataxia, and retardation. *Neurology* 1969; **19(9)**: 813–25.

67. Kendall B, Kingsley D, Lambert SR, Taylor D, Finn P. Joubert syndrome: a clinico-radiological study. *Neuroradiology* 1990; **31(6)**: 502–6.

68. Maria BL, Boltshauser E, Palmer SC, Tran TX. Clinical features and revised diagnostic criteria in Joubert syndrome. *J Child Neurol* 1999; **14(9)**: 583–90; discussion, pp. 580–1.

69. Maria BL, Quisling RG, Rosainz LC *et al.* Molar tooth sign in Joubert syndrome: clinical, radiologic, and pathologic significance. *J Child Neurol* 1999; **14(6)**: 368–76.

70. Doherty D, Glass IA, Siebert JR *et al.* Prenatal diagnosis in pregnancies at risk for Joubert syndrome by ultrasound and MRI. *Prenat Diagn* 2005; **25(6)**: 442–7.

71. Bromley B, Nadel AS, Pauker S, Estroff JA, Benacerraf BR. Closure of the cerebellar vermis: evaluation with second trimester US. *Radiology* 1994; **193(3)**: 761–3.

72. Haimovici JA, Doubilet PM, Benson CB, Frates MC. Clinical significance of isolated enlargement of the cisterna magna (>10 mm) on prenatal sonography. *J Ultrasound Med* 1997; **16(11)**: 731–4; quiz 735–6.

73. Tortori-Donati P, Fondelli MP, Rossi A, Carini S. Cystic malformations of the posterior cranial fossa originating from a defect of the posterior membranous area. Mega cisterna magna and persisting Blake's pouch: two separate entities. *Childs Nerv Syst* 1996; **12(6)**: 303–8.

74. Stein SC, Schut L. Hydrocephalus in myelomeningocele. *Childs Brain* 1979; **5(4)**: 413–19.

75. La Marca F, Herman M, Grant JA, McLone DG. Presentation and management of hydromyelia in children with Chiari type-II malformation. *Pediatr Neurosurg* 1997; **26(2)**: 57–67.

76. McLone DGDL, Kaplan WE, Sommers MW. Concepts in the management of spina bifida. *Concepts Pediatr Neurosurg* 1985; **5**: 97–106.

77. Worley G, Schuster JM, Oakes WJ. Survival at 5 years of a cohort of newborn infants with myelomeningocele. *Dev Med Child Neurol* 1996; **38(9)**: 816–22.

78. Charney EB, Rorke LB, Sutton LN, Schut L. Management of Chiari II complications in infants with myelomeningocele. *J Pediatr* 1987; **111(3)**: 364–71.

79. Mahapatra AK, Agrawal D. Anterior encephaloceles: a series of 103 cases over 32 years. *J Clin Neurosci* 2006; **13(5)**: 536–9.

80. Braithwaite JM, Economides DL. First-trimester diagnosis of Meckel-Gruber syndrome by transabdominal sonography in a low-risk case. *Prenat Diagn* 1995; **15(12)**: 1168–70.

81. Brown MS, Sheridan-Pereira M. Outlook for the child with a cephalocele. *Pediatrics* 1992; **90(6)**: 914–19.

82. Becker R, Novak A, Rudolph KH. A case of occipital encephalocele combined with right lung aplasia in a twin pregnancy. *J Perinat Med* 1993; **21(3)**: 253–8.

83. Gambello MJ, Darling DL, Yingling J, Tanaka T, Gleeson JG, Wynshaw-Boris A. Multiple dose-dependent effects of Lis1 on cerebral cortical development. *J Neurosci* 2003; **23(5)**: 1719–29.

84. Kitamura K, Yanazawa M, Sugiyama N *et al.* Mutation of ARX causes abnormal development of forebrain and testes in mice and X-linked lissencephaly with abnormal genitalia in humans. *Nat Genet* 2002; **32(3)**: 359–69.

85. Fong KW, Ghai S, Toi A, Blaser S, Winsor EJ, Chitayat D. Prenatal ultrasound findings of lissencephaly associated with Miller-Dieker syndrome and comparison with pre- and postnatal magnetic resonance imaging. *Ultrasound Obstet Gynecol* 2004; **24(7)**: 716–23.

86. Toi A, Lister WS, Fong KW. How early are fetal cerebral sulci visible at prenatal ultrasound and what is the normal pattern of early fetal sulcal development? *Ultrasound Obstet Gynecol* 2004; **24(7)**: 706–15.

87. Granata T, Farina L, Faiella A *et al.* Familial schizencephaly associated with EMX2 mutation. *Neurology* 1997; **48(5)**: 1403–6.

88. Denis D, Chateil JF, Brun M *et al.* Schizencephaly: clinical and imaging features in 30 infantile cases. *Brain Dev* 2000; **22(8)**: 475–83.

89. Granata T, Freri E, Caccia C, Setola V, Taroni F, Battaglia G. Schizencephaly: clinical spectrum, epilepsy, and pathogenesis. *J Child Neurol* 2005; **20(4)**: 313–18.

90. Granata T, Battaglia G, D'Incerti L *et al.* Schizencephaly: neuroradiologic and epileptologic findings. *Epilepsia* 1996; **37(12)**: 1185–93.

91. Barkovich AJ, Kjos BO. Schizencephaly: correlation of clinical findings with MR characteristics. *AJNR Am J Neuroradiol* 1992; **13(1)**: 85–94.

92. Aniskiewicz AS, Frumkin NL, Brady DE, Moore JB, Pera A. Magnetic resonance imaging and neurobehavioral correlates in schizencephaly. *Arch Neurol* 1990; **47(8)**: 911–16.

93. Barkovich AJ, Rowley H, Bollen A. Correlation of prenatal events with the development of polymicrogyria. *AJNR Am J Neuroradiol* 1995; **16(4 Suppl)**: 822–7.

94. Ferrer I, Catala I. Unlayered polymicrogyria: structural and developmental aspects. *Anat Embryol (Berl)* 1991; **184(5)**: 517–28.

95. de Vries LS, Gunardi H, Barth PG, Bok LA, Verboon-Maciolek MA, Groenendaal F. The spectrum of cranial ultrasound and magnetic resonance imaging abnormalities in congenital cytomegalovirus infection. *Neuropediatrics* 2004; **35(2)**: 113–19.

96. Barkovich AJ, Kjos BO. Nonlissencephalic cortical dysplasias: correlation of imaging findings with clinical deficits. *AJNR Am J Neuroradiol* 1992; **13(1)**: 95–103.

97. Baker EM, Khorasgani MG, Gardner-Medwin D, Gholkar A, Griffiths PD. Arthrogyrposis multiplex congenita and bilateral parietal polymicrogyria in association with the intrauterine death of a twin. *Neuropediatrics* 1996; **27(1)**: 54–6.

98. Glenn OA, Norton ME, Goldstein RB, Barkovich AJ. Prenatal diagnosis of polymicrogyria by fetal magnetic resonance imaging in monochorionic cotwin death. *J Ultrasound Med* 2005; **24(5)**: 711–16.

99. Fogliarini C, Chaumoitre K, Chapon F *et al.* Assessment of cortical maturation with prenatal MRI. Part II: abnormalities of cortical maturation. *Eur Radiol* 2005; **15(9)**: 1781–9.

100. Jan W, Lacey NA, Langford KS, Bewley SJ, Maxwell DJ. The antenatal diagnosis of migration disorders: a series of four cases. *Clin Radiol* 2003; **58(3)**: 247–50.

101. Righini A, Zirpoli S, Mrakic F, Parazzini C, Pogliani L, Triulzi F. Early prenatal MR imaging diagnosis of polymicrogyria. *AJNR Am J Neuroradiol* 2004; **25(2)**: 343–6.

102. Delle Urban LA, Righini A, Rustico M, Triulzi F, Nicolini U. Prenatal ultrasound detection of bilateral focal polymicrogyria. *Prenat Diagn* 2004; **24(10)**: 808–11.

103. Parazzini C, Righini A, Lalatta F, Bianchini E, Triulzi F. Frontal bilateral megalencephaly: fetal and autopsy MR evaluation of an unclassified malformation. *Prenat Diagn* 2005; **25(6)**: 489–91.

104. Becker R, Stiemer B, Patt S, Vogel M, Sperner J. [Prenatal diagnosis of fetal polymicrogyria – case report.] *Ultraschall Med* 1993; **14(1)**: 32–4.

105. Girard N, Gire C, Sigaudy S *et al.* MR imaging of acquired fetal brain disorders. *Childs Nerv Syst* 2003; **19(7–8)**: 490–500.

106. Soussotte C, Maugey-Laulom B, Carles D, Diard F. Contribution of transvaginal ultrasonography and fetal cerebral MRI in a case of congenital cytomegalovirus infection. *Fetal Diagn Ther* 2000; **15(4)**: 219–23.

107. Barkovich AJ, Kuzniecky RI. Neuroimaging of focal malformations of cortical development. *J Clin Neurophysiol* 1996; **13(6)**: 481–94.

108. Lam YH, Tang MH. Serial sonographic features of a fetus with hydranencephaly from 11 weeks to term. *Ultrasound Obstet Gynecol* 2000; **16(1)**: 77–9.

109. Gosalakkal JA. Intracranial arachnoid cysts in children: a review of pathogenesis, clinical features, and management. *Pediatr Neurol* 2002; **26(2)**: 93–8.

110. Wang PJ, Lin HC, Liu HM, Tseng CL, Shen YZ. Intracranial arachnoid cysts in children: related signs and associated anomalies. *Pediatr Neurol* 1998; **19(2)**: 100–4.

111. Pierre-Kahn A, Sonigo P. Malformative intracranial cysts: diagnosis and outcome. *Childs Nerv Syst* 2003; **19**(7-8): 477-83.

112. Lena G, van Calenberg F, Genitori L, Choux M. Supratentorial interhemispheric cysts associated with callosal agenesis: surgical treatment and outcome in 16 children. *Childs Nerv Syst* 1995; **11**(10): 568-73.

113. Schievink WI, Huston J 3rd, Torres VE, Marsh WR. Intracranial cysts in autosomal dominant polycystic kidney disease. *J Neurosurg* 1995; **83**(6): 1004-7.

114. Mazurkiewicz-Beldzinska M, Dilling-Ostrowska E. Presentation of intracranial arachnoid cysts in children: correlation between localization and clinical symptoms. *Med Sci Monit* 2002; **8**(6): CR462-5.

115. Boltshauser E, Martin F, Altermatt S. Outcome in children with space-occupying posterior fossa arachnoid cysts. *Neuropediatrics* 2002; **33**(3): 118-21.

116. Pierre-Kahn A, Hanlo P, Sonigo P, Parisot D, McConnell RS. The contribution of prenatal diagnosis to the understanding of malformative intracranial cysts: state of the art. *Childs Nerv Syst* 2000; **16**(10-11): 619-26.

117. Carstensen H, Juhler M, Bogeskov L, Laursen H. A report of nine newborns with congenital brain tumours. *Childs Nerv Syst* 2006; **22**(11): 1433.

118. Campi A, Scotti G, Filippi M, Gerevini S, Strigimi F, Lasjaunias P. Antenatal diagnosis of vein of Galen aneurysmal malformation: MR study of fetal brain and postnatal follow-up. *Neuroradiology* 1996; **38**(1): 87-90.

119. Sepulveda W, Platt CC, Fisk NM. Prenatal diagnosis of cerebral arteriovenous malformation using color Doppler ultrasonography: case report and review of the literature. *Ultrasound Obstet Gynecol* 1995; **6**(4): 282-6.

120. Lylyk P, Vinuela F, Dion JE *et al.* Therapeutic alternatives for vein of Galen vascular malformations. *J Neurosurg* 1993; **78**(3): 438-45.

121. Borthne A, Carteret M, Baraton J, Courtel J, Brunelle F. Vein of Galen vascular malformations in infants: clinical, radiological and therapeutic aspect. *Eur Radiol* 1997; **7**(8): 1252-8.

122. Mitchell PJ, Rosenfeld JV, Dargaville P *et al.* Endovascular management of vein of Galen aneurysmal malformations presenting in the neonatal period. *AJNR Am J Neuroradiol* 2001; **22**(7): 1403-9.

Chapter 13 | The baby with a suspected infection

ANDREW B. KAPETANAKIS,
CORNELIA F. HAGMANN, *and*
JANET M. RENNIE

Introduction

Viral and bacterial infections of the central nervous system (CNS) are not a common problem in the neonatal intensive care unit, but they are an important cause of mortality and morbidity. In a recent study of babies with bacterial infection of the CNS the mortality was reported to be as high as 43% (1). The mortality was higher for preterm compared to term infants (50% compared to 30%) [1,2]. Thorough evaluation of affected babies is essential in order to establish the correct diagnosis, institute prompt and effective treatment, and evaluate the prognosis.

Infections of the CNS include bacterial, fungal meningitis and viral meningitis, together with meningoencephalitis and cerebral abscess. Perinatal CNS infection can occur antenatally or postnatally, and is often part of the TORCH (Toxoplasmosis, Other agents, Rubella, Cytomegalovirus, Herpes simplex) spectrum. Infections during the first trimesters can also lead to disruption of normal brain development [3].

In this chapter we describe the approach to the infant with infections of the CNS, including specific advice on the interpretation of CNS investigations.

Clinical presentation of neonatal sepsis involving the central nervous system

History

Family history, past obstetric history

As ever, we cannot overstress the importance of starting with a good history. Several viral infections can occur when there is reactivation of a dormant maternal viral infection, and management of the mother whose previous child was affected by group B streptococcal infection is well described elsewhere. A history of vaginal herpes infection should trigger discussion regarding the mode of delivery, and in maternal human immunodeficiency virus/acquired immunodeficiency syndrome (HIV/AIDS) there should be a treatment plan for the baby. Sometimes the history taking has to be tailored to the clinical problem as it unfolds; it would not be routine practice to ask about cold sores in the family, or the ingestion of undercooked meat or unpasteurized cheese, or to enquire about whether a family kept cats, but all these are risk factors for perinatal infection.

Pregnancy

Many viral infections are asymptomatic but a history of a flu-like illness or an exanthematous rash may be the only clue to a mild maternal viral infection which nevertheless has devastating consequences for the fetus. Recurrent maternal vaginal *Candida*, especially if there is a cervical suture or a retained intrauterine contraceptive device in place, increases the risk of congenital candidiasis (which is nevertheless rare). Membrane rupture clearly increases the risk of ascending infection, but some agents are transmitted via the maternal bloodstream.

The neonatologist needs to appraise herself of the results obtained by colleagues in obstetrics and fetal medicine. There may be results of amniotic fluid culture, including viral DNA studies, viral load, viral avidity testing, results of maternal serology, and even results from invasive testing of the fetal blood.

Labor and delivery

The cardiotocograph
During labor, a baseline fetal tachycardia is an important pointer towards fetal infection. No cardiotocograph (CTG) abnormality is specific for fetal sepsis, but the presence of a fetal tachycardia in a pyrexial woman with prolonged membrane rupture should trigger investigation and treatment. There is an opportunity for intrapartum antibiotic treatment in this situation to benefit the fetus.

Maternal pyrexia
The definition of maternal pyrexia varies, but is usually a temperature of more than 38 °C for more than 2 hours. Units with a high epidural rate will report a higher incidence of maternal pyrexia, because when an epidural is in place maternal core temperature steadily rises.

Neonatal Cerebral Investigation, eds. Janet M. Rennie, Cornelia F. Hagmann and Nicola J. Robertson. Published by Cambridge University Press. © Cambridge University Press 2008.

Cord and placenta; funisitis and chorioamnionitis

Histological examination of the placenta gives important information when assessing a case of probable neonatal infection. Cytokines are released as part of the systemic inflammatory response to infection, and there is now a wealth of evidence that these are brain damaging. The evidence comes from laboratory experiments with animal models, epidemiological studies, and clinical observations. When the fetal membranes are involved (funisitis) the risk is greater than when there is chorioamnionitis alone (see Chapter 9).

Examination

When CNS infection is suspected, repeated neurological examination is essential and hopefully it goes without saying that this should include estimation of fontanelle tension and head circumference.

Laboratory tests

Laboratory tests can help establish whether there is a systemic inflammatory response. Important tests include a differential white cell count, the platelet count, blood gas estimation, and measurement of the C-reactive protein. A high fetal/neonatal immunoglobulin M level shows that the fetus has reacted to an infectious stimulus. Bacterial and viral cultures should be set up with the aim of identifying organisms in normally sterile body fluids, and the predominant flora from non-sterile areas.

Specific tests should also be requested, targeted on the basis of a history or clinical presentation, e.g., herpes virus polymerase chain reaction (PCR) in cerebrospinal fluid (CSF), or DNA testing for cytomegalovirus in urine (which is now replacing the former detection of early antigen fluorescent foci (DEAFF) test).

Lumbar puncture

There is no substitute for the laboratory examination of CSF obtained from lumbar puncture (LP). There has been an increasing reluctance to perform LPs in sick babies, driven by reports of young children with meningitis who coned as a result of the investigation. However, it is extremely rare for newborn babies to cone, because their heads are expansile. Sick newborn babies who are not ventilated sometimes do tolerate LP poorly, becoming apneic and/or cyanosed, but in skilled hands the procedure is quick and is not associated with any significant complications. The major contraindication to LP is a low platelet count or significant coagulopathy, because of the risk of a spinal epidural hematoma. The downside of omitting LP is that a diagnosis of meningitis will be missed altogether, or the organism never identified because the specimen is collected after treatment has been started, making treatment planning more difficult.

Performing LP at a level superior to the conus carries a risk of penetration of the spinal cord itself, if the needle is passed too deep. The standard position for LP, at the spinal level of L3/4, may be at a level superior to the conus in some very premature babies. Tubbs *et al.* describe a 22-week-gestation baby who developed a hematoma of the conus after LP which was said to have been carried out at the L4/5 level [4]. These authors speculate that the adult position of the conus may only be reached after 2 months in term babies, and that the conus may not be below L3/4 in very preterm babies. Others have described the position of the conus with ultrasound, and found the tip to be between L1 and L2 in 90% of both term and preterm babies [5,6].

There are more white cells present in the normal neonatal CSF than in the CSF of adults, and this has been ascribed to a "leaky" blood–brain barrier. However, over the years the "acceptable" number of white cells has reduced; this is almost certainly because the early series on which normal ranges were based included many babies with undiagnosed intracranial hemorrhage. With the advent of cranial ultrasound scanning, normal ranges are available from babies with normal cranial ultrasound scans. In our view, the upper limit of normal white cell count at term should probably be set at 21 cells per cubic millimeter; this is slightly lower than the previously published recommended range of up to 30 [7] (Table 13.1). An elevated CSF white cell count in a specimen obtained from an untreated baby in which no organisms are seen on Gram stain should raise a strong suspicion of viral meningitis, and in this situation we would recommend that aciclovir treatment is begun whilst the specific result of herpes virus PCR is awaited.

Repeated LP, or ventricular taps, may be necessary for monitoring treatment of meningitis. In our view there should be no hesitation in repeating a LP if a baby is failing to respond to treatment.

Table 13.1. Normal CSF values in the newborn. Modified from [7]. Suggested normal values for CSF in neonates established from literature reviews cited and from personal experience. All values are given as mean and range. Take blood for plasma glucose *before* doing the lumbar puncture (stress raises the serum glucose).

Type of infant	Red cell count (mm³)	White cell count (mm³)	Protein (g/l)	Glucose (mmol/l)
Preterm <7 days	30 (0–333)	9 (0–30)	1 (0.5–2.9, but mostly <2 g/l)	3 (1.5–5.5)‡
Preterm >7 days	30	12 (2–70)	0.9 (0.5–2.6 mostly <1.5)	3 (1.5–5.5)‡
Term <7 days	9 (0–50)	5 (0–21)[a]	0.6 (0.3–2.5)	3 (1.5–5.5)‡
Term >7 days	<10	3 (0–10)	0.5 (0.2–0.8)	3 (1.5–5.5)‡

[a] Revised down to 5 (0–21) in 2006 on the basis of further clinical experience and publications [8].

The electroencephalogram

The electroencephalogram (EEG) is not diagnostic in meningitis, but an EEG is helpful in order to show whether seizures are present. The EEG can assist in prognosis [9].

Cranial ultrasound

Cranial ultrasound provides very useful diagnostic and prognostic information in babies with suspected cerebral infection. Increased echogenicity seems to be the most common ultrasound finding [1]. Ventricular dilatation and abscess formation are complications of meningitis, and both can be detected by ultrasound [1,10]. Calcification, lenticulostriate vasculopathy, and subependymal cysts, common findings in congenital infections, are better detected by ultrasound than magnetic resonance imaging (MRI) [1,11].

Magnetic resonance imaging

Magnetic resonance imaging is very helpful and is complementary to cranial ultrasound; it is superior to ultrasound in the detection of abscess formation; it can accurately delineate the severity and extent of the abnormalities; and it is superior to ultrasound in detecting lesions in the posterior fossa, brainstem, and in diagnosing abnormal brain development, especially white matter, gyral, and cerebellar abnormalities [1,3,10,12]. Diffusion-weighted imaging is useful in demonstrating acute infectious disease processes earlier than conventional MRI [13,14,15]. Diffusion-weighted imaging becomes less sensitive if there is a time delay between onset of illness and imaging that is more than 7 days [13,14]. In recent reports, diffusion-weighted imaging was shown to make the diagnosis of herpes encephalitis and ischemic infarctions earlier than conventional MRI [13,14,16].

Diagnostic categories resulting from investigation of the baby with CNS infection

Congenital infection

Cytomegalovirus

Natural history of cytomegalovirus infection

Congenital cytomegalovirus (CMV) infection is present in about 0.5%–2.5% of all live-born infants and is the most common viral infection known to be transmitted in utero [17,18]. In the developed world about 40% of women of childbearing age are susceptible to the infection, and about 1% will seroconvert during pregnancy. Approximately 30%–40% of infants whose mothers are primarily infected during pregnancy develop congenital infection [19]. Of those, about 7% have signs of infection at birth [17,20], and a further 7% have no signs of overt infection but develop CMV-related problems later on, such as deafness or learning difficulties. Amongst the babies who present clinically in the neonatal period with congenital CMV infection the mortality is 30% [21]. Babies may be of low weight for gestational age and present with jaundice, thrombocytopenia, hepatosplenomegaly, and petechiae [20,22]. Specific neurological signs at birth include microcephaly (an ominous sign), seizures, feeding difficulties, and abnormal neurological examination. Ocular abnormalities, including chorioretinitis, optic atrophy and retinal scars, may be present at birth [23].

Neurological sequelae develop in about 80% of infants who have overt signs of infection in the neonatal period, whereas, as discussed, those who are infected but not ill can also develop sequelae later on. It is estimated that around 7% (range 5%–17%) suffer neurological sequelae [17]. Long-term sequelae include sensorineural hearing loss, mental retardation, cerebral palsy, and visual impairments [21,22,24,25,26,27,28,29].

A wide range of cerebral abnormalities is found with CMV infection: meningoencephalitis, calcifications, microcephaly, germinal matrix cysts, ventriculomegaly, white matter abnormalities, cerebellar hypoplasia, and disorders of cortical development [1,3,10,11,30,31,32]. Barkovich and Lindan postulated that in infants with lissencephaly the injury due to CMV infection occurred before 16 and 18 weeks of gestational age, whereas in those with polymicrogyria it occurred between 18 and 24 weeks of gestation [3].

On delivery, a urine sample should be sent to the virology laboratory for CMV DNA testing in order to confirm infection. In addition, a neonatal EDTA blood sample should be sent for CMV IgM and CMV viral load as these tests are of prognostic value [31].

Imaging findings

Ultrasound On antenatal ultrasound abnormal periventricular signal, intraparenchymal echogenic foci, intraventricular adhesions, ventriculomegaly, abnormal sulcation, and gyral patterns and cerebellar abnormalities should be an indication for TORCH screening [34]. Ultrasound findings in infants with congenital CMV infection are ventricular dilatation, lenticulostriate vasculopathy (see Chapter 10), periventricular cysts, periventricular calcification, and cerebellar lesions such as hypoplasia and hyperechogenicity [1,3,10,11] (Fig. 13.1). Figure 13.1 is an example of acoustic shadow behind the calcification.

Magnetic resonance imaging Ultrasound seems superior to MRI in identifying lenticulostriate vasculopathy, germinal matrix cysts, and calcifications [1,11] (Fig. 13.2). Magnetic resonance imaging has proven to be of particular value in assessing cortical abnormalities such as polymicrogyria and lissencephaly, cerebellar abnormalities, hippocampal dysplasia, and white matter abnormalities [1,3,10,11,30,31,35].

Computerized tomography Computerized tomography has been commonly performed to detect the calcifications and to predict outcome [10,32,35]. But cranial ultrasound can reliably detect the calcifications [1,11] and MRI gives more details about the white matter and cortical abnormalities. We suggest a combination of ultrasound and MRI in infants with congenital CMV infection.

Prognosis and counseling

Neurological sequelae occur in as many as 80% of infants with symptoms at birth, whereas 5%–15% of asymptomatic infants will develop either audiological or developmental impairment

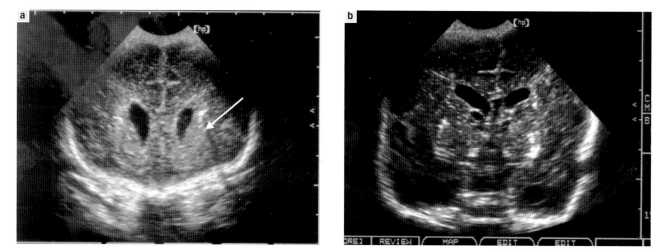

Fig. 13.1.a,b. **Coronal ultrasound images showing calcification and subependymal cyst formation in a baby with congenital cytomegalovirus (CMV) infection. There is an acoustic shadow behind a calcified area in the left-hand image (arrowed).**

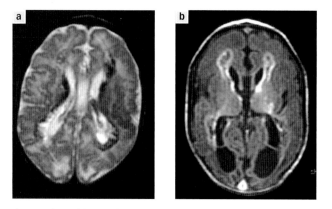

Fig. 13.2.a,b. **Axial T_2- and T_1-weighted MR images show ventricular dilatation due to white matter damage, with septation. There are multiple calcified hemorrhagic lesions adjacent to the ependyma and within the periventricular white matter. There is bilateral peri-Sylvian polymicrogyria.**

neurological abnormalities at birth or in early infancy, and abnormal cranial ultrasound and/or MRI within the first month of life [27,29,37].

The neurological outcome is especially poor in infants diagnosed with polymicrogyria and/or cerebellar hypoplasia [11]. Normal imaging at term in symptomatic congenital infection seems to predict good long-term neurological outcome [10,32]. Petechiae and intrauterine growth restriction were reported to be the only factors that were independently predictive for hearing loss [29].

In asymptomatic infants
Approximately 10% of asymptomatic infants will develop bilateral sensorineural hearing loss, about 5% develop microcephaly and neuromuscular defects, and 2% chorioretinitis [42]. If normal development is present at 1 year of age, subsequent neurodevelopmental or intellectual impairment is unlikely [40]. Predictors for adverse outcome in asymptomatic infants have not been defined. This inability to identify infants at risk for hearing loss and neurodevelopmental impairment enhances the importance of monitoring and follow-up of such infants.

Toxoplasmosis
The incidence of congenital toxoplasmosis infection is 1.5 per 1000 live births [43]. Only about 20%–25% of infants will be infected if the maternal infection occurs in the first or second trimester versus approximately 65% if maternal infection occurs in the third trimester [44]. But the earlier the infection occurs the more severe are the manifestations and the prognosis [44,45,46]. The clinical signs of congenital toxoplasmosis are chorioretinitis, hydrocephalus, and neonatal seizures. Hydrocephalus is thought to be the consequence of an aqueductal block. It is believed that the organisms enter the ventricular system from the parenchymal lesions, disseminate there and cause additional necrosis and ependymitis, which lead to aqueductal block [47]. Although hydrocephalus is a

in the first year of life [36,37,38,39,40]. Recently, viral load studies have proved to be an independent predictive factor for outcome in symptomatic and asymptomatic infants; one study showed that 19/20 babies whose viral load was quantified as less than 1000 copies per 10^5 polymorphonuclear leukocytes did not develop sequelae; a negative predictive factor for outcome of 95% [33]. There were only three babies with a viral load of more than 10 000 copies, and two of these did develop sequelae.

In symptomatic infants
Recent studies have shown that fewer than 5% of symptomatic infants will die in the neonatal period [17,21,41]. About half of the surviving symptomatic infants will develop sensorineural hearing loss, mental retardation with IQ <70, and microcephaly [21,24,27]. Predictors for adverse neurological outcome include microcephaly, chorioretinitis, the presence of other

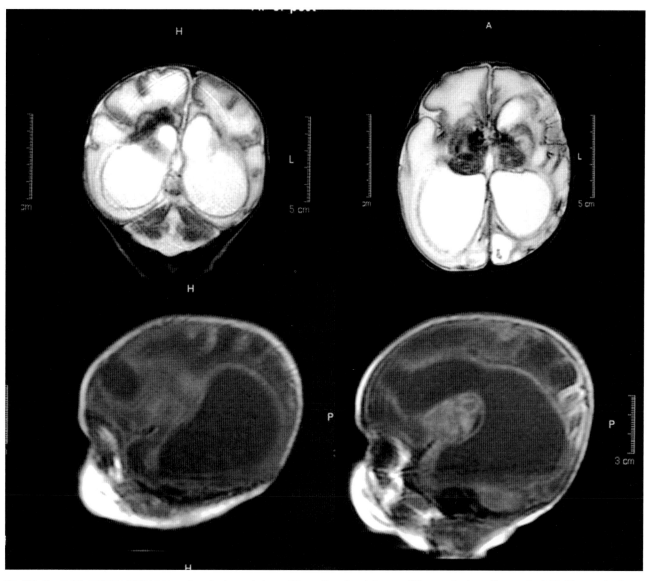

Fig. 13.3. **T$_1$- and T$_2$-weighted MR images show hydrocephalus, white matter signal abnormalities, cerebral swelling, and calcified/hemorrhagic lesions in the deep gray matter in congenital toxoplasmosis.**

more common result of toxoplasmosis infection, micro-cephaly does occur in 15%–26% of infants with congenital tox-oplasmosis [47,48]. Most infected infants have no symptoms at birth, but 40% will show abnormalities on cranial ultrasound and ophthalmologic examination [49].

Imaging

Ultrasound Typical ultrasound findings for congenital toxo-plasmosis infection are ventricular dilatation, calcifications in the basal ganglia, cortex, and periventricular white matter. The calcifications can resolve with treatment [48].

Magnetic resonance imaging In comparison with congenital CMV infection, toxoplasmosis is not associated with corti-cal abnormalities such as polymicrogyria or lissencephaly. Nevertheless, MRI is indicated to assess the development

and maturation of the brain and the hydrocephalus, especi-ally if shunt surgery is being considered. Figure 13.3 shows the typical MRI findings in a case of congenital toxoplasmosis.

Prognosis/Counseling

If the antenatal cranial ultrasound remains normal then the outcome for those infants is good [50]. Most babies with con-genital toxoplasmosis develop normally [51], but up to 4% die [49,52] or have evidence of long-term neurological sequelae or bilateral visual impairment during the first years of life [49,53,54,55].

Babies without hydrocephalus at birth seem to have an excellent neurodevelopmental and cognitive prognosis; those with late-developing or shunt-responsive hydrocephalus have an encouraging prognosis (75% normal outcome), whereas those with hydrocephalus at birth have a guarded prognosis (only 20% were normal or had mild neurological abnormalities) [48]. Treated infants seem to have a significantly better outcome than untreated infants [48,56,57]. While it is not certain whether the anti-parasitic treatment given early in pregnancy reduces the transplacental transmission [58], it seems that such treatment reduces the frequency of severe congenital toxoplasmosis [46,48,59,60]. With particularly severe, diffuse, and destructive disease porencephalic cysts or hydranencephaly can develop [46].

Rubella

As with CMV and toxoplasmosis the neuropathology of congenital rubella infection is characterized by inflammation and tissue necrosis; in addition, rubella seems to interfere with cellular proliferation in the developing brain resulting in microcephaly and delayed myelination. The absences of prominent cerebral calcifications, hydrocephalus, overt microcephaly, and vesicular rash are the clinical features that best differentiate congenital rubella from congenital CMV and toxoplasmosis infection.

Syphylis

In a recent surveillance report new diagnoses of syphilis increased eightfold in the UK between 1997 and 2002 [61]. This reflects worldwide trends [62,63,64]. Congenital syphilis is a multiorgan infection that can cause neurological or musculoskeletal disabilities or death in the fetus and newborn. However, when mothers with syphilis are treated early in pregnancy, congenital disease is almost entirely preventable [64]. Congenital syphilis usually occurs after infection that is acquired in the second and third trimesters. Central nervous system manifestations of congenital syphilis infection include meningitis, cranial neuropathies, hydrocephalus, infarction, and seizures. Congenital syphilis is likely to be asymptomatic within the neonatal period and neurological signs are unusual in the first week of life [65,66]. Hence, the diagnosis of congenital syphilis in the neonate based on clinical signs can be difficult to establish. Even a combination of CSF tests (protein, VDRL, white cell count) has suboptimal sensitivity and specificity [67]. However, a normal physical examination and normal results on conventional evaluations (umbilical-cord VDRL, radiographs of long bones, cell count and protein measurements in CSF) have good negative predictive values of 96% and 97% respectively [67]. The best predictors of CNS infection seem to be the umbilical-cord VDRL test and the serum or blood PCR assay [67].

Signs of late congenital syphilis are abnormalities in teeth, interstitial keratitis, optic atrophy, sensorineural hearing loss, general paresis, and tabes dorsalis.

Human immunodeficiency virus/acquired immunodeficiency syndrome

Central nervous system involvement in congenital HIV infection includes abnormalities such as meningoencephalitis, cerebral atrophy, cerebral calcifications in basal ganglia and white matter, and delayed myelination [68,69]. Cerebral atrophy, secondary to loss both of neurons and myelin, is a prominent feature of the HIV infection [70]. Infants who are not infected with HIV, born to seropositive mothers and perinatally exposed to zidovudine, can have persistent mitochondrial dysfunction and present with neurological symptoms [71,72]. The most frequent abnormalities seen on MRI in infants exposed to zidovudine in utero and perinatally consisted of hyperintensity in the central white matter and in the tegmentum pons [73].

Meningitis

A national cohort study of meningitis from England and Wales showed an incidence of 0.32 per 1000 live births with an incidence for bacterial meningitis of around 0.22 per 1000 live births [2,74]. Despite the dramatic decrease of mortality from meningitis in England and Wales (to 6.6% from 22% in 1985–87), bacterial meningitis remains a significant cause of long-term disability: 23.5% (compared to 25.5% in 1985–87) of infants with bacterial meningitis in this large national cohort study showed severe to moderate disability at 5 years of age [2]. Other studies have reported higher mortality (43%) which was particularly high in preterm babies (50%) compared to those born at term (30%) [1]. Group B streptococci and *Escherichia coli* remain the most commonly cultured organism in neonatal CSF [2,75]. Cerebral meningitis caused by coagulase-negative staphylococci is rare [1,76]. An estimate of the true incidence of viral meningitis remains elusive, but was reported as 0.05/1000 live births in one study [2]. The main pathogens are Enterovirus, Echovirus and Herpes virus and the clinical presentation is usually that of a meningoencephalitis.

Fungal meningitis can occur in up to 25% of newborn infants with invasive fungal infection [77]. Invasive fungal infections occur in either extremely premature infants or in term infants with predisposing factors such as central venous catheters, congenital immunodeficiencies and prolonged antibiotic treatment [77,78]. The most common fungal organism is *Candida* species with *Candida albicans* the most predominant.

Brain abscess is an uncommon but serious complication of bacterial meningitis [79,80]. Gram-negative organisms have been implicated most often, especially *Citrobacter*, but also *Proteus*, *Enterobacter*, *Serratia*, and other coliform pathogens [80,81,82,83,84]. Approximately 70% of the neonatal brain abscesses appear in the frontal lobes [79].

Bacterial meningitis and ventriculitis

Ultrasound

Increased echogenicity was the most common ultrasound finding in infants with bacterial meningitis; this could develop and become more extensive within 12–24 hours and then either resolve or evolve into cystic lesions [1] (Fig. 13.4).

Ventricular dilatation can occur many weeks after the original infection [1,85,86,87,88]; hence, close monitoring of head circumference and repeated ultrasound imaging are indicated. In ventriculitis strands forming intraventricular septa, increased echogenicity of the CSF and echogenic material can be seen in the ventricular cavity [89,90]. Brain

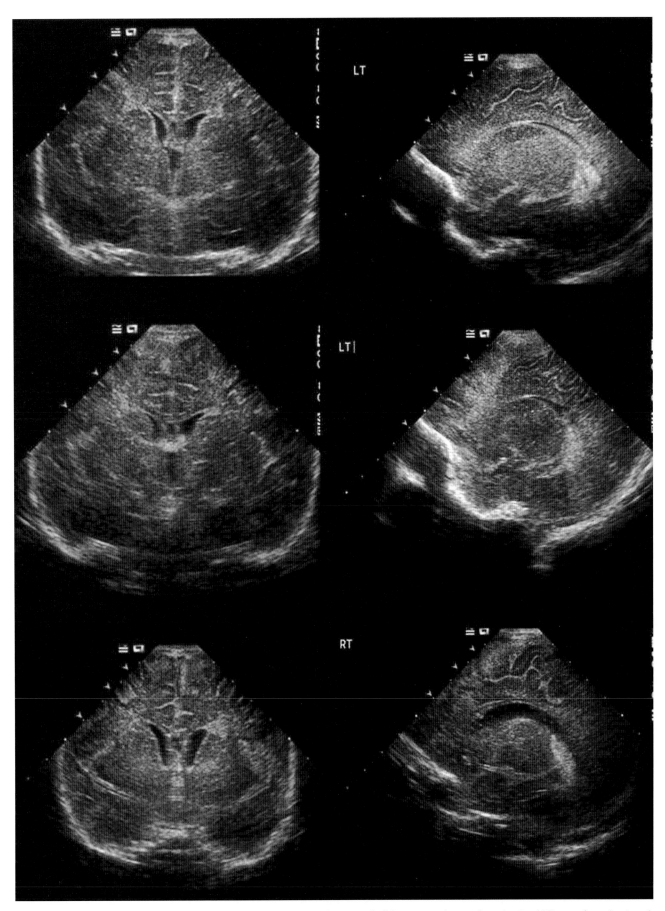

Fig. 13.4. **Ultrasound imaging in a baby with group B streptococcal meningoencephalitis. Top row: images from day 2; middle row: from day 6; and bottom row: from day 11 of life. There is progressive ventricular enlargement, and on day 6 in particular there is a patchy increase in echogenicity in the white matter.**

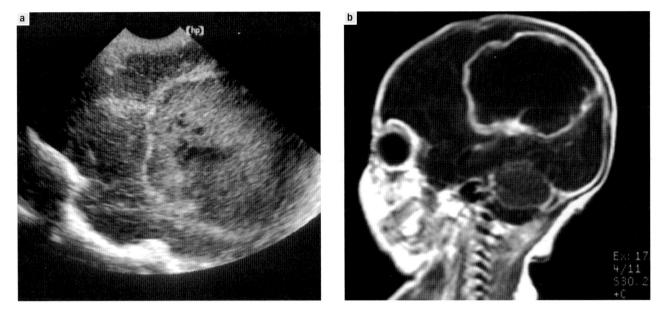

Fig. 13.5.a,b. **Parasagittal images showing the appearances of a large abscess. (a) The ultrasound appearances with cavitation in the occipito-parietal lobe. (b) Parasagittal T$_1$-weighted post contrast image shows a rim-enhancing lesion with necrotic center consistent with an abscess.**

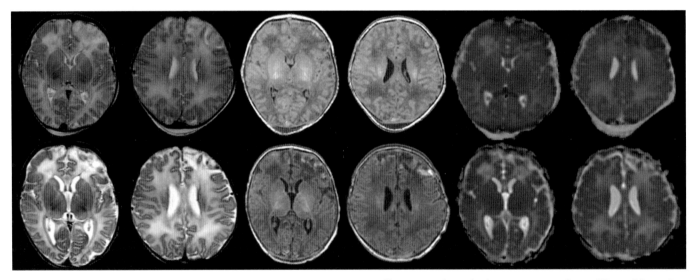

Fig. 13.6. **MR images of the baby with meningoencephalitis whose ultrasound images are shown in Fig. 13.4. Top row shows diffuse white matter signal abnormalities and cortical swelling particularly in the frontal lobe. There is restricted diffusion in the frontal lobe and cortex in the ADC map. Bottom row shows maturing of the areas of cerebral damage with gyral hemorrhage, and increased diffusion on the ADC map. These images were taken on day 13 after birth.**

abscess on ultrasound can present as hypoechogenic with a hyperechogenic rim or small round echogenic structures (Fig. 13.5a).

Magnetic resonance imaging
Magnetic resonance imaging is indicated in all babies who are suspected to have an abscess in order to confirm or refute the diagnosis, assess the exact localization of the abscess [1] (Fig. 13.5b), and define any associated white matter injury (Fig. 13.6) [91]. Contrast is useful for better

delineation of the abscess and meningitis. Diffusion-weighted imaging has shown to be helpful in outlining areas of necrosis and early detection of white matter injury (Fig. 13.6) [1,91,92].

Fungal meningitis

Ultrasound
Two distinct pattern of CNS candidiasis have been described on ultrasound: these are the patterns of parenchymal and

ventricular involvement, with parenchymal being the more common form [12].

The most common ultrasound findings are small, echogenic rim-like microabscesses, which can be symmetrically scattered in the subcortical, periventricular white matter, and basal ganglia (Fig. 13.7a). These lesions show irregular hyperechogenic borders and hypoechogenic centers. Evolution of confluent macroabscess formation may occur and they present echogenic mass-like lesions. Ventricular dilatation with increased ependymal thickness and echogenicity with or without ventricular nodularity and hyperechogenicity in the white matter are additional ultrasound findings [12].

Magnetic resonance imaging
Magnetic resonance imaging has been shown to be very useful in demonstrating microabscesses in the brainstem, and in the cerebellum; those lesions would have been missed by ultrasound [12] (Fig. 13.7b).

Viral meningitis/meningoencephalitis

Ultrasound
Diffuse mild echogenicity of the periventricular and deep white matter has been described [1]. This echogenicity may evolve into cystic lesions or resolve [1,93].

Magnetic resonance imaging
Magnetic resonance imaging and especially diffusion-weighted imaging are helpful in defining the extent and severity of the white matter involvement. Diffusion-weighted imaging can detect white matter involvement as early as within hours of onset of illness when conventional T_1- and T_2-weighted images might still be normal. Hence, diffusion-weighted imaging is very useful in detecting and diagnosing encephalitis at an early stage [13,15,16]. Using diffusion-weighted imaging, it was shown that the corpus callosum can be affected in viral meningoencephalitis [1,93].

Prognosis
Survivors of neonatal bacterial meningitis have an increased risk of disability such as severe neuromotor impairment, hearing impairment, learning difficulties, behavioral problems such as attention deficits, and seizures [79,94,95,96]. Hydrocephalus and mental retardation seem to be significantly correlated [79].

Survivors (infants born with birth weight <1000 g) of candidiasis are more likely to have Bayley mental and psychomotor developmental index scores <70, are more likely to have moderate or severe cerebral palsy, and are more likely to be blind or deaf than are the survivors without candidiasis at 18–22 months of age [77].

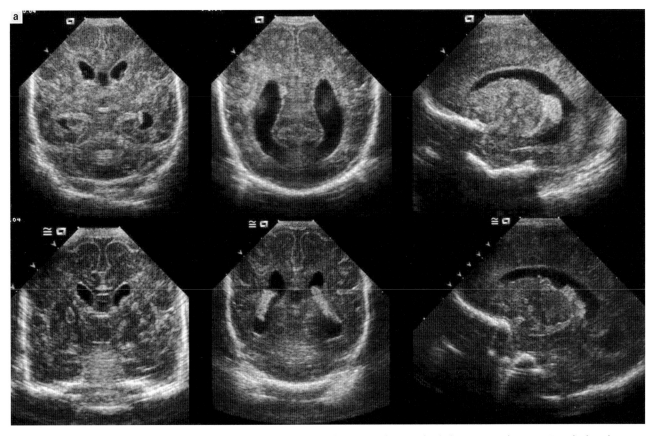

Fig 13.7.a,b. **(a) Ultrasound images in a case of fungal meningoencephalitis in a 27-week- gestation baby. Top row shows scattered microabcesses and mild ventriculomegaly. Bottom row shows the imaging appearances 1 week later. (b) MRI made at term in the baby whose ultrasound images are shown in (a). There are multiple small foci of T_1 shortening (microhemorrhages or calcification) and regions of white matter edema.**

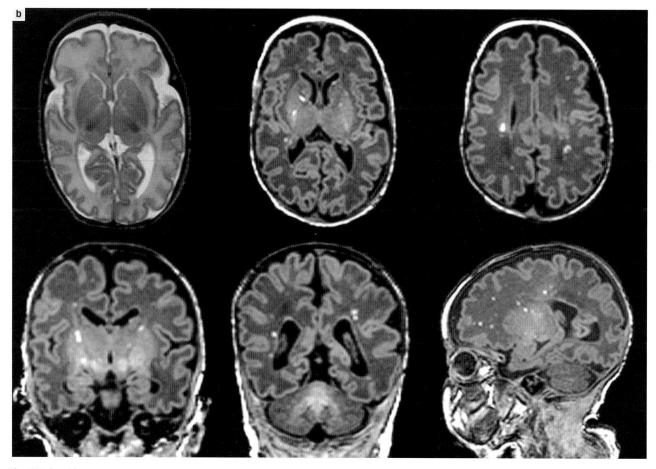

Fig. 13.7. **(cont.)**

References

1. de Vries LS, Verboon-Maciolek MA, Cowan FM, Groenendaal F. The role of cranial ultrasound and magnetic resonance imaging in the diagnosis of infections of the central nervous system. *Early Hum Dev* 2006; **82**(12): 819–25.

2. Holt DE, Halket S, de Louvois J, Harvey D. Neonatal meningitis in England and Wales: 10 years on. *Arch Dis Child Fetal Neonatal Ed* 2001; **84**(2): F85–9.

3. Barkovich AJ, Lindan CE. Congenital cytomegalovirus infection of the brain: imaging analysis and embryologic considerations. *AJNR Am J Neuroradiol* 1994; **15**(4): 703–15.

4. Tubbs RS, Smyth MD, Wellons JC, 3rd, Oakes WJ. Intramedullary hemorrhage in a neonate after lumbar puncture resulting in paraplegia: a case report. *Pediatrics* 2004; **113**(5): 1403–5.

5. Unsinn KM, Geley T, Freund MC, Gassner I. US of the spinal cord in newborns: spectrum of normal findings, variants, congenital anomalies, and acquired diseases. *Radiographics* 2000; **20**(4): 923–38.

6. Sahin F, Selcuki M, Ecin N *et al.* Level of conus medullaris in term and preterm neonates. *Arch Dis Child Fetal Neonatal Ed* 1997; **77**(1): F67–9.

7. Rennie. JM. *Roberton's Textbook of Neonatology*, 4th edn. London, Churchill Livingstone, 2005.

8. Garges HP, Moody MA, Cotten CM *et al.* Neonatal meningitis: what is the correlation among cerebrospinal fluid cultures, blood cultures, and cerebrospinal fluid parameters? *Pediatrics* 2006; **117**: 1094–110.

9. Chequer RS, Tharp BR, Dreimane D, Hahn JS, Clancy RR, Coen RW. Prognostic value of EEG in neonatal meningitis: retrospective study of 29 infants. *Pediatr Neurol* 1992; **8**(6): 417–22.

10. Ancora G, Lanari M, Lazzarotto T *et al.* Cranial ultrasound scanning and prediction of outcome in newborns with congenital cytomegalovirus infection. *J Pediatr* 2007; **150**(2): 157–61.

11. de Vries LS, Gunardi H, Barth PG, Bok LA, Verboon-Maciolek MA, Groenendaal F. The spectrum of cranial ultrasound and magnetic resonance imaging abnormalities in congenital cytomegalovirus infection. *Neuropediatrics* 2004; **35**(2): 113–19.

12. Huang CC, Chen CY, Yang HB, Wang SM, Chang YC, Liu CC. Central nervous system candidiasis in very low-birth-weight premature neonates and infants: US characteristics and histopathologic and MR imaging correlates in five patients. *Radiology* 1998; **209**(1): 49–56.

13. Teixeira J, Zimmerman RA, Haselgrove JC, Bilaniuk LT, Hunter JV. Diffusion imaging in pediatric central nervous system infections. *Neuroradiology* 2001; **43**(12): 1031–9.

14. Kuker W, Nagele T, Schmidt F, Heckl S, Herrlinger U. Diffusion-weighted MRI in herpes simplex encephalitis: a report of three cases. *Neuroradiology* 2004; **46**(2): 122–5.

15. Kubota T, Ito M, Maruyama K *et al.* Serial diffusion-weighted imaging of neonatal herpes encephalitis: a case report. *Brain Dev* 2007; **29**(3): 171–3.

16. Dhawan A, Kecskes Z, Jyoti R, Kent AL. Early diffusion-weighted magnetic resonance imaging findings in neonatal herpes encephalitis. *J Paediatr Child Health* 2006; **42**(12): 824–6.

17. Demmler GJ. Infectious Diseases Society of America and Centers for Disease Control. Summary of a workshop on surveillance for congenital cytomegalovirus disease. *Rev Infect Dis* 1991; **13**(2): 315–29.

18. Azam AZ, Vial Y, Fawer CL, Zufferey J, Hohlfeld P. Prenatal diagnosis of congenital cytomegalovirus infection. *Obstet Gynecol* 2001; **97**(3): 443–8.

19. Remington JS. Klein JO. *Infectious Diseases of the Fetus and Newborn Infant*, 6th edn. Philadelphia, WB Saunders, 2006.
20. Dobbins JG, Stewart JA, Demmler GJ. Surveillance of congenital cytomegalovirus disease, 1990-1991. Collaborating Registry Group. *MMWR CDC Surveill Summ* 1992; **41**(2): 35-9.
21. Boppana SB, Pass RF, Britt WJ, Stagno S, Alford CA. Symptomatic congenital cytomegalovirus infection: neonatal morbidity and mortality. *Pediatr Infect Dis J* 1992; **11**(2): 93-9.
22. Kylat RI, Kelly EN, Ford-Jones EL. Clinical findings and adverse outcome in neonates with symptomatic congenital cytomegalovirus (SCCMV) infection. *Eur J Pediatr* 2006; **165**(11): 773-8.
23. Coats DK, Demmler GJ, Paysse EA, Du LT, Libby C. Ophthalmologic findings in children with congenital cytomegalovirus infection. *J AAPOS* 2000; **4**(2): 110-16.
24. Conboy TJ, Pass RF, Stagno S et al. Early clinical manifestations and intellectual outcome in children with symptomatic congenital cytomegalovirus infection. *J Pediatr* 1987; **111**(3): 343-8.
25. Fowler KB, Boppana SB. Congenital cytomegalovirus (CMV) infection and hearing deficit. *J Clin Virol* 2006; **35**(2): 226-31.
26. Madden C, Wiley S, Schleiss M et al. Audiometric, clinical and educational outcomes in a pediatric symptomatic congenital cytomegalovirus (CMV) population with sensorineural hearing loss. *Int J Pediatr Otorhinolaryngol* 2005; **69**(9): 1191-8.
27. Williamson WD, Desmond MM, LaFevers N et al. Symptomatic congenital cytomegalovirus. Disorders of language, learning, and hearing. *Am J Dis Child* 1982; **136**(10): 902-5.
28. Pass RF, Stagno S, Myers GJ, Alford CA. Outcome of symptomatic congenital cytomegalovirus infection: results of long-term longitudinal follow-up. *Pediatrics* 1980; **66**(5): 758-62.
29. Rivera LB, Boppana SB, Fowler KB, Britt WJ, Stagno S, Pass RF. Predictors of hearing loss in children with symptomatic congenital cytomegalovirus infection. *Pediatrics* 2002; **110**(4): 762-7.
30. Hayward JC, Titelbaum DS, Clancy RR, Zimmerman RA. Lissencephaly-pachygyria associated with congenital cytomegalovirus infection. *J Child Neurol* 1991; **6**(2): 109-14.
31. van der Knaap MS, Vermeulen G, Barkhof F, Hart AA, Loeber JG, Weel JF. Pattern of white matter abnormalities at MR imaging: use of polymerase chain reaction testing of Guthrie cards to link pattern with congenital cytomegalovirus infection. *Radiology* 2004; **230**(2): 529-36.
32. Boppana SB, Fowler KB, Vaid Y et al. Neuroradiographic findings in the newborn period and long-term outcome in children with symptomatic congenital cytomegalovirus infection. *Pediatrics* 1997; **99**(3): 409-14.
33. Lanari M, Lazzarotto T, Venturi V et al. Neonatal cytomegalovirus blood load and risk of sequelae in symptomatic and asymptomatic congenitally infected newborns. *Pediatrics* 2006; **117**(1): e76-83.
34. Malinger G, Lev D, Zahalka N et al. Fetal cytomegalovirus infection of the brain: the spectrum of sonographic findings. *AJNR Am J Neuroradiol* 2003; **24**(1): 28-32.
35. Steinlin MI, Nadal D, Eich GF, Martin E, Boltshauser EJ. Late intrauterine cytomegalovirus infection: clinical and neuroimaging findings. *Pediatr Neurol* 1996; **15**(3): 249-53.
36. Stagno S, Pass RF, Cloud G et al. Primary cytomegalovirus infection in pregnancy. Incidence, transmission to fetus, and clinical outcome. *J Am Med Assoc* 1986; **256**(14): 1904-8.
37. Saigal S, Lunyk O, Larke RP, Chernesky MA. The outcome in children with congenital cytomegalovirus infection. A longitudinal follow-up study. *Am J Dis Child* 1982; **136**(10): 896-901.
38. Williamson WD, Percy AK, Yow MD et al. Asymptomatic congenital cytomegalovirus infection. Audiologic, neuroradiologic, and neurodevelopmental abnormalities during the first year. *Am J Dis Child* 1990; **144**(12): 1365-8.
39. Fowler KB, McCollister FP, Dahle AJ, Boppana S, Britt WJ, Pass RF. Progressive and fluctuating sensorineural hearing loss in children with asymptomatic congenital cytomegalovirus infection. *J Pediatr* 1997; **130**(4): 624-30.
40. Ivarsson SA, Lernmark B, Svanberg L. Ten-year clinical, developmental, and intellectual follow-up of children with congenital cytomegalovirus infection without neurologic symptoms at one year of age. *Pediatrics* 1997; **99**(6): 800-3.
41. Ahlfors K, Ivarsson SA, Harris S. Report on a long-term study of maternal and congenital cytomegalovirus infection in Sweden. Review of prospective studies available in the literature. *Scand J Infect Dis* 1999; **31**(5): 443-57.
42. Ross SA, Boppana SB. Congenital cytomegalovirus infection: outcome and diagnosis. *Semin Pediatr Infect Dis* 2005; **16**(1): 44-9.
43. Mombro M, Perathoner C, Leone A et al. Congenital toxoplasmosis: 10-year follow up. *Eur J Pediatr* 1995; **154**(8): 635-9.
44. Dunn D, Wallon M, Peyron F, Petersen E, Peckham C, Gilbert R. Mother-to-child transmission of toxoplasmosis: risk estimates for clinical counselling. *Lancet* 1999; **353**(9167): 1829-33.
45. Boyer KM. Diagnosis and treatment of congenital toxoplasmosis. *Adv Pediatr Infect Dis* 1996; **11**: 449-67.
46. Hohlfeld P, Daffos F, Thulliez P et al. Fetal toxoplasmosis: outcome of pregnancy and infant follow-up after in utero treatment. *J Pediatr* 1989; **115**(5 Pt 1): 765-9.
47. Volpe J. *Neurology of the Newborn*, 4th edn. Philadelphia, Saunders, 2001.
48. Roizen N, Swisher CN, Stein MA et al. Neurologic and developmental outcome in treated congenital toxoplasmosis. *Pediatrics* 1995; **95**(1): 11-20.
49. Guerina NG, Hsu HW, Meissner HC et al. Neonatal serologic screening and early treatment for congenital *Toxoplasma gondii* infection. The New England Regional Toxoplasma Working Group. *N Engl J Med* 1994; **330**(26): 1858-63.
50. Berrebi A, Bardou M, Bessieres MH et al. Outcome for children infected with congenital toxoplasmosis in the first trimester and with normal ultrasound findings: A study of 36 cases. *Eur J Obstet Gynecol Reprod Biol* 2007; **135**(1): 53-7.
51. Salt A, Freeman K, Prusa A et al. Determinants of response to a parent questionnaire about development and behaviour in 3 year olds: European multicentre study of congenital toxoplasmosis. *BMC Pediatr* 2005; **5**: 21.
52. Gras L, Wallon M, Pollak A et al. Association between prenatal treatment and clinical manifestations of congenital toxoplasmosis in infancy: a cohort study in 13 European centres. *Acta Paediatr* 2005; **94**(12): 1721-31.
53. Koppe JG, Loewer-Sieger DH, de Roever-Bonnet H. Results of 20-year follow-up of congenital toxoplasmosis. *Lancet* 1986; **1**(8475): 254-6.
54. Wilson CB, Remington JS, Stagno S, Reynolds DW. Development of adverse sequelae in children born with subclinical congenital *Toxoplasma* infection. *Pediatrics* 1980; **66**(5): 767-74.
55. Saxon SA, Knight W, Reynolds DW, Stagno S, Alford CA. Intellectual deficits in children born with subclinical congenital toxoplasmosis: a preliminary report. *J Pediatr* 1973; **82**(5): 792-7.
56. McLeod R, Boyer K, Karrison T et al. Outcome of treatment for congenital toxoplasmosis, 1981-2004: the National Collaborative Chicago-Based, Congenital Toxoplasmosis Study. *Clin Infect Dis* 2006; **42**(10): 1383-94.
57. Couvreur J, Nottin N, Desmonts G. [Treatment of congenital toxoplasmosis. Clinical and biological results (author's transl).] *Ann Pediatr (Paris)* 1980; **27**(10): 647-52.
58. Gilbert R, Gras L. Effect of timing and type of treatment on the risk of mother to child transmission of Toxoplasma gondii. *Br J Obstet Gynaecol* 2003; **110**(2): 112-20.
59. Couvreur J, Thulliez P, Daffos F et al. [Fetal toxoplasmosis. In utero treatment with pyrimethamine sulfamides.] *Arch Fr Pediatr* 1991; **48**(6): 397-403.
60. Bessieres MH, Berrebi A, Rolland M et al. Neonatal screening for congenital toxoplasmosis in a cohort of 165 women infected during pregnancy and influence of in utero treatment on the results of neonatal tests. *Eur J Obstet Gynecol Reprod Biol* 2001; **94**(1): 37-45.

61. Brown AE, Sadler KE, Tomkins SE *et al.* Recent trends in HIV and other STIs in the United Kingdom: data to the end of 2002. *Sex Transm Infect* 2004; **80**(3): 159–66.

62. Chen ZQ, Zhang GC, Gong XD *et al.* Syphilis in China: results of a national surveillance programme. *Lancet* 2007; **369**(9556): 132–8.

63. Hopkins S, Lyons F, Mulcahy F, Bergin C. The great pretender returns to Dublin, Ireland. *Sex Transm Infect* 2001; **77**(5): 316–18.

64. Gust DA, Levine WC, St Louis ME, Braxton J, Berman SM. Mortality associated with congenital syphilis in the United States, 1992–1998. *Pediatrics* 2002; **109**(5): E79.

65. Rawstron SA, Jenkins S, Blanchard S, Li PW, Bromberg K. Maternal and congenital syphilis in Brooklyn, NY. Epidemiology, transmission, and diagnosis. *Am J Dis Child* 1993; **147**(7): 727–31.

66. Srinivasan G, Ramamurthy RS, Bharathi A, Voora S, Pildes RS. Congenital syphilis: a diagnostic and therapeutic dilemma. *Pediatr Infect Dis* 1983; **2**(6): 436–41.

67. Michelow IC, Wendel GD, Jr, Norgard MV *et al.* Central nervous system infection in congenital syphilis. *N Engl J Med* 2002; **346**(23): 1792–8.

68. Kauffman WM, Sivit CJ, Fitz CR, Rakusan TA, Herzog K, Chandra RS. CT and MR evaluation of intracranial involvement in pediatric HIV infection: a clinical-imaging correlation. *AJNR Am J Neuroradiol* 1992; **13**(3): 949–57.

69. Spreer J, Enenkel-Stoodt S, Funk M, Fiedler A, de Simone A, Hacker H. [Neuroradiological findings in perinatally HIV-infected children.] *Rofo* 1994; **161**(2): 106–12.

70. Kozlowski PB, Brudkowska J, Kraszpulski M *et al.* Microencephaly in children congenitally infected with human immunodeficiency virus – a gross-anatomical morphometric study. *Acta Neuropathol (Berl)* 1997; **93**(2): 136–45.

71. Blanche S, Tardieu M, Rustin P *et al.* Persistent mitochondrial dysfunction and perinatal exposure to antiretroviral nucleoside analogues. *Lancet* 1999; **354**(9184): 1084–9.

72. Barret B, Tardieu M, Rustin P *et al.* Persistent mitochondrial dysfunction in HIV-1-exposed but uninfected infants: clinical screening in a large prospective cohort. *Aids* 2003; **17**(12): 1769–85.

73. Tardieu M, Brunelle F, Raybaud C *et al.* Cerebral MR imaging in uninfected children born to HIV-seropositive mothers and perinatally exposed to zidovudine. *AJNR Am J Neuroradiol* 2005; **26**(4): 695–701.

74. de Louvois J, Halket S, Harvey D. Neonatal meningitis in England and Wales: sequelae at 5 years of age. *Eur J Pediatr* 2005; **164**(12): 730–4.

75. Francis BM, Gilbert GL. Survey of neonatal meningitis in Australia: 1987–1989. *Med J Aust* 1992; **156**(4): 240–3.

76. Isaacs D. A ten year, multicentre study of coagulase negative staphylococcal infections in Australasian neonatal units. *Arch Dis Child Fetal Neonatal Ed* 2003; **88**(2): F89–93.

77. Benjamin DK, Jr, Stoll BJ, Fanaroff AA *et al.* Neonatal candidiasis among extremely low birth weight infants: risk factors, mortality rates, and neurodevelopmental outcomes at 18 to 22 months. *Pediatrics* 2006; **117**(1): 84–92.

78. Fernandez M, Moylett EH, Noyola DE, Baker CJ. Candidal meningitis in neonates: a 10-year review. *Clin Infect Dis* 2000; **31**(2): 458–63.

79. Renier D, Flandin C, Hirsch E, Hirsch JF. Brain abscesses in neonates. A study of 30 cases. *J Neurosurg* 1988; **69**(6): 877–82.

80. Sutton DL, Ouvrier RA. Cerebral abscess in the under 6 month age group. *Arch Dis Child* 1983; **58**(11): 901–5.

81. Basu S, Mukherjee KK, Poddar B, Goraya JS, Chawla K, Parmar VR. An unusual case of neonatal brain abscess following *Klebsiella pneumoniae* septicemia. *Infection* 2001; **29**(5): 283–5.

82. Graham DR, Anderson RL, Ariel FE *et al.* Epidemic nosocomial meningitis due to *Citrobacter diversus* in neonates. *J Infect Dis* 1981; **144**(3): 203–9.

83. Graham DR, Band JD. *Citrobacter diversus* brain abscess and meningitis in neonates. *J Am Med Assoc* 1981; **245**(19): 1923–5.

84. Burdette JH, Santos C. *Enterobacter sakazakii* brain abscess in the neonate: the importance of neuroradiologic imaging. *Pediatr Radiol* 2000; **30**(1): 33–4.

85. Hung KL. Cranial ultrasound in the detection of postmeningitic complications in the neonates. *Brain Dev* 1986; **8**(1): 31–6.

86. Han BK, Babcock DS, McAdams L. Bacterial meningitis in infants: sonographic findings. *Radiology* 1985; **154**(3): 645–50.

87. Edwards MK, Brown DL, Chua GT. Complicated infantile meningitis: evaluation by real-time sonography. *AJNR Am J Neuroradiol* 1982; **3**(4): 431–4.

88. Perlman JM, Rollins N, Sanchez PJ. Late-onset meningitis in sick, very-low-birth-weight infants. Clinical and sonographic observations. *Am J Dis Child* 1992; **146**(11): 1297–301.

89. Reeder JD, Sanders RC. Ventriculitis in the neonate: recognition by sonography. *AJNR Am J Neuroradiol* 1983; **4**(1): 37–41.

90. Brown BS, Thorp P. The ultrasonographic diagnosis of bacterial meningitis and ventriculitis in infancy: six case reports. *J Can Assoc Radiol* 1984; **35**(1): 47–51.

91. Shah DK, Daley AJ, Hunt RW, Volpe JJ, Inder TE. Cerebral white matter injury in the newborn following *Escherichia coli* meningitis. *Eur J Paediatr Neurol* 2005; **9**(1): 13–17.

92. Messerschmidt A, Prayer D, Olischar M, Pollak A, Birnbacher R. Brain abscesses after *Serratia marcescens* infection on a neonatal intensive care unit: differences on serial imaging. *Neuroradiology* 2004; **46**(2): 148–52.

93. Verboon-Maciolek MA, Groenendaal F, Cowan F, Govaert P, van Loon AM, de Vries LS. White matter damage in neonatal enterovirus meningoencephalitis. *Neurology* 2006; **66**(8): 1267–9.

94. Stevens JP, Eames M, Kent A, Halket S, Holt D, Harvey D. Long term outcome of neonatal meningitis. *Arch Dis Child Fetal Neonatal Ed* 2003; **88**(3): F179–84.

95. Grimwood K, Anderson P, Anderson V, Tan L, Nolan T. Twelve year outcomes following bacterial meningitis: further evidence for persisting effects. *Arch Dis Child* 2000; **83**(2): 111–16.

96. Bedford H, de Louvois J, Halket S, Peckham C, Hurley R, Harvey D. Meningitis in infancy in England and Wales: follow up at age 5 years. *Br Med J* 2001; **323**(7312): 533–6.

Chapter 14 | Postmortem imaging

CORNELIA F. HAGMANN,
NICOLA J. ROBERTSON, *and*
JANET M. RENNIE

Introduction to the clinical problem

Establishing the cause of perinatal death has a particularly valuable role in the counseling of the parents after a loss of a baby. Assigning a cause of death can help parents in the grieving process, improve parental and professional understanding, and address any concerns they may have that prenatal events such as maternal illness or maternal use of medication might have contributed to the death of their baby [1,2,3,4]. After termination, confirmation of the prenatal diagnosis is vitally important information when counseling for future pregnancies.

Despite the recognized value of autopsy, perinatal autopsy rates have declined significantly in recent years [2,3,5]. Studies in both Europe and the United States indicate that as many as 40% of all perinatal deaths are not submitted for autopsy [6,7,8]. There is no obvious single explanation for the decline in autopsy rates but possible influences include a shift in attitude of clinicians towards autopsies and a change in the public's willingness to grant permission [3].

This decline in consent for autopsy leads to a reduction in the information available to parents about the risk for future pregnancies. The Chief Medical Officer of the United Kingdom issued two reports in 2000 and 2001 [9,10] recommending the assessment of less invasive forms of postmortem examination. After wide consultation with interested parties and faith groups, Alistair Parker produced a document (on behalf of the Department of Health) entitled *Less Invasive Autopsy: The Place of MR Imaging* in 2004 [11]. Recommendations included setting up comparative studies of postmortem magnetic resonance imaging (MRI) against conventional autopsies for adults, infants, and fetuses separately [11]. Funding for the Department of Health study was awarded to University College London Hospitals, and the work started in 2007.

Current autopsy

Currently, non-invasive tests and invasive tests are part of the autopsy. The non-invasive tests include review of medical records (including imaging), external examination, examination of placenta, cord, fetal skin scraping, cytogenetic and metabolic laboratory investigations of cord and placental blood, imaging (photography, x-ray), and microbiology. These are followed by the invasive tests, which include the examination and dissection of internal organs and subsequent histology.

Postmortem MRI magnetic resonance imaging

In the early 1990s, the first experiences with MRI as an alternative for autopsy in postmortem examinations of adults, fetuses, and neonates were published [12,13]. The use of MRI as an adjunct and possible alternative to the internal examination of perinatal necropsy was first proposed by Ros *et al.* in 1990 [13]. They examined the bodies of three stillbirths, one neonatal death, and two adults with a 0.1-T resistive magnet, and found that gross abnormalities were clearly demonstrated and MRI was superior to conventional methods for demonstrating air and fluid in undisturbed body spaces [13]. In 1996 Brookes *et al.* published the first 20 cases of fetal and perinatal non-invasive necropsy by MRI [14]. They systematically compared postmortem fetal MRI findings with matched necropsy results and reported a 90% agreement; in four cases MRI provided more information when compared with autopsy [14]. Early in 1997, Woodward *et al.* published a similar comparative series of 26 matched postmortem fetal MRI examinations with necropsy [15]. They found that with regard to major malformations demonstrated, the information given to parents regarding fetal anomalies would have been essentially the same as that provided by autopsy [15]. Magnetic resonance imaging was particularly useful for examination of the brain and spine [15]. Two similar studies confirmed these results [16,17].

Postmortem MRI of fetal and neonatal brain

Dissection of the fetal brain at autopsy can be very difficult, and after maceration it can be impossible. Fixation can take up to 4 weeks. Magnetic resonance imaging provides a non-invasive examination of the fetal brain in situ (Fig. 14.1). Griffiths and his co-workers in Sheffield examined 40 fetal brains with MRI and subsequently at autopsy [18]. In eight

Neonatal Cerebral Investigation, eds. Janet M. Rennie, Cornelia F. Hagmann and Nicola J. Robertson. Published by Cambridge University Press. © Cambridge University Press 2008.

In conclusion, postmortem MRI has been shown to be especially advantageous in the evaluation of the fetal and neonatal brain; the ability to image the brain in situ is a particular advantage. Results from the Department of Health trial of less invasive autopsy are awaited for further clarification of the role of postmortem MRI in the perinatal postmortem examination. Nevertheless, we currently advise the following:

- If the parents consent to an autopsy, we ask permission to perform a postmortem brain MRI as adjunct to the autopsy.
- If the parents do not give consent to autopsy we suggest a whole-body MRI to the parents, especially if brain malformations or brain injuries are suspected.

References

1. Wright C, Lee RE. Investigating perinatal death: a review of the options when autopsy consent is refused. *Arch Dis Child Fetal Neonatal Ed* 2004; **89(4)**: F285-8.
2. Kumar P, Angst DB, Taxy J, Mangurten HH. Neonatal autopsies: a 10-year experience. *Arch Pediatr Adolesc Med* 2000; **154(1)**: 38-42.
3. Brodlie M, Laing IA, Keeling JW, McKenzie KJ. Ten years of neonatal autopsies in tertiary referral centre: retrospective study. *Br Med J* 2002; **324(7340)**: 761-3.
4. Laing IA. Clinical aspects of neonatal death and autopsy. *Semin Neonatol* 2004; **9(4)**: 247-54.
5. Okah FA. The autopsy: experience of a regional neonatal intensive care unit. *Paediatr Perinat Epidemiol* 2002; **16(4)**: 350-4.
6. Craven CM, Dempsey S, Carey JC, Kochenour NK. Evaluation of a perinatal autopsy protocol: influence of the Prenatal Diagnosis Conference Team. *Obstet Gynecol* 1990; **76(4)**: 684-8.
7. Cartlidge PH, Dawson AT, Stewart JH, Vujanic GM. Value and quality of perinatal and infant postmortem examinations: cohort analysis of 400 consecutive deaths. *Br Med J* 1995; **310(6973)**: 155-8.
8. Saller DN, Jr, Lesser KB, Harrel U, Rogers BB, Oyer CE. The clinical utility of the perinatal autopsy. *J Am Med Assoc* 1995; **273(8)**: 663-5.
9. Chief Medical Officer. Report of a consensus of organs and tissues retained by pathology services in England. London, Stationery Office, 2000.
10. Chief Medical Officer. The removal, retention and use of human organs and tissues from post mortem examination. London, Stationery Office, 2001.
11. Parker. A. Less invasive autopsy: the place of magnetic resonance imaging. February, 2004. www.dh.gov.uk.
12. Roberts IS, Benbow EW, Bisset R *et al.* Accuracy of magnetic resonance imaging in determining cause of sudden death in adults: comparison with conventional autopsy. *Histopathology* 2003; **42(5)**: 424-30.
13. Ros PR, Li KC, Vo P, Baer H, Staab EV. Preautopsy magnetic resonance imaging: initial experience. *Magn Reson Imaging* 1990; **8(3)**: 303-8.
14. Brookes JA, Hall-Craggs MA, Sams VR, Lees WR. Non-invasive perinatal necropsy by magnetic resonance imaging. *Lancet* 1996; **348(9035)**: 1139-41.
15. Woodward PJ, Sohaey R, Harris DP *et al.* Postmortem fetal MR imaging: comparison with findings at autopsy. *AJR Am J Roentgenol* 1997; **168(1)**: 41-6.
16. Huisman TA, Wisser J, Stallmach T, Krestin GP, Huch R, Kubik-Huch RA. MR autopsy in fetuses. *Fetal Diagn Ther* 2002; **17(1)**: 58-64.
17. Alderliesten ME, Peringa J, van der Hulst VP, Blaauwgeers HL, van Lith JM. Perinatal mortality: clinical value of postmortem magnetic resonance imaging compared with autopsy in routine obstetric practice. *Br J Obstet Gynaecol* 2003; **110(4)**: 378-82.

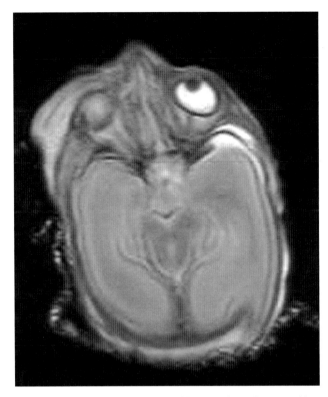

Fig. 14.1. Previous sibling diagnosed with Joubert's syndrome. In this pregnancy the antenatal ultrasound at 20 weeks of gestation showed abnormal posterior fossa. Fetal MRI at 20 weeks showed mild ventriculomegaly, small cerebellar vermis, small cerebellar hemisphere, and excessive fluid around the cerebellum. Given the previous history of Joubert's syndrome of the sibling, Joubert's syndrome was suspected. Postmortem MRI at 24 weeks confirmed the suspected diagnosis with the appearance of the molar tooth sign.

cases, the autopsy did not provide structural information of the brain or spine because assessment of the unfixed brain was impossible; leaving 32 cases in which a formal comparison between autopsy and MRI findings could be made. In 88% there was complete agreement between autopsy and MRI findings [18]. These authors reported a sensitivity of 100%, specificity of 92%, positive predictive value (PPV) of 95%, and negative predictive value (NPV) of 100% for postmortem brain MRI [18].

Whole-body postmortem MRI

Postmortem imaging of the body systems apart from the brain has been less well documented. Cardiac MRI has not performed well so far according to the published postmortem MRI studies, but recent advances in MRI techniques have improved the accuracy of diagnosis in congenital cardiac malformation [19,20]. Renal abnormalities were easily identified by postmortem MRI [15,16,21]. The structures of the gastrointestinal system from the lower esophagus to the rectum are also well demonstrated. Large anomalies (e.g., diaphragmatic hernia, herniated organs, and malrotation of the gut) are more accurately reported than more subtle anomalies, such as ileocecal atresia [14,15].

18. Griffiths PD, Variend D, Evans M *et al.* Postmortem MR imaging of the fetal and stillborn central nervous system. *AJNR Am J Neuroradiol* 2003; **24(1)**: 22–7.

19. Brookes JA, Deng J, Wilkinson ID, Lees WR. Three-dimensional imaging of the postmortem fetus by MRI: early experience. *Fetal Diagn Ther* 1999; **14(3)**: 166–71.

20. Razavi RS, Hill DL, Muthurangu V *et al.* Three-dimensional magnetic resonance imaging of congenital cardiac anomalies. *Cardiol Young* 2003; **13(5)**: 461–5.

21. Hagmann CF, Robertson NJ, Sams VR, Brookes JA. Postmortem MRI as an adjunct to perinatal autopsy for renal tract abnormalities. *Arch Dis Child Fetal Neonatal Ed* 2007; **92(3)**: F215–18.

Index

Note: page numbers in *italics* refer to figures and tables